The Anaesthesia Science Viva Book
Third Edition

The Anaesthesia Science Viva Book

THIRD EDITION

Clinical Science as Applied to Anaesthesia,
Intensive Therapy and Chronic Pain
A Guide to the Oral Questions

SIMON BRICKER
The Countess of Chester Hospital,
Chester, UK

Medical illustrations by
CELYN BRICKER

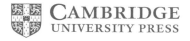
CAMBRIDGE
UNIVERSITY PRESS

CAMBRIDGE
UNIVERSITY PRESS

University Printing House, Cambridge CB2 8BS, United Kingdom

One Liberty Plaza, 20th Floor, New York, NY 10006, USA

477 Williamstown Road, Port Melbourne, VIC 3207, Australia

314-321, 3rd Floor, Plot 3, Splendor Forum, Jasola District Centre, New Delhi - 110025, India

79 Anson Road, #06-04/06, Singapore 079906

Cambridge University Press is part of the University of Cambridge.

It furthers the University's mission by disseminating knowledge in the pursuit of
education, learning and research at the highest international levels of excellence.

www.cambridge.org
Information on this title: www.cambridge.org/9781316608814
DOI: 10.1017/9781316651841

First edition © Greenwich Medical Media 2004
Second edition © Simon Bricker 2009
Third edition © Simon Bricker 2017

First published 2004
Second edition 2009
Third edition 2017

A catalogue record for this publication is available from the British Library

Library of Congress Cataloging in Publication data
Names: Bricker, Simon, author.
Title: The anaesthesia science viva book : clinical science as applied to anaesthesia, intensive therapy,
and chronic pain : a guide to the oral questions / Simon Bricker ; medical illustrations by Celyn Bricker.
Description: Third edition. | Cambridge ; New York, NY : Cambridge University Press, 2017. |
Includes bibliographical references and index.
Identifiers: LCCN 2017019176 | ISBN 9781316608814 (pbk. : alk. paper)
Subjects: | MESH: Anesthesia | Clinical Medicine | Study Guide
Classification: LCC RD82.3 | NLM WO 18.2 | DDC 617.9/6076–dc23
LC record available at https://lccn.loc.gov/2017019176

ISBN 978-1-316-60881-4 Paperback

....

To Imogen

Contents

Contents

Preface to the Third Edition

The syllabus for the Final FRCA exam is dauntingly wide, and a book such as this could never claim to be comprehensive. There are nonetheless a number of subjects which do reappear in the oral part of the exam, and it is some of these core topics that this third edition aims to identify. In previous editions I did make some attempt to second-guess the examiners by suggesting in which direction the questioning might lead. However the increasingly structured nature of the exam makes this approach less suitable, and so the topics have now been divided into 'core' and 'supplementary' information, including clinical considerations where appropriate. This may not necessarily be the order in which the subject is introduced during the oral, but there should be sufficient information in both these sections to ensure that you pass. The pace of change in medical knowledge is such that it is inevitable that some of the material in this book will date. However, there is usually a lag time before advances in information or changes in practice become incorporated into the exam itself, and so in some instances it may not matter, particularly if you are able to revert to first principles as you give your answers. Although it now extends to more than 500 pages, I would emphasize that this is not an anaesthetic textbook as such, and although some of the topics are dealt with in some detail, there is considerable simplification of what can be very complex areas. There is now much more known, for example, about cell signalling and gene expression than realistically could be encompassed within the short time frame of the viva. So the primary aim of the book remains that of helping you towards success in the exam; yet I would also hope finally that at least some of the information it contains will be of value in your clinical practice once you have left the Final FRCA far behind.

Preface to the Second Edition

The emphasis, if not the content, of the Final FRCA science viva is changing. In response to muted criticism that an otherwise good exam has been diminished by a basic science viva that at times seemed to be little more than 'Primary Lite', the College has introduced greater clinical focus. This has meant that many of the answers that appeared in the first edition needed some reorientation. Yet, as before, this book's prime purpose remains to give you a wide range of potential questions presented in a way that is relevant to the exam that you are facing, and organized so that the information is manageable. As before, the introduction still aims to give you some insight into how the clinical science viva works, together with some revised general guidance as to how to improve your chances of success.

The examination questions continue to be divided broadly into the four subject areas of anatomy, physiology, pharmacology and physics, although the increased clinical emphasis can mean that the distinction between the subject areas can be somewhat blurred. The anatomy question on the internal jugular vein, for example, may well include some discussion of the physiology of central venous pressure. Equally, some questions on pharmacology may encompass aspects of physiology with which there is obvious potential for overlap. This means that you may not always find all the necessary information within one single answer, but should find most of it covered in other sections. The basic format of the book remains unchanged, although the content has been updated where appropriate. A new feature of this edition is the inclusion of some illustrations and diagrams which should make the material more accessible.

My family, as always, offered no objection to the project; and, as always, my thanks and love to them for their support. The anatomical drawings were produced by a student who is studying Fine Art at Edinburgh University and who happens to be my eldest son Celyn. To him are due especial thanks.

Preface to the First Edition

The Final FRCA examination has a daunting syllabus which is tested by a multiple-choice paper, by written short-answer questions, by one oral examination in clinical anaesthesia, and finally by another in applied basic clinical science. This book is intended to give you some insight into how the clinical science viva works, along with some general guidance as to how to improve your chances of passing. More importantly it aims to provide you with a wide range of potential questions that contain, nonetheless, a manageable amount of information.

The introduction explains the format of the viva, outlines how the questions are constructed, conducted and marked, and offers some advice about technique. The questions which then follow, which are typical of those which have appeared, are divided broadly into the four areas which the exam is designed to cover, namely applied anatomy, physiology, pharmacology and clinical measurement. One section, entitled 'Miscellaneous Science and Medicine', includes a number of subjects which do not fall readily into any of the other categories.

You may notice that there is some overlap in content with the companion volume, 'Short Answer Questions in Anaesthesia'. Where this has happened I have reworked the answers both to give more detail and to focus the topic more specifically towards the oral part of the exam, but a degree of duplication in one or two of the questions is inevitable.

The answers have been constructed to provide you with enough information to pass the viva, but as I have had to be selective in the detail that has been included, they do not claim to be complete accounts of the subjects. This means that in some areas you may notice various omissions, but none I hope so egregious that your chances of success will be ruined. Each of the questions is prefaced by a short commentary on the relevance (or otherwise) of the subject that is being asked. There follows the body of the answer to the likely areas of questioning. This is presented mainly in the form of bulleted but detailed points which include supporting explanation. These are written in text rather than as lists, because I felt that this format would make the book easier to read. If some of the questions seem long, then it is either because the background information is complex, or because they contain enough material for more than one viva topic.

Even in a structured examination a viva may take an unforeseen course, and so the answers also include some possible directions which the questioning might follow. Although each one is intended to provide background details more than sufficient to allow you to pass, in many cases they are simplified, and it is always possible that some examiners may ask at least part of the question in more depth than can be covered in a book of this size. There are 150 specimen questions in this book, and on the day of the exam you will be asked only four. Odds of about 40 to 1 or less do not provide a huge incentive for study, but I should hope that at least some of the material would be relevant to your anaesthetic practice. The material that is irrelevant, and there is certainly some, may at least prove of some future use as in due course you guide less experienced colleagues through the FRCA.

I promised my family that I would never again succumb to the temptation of writing a book. I lied. To my wife and three boys, therefore, my love and thanks for their unfailing patience and support.

Advice on Answering Clinical Science Viva Questions

The Clinical Science Viva (Structured Oral Examination)

Although the Final FRCA examination has undergone a degree of evolution since its inception in 1996, its basic format has remained broadly unchanged, and the clinical science viva continues to test 'the understanding of basic science to the practice of anaesthesia, intensive therapy and pain management'. The term 'viva' is now officially obsolete, and this part of the examination is now referred to as the 'Structured Oral Examination' or SOE. In colloquial reference, however, anaesthetists still talk about 'vivas', and so the word still appears in the title of this book, the first edition of which predated the change in terminology. In the text it has been replaced by the word 'oral'. The College has always included the proviso that 'it is accepted that candidates will not have acquired a detailed knowledge of every topic during the period of recognised training', but this has on occasion contrasted uneasily with the bitter perception of at least some candidates that they had been examined almost to destruction on scientific minutiae. This perception, against a background of muted unease about this section of the exam, was acknowledged by the College, which decided therefore to introduce greater clinical emphasis into the science oral. The change of emphasis is relatively subtle, because both the College and its examiners remain reluctant to dilute the rigour of what for most candidates will be the last examination in anaesthesia that they are likely to take. Nevertheless, the tenor of many of the questions is now such that the clinical applications of the underlying science have more prominence than hitherto. The questions continue to have two parts – the basic scientific principles and their clinical application – but many of the topics will include clinically orientated questions that are intended to reassure you that they do have anaesthetic relevance. The clinical applications may introduce the topic or may follow the basic science according to the nature of the subject. The oral lasts a total of 30 minutes, during which time you will be asked questions on four different and unrelated subjects. The time spent on each should be around 7–8 minutes.

As the name of this part of the exam implies, the FRCA has a highly structured format. The material on which candidates are to be tested is made available to the examiners only on each morning of the exam. The questions are changed after each session to avoid any possibility of later candidates obtaining unfair advantage. Each pair of examiners will decide between themselves which two of the four questions they are going to ask. This is largely the extent of the choice that they are able to make, because the scope of each question is limited both by the guidance answer and by the relatively short time available for each topic. The first examiner will spend 7 or 8 minutes on the first subject before changing to the second. At the first bell (after 15 minutes), the other examiner will repeat the process. The examiner who is not asking questions will usually be making detailed notes which inform the marking process. At the end of the oral each examiner will mark each of the four questions entirely independently, without conferring and without discussion. (This removes any accusation that one examiner may exert undue pressure on the other during the marking process.)

The Marking System

The examiners can each give a mark of 0, 1 or 2 to each of the four questions, which means that a total of 16 marks is available to add to the 24 that can be achieved in the clinical section of the exam. This distribution of marks is of some importance because it means that you can perform very poorly in one or more of the questions yet still achieve the 32 marks that you need to pass the exam overall. Let us assume for the sake of argument that your clinical anaesthesia is stronger than your basic science and that you have obtained all 24 marks going forward. The first science question is, say, the anatomy of the coeliac plexus, followed by a discussion in the physiology section about cytochrome P450. You are then asked rather more forgiving questions about propofol and the safety features of the anaesthetic machine. In theory you could actually respond to the first two questions with complete silence (and be awarded four 0's) before dealing confidently with the second two questions, receive a total of 8 marks and pass the overall exam. It is an improbable scenario, but it does make the point that even if you feel that you have done really badly on a particular question (and you may have performed better than you think, because most candidates are notoriously pessimistic when assessing their own performance), you must not let it affect your approach to the next topic. If you allow yourself to become demoralized, then you will enter a downward spiral from which it may be difficult to recover. You must leave the question behind you, cognizant of the fact that the four subjects are unrelated and that your other answers may well redeem it. (In that respect it is not unlike the short-answer question paper, in which a good answer can outweigh a poor one.)

Appearance and Affect

You cannot fail the Final FRCA because of your appearance or because of poor taste in clothes, and most examiners will be able to recollect candidates whose personal presentation could at best be described as unconventional. It never matters. At worst, however, an unkempt or casual appearance may convey the subliminal impression that you are unprofessional, and at the least it is likely to be a distraction. You should therefore wear something neutral and reasonably smart, which is comfortable and which you have worn before. The examination areas can be hot, and there is no need to increase your stress levels further by forcing yourself into a three-piece suit or other outfit that sees the light of day only rarely.

Nor can you fail the FRCA because of inappropriate behaviour alone. Examiners are well aware of the stress that candidates are enduring, and most will make every attempt to put you at your ease. They are also likely to assume that aggressive or facile responses are a manifestation of stress and will make allowances accordingly. Examiners have been answered with hostility: 'For God's sake don't ask me that – I've never even thought about it'; and with fatuity: 'I'll probably know the answer when you tell it to me.' They have also been subject to what might be described as the Bertie Wooster approach: the candidate didn't quite call the examiner Jeeves but did say that 'it blocks the 1,2 hydroxy-whatsit, oh I don't know, you give the stuff and the atom bings off.' They have been patronized – 'Forgive me, but what I think that you are trying to ask is' – and have even had to resist the obvious retort to the candidate who asks: 'Can I interest you in the concept of context-sensitive half-time?' None of it much matters. Yet examiners can be indulgent only up to a point, and the overall impression that you are creating will not be reassuring. If an inappropriate manner is also accompanied by a weak perform-ance, then you will stand little chance of being given the benefit of the doubt. Take issue with examiners, by all means – it is stimulating for both sides to develop a considered discussion of a topic – but avoid getting into an argument. Unfair though it may seem, the rules of this particular enterprise are not written in your favour.

Oral Questions

On average, you will have about 7 minutes on the topic. Should a question have somewhat limited scope, or if your knowledge is thin, you may spend a bit less time on it, but consistency and fairness demand that the examiners divide the time more or less equally. As explained earlier, these orals are structured, and the examiners have no choice of question. Although it would be logical, given the avowed purpose of the clinical science oral, to subdivide the questions into anaesthesia, intensive therapy and pain management, in practice they do not fit readily into these categories. In the past, the four questions could be somewhat random; it is now usual to have one question which relates to applied anatomy, one to physiology, one to pharmacology and one to physics, clinical measurement, equipment and statistics. This classification is not absolute (topics such as jaundice or latex allergy do not fit strictly into any one of these groups), but it does indicate the broad division of the available questions. The structured nature of the exam minimizes the likelihood of an examiner being able to question you in excessive depth on a subject which happens to be an area of special interest or expertise. It also increases the likelihood of an examiner having to ask questions about a subject in which they do not even have a current generalist interest.

The sub-specialty interests of examiners change as retiring examiners are replaced, but, at any one time, only about 15–20% will have an interest in intensive care medicine, in paediatric anaesthesia or in neuroanaesthesia, and a much smaller number will work in chronic pain management. Thus a paediatric cardiac anaesthetist may have to ask about adult ophthalmic applied anatomy, a neuroanaesthetist about neonatal fluid requirements or an obstetric anaesthetist about intensive therapy ventilatory strategies. These examiners will not necessarily be ignorant on these topics, but it is certainly possible that your own clinical experience will be more recent and well informed than theirs. This should give you confidence, and you should not let the stress of the exam situation override it. Many candidates, for example, will have performed percutaneous tracheostomies in intensive care. Unless your examiner is an intensivist, however, it is possible (if not probable) that he or she has performed not even one, and so your own clinical experience in this area is already much wider than his or hers. Draw confidence from this, and do not be intimidated. The examiner guidance may even be dated and, say, for instance, that the approach should be through the first and second tracheal rings, whereas your own experience may reflect the common practice of siting the tracheostomy lower, between the second and third. So, if you do get the sense that the examiner is unhappy with your answer mainly because it does not accord with what is written on the sheet, then have the confidence to explain the current thinking. Do not be argumentative but simply offer your considered reasoning of the issue. This is likely to increase your own credibility while perhaps denting that of the examiner. So, if you have recently seen an innovative technique used in the operating theatre, in the chronic pain clinic or in critical care, do not be hesitant about citing it during the discussion.

The other consequence of the format of the structured oral is that it may lack fluency. It is partly a reflection of examining technique. Some examiners simply introduce the question before initiating a discussion, with only occasional reference to their paper-work. This is usually because they are familiar with the material and can allow the oral to run a more spontaneous course because they have confidence enough in their own ability to assess the answers. An examiner who is less comfortable with the topic and who is less certain of the criteria against which the answers are to be judged is likely to spend much more time referring to the answer sheet. Alternatively, of course, they might just be particularly pedantic in their interpretation of how the structured oral should be conducted. You may get a clue as to which of these you are facing by the way that they introduce the topic. The one type of examiner will try to put you more at ease by phrasing the question in a way which emphasizes the clinical context. Other examiners may simply look down at the sheet and intone, 'What is an inotrope?' This second examiner is likely to want facts, and ideally the facts that are listed on the answer paper. He or she clearly has not realized that you are not telepathic. If, however, you have some confidence both in your knowledge and in your clinical experience, you may be able to get him or her on the defensive. Remember that such an examiner may never have initiated the use of dopexamine or enoximone, and if you sense a slight uncertainty which confirms that suspicion, then expound as freely as they will let you. Remember also that this may be the limit of the manipulation that you are able to employ, unless you can muster the bravado of the candidate who, when his examiner tried to interrupt his fluent and detailed answer, paused briefly to announce, 'No, thank you, but I wish to finish.' The examiner, by his own confession somewhat intimidated by the intellectual onslaught, allowed the candidate to continue to the bell. That candidate passed. This is not, however, a strategy for the faint-hearted.

What you may be able to do, however, is to refine your technique to improve the overall impression that you create. Take, for example, two imaginary candidates who have been asked about the Poiseuille–Hagen equation. The examiner initiates the questioning: 'Does this have any clinical relevance?' Candidate: 'Yes.' Examiner: 'Can you give me some examples?' Candidate: 'It affects fluid flow through tubes.' Examiner: 'In what way?' Candidate: 'If you increase the driving pressure, then you increase the flow' . . . and so it goes on, with more abbreviated answers prompted by the examiner from a candidate who gives no real sense of mastery of the subject. Could it be done better? The examiner asks the same question: 'Does this have any clinical relevance?' Candidate: 'The equation strictly applies only to Newtonian or ideal fluids, but in practice it still has cardiorespiratory implications. The relationship means that gas or liquid flowing through a tube is inversely proportional to the length and viscosity of the fluid, and is directly proportional to the pressure gradient down the tube and, crucially, to the fourth power of its diameter.' This candidate, in contrast, requires no prompting, but demonstrates instead an orderly and logical approach that conveys the impression of obvious understanding of the topic. Only the occasional candidate achieves the fluency of the second example, whereas rather more candidates behave like the first and require a little help. Yet if you do have some knowledge of the subject asked, you can train yourself, with practice, to deliver the information both with more facility and more enthusiasm. This applies particularly to the clinical aspects in respect of which you can make your experience count. The structured nature of the examination question and marking system, however, does mean that you may get no chance to exhibit that fluency, and the oral may have a very staccato and rather disjointed feel as the examiners move rapidly on to the next part of the topic. Do not be disconcerted by this; it does not mean that you are doing poorly. It simply reflects the marking system, and so it is much more likely that you are doing well as the examiner in effect ticks off the question that has been answered and goes on to the next.

You do not need to worry about trying to pace the oral. It is the responsibility of the examiners to ensure that the requisite points are covered, and the guided answer sheets from which they are working contain more information than all but the most excep-tional candidate will cover in the time. The clinical science questions continue broadly to have two parts, the basic science and its clinical application. Nonetheless, this is still a science oral, and, despite the aspiration to increase the clinical relevance, the reality remains that in many of the questions it is the basic science that will be seen as the more important. Take, for example, the humidification of inspired gases. The clinical benefits of humidification are obvious: inhaled dry gases inspissate secretions, affect ciliary function and may cause impaired gas exchange due to atelectasis. However, these benefits can be summarized in a sentence – a sentence, moreover, that does not contain concepts that are especially complex. In contrast, the physical principles of latent heat of vaporization and saturated vapour pressure (which may be introduced by the subject of humidification) are topics which may warrant more detailed discussion. Equally, the anatomy of the nerves supplying the lower abdominal wall will take much longer to discuss than the description of a field block or a TAP block.

The questioning on each subject lasts less than 8 minutes. The examiner will take up at least 20% of this time in framing the questions. That leaves you, therefore, with only about 5 or 6 minutes during which to talk. Were you to read out steadily, fluently and without hesitation one of the average length answers in this book, it would probably take you twice that long. There are few candidates, moreover, who can answer questions as rapidly as they can read. You should find this reassuring, because it means that you cannot be expected to convey more than a proportion of the information that appears in each of the specimen questions.

Why Do They Have to Ask These Kinds of Question?

When your examiner looks up with an air of benign amusement from the question paper and invites you to discuss 'cytochrome P450' or 'chirality', your initial instinct may be to leap across the table to transfix them with your free Royal College examinations pencil. Some examiners will ask these questions with at least a hint of apology, which may raise your spirits marginally as you sense that these individuals might be on your side. Other examiners, alas, will be completely bereft of irony.

The difference between them should be obvious, but it might be of interest, if little consolation, were you to be aware of some of the reasons why such questions can arise.

A Brief History of Anaesthesia's Inferiority Complex

Anaesthesia had its humble origins in mid-nineteenth-century dentistry, and although hospital-based anaesthesia did become more sophisticated, in the early twentieth century simple general anaesthesia in the United Kingdom was still being delivered by individuals who were not only without medical qualifications but in many instances without even a rudimentary education. In contrast, however, physicians and surgeons of that era had high social and intellectual standing that had been established for centuries. As the specialty evolved over succeeding decades, it continued to enjoy only very modest status. There were, however, some politically astute anaesthetists, such as Robert Macintosh and Ivan Magill, who recognized the potential perils of anaesthetic humility and who thought it unwise to succumb to anaesthesia's inferiority complex. In particular they recognized the truth that anaesthetists could achieve equality of status with surgeons only if they had a qualification that was equivalent to the Fellowship of the Royal College of Surgeons, the FRCS. It was this realization which explained the early two-part exams, first the Diploma of Anaesthesia and then the FFARCS, which was the immediate forerunner of the FRCA. These examinations were modelled on the FRCS, had a low pass mark in the region of 25–30% and, by including in the syllabus detailed anatomy and pathology, established the precedent for rigour in the basic sciences.

The establishment of a difficult anaesthetic exam with a low pass rate actually played a crucial role in the development of the specialty. When you are tempted, therefore, to curse the College for erecting the hurdles of the Primary and Final FRCA, you could at least reflect that the difficulty of these examinations may in some oblique way ensure that you get paid the same as your colleagues in surgery and medicine. Anaesthesia has a reputation for having amongst the most difficult postgraduate exams, and, superficial though this may sound, it does remain one of the ways in which the specialty safeguards its standing.

Did this attempt to mirror the FRCS take the process too far? At times it can certainly seem so, and you may have to console yourself with the familiar, yet no less true, observation that 'Examinations are formidable even to the best prepared . . . for the greatest fool may ask more than the wisest man can answer' (Rev. Charles Colton [1780–1832]). A more recent perspective was provided by a distinguished professor of medicine and scientist from Oxford. During his valedictory speech to the faculty of medicine, he commented that in 30 years of clinical medicine his intimate knowledge of the Krebs cycle had influenced his management 'of not one single patient'. Medicine is as often pragmatic and empirical as it is intellectual. Some, but not all, examiners agree with that view, and do not accept that a detailed knowledge of scientific minutiae is necessary for the safe and effective practice of clinical anaesthesia. It may be obvious at your oral into which category the examiner falls.

Strategies for Answering Clinical Science Questions

Anatomy

Some candidates demonstrate a very detailed knowledge of areas of human anatomy, which allows them to embark on a thorough description of all the relevant structures and their immediate relations. Others have a more modest working knowledge, and then there is a final group which includes candidates who are able to demonstrate only a very vague idea of where these structures lie. You will know as soon as the question is asked of you which of these types you most closely match. One obvious strategy for passing questions on applied anatomy is just to learn it, or at least to develop enough confidence to be able to launch into a rapid account of the area in question. The speed of delivery is of some importance. Not every examiner will be able to recall the precise anatomical details that are found in the questions in this book. This means that they will probably have to make repeated reference to their answer sheet to check that what you are saying is true. Yet if they were to ask you to clarify more than one or two of your descriptions, then too much of the time in the oral would be lost. There is a tendency, therefore, for the examiner to listen to what you are saying, rather than making frequent interruptions. At the end of your account he or she may simply judge their overall impression of its accuracy. Confident presentation may, in this instance, allow you to mask some gaps in your knowledge.

What if you are the candidate whose recollection of an area is vague? Your chances of success in the question will depend on whether it is what could be termed 'theoretical anatomy' or 'practical anatomy'. The coronary arterial and venous circulation is an example of theoretical anatomy. It is not theoretical in the sense that it may be hypothetical. It is clearly of central importance, and anaesthesia may influence it, but it remains a construct which is visualized but neither seen nor felt. (To visualize means to construct a mental image of something, and is not a synonym for 'to see'.) The same can be said to apply to the cerebral circulation and the blood supply to the spinal cord. In contrast, the brachial plexus can be seen on ultrasound as you advance towards it with a regional block needle, and the structures of the posterior lumbar spine can be felt and visualized as you introduce your needle into the epidural or subarachnoid spaces. One tactic, which may salvage something from this part of the oral, is to move swiftly to the functional anatomy of the circulation. 'The main importance for anaesthetists of the right and left coronary circulations', you could state airily, 'lies in the way that we can influence oxygen supply and demand.' The examiner will take you back to check that you are indeed ignorant of the anatomy, but you will at least have initiated the physiological discussion which is the clinical part of the question and which may generally be of greater interest to candidates and examiners alike. Questions on 'practical anatomy' should be rather easier to handle because they relate to areas such as the internal jugular vein and the brachial plexus, detailed knowledge of which is of direct and self-evident importance. You can also reinforce this knowledge by disciplining yourself to visualize the relevant structures each time that you perform or observe a procedure relating to such an area. If you rehearse in your mind the nerves that are being blocked for an awake carotid endarterectomy as you see it being done, or describe the anatomy of the sacrum to a less-experienced colleague to whom you are teaching a caudal block, it will not be long before the details are secure in your mind without recourse to yet more evening study. In other words, you can revise for the Final FRCA during the course of your daily work. This does not apply only to anatomy, of course; it is true of other areas of the examination as well.

The examiner may ask you if you have performed a particular procedure, or may even give you a question that allows you to discuss, for example, an upper or lower limb block of your choosing. In respect of practical procedures that you claim to have undertaken, you should be aware that the threshold for a pass shifts sharply upwards. If you say that you regularly perform caudal blocks in children or interscalene blocks in adults, but then go on to reveal that your knowledge either of the anatomy or of the appropriate drug doses is at best hazy, then you are likely to be penalized accordingly. In examination anaesthesia, as in real-life anaesthesia, whenever you are in any doubt, you should choose the safest option. Better in both situations to admit that you have done very few caudal or interscalene blocks and that you would seek experienced help.

Finally, anatomy questions do lend themselves readily to diagrammatic answers. Many candidates seem to benefit from being allowed to describe the anatomy while they draw; producing the diagram acts as a stimulus to recollection. It is worth practising this technique because the number of anatomy topics is relatively small and it is almost certain that one of the accounts below will appear as a question.

Physiology

Anatomy, pharmacology and physics are all large scientific disciplines, yet in the context of the Final FRCA their scope is restricted, and the areas of specific relevance to anaesthetic practice are finite. Physiology, in contrast, is very wide-ranging, and questions appear which are related to all the systems, including renal, gastrointestinal and endocrine.

When the oral was marked as a whole entity, it was almost inevitable that examiners would give more weight to core topics related to respiratory and cardiac physiology. The change in the marking system is probably intended to mean that this is no longer the case, with topics such as 'plasma proteins' and 'thyroid hormones' ranked equally with 'oxygen delivery' and 'pulmonary oedema'. However, it is possible that examiners may mark less stringently those subjects which they do not regard as central. You may need to do less, in other words, to pass a question on gut hormones than on assessment of cardiac function. So, as before, what this means in practice is that your grasp of core areas needs to be more secure than your knowledge of more peripheral aspects of physiology. It is not that you will not get asked a question on the latter but rather that you will disadvantage yourself much more by ignorance of the former.

Pharmacology

The number of core anaesthetic drugs is limited. The sum of the regularly used induction agents, neuromuscular blockers, volatiles, analgesic drugs and local anaesthetics barely exceeds 20. The pharmacology of these substances is almost by definition applied science, and so you will find examiners much less forgiving of deficiencies in anaesthetic pharmacological knowledge than they would be of ignorance of lasers or medical statistics. You may feel somewhat aggrieved if the oral concentrates on chirality or GABA/NMDA receptor theory, but you should recognize that there is only so far that such a topic can be pursued, and you should be able to acknowledge finally that questioning about the scientific foundation of your everyday anaesthetic practice is a legitimate area of enquiry. Given the restricted numbers of drugs, however, it should not be an insuperable task to acquire the necessary amount of information. Some of the questions can be straightforward and lend themselves readily to a structured answer that you can adapt across the range of anaesthetic drugs. One such question, for instance, may ask you to enumerate the properties of an ideal volatile agent, and then to compare desflurane and sevoflurane against that ideal. You will see that this same question could be asked of local anaesthetics, neuromuscular blockers, inotropes, anti-emetics and any number of classes of agents. You will also need to have some understanding of subjects such as pharmacokinetics and receptor theory. Other areas of relevance to anaesthetists are the non-anaesthetic drugs that patients may commonly be taking. The potential list is quite long and includes anti-hypertensive agents, antibiotics, drugs to treat asthma, drugs to treat diabetes and drugs which affect mood. Much of the knowledge that you may have acquired in working for the Primary FRCA will stand you in good stead for the Final. One final piece of advice: if you are asked the dose of a drug and you are unsure, then do not guess. Both in anaesthetic exams and in anaesthetic practice it is safer by far to admit that you would look it up.

Clinical Measurement and Equipment

You might have hoped to have left much of the physics and clinical measurement behind, but as also applies to pharmacology questions, much of the knowledge that you may have acquired in working for the Primary FRCA will be helpful for the Final. Some

Final examiners are mesmerized by the physics involved in some of the questions that appear; others are less beguiled. If you are examined by one of the former group, then expect to be asked to define, for example, the SI units that are appropriate to the particular question, and try not to worry if you get so immersed in the science that you only touch briefly on its clinical application. This is less likely than once it was, now that there is an explicit emphasis on the clinical applications. At the other extreme lies the examiner who takes the view that complex anaesthetic devices are essentially black boxes whose inner workings can safely be left a mystery. In this case the oral may follow a rather different course, and it is probable that the emphasis will be more on clinical uses and on sources of error in interpretation of the information that is delivered. You will still need, therefore, to be prepared for both. Yet even those examiners who have considerable enthusiasm for this subject will recognize that there is a limit to how far it can reasonably be taken. The detailed physics underlying magnetic resonance imaging, for example, is too formidable to be covered in an oral such as this. If you can articulate the basic principles of the topic, whether it be magnetic resonance scanning or lasers, and if you can demonstrate that you are aware of its clinical and safety implications, then in most cases that should be enough to ensure you a pass.

Statistics

There are doctors who have an intuitive gift for statistics, which is a subject that they find very straightforward. Included amongst such doctors are some examiners and some candidates, and they do not therefore understand the collective groan that goes up when the prospect emerges either of having to ask or to answer a question on medical statistics. The fact remains, however, that the topic is unpopular with the majority of anaesthetists. Yet paradoxically this may be of some benefit to those who are uncomfortable with the concepts. Most examiners are conditioned by their own experience of asking about statistics to expect less than brilliant answers. What this means in practice is twofold. First, the questions should not be especially demanding, and, second, as long as you are able to enunciate some basic principles and definitions, then you are more likely to get a bare pass than you would were you to offer the same level of information about, say, the anatomy of the epidural space. So, as a minimum make sure, for example, that you know the difference between parametric and non-parametric data and tests, between paired and unpaired *t*-tests, about degrees of freedom and about the null hypothesis. Be prepared to discuss briefly the principles which underlie meta-analysis and systematic reviews and the differences between them, and ensure that you have some familiarity with the results of at least one systematic review or meta-analysis of clinical importance, ideally one that is recent and therefore topical. Questions on statistics are unlikely now to stand alone but may be linked to subjects such as the design of clinical trials.

And Finally: Information, Understanding and 'Buzzwords'

It is only a few years since one particularly ferocious examiner, having encountered some hapless candidate or other, argued that no one should be allowed to pass the

FRCA if they did not know the structure of ether. Although she said 'structure', it is likely that she really meant 'formula' (which as it happens is $CH_3-CH_2-O-CH_2-CH_3$). Either way, the proposition is absurd. Yet it does raise interesting issues in relation to postgraduate examinations. What is their primary purpose? What are they actually for?

Some have argued that, in addition to providing a test of knowledge and a core syllabus, examinations also act as an incentive to learn and, perhaps less urgently, as an incentive to teach. They are used as a hurdle to promotion, and success indicates to colleagues that a standard of training has been achieved. This may also offer a measure of reassurance to an increasingly suspicious public, particularly if the examination is perceived as conferring a title of distinction.

Only two of these functions are of immediate relevance to you. The first is the suggestion that the possession of the diploma of FRCA is a title of distinction. That may sound somewhat grandiose, but in fact it is in everyone's interest that it should be such. The diploma should not be easily won; it should feel like an exam that is difficult to pass yet one that is worth passing. Were it not so, then examiners and candidates alike would rapidly become demotivated and the standing of the specialty would slide. This thought may offer some solace as you lose many months of your life to the bookwork that is necessary. The second relevant factor is the exam's function as a test of knowledge. It is relatively simple to test for information, harder to assess understanding and more difficult still to provide an objective test of judgement. Hence, as a particular exam evolves, its structure and content elide to create what in effect becomes an examination game. Yet it is a game whose rules curiously do seem to become clear both to candidates and to examiners, as independently they develop a broad appreciation of the level of knowledge that the exam expects.

This is partly because with many topics which appear as examination questions, there is what could be described as a hierarchy of information. Take, for instance, 5-hydroxytryptamine (5-HT). At one end of its continuum of knowledge is the straightforward fact that it is an aminergic neurotransmitter. At the more difficult end are details such as the significance of the inositol triphosphate pathway for $5-HT_2$ receptor function. In between these two extremes is the information about drugs which act at 5-HT receptors, the classes of 5-HT receptors, the subsets of those receptors and the physiological functions that they mediate. Somewhere along that scale is the boundary between a pass and a fail. So how much do you have to know about 5-HT to pass the question? Ask yourself. Should you know that ondansetron is a $5-HT_3$ antagonist? Probably. Should you know the exact details of the fourteen 5-HT receptors that have been identified? Probably not, particularly as their functions have not been fully elaborated. Should you know that all bar $5-HT_3$ receptors are coupled to G proteins? Possibly. Should you know that cerebrospinal fluid production is mediated via $5-HT_{2C}$ receptors? Not unless you are heading for the prize. Strange to say most examiners would probably give much the same replies. Both parties seem to understand the rules which dictate that the oral will start at the simpler end of the spectrum and move towards that fail/pass boundary. It is inevitable that it will take some time to cover the basic information, so how do you then convince the examiners that you deserve to pass? Facile though it may seem, some of the time you do it by producing the appropriate buzzwords. They can be described as buzzwords because, unless you are a potential prizewinner who has swept the core knowledge aside, there is unlikely to be much time to discuss the more complex information in any detail. By producing the key words and phrases, however, you will have given the examiner at least the subliminal impression that you know more about the subject than just basic information. So, what are the buzzwords in the example above? One of them would be G protein-coupling. This has a nice echo of Primary FRCA basic science about it, and its mention alone may well satisfy the examiner who is unlikely then to explore your knowledge of ligand-gated ion channels. Similarly, it might help were you to mention that there were seven main 5-HT receptor types. What about a question, say, on atracurium or sevoflurane – how much should you know? Clearly you will have to display sufficient knowledge to show that your use of these agents is safe and effective. But beyond that, it will help if you happen to refer to atracurium as a 'benzylisoquinolinium' and sevoflurane as a 'halogenated ether'. The examiners are not going to start asking about benzylisoquino-linium chemistry, although they might perhaps want to know what you mean by a 'halogenated ether'. Were you to reply that it is a hexafluorinated methyl isopropyl ether, then that line of questioning would end. That is because it is actually a complete dead end down which, were you to have the knowledge, you could continue with the information that sevoflurane is fluoromethyl 1,1,1,3,3,3–hexafluoroisopropyl ether, and that it can be synthesized by a reaction that involves formaldehyde and hydrogen fluoride. By this point even the most astringent examiner would recognize that you had both left anaesthesia far behind in the hot pursuit of irrelevant facts. So, as you revise topics, it is worth bearing this advice in mind because it should not be too difficult to identify those small additional pieces of information that may add further credibility to your answers. This analysis may seem dispiritingly reductive, if not intellectually disreputable, but it is an inevitable consequence of the nature of a standardized exam in which knowledge of the relevant basic sciences has to be explored in a relatively rigid way. If, however, your grasp of that basic knowledge is sound, then you deserve to pass, and it would be unfortunate to fail the examination for want of a few of these simple strategies. So finally –

The best of luck.

Anatomy and Its Applications

The Cerebral Circulation

Commentary

This is a standard question, but one which contains a lot of anatomical detail. It may be helpful to practise drawing a simple explanatory diagram. The oral may be linked to intracranial aneurysms and their management, and it may also include physiological aspects of cerebral perfusion, on the problem of cerebral vasospasm following subarachnoid haemorrhage or briefly on the subject of intracranial pressure.

Core Information

The arterial supply to the brain. The venous drainage is included in the following but is less likely to feature as prominently.

Arterial Supply (Figure 2.1)

- The brain is supplied by four major vessels: two internal carotid arteries which provide two-thirds of the arterial supply, and the two vertebral arteries which deliver the remaining third. (Some texts quote an 80:20 distribution.)
- The vertebral arteries give off the posterior inferior cerebellar arteries, before joining to form the basilar artery. This also provides the anterior inferior cerebellar and the superior cerebellar arteries.
- The basilar artery then gives off the two posterior cerebral arteries, which supply the medial side of the temporal lobe and the occipital lobe.
- The artery then anastomoses with the carotid arteries via two posterior communicating arteries.
- The internal carotid arteries meanwhile give rise to the middle cerebral arteries which supply the lateral parts of the cerebral hemispheres. They also provide much of the supply to the internal capsule, through which pass a large number of cortical afferent and efferent fibres.

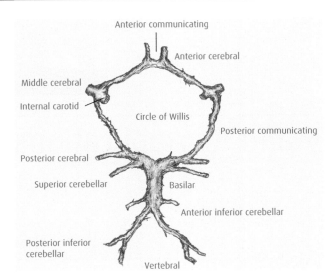

Fig. 2.1 Arterial supply of the brain.

- The carotids also give rise to the anterior cerebral arteries, which are connected by the anterior communicating artery and which supply the medial and superior aspects of the hemispheres.
- The three arterial stems (basilar and carotid arteries), linked by the anterior and posterior communicating arteries, comprise the arterial circle of Willis. This is said to be incomplete in up to 15% of normal asymptomatic subjects.

Venous System

- The cerebral and cerebellar cortices, which are relatively superficial structures, drain into the dural sinuses. These venous sinuses lie between the two layers of the cranial dura mater. The superior sagittal sinus lies along the attached edge of the falx cerebri, dividing the hemispheres, and usually drains into the right transverse sinus. The inferior sagittal sinus lies along the free edge of the falx and drains via the straight sinus into the left transverse sinus. (The straight sinus lies in the tentorium cerebelli.) The transverse sinuses merge into the sigmoid sinuses before emerging from the cranium as the internal jugular veins.
- Deeper cranial structures drain via the two internal cerebral veins, which join to form the great cerebral vein (of Galen). This also drains into the inferior sagittal sinus.
- The cavernous sinuses lie on either side of the pituitary fossa and drain eventually into the transverse sinuses.

Supplementary and Clinical Information

Aneurysmal Subarachnoid Haemorrhage

- Intracranial aneurysms account for about 85% of cases of spontaneous SAH; the incidence is 1 in 10–12,000 persons per year. The overall mortality rate approaches 50%, and morbidity amongst survivors is high.
- Aneurysms are associated with a weakening of the tunica media of the arterial wall and develop most commonly at vascular bifurcations. Only 10–20% of aneurysms

form in the posterior vertebrobasilar circulation. Most are found in the anterior carotid circulation, in the middle cerebral artery and in the anterior and posterior communicating arteries.

- Initial management is as for any other acute cerebral injury, with the emphasis on cardiorespiratory stabilization and the prevention of secondary brain injury. Treatment is either with endovascular occlusion using coils or by aneurysm clipping via a direct neurosurgical approach. The cumulative risk of rebleeding approaches 20% at 14 days.
- **Cerebral vasospasm:** this is the major cause of morbidity and mortality following SAH, and occurs in up to 70% of cases. It is a cause of delayed cerebral ischaemia (DCI). Its peak onset is at 7–10 days, may manifest as early as day 3 and usually resolves by 21 days. There are various theories for its aetiology on which the oral may touch, but their complexity precludes excessive detail. Acutely there is an increase in intracellular calcium which follows exposure to haemoglobin and which produces contraction (via phosphorylation of myosin light chains). However, prolonged vasoconstriction is independent of intracellular calcium levels, but it may be due to an increase in calcium responsiveness induced by endothelin. Endothelin-1 (ET-1) is a potent vasoconstrictor whose receptors are upregulated in response to cerebral ischaemia. There is also a general increase in the density both of ET-1 and 5-HT$_{1B}$ receptors. Other factors include the production of reactive oxygen species and lipid peroxidation secondary to haemoglobin autoxidation and changes in the scavenging or production of nitric oxide. A large volume of subarachnoid blood (as seen on CT) is a consistent predictor of the development of vasospasm.
- **Prevention and management:** there is unlikely to be time to cover this in any detail, so an understanding of the broad principles should suffice. There is good evidence to support the prophylactic use of the dihydropyridine calcium channel blocker nimodipine which improves outcome (typical dose regimen is 60 mg 4 hourly for 21 days). Nimodipine blocks the slow calcium channel of vascular smooth muscle and cardiac muscle but has no effect on skeletal muscle. The British aneurysm trial demonstrated a 40% reduction in poor outcomes (mortality and neurodisability). Established or incipient cerebral vasospasm can be managed with so-called triple-H therapy, or **H**ypertension, **H**ypervolaemia and **H**aemodilution, the combination of which aims to increase perfusion pressure, decrease blood viscosity and maximize cerebral blood flow. While it is important to avoid hypotension, hypovolaemia and haemoconcentration, triple-H therapy lacks evidence from controlled trials and its use remains contentious. A low haematocrit, for example, may improve cerebral blood flow but may reduce oxygen delivery.

The direct anaesthetic implications of the anatomy described here are modest. Further discussion may include cerebral perfusion (See under 'Cerebral Blood Flow' in Chapter 3) or intracranial pressure (see under 'Intracranial Pressure' in Chapter 3). Following are some miscellaneous facts which may also prove useful.

- The circle of Willis provides effective collateral blood supply in the presence of arterial occlusion. Three out of four of the main arteries can be occluded as long as the process is gradual, without producing cerebral ischaemia. The normal intracranial blood volume is around 100–130 ml.

- The middle cerebral artery has been described as 'the artery of cerebral haemorrhage'. This is mainly because it supplies the internal capsule, where a large number of important cortical afferent and efferent fibres congregate.
- The superficial areas of the cerebral (and cerebellar) cortex drain to the venous sinuses via thin-walled veins. These are vulnerable to rupture, with the formation of subdural haematomas, particularly in the elderly in whom there is a loss of brain mass.
- Other potential intracranial catastrophes include cavernous sinus thrombosis, sagittal sinus thrombosis and cortical vein thrombosis (CVT). CVT is particularly associated with pregnancy, and is reported as occurring in between 1 in 3,000 and 1 in 6,000 deliveries. If this figure is accurate, then CVT is being under-diagnosed, because very few obstetric anaesthetists in an average-sized maternity unit encounter the one or two cases a year that this incidence would suggest. It should always be included in the differential diagnosis of peri-partum headache.

Brain Stem Death Testing

Commentary

Testing for brain stem death is long established, but still excites debate. The residual controversy can greatly trouble the relatives of a patient who may be brain-dead, and so it is of crucial importance that you understand the neurological basis of the tests sufficiently well to be able to answer any question that they might wish to ask. This is not a pure anatomy question, and as it is the cranial nerve reflexes that are the underlying basis of the tests, it may appear in either the anatomy or physiology part of the oral.

Core Information

Established Criteria for Brainstem Death Testing

- **Definition:** brain death describes the situation in which a patient has undergone the irreversible loss of any capacity for consciousness, together with the irreversible loss of the ability to breathe.
- **Preconditions:** before testing can be considered, there are preconditions that must be satisfied, the most important of which is that there must be a definitive diagnosis of the cause of the brain damage. The patient should also be in an apnoeic coma, with a Glasgow Coma Score of 3 (no eye opening, no verbal response and no localization of pain).
- **Children:** theoretically, the clinical criteria are the same in children, although there are enough concerns about their applicability to make this a very difficult area. In neonates, for example, CNS immaturity raises doubts about the validity of brain stem death tests, and there is much anecdotal evidence of children who have recovered substantial neurological function despite severe insult and prolonged coma.
- **Exclusions: Temperature:** this must be at least 35 °C. **Sedatives:** There should be no residual depressant drugs in the system, which in practice may mean substantial delay until clearance can be assured. Such patients are usually sedated with

short-acting agents whose elimination can be predicted with some confidence. (Observation over four elimination half-lives is commonly recommended). If, however, they have received longer-acting drugs, such as barbiturates (e.g. thiopental) to control convulsive activity, or if there is a suspicion of illicit drug use then the situation can be more difficult. Plasma determinations may be indicated, but if the intracranial catastrophe is obvious and extreme, some clinicians do not believe them to be necessary. **Neuromuscular blockade**: This should be excluded (where appropriate) by using a peripheral nerve stimulator. **Metabolic derangement**: There must be no endocrine or metabolic disturbance that may contribute to continued coma, and there should be no possibility that impaired circulatory function is compromising cerebral perfusion. **Normocapnia**: A high $PaCO_2$ can obtund cerebral function and so must be kept normal (for that patient).

- **The tests:** these are carried out by two doctors, both of whom have been registered for more than 5 years, and one of whom must be a consultant. Two sets of tests are performed, although there is no set interval between them. In practice, they are usually done a few hours apart. There has never been a reported case of a patient who initially satisfied the criteria for brain stem death and who subsequently failed to do so. The tests aim to confirm the absence of brain stem reflexes and examine those cranial nerves which are amenable to testing.

- **The cranial nerve reflexes**
  - *I*: the first nerve (olfactory) cannot be tested.
  - *II*: the second nerve (optic), together with the parasympathetic constrictor outflow, is tested by pupillary responses to light (direct and consensual). Pupillary size is not important.
  - *III, IV, VI*: the third, fourth and sixth nerves (oculomotor, trochlear and abducens) are not tested.
  - *V, VII*: the fifth (trigeminal) and seventh (facial) nerves are tested first by the corneal reflex, and then by the response to painful stimuli applied to the face (supraorbital or infraorbital pressure), to the limbs (nail bed pressure) and to the trunk (sternal stimulation). It is because of the possibility of tetraplegia that a stimulus should be applied above the neck.
  - *VIII*: the eighth nerve (auditory/vestibular) is examined by caloric testing. It is important to establish that both drums are visible and intact, after which 30 ml of ice-cold water is instilled via a syringe. Nystagmus is absent if the patient is brain-dead. The assessment of doll's eye movements, to test whether the eyes move with the head (which is abnormal) instead of maintaining central gaze, is not part of the brain stem death tests as performed in the UK.
  - *IX, X*: the ninth (glossopharyngeal) and tenth (vagus) nerves are tested by stimulating the pharynx, larynx and trachea. The patient should neither gag nor cough.
  - *XI, XII*: the eleventh (accessory) and twelfth (hypoglossal) nerves are not tested.

- **Apnoea testing:** after ventilation with 100% oxygen for 10 minutes, the patient is disconnected from the ventilator. Oxygen saturation is maintained thereafter by apnoeic oxygenation via a tracheal catheter. In the apnoeic patient, arterial CO_2 rises at a rate of about 0.40–0.80 kPa per minute, depending on the metabolic rate, and so it may take some time to reach the arterial blood gas level of 6.65 kPa required by the testing criteria.

Supplementary Information

Potential Pitfalls

- With the preconditions satisfied and the tests performed with scrupulous care, there should be none. There are, however, some conditions of which those carrying out the tests should be aware.
- There are a number of lesions of the brain stem which may closely mimic irreversible brain death. These include severe Guillain–Barré and Miller–Fisher syndromes, Bickerstaff's brain stem encephalitis and ventral pontine infarction associated with the 'locked-in syndrome'. Brain stem encephalitis is characterized by acute progressive cranial nerve dysfunction associated with ataxia, coma and apnoea. There is no structural abnormality of the brain, but the picture is one of brain stem death. It is reversible. Bilateral ventral pontine lesions may involve both corticospinal and corticobulbar tracts, leading to tetraplegia and the locked-in syndrome. Patients are unable to speak or produce facial movements. They can usually blink and move their eyes vertically, and because the tegmentum of the pons is spared, they remain sensate, fully conscious and aware. It is the stuff of nightmares, and meaningful recovery from the locked-in syndrome is extremely rare.

Further Confirmatory Tests That Can Be Undertaken

- Auditory, visual and somatosensory evoked potentials can be used, as can the EEG and cerebral angiography. None of these is required in the UK.
- Management of the ASA 6 patient for organ retrieval. Clearly the potential donor organs must be oxygenated and well perfused, and this may require some haemodynamic manipulation. The problem arises with the question of 'anaesthesia'. The legal time of death occurs when brain stem death is confirmed, and so logically a dead patient cannot require anaesthesia (except perhaps for muscle relaxants to prevent spinal reflexes). There are, however, those who believe brain stem death testing to be little more than a pragmatic way of providing donor organs for transplant, and some anaesthetists appear to share enough residual unease about the process to make them give a general anaesthetic. The philosophical questions that this raises are interesting and important, but the clinical science oral is probably not the best place to explore them.

Pupillary and Eye Signs (in General)

- **Pupillary signs:** lateral herniation of the tentorium as a result of increased intracranial pressure (ICP) can compress the oculomotor (III) nerve with ipsilateral papillary dilatation. This may also be accompanied by ptosis and motor paralysis of the extraocular muscles (apart from the superior oblique and lateral rectus muscles which are supplied by cranial nerves IV and VI, respectively). Central tentorial herniation can cause miosis (due to diencephalic damage). If there is midbrain compression, the size of the pupils may remain in the mid-range, but they are unresponsive. Pinpoint and unreactive pupils may signify pontine haemorrhage.
- **Eye signs:** raised ICP obstructs cerebrospinal fluid (CSF) flow in the optic nerve sheath with the development of papilloedema. The lateral rectus is also affected because of the displacement of the sixth cranial nerve (abducens) during its long intracranial course. (As it leaves the posterior margin of the pons, it is crossed by the

anterior inferior cerebellar artery. Cerebellar displacement may cause compression of the nerve, paresis and failure of lateral gaze.)

- **Cranial nerves XIII and XIV:** it is unlikely to come from the examiners, but they may well be impressed if you impart information about these two extra cranial nerves which have long been identified but which have not routinely been described in medical texts. (You could mention, e.g., that 'cranial nerves XIII and XIV are of course not tested as part of brain stem function'.) The thirteenth cranial nerve, also known as Nerve Zero (because it lies more rostrally than the other cranial nerves) or the Nervus Terminalis, has its origins close to the olfactory bulb but is not part of it. It appears to mediate the release of luteinizing hormone and is thought therefore to have some role in the regulation of reproductive behaviour. This hypothesis is reinforced by its projections to septal nuclei and the preoptic areas of the brain, which in mammals are associated with sexual behaviour, including the response to pheromones. The fourteenth cranial nerve is also known as the Nervus Intermedius and has usually been considered to be part of the 7th cranial nerve, the facial nerve. It lies between this nerve and the superior part of the 8th cranial nerve, the vestibulo-cochlear. However, it has a different origin in the brain and subserves different functions, including taste; the sensory innervation of part of the outer ear, the nose and the mouth; and lacrimation and salivation. Its motor functions include contraction of the orbicularis oris muscle.

The Internal Jugular Vein

Commentary
The right internal jugular vein is the first site of choice for short-term central venous cannulation, although the subclavian route is preferred by many for longer-term central access. The internal jugular vein is readily accessible and the technique has a relatively low complication rate. The ability to cannulate the vessel is a core skill.

Core Information
The anatomy of the **internal jugular vein (Figure 2.2)**.

- The internal jugular vein originates at the jugular foramen in the skull (the foramen drains the sigmoid sinus) and is a continuation of the jugular bulb.
- It follows a relatively straight course in the neck to terminate behind the sterno-clavicular joint, where it joins the subclavian vein.
- Throughout its course it lies with the carotid artery and the vagus nerve within the carotid sheath, but it changes position in relation to the artery, lying first posteriorly before moving laterally and then anterolaterally.
- The vein is superficial in the upper part of the neck and then descends deep to the sternocleidomastoid muscle. The structures through which a cannulating needle passes are skin and subcutaneous tissue, the platysma muscle, sternocleidomastoid (in the lower neck) and the loose fascia of the carotid sheath.

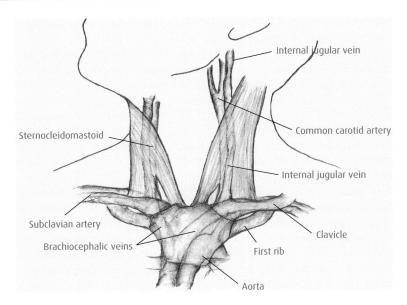

Fig. 2.2 The great veins of the neck.

- Anterior to the vein at the top of its course lie the internal carotid artery and the vagus nerve.
- Posterior to the vein (from above downwards) are the lateral part of C_1, the prevertebral fascia and vertebral muscles, the cervical transverse processes, the sympathetic chain and, at the root of the neck, the dome of the pleura. On the left side, the jugular vein lies anterior to the thoracic duct.
- Medial to the vein are the carotid arteries (internal and common) and four cranial nerves: the ninth (glossopharyngeal, IX), the tenth (vagus, X), the eleventh (accessory, XI) and the twelfth (hypoglossal, XII).

Supplementary and Clinical Information

The Principles of, and Indications for, Central Venous Cannulation

- **Principle:** the central venous pressure (CVP) gives information both about a patient's volaemic status and about the function of the right ventricle.
- **Intravascular volume:** the CVP is the hydrostatic pressure generated by the blood within the right atrium (RA) or the great veins of the thorax. It provides an indication of volaemic status because the capacitance system, which includes all the large veins of the thorax, abdomen and proximal extremities, forms a large compliant reservoir for two-thirds of the total blood volume.
- **Right ventricular function:** CVP measurements also provide an indication of right ventricular (RV) function. Any impairment of RV function will be reflected by the higher filling pressures that are needed to maintain the same stroke volume (SV).
- **Normal values:** the normal range is 0–8 mmHg, measured at the level of the tricuspid valve. The tip of the catheter should lie just above the right atrium in the superior vena

cava. CVP measurements are sometimes recorded as negative values. Sustained mean negative values can occur only if the transducer has been placed above the level of the right atrium. Transient negative values may be recorded in conditions such as severe acute asthma in which partial respiratory obstruction generates high negative intrathoracic pressures which are transmitted to the central veins.

- **Indications:** CVP catheters are used for the monitoring of CVP, for the insertion of pulmonary artery catheters (much less commonly in current practice) and to provide access for haemofiltration and transvenous cardiac pacing. They also allow the administration of drugs that cannot be given peripherally, such as inotropes and cytotoxic agents, and the infusion of total parenteral nutrition. In massive air embolism they can be used to aspirate air from the right side of the heart, although few anaesthetists have ever used them for this purpose.

Technique(s) for Insertion of a Central Venous Catheter (CVC)

You will have had experience of this technique, many variations of which have been described. Outline the one with which you are most familiar. The use of ultrasound-guided cannulation is now more or less universal, but this does not absolve you of the need to know the basic anatomy (for the 'landmark' approach). Landmark approaches are associated with failure and complication rates of around 10%.

- An example would be the high approach. A fine 'seeking' needle (25G or similar) is inserted at the level of the superior border of the thyroid cartilage (at about C_4) and on the medial border of sternocleidomastoid.
- The needle is directed caudally at an angle of 30° in the direction of the ipsilateral nipple. The vein is usually quite superficial, although this will depend on the body habitus of the patient.
- Once the vein is located, the Seldinger technique (catheter over guidewire) can be used to establish definitive central access.

There are alternative sites, should internal jugular cannulation be impossible (for example, in major head and neck surgery or in patients with neck and facial burns).

- These alternatives are the **subclavian**, **femoral** and the **median cubital** and **basilic** veins of the antecubital fossa. A peripheral long line can be inserted via the latter. This technique has few complications, but the catheter tip may fail to pass beyond the acute curve at the clavipectoral fascia and the catheter length means that fluid cannot be infused rapidly. The femoral vein is commonly overlaid by the superficial femoral artery and the variable anatomy means that femoral access can sometimes be difficult. The route is used commonly in children but is more of a last resort in adults, in whom the subclavian veins are usually a better alternative.
- **Anatomy of the subclavian veins:** the right and left subclavian veins are relatively short, extending from the outer border of the first rib to the medial border of the scalenus anterior muscle. Here they unite with the internal jugular veins to form the brachiocephalic veins. The important relations are anteriorly – the clavicle; posteriorly – the subclavian artery; inferiorly – the dome of the pleura. The insertion point of the cannula is usually 1 cm below the clavicle at its midpoint, directed towards the suprasternal notch.

Complications Associated with the Technique

Following is a compilation of the most common; the literature is full of others which range from spinal accessory nerve injury to cardiac tamponade.

- **Complications:** many of these can be minimized by the use of an ultrasound-guided needle. The National Institute of Clinical Excellence (NICE) report of September 2002 recommended the routine use of ultrasound for locating the internal jugular vein. The vessel is not always present, is not always located in the textbook anatomical position and is not always patent. Experienced has widened to the point at which ultrasound-guided cannulation is now routine, if not mandatory.
- **Carotid artery puncture or cannulation:** the risk is reduced if the artery is palpated continuously throughout cannulation, and as for the preceding example is minimized by the use of ultrasound.
- **Pneumothorax (and haemothorax):** this is less likely if a high approach is used which avoids the dome of the pleura.
- **Thoracic duct injury (chylothorax):** the thoracic duct cannot be damaged if the left side is not used. Otherwise the risk is again minimized by using a high approach.
- **Intrapleural placement:** here too the risk is attenuated by using a high approach which avoids the pleura. A check X-ray (which is mandatory following central venous cannulation) will prevent inadvertent intrapleural infusion.
- **Air embolism:** positioning the patient head down during insertion (and removal) decreases the risk.
- **Cardiac arrhythmias:** these may occur should the guidewire or catheter reach the heart.
- **Infection:** central line infection can be disastrous. Significant infection is said to occur in around 12% of insertions, although some degree of bacterial colonization, both intra- and extra-luminal, probably occurs in every placement. Both external and endoluminal surfaces of any intravascular catheter rapidly become coated with plasma proteins, which in turn become colonized by bacteria which migrate down from the skin. This process occurs within hours. Once a threshold number of organisms is reached, symptomatic bacteraemia will follow. This process usually takes 3 to 4 days, and the commonest organisms implicated are coagulase-negative staphylococci and staphylococcus aureus (together these account for around 60% of the total). Other species include enterococci and pseudomonas. Catheter-related sepsis has a mortality that has been reported as high as 25%. The risks are reduced by scrupulous aseptic technique as well as meticulous aftercare. The insertion site is also significant: subclavian CVCs have the lowest rates of infection.

Ocular Anatomy

Commentary

Questions on the eye seem to be over-represented in the Final FRCA. It may be owing to the fact that considerable anatomical detail is concentrated in a small well-circumscribed area, and that the oral can go in a number of directions, including pupillary and eye signs and intraocular pressure.

Core Information

The Anatomy of the Orbit

- The bony orbit has been described variously as a pyramid whose apex is directed inwards and upwards, as a cone and as a pear whose stem points towards the optic canal. Its roof consists of the orbital plate of the frontal bone, with the anterior cranial fossa above, while its floor is formed by the zygoma and the maxilla, with the maxillary sinus beneath. Its medial wall is formed by parts of the maxilla, lacrimal bone, ethmoid and sphenoid, and beyond it lie the ethmoid air cells and the nasal cavity. The zygoma and the greater wing of the sphenoid make up its lateral wall.
- The bony orbit contains the globe, together with the muscles, nerves and blood vessels that subserve the normal functions of the eye.
- The normal globe has an axial length of around 24 mm (as measured in the anteroposterior diameter). An eye longer than 26 mm is usually myopic. Its outer layer comprises sclera and cornea; the middle vascular layer contains the choroid, the ciliary body and the iris; and the innermost layer comprises neural tissue in the form of the retina.
- The movements of the globe are controlled by the six extraocular striated muscles. The four recti (lateral, medial, superior and inferior) originate from the annulus of Zinn, the tendinous ring which encircles the optic foramen, and insert beyond the equator of the globe. The lateral and medial recti have two heads. The superior oblique muscle originates above and medial to the annulus, curves round the trochlea (which acts like a pulley), before inserting behind the equator and beneath the superior rectus. The inferior oblique originates from the lacrimal bone and inserts posterolaterally on the globe, having passed beneath the inferior rectus muscle.
- **Motor innervation:** the lateral rectus is supplied by the sixth cranial nerve, the abducens (VI), and the superior oblique is supplied by the fourth, the trochlear (IV). The remaining muscles are supplied by the third cranial nerve, the oculomotor (III). (This also supplies levator palpebrae superioris, which elevates the eyelid).
- **Autonomic innervation:** sympathetic innervation is by the long and short ciliary nerves via the superior cervical ganglion. Nerve impulses dilate the pupil via the dilators of the iris. Parasympathetic innervation is by the short postganglionic ciliary nerves via the ciliary ganglion. The pre-ganglionic supply comes from the oculomotor nerve, and its impulses constrict the pupil.
- **Sensory supply:** this is derived mainly from the ophthalmic branch of the fifth cranial nerve, the trigeminal (V), although branches of the maxillary division make some contribution to lateral structures and to the nasolacrimal apparatus. There are a large number of sensory nerves for such an anatomically confined area. The examiner is unlikely to dwell on these in any detail but, in summary, the innervation that may have relevance for ocular surgery can be outlined as follows. The ophthalmic division V^1 branches into the frontal nerve, which then subdivides into the supratrochlear nerves (medial upper conjunctiva), the supraorbital nerve (upper conjunctiva)

and the long ciliary nerve (cornea, iris and ciliary muscle). V^1 also forms the nasociliary nerve, which in turn branches into the infratrochlear nerve (inner canthus and lacrimal sac) and the long sensory root to the ciliary ganglion (thence to the cornea and iris). The lacrimal branch of V^1 supplies the rest of the conjunctiva.

- **Foramina:** the orbit contains nine fissures and foramina, of which three are particularly important: the optic foramen (canal), and the superior and inferior orbital fissures.
- **Optic canal.** The optic nerve and ophthalmic artery traverse the optic foramen.
- **Superior orbital fissure:** through this fissure run the oculomotor, trochlear and abducens nerves to the extraocular muscles, together with the frontal, nasociliary and lacrimal nerves and the superior and inferior ophthalmic veins. The oculomotor, abducens and nasociliary nerves traverse the lower part of the fissure and enter the muscular cone between the two heads of the lateral rectus. The trochlear, frontal and lacrimal nerves remain outside the cone.
- **Inferior orbital fissure:** through the inferior fissure run the zygomatic and infraorbital nerves (branches of V^2), the infraorbital artery and the inferior ophthalmic vein.

Supplementary and Clinical Information

Ophthalmic Reflexes

- **Corneal reflex:** this is the normal blink reflex but is used as part of brain stem death testing. Stimulation should provoke both a direct and a consensual reflex. The afferent pathway from the nasociliary branch of the ophthalmic division of the trigeminal nerve (V_1) leads to the trigeminal sensory nucleus in the medulla oblongata. Interneurons connect to the facial motor nucleus which mediates the motor response (contraction of the orbicularis oculi muscles) via the temporal and zygomatic branches of the facial (seventh cranial) nerve.
- **Pupillary reflexes: constriction (miosis).** These are essentially photopupillary responses to the intensity of ambient light. In health, this reflex is also consensual; thus stimulation of one pupil elicits the same response in the other. The sensory afferent apparatus consists of photosensitive cells in the retina, the optic nerve and the pretectal nucleus in the midbrain. Efferents from the pretectal nucleus pass to the ipsilateral and contralateral Edinger-Westphal nuclei (also in the midbrain). From these nuclei project preganglionic parasympathetic fibres which run with the oculomotor (third cranial) nerve to synapse with post-ganglionic neurons in the ciliary ganglion. The short ciliary nerves (around 6–10 in number) project from this ganglion to innervate the sphincter pupillae of the iris. Stimulation of this muscle results in pupillary constriction (miosis).
- **Pupillary reflexes: dilation (mydriasis).** Afferents from the retina and optic nerve terminate in the hypothalamus, from whence neurons project to sympathetic preganglionic neurons in the lateral horn of the spinal cord at the level of T_1, T_2 and T_3. From these ganglia project neurons to the superior cervical ganglion and from there sympathetic postganglionic axons run in the long ciliary nerve to innervate the dilator pupillae of the iris.
- **Abnormal pupillary signs.** These are many in number and include eponymous rarities such as the Holmes-Adie syndrome (sluggish pupillary reflexes secondary to denervation in postganglionic parasympathetic nerves) and the Argyll-Robertson

pupil of tertiary syphilis (no constriction in response to light, but constriction in response to accommodation). These are more frequently asked about than seen in clinical practice. Otherwise knowledge of the basic anatomy should allow you to work out from basic principles the site of a possible lesion. For example, if a patient complains of unilateral eye pain with a dilated unreactive pupil, and a contralateral pupil that constricts directly and consensually (with no other signs), then it is possible to deduce that the problem involves motor innervation at the level of the ipsilateral ciliary ganglion or short ciliary nerves. The oculomotor nucleus and nerve are not involved because normal eye movements are not affected.

Local Anaesthesia for Eye Surgery

You may be asked about methods of anaesthetizing the eye for intraocular surgery. Although retrobulbar and peribulbar blocks are being supplanted by sub-Tenon's block and by topical local anaesthesia, they allow some discussion of the anatomy. You will only have to discuss one or two of these methods, usually the one(s) with which you are familiar, and so there is more detail in what follows than you will need.

- **Topical:** the anterior structures can be anaesthetized using topical amethocaine 0.5% or 1.0%, oxybuprocaine 0.4% and proxymetacaine 0.5%. Topical anaesthesia is simple and (mostly) safe and effective, although the lack of akinesia of the eye and eyelids means that the surgeon has to control eye movement via the intraocular instruments. Anaesthesia can be supplemented by the addition of lignocaine to the irrigation fluid, or by further instillation of drops. These can cause oedema of the cornea, and excessive doses may exacerbate the problem.
- **Retrobulbar block:** this is performed by a single injection that is made either percutaneously or transconjunctivally. The axial length of the eye gives a guide to needle depth and, if the percutaneous approach is used, a 25-mm needle is long enough to reach the retrobulbar muscular cone. The injection (3–4 ml) is made at the junction of the lateral and middle thirds of the orbital margin in the inferotemporal quadrant. Complications (which are more common in myopic eyes with increased axial lengths) include retrobulbar haemorrhage, penetration of the globe, damage to the optic nerve or ophthalmic vessels and central spread of local anaesthetic (quoted as 1 in 500). Retrobulbar block is very effective, but potential complications have led most ophthalmic surgeons and anaesthetists to abandon it in favour of other techniques.
- **Peribulbar block:** this has been cited as a safe and effective alternative to retrobulbar block, but it too is not without its problems. Larger volumes of local anaesthetic are required (8–10 ml), which increases the intraorbital pressure and causes periorbital chemosis. The onset of block is also considerably slower and the failure rate higher. The risk of scleral perforation is not removed because the technique requires one inferotemporal and one superonasal injection, both of which are directed beyond the equator of the globe. (Some include a third injection, made at the extreme medial side of the palpebral fissure).
- **Sub-Tenon's block:** the popularity of this technique has increased because it is viewed as safer than the sharp needle approaches. It is, however, more invasive, in that a modest amount of surgical dissection is necessary. After topical anaesthesia to

the conjunctiva the patient is asked to look upwards and outwards (in the direction of the operator). This improves access to the inferonasal quadrant where the injection is made, as posteriorly as possible. A fold of conjunctiva is drawn upwards with forceps. A small nick at the base of this fold with surgical scissors opens the sub-Tenon's fascia. A blunt cannula is then inserted gently into this space and guided backwards following the contour of the globe. Injection of 4–5 ml of local anaesthetic solution will provide analgesia and adequate akinesia. This injection requires pressure to distend the space and some patients find this very uncomfortable. The globe can in theory be perforated, and central spread of local anaesthetic has been described, but these complications are sufficiently rare for sub-Tenon's block to be considered suitable for administration by trained, but non-medical, practitioners.

- **Intraocular pressure:** see under 'Intraocular Pressure' in Chapter 3.

The Pituitary

Commentary
The anatomy of the pituitary gland is less complicated than its numerous endocrine functions and the rare but important medical conditions that follow pituitary dysfunction. Its surgical accessibility via the trans-sphenoidal approach gives this topic direct anaesthetic relevance.

Core Information

The Anatomy of the Pituitary Gland
- The pituitary (hypophysis) is located within the hypophyseal fossa in the sphenoid bone at the base of the skull. The fossa and its boundaries comprise the sella turcica within which the pituitary sits. The sella turcica is a small, saddle-shaped structure (hence its name, 'Turkish saddle') that accommodates the gland, which weighs only between 500 and 900 mg and has typical dimensions in the adult of $1.5 \times 1.0 \times 0.5$ cm.
- The anterior and inferior boundaries of the fossa are formed by the sphenoidal sinuses; while the posterior boundary is formed by the clivus of the sphenoid bone. Superiorly there is a fold of dura mater, the diaphragma sellae, through which passes the infundibulum (the neural component which connects the hypothalamus to the posterior pituitary) and the stalk of the pituitary of which it is part. This dural fold separates the subarachnoid space, with its cerebrospinal fluid, from the bulk of the pituitary itself which is therefore outside the blood–brain barrier.
- Immediately superior to the pituitary is the optic chiasma with the decussating optic nerves. Laterally lie the cavernous sinuses which contain cranial nerves: the oculomotor (III), trochlear (IV) and abducens (VI), and below these the ophthalmic (V1) and maxillary (V2) branches of the trigeminal (V) nerve. Medial to these nerves in each cavernous sinus is the internal carotid artery. All these structures are potentially at risk from pituitary surgery.

- The pituitary consists of two main lobes: the adenohypophysis (anterior pituitary) and the neurohypophysis (posterior pituitary). The anterior pituitary accounts for up to 80% of the total size and is further subdivided into the pars distalis, which is the area that contains the specialized secretory cells, the pars tuberalis and the pars intermedia. The posterior pituitary consists of the pars nervosa and the infundibulum.
- The anterior pituitary contains hormone-secreting epithelial cells that synthesize a large number of peptides and whose release into the systemic circulation is mediated by neurohormones produced by the hypothalamus (such as growth hormone releasing hormone, GHRH; thyroid releasing hormone, TRH; and corticotropin releasing hormone, CRH). The posterior pituitary in contrast contains unmyelinated secretory neurons which are anatomically continuous with the hypothalamus. It does not itself produce hormones; these are synthesized in the supraoptic and paraventricular nuclei of the hypothalamus before being stored in neurohypophyseal terminal axons.
- **Regulation of pituitary function**. The pituitary is under the direct control of the hypothalamus which produces a number of stimulatory tropic hormones. Release is controlled by a negative feedback mechanism, such, for example, that circulating thyroid hormones inhibit the release both of TRH and TSH.
- **Blood supply**. The pituitary receives arterial blood from branches of the internal carotid artery (via superior and inferior hypophyseal arteries). The arterial supply to the hypothalamus comes from the circle of Willis. The superior hypophyseal artery forms a primary capillary plexus in the hypothalamus which then drains into the hypophyseal portal veins. These form the secondary capillary plexus that surrounds the pars distalis. In this way, the hypothalamic neurohormones are delivered to the adenohypophysis, and the hormones that are secreted in response to these releasing factors are then delivered into the systemic venous circulation. Hormones produced by the neurohypophysis drain directly into the pituitary venous circulation. This hypothalamo-hypophyseal portal circulation is one of only two that exist in humans.
- **Portal circulation**. This can be defined as 'any part of the systemic circulation in which blood draining from the capillary bed of one structure flows through a larger vessel or vessels to supply the capillary bed of another structure'. The classic example is the hepatic portal circulation in which the capillaries of the gastrointestinal tract and spleen merge to form the portal vein which, as per the definition, enters the liver and forms portal capillaries.

Endocrine Functions of the Pituitary Gland
Anterior Pituitary Hormones and Their Primary Functions
- Adrenocorticotrophic hormone (ACTH): acts on the adrenal glands to produce glucocorticoids (cortisol, cortisone) and mineralocorticoids (aldosterone).
- Beta-melanocyte stimulating hormone: influences skin pigmentation.
- Endorphins/enkephalins: endogenous opioid ligands which inhibit nociception.
- Follicle stimulating hormone (FSH): ovarian stimulation to produce oocytes and in the male, stimulation of sperm production.
- Growth hormone (GH, also known as somatotropin): has marked anabolic effects on bone and muscle. This is mediated via hepatic insulin-like growth factor (IGF-1).
- Luteinising hormone (LH): similar action to FSH.

- Prolactin: this stimulates milk production and inhibits ovarian function by antagonizing the actions of gonadotrophins.
- Thyroid stimulating hormone (TSH): stimulates production of thyroid hormones.

Posterior Pituitary Hormones and Their Primary Function

- Antidiuretic hormone (ADH, arginine vasopressin): this increases the permeability to water of the renal collecting ducts thereby preventing water loss; it also increases peripheral vascular resistance.
- Oxytocin: this peptide stimulates contraction of uterus during puerperium and the contraction of milk ducts in lactation.

Supplementary and Clinical Information

Disorders of Pituitary Function

These can be separated into the effect of hypersecretion, of hyposecretion and of mass effects secondary to an increase in glandular size.

Hypersecretion

- **Microadenomas** (<1.0 cm in diameter) exert their effects by excessive secretion of hormones. None is that common (acromegaly has a population prevalence of 60 per million, and an incidence of 3–4 million per year), but they can be dramatic conditions with clinical features therefore that are well known.
- **Cushing's Disease.** This is due to hypersecretion of ACTH with a consequent rise in plasma glucocorticoid concentrations. Clinical features are all those of chronic corticosteroid excess and include hyperglycaemia, refractory hypertension, central obesity with abnormal fat deposition (giving rise to the typical 'buffalo hump'), hirsutism, skin fragility, osteoporosis, peptic ulceration and immuno-compromise with recurrent infection. There may be cognitive disturbances, but patients do not usually exhibit the 'steroid psychosis' which can, in other situations, accompany sudden large increases in plasma corticosteroid levels.
- **Acromegaly.** This is due to hypersecretion of growth hormone, with a resultant increase in pre-pubertal individuals of height and muscle mass, and in adults, stimulation of tissue leading to the characteristic facies. Affected patients have enlarging hands and feet, macrognathia, macroglossia and upper airway soft tissue hypertrophy. As a consequence, they may have obstructive sleep apnoea and also may develop hypertension and ischaemic heart disease. Medical management includes treatment with bromocriptine or cabergoline, which reduce growth hormone secretion. (Bromocriptine is a semi-synthetic derivative of an ergot alkaloid, which acts as a dopamine agonist but which also has actions at serotoninergic and adrenergic receptors. Cabergoline is also an ergot alkaloid derivative but with greater specific agonism at the dopamine D_2 receptor).
- **Prolactinomas.** These microadenomas cause galactorrhoea and menstrual dysfunction in females and secondary hypogonadism in males. The first line of management is also with bromocriptine or cabergoline.

Hyposecretion

- **Hypopituitarism.** Panhypopituitarism with global deficiency is less common than deficiencies in separate adenohypophyseal hormones. An exception is so-called pituitary apoplexy secondary to ischaemia or acute haemorrhage into the gland. The classic example is the acute haemorrhagic infarction of Sheehan's syndrome, which is associated particularly with peripartum haemorrhage. During pregnancy, there is pituitary hypertrophy and an increased susceptibility to vascular spasm and compromised blood flow. Other causes include trauma, major surgical stress and sickle cell crisis. It presents with failure of all the hormones of the anterior pituitary. Treatment includes immediate hormone replacement and in some cases emergency transsphenoidal decompression.

- **Hormone deficiencies**. In most cases, more than one of the pituitary hormones is deficient, and the clinical presentation can be predicted from their primary actions. Deficiency of thyroid stimulating hormone, for example, will lead to the well-known features of hypothyroidism. ACTH deficiency may result in more equivocal symptoms of low glucocorticoid concentrations such as anorexia, fatigue, weakness and lassitude. Mineralocorticoids are not affected, as the renin-angiotensin-aldosterone system remains unimpaired. Serum potassium levels therefore are usually unchanged (in contrast to primary adrenal insufficiency, in which the loss of aldosterone leads to hyperkalaemia). Neurogenic diabetes insipidus secondary to failure of ADH secretion has numerous causes, including trauma, which is the aetiology most familiar to critical care anaesthetists, although up to 50% of cases are idiopathic. Acute treatment is with the ADH analogue DDAVP (desmopressin) in a typical intravenous dose of 0.5–1.0 micrograms.

Mass Effects

- An enlarging macroadenoma (>1.0 cm in diameter) may lead to the typical general sequelae of any intracranial space-occupying lesion. Given the proximity of the pituitary to the optic chiasm, however, there may also be visual field disturbances – classically a bitemporal hemianopia caused by pressure on fibres from the nasal retina as they cross the chiasm.

Anaesthesia for Pituitary Surgery

- **Transsphenoidal hypophysectomy**. The favoured surgical approach to the pituitary is extracranial. Pre-operative evaluation must include assessment of the patient's endocrine status and of physical and physiological changes of relevance to anaesthesia. The transsphenoidal approach involves fracturing the nasal septum, and so there may be associated bleeding. The operation is usually carried out in the sitting position with the risk (rare in practice) of venous air embolism. The surgical field is restricted and it may be necessary to reduce intracranial pressure to allow the tumours to descend. This may be possible by reducing the P_aCO_2 by hyperventilation, but on occasion lumbar cerebrospinal fluid (CSF) drainage may be indicated. Otherwise the management is largely generic as for any major case, with the maintenance of cerebral oxygenation, haemodynamic stability and normothermia. Direct intra-arterial blood pressure monitoring is recommended. Rapid emergence from anaesthesia is ideal because this allows early assessment of neurological status. (Surgical complications include CSF rhinorrhoea with the risk of meningitis; vascular and nerve damage given the proximity of cranial nerves in the cavernous sinuses, cerebral vasospasm, diabetes insipidus and panhypopituitarism.)

- **Gamma knife radiosurgery**. This is a technique of delivering highly focused radiation to intracerebral tumours, including pituitary adenomas. MR scanning allows the exact 'surgical' field to be plotted, and a stereotactic frame ensures precise delivery. If the targeting is not highly accurate, then structures such as the optic chiasm and the hypothalamus are at risk. This procedure does not require anaesthesia.

The Autonomic Nervous System

Commentary

This potentially is a large question which, were you to address it in even moderate detail, would exceed the time available. The following account is simplified, but it should prove adequate. Discussion of the core anatomy may be followed or preceded by a more clinically orientated question on, for example, autonomic neuropathy. Other topics may include sympathetic blocks, vagal reflexes or sympathetically maintained pain.

Core Information

The Anatomy of the Autonomic Nervous System

Sympathetic Division

- Pre-ganglionic myelinated efferents from the hypothalamus, medulla oblongata and spinal cord leave the cord with the ventral nerve roots of the first thoracic nerve down to the second, third and, in some subjects, the fourth lumbar spinal nerves (T_1–L_{2-4}).
- These efferents pass via the white rami communicantes to synapse in the sympathetic ganglia lying in the paravertebral sympathetic trunk, which is closely related throughout its length to the spinal column.
- They synapse with post-ganglionic neurons, usually non-myelinated, some of which pass directly to viscera. Others pass back via the grey rami communicantes to rejoin the spinal nerves with which they travel to their effector sites. A number of preganglionic fibres (from T_5 and below) synapse in collateral ganglia which are close to the viscera that they innervate. These collateral ganglia include the coeliac ganglion (receiving fibres from the greater and lesser splanchnic nerves) and the superior and inferior mesenteric ganglia. The adrenal medulla is innervated directly by pre-ganglionic fibres via the splanchnic nerves, which pass without relay through the coeliac ganglion.
- The sympathetic supply to the head originates from three structures: the superior cervical ganglion, the middle cervical ganglion and the stellate ganglion.
- Distribution of the sympathetic supply to the viscera occurs via a series of sympathetic plexuses. The main three are the cardiac, the coeliac and the hypogastric plexuses.
- The segmental sympathetic supply to the head and neck is from T_1 to T_5, to the upper limb from T_2 to T_5, to the lower limb from T_{10} to L_2 and to the heart from T_1 to T_5.

- The anatomy of the sympathetic division is such that it can function better as a mass unit. The parasympathetic division, in contrast, comprises relatively independent components.

Parasympathetic Division

- The parasympathetic nervous system has a cranial and a sacral outflow. The cranial efferents originate in the brain stem and travel with the third (oculomotor), seventh (facial) and ninth (glossopharyngeal) cranial nerves. These pass via the ciliary, sphenopalatine, submaxillary and otic ganglia to subserve parasympathetic function in the head. The most important cranial efferent is the tenth (vagus) cranial nerve, which supplies the thoracic and abdominal viscera. Its fibres synapse with short post-ganglionic neurons that are on or near the effector organs.
- The sacral outflow originates from the second, third and fourth sacral spinal nerves to supply the pelvic viscera. As with the vagus nerve, the fibres synapse with short post-ganglionic neurons that are close to the effector organs.

Autonomic Afferents

- These mediate the afferent arc of autonomic reflexes and conduct visceral pain stimuli. The vagus has a substantial visceral afferent component, the importance of which is well recognized by anaesthetists who commonly have to deal with vagally mediated bradycardia or laryngeal spasm. Sympathetic afferent fibres are also involved in the transmission of visceral pain impulses, including those originating from the myocardium. This is the rationale for using stellate ganglion block to treat refractory angina pectoris. Sympathetic afferents are also involved in sympathetically maintained pain states such as the complex regional pain syndrome. There is usually no direct communication between afferent neurons and sympathetic post-ganglionic fibres, but following injury there is some form of sympathetic–afferent coupling.

Neurotransmitters

- **Sympathetic:** acetylcholine is the neurotransmitter at sympathetic pre-ganglionic fibres (at nicotinic receptors). Noradrenaline is the neurotransmitter at most post-ganglionic fibres, apart from those to sweat glands and to some vasodilator fibres in skeletal muscle.
- **Parasympathetic:** acetylcholine is the neurotransmitter throughout the parasympathetic division, acting at nicotinic receptors in autonomic ganglia, and at muscarinic post-ganglionic receptors thereafter.

Supplementary and Clinical Information

- **Autonomic neuropathy:** this may be associated with conditions such as diabetes, chronic alcoholism, nutritional deficiency, Guillain–Barré syndrome, Parkinson's disease and AIDS. Rarely, it is seen as a primary condition in the Shy–Drager syndrome or familial dysautonomia. Its clinical features include disordered cardio-vascular responses and orthostatic hypotension, the absence of sinus arrhythmia and inability to compensate during the Valsalva manoeuvre. Patients may complain of flushing, erratic temperature control with night sweats, episodic diarrhoea and nocturnal diuresis. The normal response to hypoglycaemia is lost, as are normal diurnal rhythms. A more recently identified form of autonomic dysfunction is the postural orthostatic tachycardia syndrome (POTS), treated by a high-salt diet and in more severe cases with mineralocorticoids.

- **Sympathetic blocks:** examples include lumbar sympathectomy, stellate ganglion block, and coeliac plexus block. Chemical or surgical sympathectomy has been used to improve the blood supply in vasospastic or atherosclerotic disorders of the peripheral circulation, to control hyperhydrosis and to treat pain associated with myocardial ischaemia. Sympathetic blocks also have a place in the management of sympathetically maintained pain (see under 'Complex Regional Pain Syndrome' in Chapter 3), although much of the evidence shows them to be no more effective than placebo.

Supplementary topics could include vagal reflexes or sympathetically maintained pain.

- **Vagal reflexes:** the nerve distributes widely, hence its name; the word 'vagus' comes from the Latin, meaning 'wandering'. (Had it been derived instead from Greek, then the nerve – improbably – would have been called the 'plankton'). Sources of stimulation that can lead to bradycardia and sometimes to asystolic cardiac arrest include the dura, the zygoma, the extraocular muscles – particularly the medial rectus – the carotid sinus, the pharynx, the glottis, the bronchial tree, the heart, the mesentery and peritoneum, the bladder and urethra, the testis, and the rectum and anus. The Brewer–Luckhardt reflex describes laryngospasm that is provoked by a distant stimulus. Vagal reflexes can be attenuated by the use of an anticholinergic such as atropine, but in low doses this paradoxically can stimulate the vagus before it blocks it (the Bezold–Jarisch reflex).
- **Sympathetically maintained pain:** in some pain syndromes, it appears that efferent noradrenergic sympathetic activity and circulating catecholamines have a role in maintaining chronic pain. There is usually no communication between sympathetic efferent and afferent fibres, but following nerve injury it is apparent that modulation of nociceptive impulses can occur not only at the site of injury but also in distal undamaged fibres and the dorsal root ganglion itself around which sympathetic axons may proliferate (see under 'Chronic Regional Pain Syndrome' in Chapter 3).

The Trigeminal Nerve

Commentary
The applied anatomy of the trigeminal nerve is relevant mainly for those working in the management of chronic pain. Trigeminal neuralgia is described classically as one of the most extreme pains in human experience, one which is reported to have driven some patients even to suicide. It is a dramatic condition, and one that is amenable to a range of treatments.

Core Information

The Anatomy of the Trigeminal Nerve

- The trigeminal (fifth cranial nerve, V) is the largest of the 12, and provides the sensory supply to the face, nose and mouth as well as much of the scalp. Its motor branches include the supply to the muscles of mastication.
- It has a single motor nucleus and three sensory nuclei in the brain. The motor nucleus is in the upper pons, and lying lateral to it is the principal sensory nucleus, which subserves touch sensation. The mesencephalic nucleus is sited in the midbrain and subserves proprioception. Pain and temperature sensation are subserved by the nucleus of the spinal tract of the trigeminal nerve. This lies deep to a tract of descending fibres which run from the pons to the substantia gelatinosa of the spinal cord.
- Sensory fibres pass through the trigeminal (Gasserian) ganglion. It is crescent-shaped (hence its alternative description as the semilunar ganglion), and lies within an invagination of dura mater near the apex of the petrous temporal bone, and at the posterior extremity of the zygomatic arch. The motor fibres of the trigeminal nerve pass below the ganglion.
- From this ganglion pass the three divisions of the nerve: the ophthalmic (V^1), which is the smallest of the three; the maxillary (V^2); and the mandibular (V^3). (This division explains the name: 'tri-gemini'; from the Latin for 'triplet').
- **Ophthalmic division V_1:** this passes along the lateral wall of the cavernous sinus before dividing just before the superior orbital fissure into the lacrimal, nasociliary and frontal branches. The frontal branch divides further into the supraorbital and supratrochlear nerves.
- **Maxillary division V_2:** This runs below the ophthalmic division before leaving the base of the skull via the foramen rotundum. It crosses the pterygopalatine fossa, giving off superior alveolar dental nerves, zygomatic nerves and sphenopalatine nerves before entering the infraorbital canal and emerging through the infraorbital foramen as the infraorbital nerve.
- **Mandibular division V_3:** this is the largest of the three branches and is the only one to have both motor and sensory components. Its large sensory root passes through the foramen ovale to join with the smaller motor root, which runs beneath the ganglion. Its branches include the sensory lingual, auriculotemporal and buccal nerves; the inferior dental nerve, which is mixed motor and sensory; and motor nerves to the muscles of mastication, the masseteric and lateral pterygoid nerves.

Supplementary and Clinical Information

Trigeminal Neuralgia: Definition, Clinical Features and Its Management

- **Definition:** trigeminal neuralgia is a severe neuropathic pain with a reputation as one of the worst pains in human experience.
- **Clinical features:** the peak onset of the condition is in middle age. The pain typically is intermittent, lancinating and of the utmost severity. Attacks are spasmodic, lasting only seconds. Patients are pain-free in the interim, but episodes may be very frequent. Pain is limited usually to one (occasionally two) of the branches of the

trigeminal nerve, which supplies sensation to the face. It occurs least commonly in the ophthalmic division, which accounts for only around 5% of cases, and more frequently in the maxillary or mandibular divisions. The distribution is always unilateral. Paroxysmal pain can be precipitated by trigger points around the face which react to the lightest of stimuli, such as a light breeze or touch, and by actions such as chewing or shaving.

- **Pathogenesis:** this remains speculative. It may be caused centrally, with abnormal neurons in the pons exhibiting spontaneous and uncontrolled discharge in the nerve. It may also be caused by peripheral factors: due either to demyelination (in younger patients, trigeminal neuralgia may be a first symptom of multiple sclerosis) or to compression by abnormal blood vessels in the posterior fossa.

- **Pharmacological treatment:** (in an anatomy oral you will probably not be asked about this in great detail; it is included in the following for completeness. This is adequate treatment for around 75% of cases, although the effectiveness of medical therapy does fade with time, with up to 50% of patients eventually experiencing breakthrough pain).

  — *Carbamazepine* is said to be effective in more than 90% of cases of true trigeminal neuralgia (100 mg b.d. up to maintenance of 600–1,200 mg day^{-1}). The full blood count must be monitored because the drug can cause bone marrow suppression.

  — *Phenytoin* is effective in a smaller proportion (around 60%) and can be given intravenously for acute intractable pain (the starting dose is 300–500 mg day^{-1}).

  — *Baclofen* is an antispasmodic γ-amino butyric acid (GABA) analogue, which binds to GABA$_B$ receptors (the dose is up to 80 mg day^{-1}).

  — *Gabapentin* is a GABA analogue, which does not, however, act on GABA receptors. Its mechanism of action is unclear. It is an anticonvulsant which clinicians increasingly are using to treat neuropathic pain. It appears to be particularly effective in patients whose trigeminal neuralgia is secondary to multiple sclerosis. The dose is titrated against response to a maximum of 1,800 mg daily.

  — *Lamotrigine* is primarily a sodium channel inhibitor and neuronal membrane stabilizer. It is also a weak 5-HT$_3$ receptor inhibiter with a secondary antiglutaminergic action. The dose is up to 400 mg day^{-1}.

Non-Pharmacological Methods of Management
Destructive

- **Radiofrequency ablation:** a needle is passed percutaneously and under X-ray control through the foramen ovale to the trigeminal ganglion. The entry point of the needle is below the posterior third of the zygoma. Chemical ablation may also be used. This technique can be complicated by anaesthesia dolorosa, in which the patient loses not only the pain, but also most of the sensation to that side of the face, which feels dead and 'woody'. The patient needs to be awake and cooperative during part of the procedure but needs to be 'deeply sedated' – transiently – for the ablation itself. This can be challenging.

- **Gamma knife surgery:** this is stereotactic radiosurgery delivered by intensely focused gamma radiation from an array of cobalt sources. It is as effective as radiofrequency ablation, although full relief may take some weeks to develop.

Surgical
- **Surgical decompression:** this is the most invasive therapeutic technique because it requires formal neurosurgical exploration of the posterior fossa to identify the aberrant vessel(s) which are compressing the nerve near its emergence from the pons.

The Nose

Commentary

The nose has never featured highly in the anatomical canon of most anaesthetists. Perhaps it deserves greater prominence, acting as it does as a conduit for devices such as nasopharyngeal airways, nasotracheal tubes, nasogastric tubes and fibreoptic broncho-scopes. Potentially this subject could incorporate a considerable amount of information which would take too long to convey, and so it is unlikely that you will be required to describe it in fine detail. The following account therefore is simplified.

Core Information

- **Framework of the nose:** the anatomy is not limited to the external nose but also includes the extensive nasal cavity which is composed of several bones of the skull. Each side of the nose comprises, in summary, the roof, medial and lateral walls, and floor.
  - *Roof*: this is formed from the nasal and frontal bones which make up the bridge of the nose: the cribriform plate of the ethmoid, which forms the middle flat section, and the body of the sphenoid, which slopes backwards and downwards to complete the posterior part of the cavity.
  - *Medial wall*: medially is the nasal septum – the lower part is cartilaginous; the upper is formed from the perpendicular plate of the ethmoid and from the vomer.
  - *Lateral wall*: this comprises the ethmoid above, the nasal maxilla below and in front, and the perpendicular plate of the palatine bone behind. This lateral wall contains the three turbinate bones, also known as the conchae (pronounced 'con-kee'). ('Turbinate' comes from the Latin word for 'spinning top', and 'concha' derives from the Latin word for 'mussel shell', reflecting the scrolled shape of the bones.) Each of the upper, middle and inferior conchae curves over a meatus. The shape of the conchae increases the flow of inspired air over as large a surface area as possible, thereby maximizing the humidifying, warming and filtering functions of the nose.
  - *Floor*: this surface is slightly curved and is formed from part of the maxilla and the palatine bone. Anteriorly is the nasal vestibule.
- **Blood supply:** the upper part of the nose is supplied by branches of the ophthalmic artery (anterior and posterior ethmoidal), and the lower is supplied by branches of the maxillary artery (sphenopalatine) and the facial artery (superior labial). Venous drainage is via the facial and ophthalmic veins, some tributaries of which drain into the cavernous sinus.
- **Olfaction:** olfactory receptors are found in a small area of the upper part of the nasal septum and the lateral walls. The fibres of the olfactory (first cranial) nerve pass

through the cribriform plate of the ethmoid bone to synapse directly with cells in the olfactory bulb. Unlike other visceral afferents, these fibres do not synapse in ganglia. As they pass through the cribriform plate, the nerve bundles become invested in a sleeve of dura, thereby providing a route of infection from the nasal cavity to the central nervous system.

- **Sensation:** branches of the trigeminal (V) nerve supply the nose. The septum is innervated mainly by the long sphenopalatine nerve (a branch of the maxillary division, V^2), with a contribution from the anterior ethmoidal nerve (a branch of the nasociliary nerve from V^1). The upper lateral wall is innervated by the short sphenopalatine nerve (also from V^2). The inferior part is innervated by the superior dental nerve and the greater palatine nerve (which are also branches of V^2).

Supplementary and Clinical Information

- **Functions:** it is the organ of olfaction. As part of the respiratory apparatus it warms and humidifies inspired gases, it has a secondary function as a resonator in speech and it filters inspired pathogens and irritants. In infants and small children, the small degree of expiratory resistance which it provides combines with partial adduction of the vocal cords during expiration to produce the continuous positive airways pressure (CPAP) which opposes premature airway closure.

- **Instrumentation:** the nose is a passage for nasotracheal tubes, nasopharyngeal airways, nasogastric tubes, fibreoptic bronchoscopes, temperature probes and oesophageal Doppler monitoring probes. The technique for their insertion does not differ: each device should be directed straight backwards along the floor of the nose and beneath the inferior concha (Figure 2.3). It is not necessary to use any force: firm pressure is the most that is needed for an appropriate-sized tube. The rich blood supply to the turbinates is under reflex control and the vessels engorge and empty in response to factors such as airflow pressure and temperature. Sustained but gentle pressure may be enough to allow vascular engorgement to subside and prevent the copious bleeding that can follow nasal instrumentation.

- **Indications for nasotracheal intubation:** nasal intubation allows surgeons optimal access to the oral cavity. Awake fibreoptic nasal intubation may be indicated in patients whose mouth opening is limited, but it is also the route preferred by most anaesthetists for cases of predicted difficult intubation. Fibreoptic intubation has superseded blind nasal intubation, which is a technique that is no longer routinely taught. Nasal tubes are used in patients who require prolonged intubation. This applies more to children than to adults in whom tracheostomy is a more common option.

- **Contraindications for nasotracheal intubation:** midface deformity, congenital or acquired, may make nasal intubation impossible. Coagulopathy may be accompanied by significant nasal haemorrhage, and traditional teaching always held, for example, that nasal intubation should be avoided in patients with haemophilia. One of the primary contraindications is basal skull fracture, the clinical features of which can include cerebrospinal fluid (CSF) rhinorrhoea, so-called raccoon eyes and mastoid bruising (Battle's sign).

- **Complications:** brisk bleeding can occur following trauma to the rich blood supply. The nasopharyngeal mucosa is not robust, and a nasal or nasogastric tube can breach the mucosa of the posterior pharyngeal wall. Nasal instrumentation is associated with

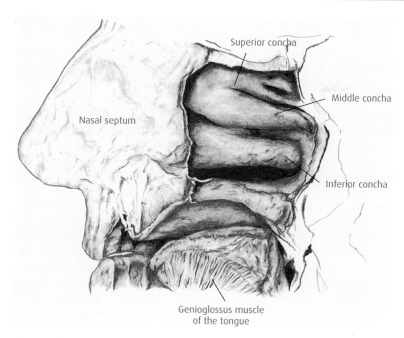

Fig. 2.3 The nose.

bacteraemia, and some anaesthetists even give prophylactic antibiotics when using a nasotracheal tube. Intracranial placement has been described following procedures such as transsphenoidal neurosurgery, which leaves a small bony defect that inadvertently can be penetrated.

- **Which nostril?** Most anaesthetists, presumably because most are right-handed, favour the right side. This is appropriate if the nares are symmetrical but more problematic if they are not. Asymmetrical nostrils indicate that the nasal septum is probably deviated. The naris that is narrower anteriorly is actually wider posteriorly, and so, paradoxically, it is the narrower nostril that should be chosen.

- **Local anaesthesia:** the nasal mucosa is most effectively and easily blocked by topical solutions of local anaesthetic. Common options are cocaine 10% and lidocaine 5%/phenylephrine 0.5% mixtures. Xylometazoline (Otrivine) is a nasal decongestant which causes vasoconstriction of mucosal blood vessels. Its effect is short-lived and it usually causes rebound hyperaemia.

The Sensory Nerve Supply to the Face

Commentary

The major sensory supply to the face is easy to describe; it is the numerous terminal branches that may present more difficulty. Equally, the examiner may not immediately be intimate with the 25 or more named nerves which originate from the trigeminal nerve, and so detailed knowledge need extend only to those branches which can be blocked with local anaesthetic to allow minor surgery on the face or to provide postoperative analgesia.

Core Information

- **Sensory supply:** the sensory supply to the face is provided mainly by the three divisions of the fifth cranial nerve, the trigeminal. (As the largest cranial nerve it also supplies much of the scalp, the mouth, teeth and the nasal cavity.) The skin over the parotid gland and the angle of the mandible is, however, supplied by the greater auricular nerve, which arises from the ventral rami of the second and third cervical nerves.
- **Trigeminal nerve divisions:** at the trigeminal (Gasserian) ganglion, the nerve separates into the ophthalmic (V^1), the maxillary (V^2) and the mandibular (V^3) divisions.
  - *Ophthalmic (V^1):* the ophthalmic nerve supplies the skin of the nose, the forehead, eyelids and the scalp. (It also supplies the globe, the lacrimal apparatus and the conjunctiva.) The nerve divides just before the superior orbital fissure into the lacrimal, nasociliary and frontal branches. The large frontal branch divides further into the supraorbital and supratrochlear nerves. The supraorbital nerve supplies the skin of the forehead and scalp, sometimes as far back as the lambdoid suture. The supratrochlear nerve supplies part of the upper eyelid and the skin of the lower part of the forehead near the midline. The lacrimal nerve supplies the skin adjacent to the medial canthus of the eye, and the nasociliary nerve and its branches supply the skin of the nose down as far as the alae nasae.
  - *Maxillary (V^2):* this runs below the ophthalmic branch before leaving the base of the skull via the foramen rotundum to divide into its various branches. The zygomatic nerve divides further on the lateral wall of the orbit into a zygomaticotemporal branch which supplies the skin of the temple, and a zygomaticofacial branch which supplies the skin over the cheekbones. The maxillary nerve proper crosses the pterygopalatine fossa to enter the infraorbital canal, from which it emerges through the infraorbital foramen as the infraorbital nerve. This supplies the skin of the lower eyelid, the cheek and upper lip.
  - *Mandibular (V^3):* its large sensory root passes through the foramen ovale with branches that include the auriculotemporal, lingual and buccal nerves. The auriculotemporal nerve emerges from behind the temporomandibular joint to supply the skin over the tragus and meatus of the ear as well as the skin over the temporal region. The mandibular division also provides the inferior dental nerve, and one of its terminal branches, the mental nerve, emerges through the mental foramen in the mandible to supply the skin of the chin and lower lip.

Supplementary and Clinical Information

Clinical applications are modest; some of the nerves of the face are at risk from pressure (such as the supraorbital nerve in the prone position), and some may be affected by disease processes such as herpes zoster (ophthalmic branch of the trigeminal nerve) or trigeminal neuralgia. The discussion may move to the provision of local anaesthesia for superficial surgery on the face. In practice the surgeon is likely to offer local infiltration, but for the purposes of the question you will need a more formal approach.

- The *supraorbital* and *supratrochlear* nerves can be blocked a few millimetres above the supraorbital ridge. If the injection is made too close to the eyebrow it increases the risk of periorbital haematoma. Alternatively, a single insertion point can be used in the midbrow region to allow bilateral blocks.
- The *infratrochlear* nerve can be blocked by a needle directed along the medial wall of the orbit via an insertion site about 1 cm above the inner canthus.
- The *infraorbital* nerve can be blocked as it exits the infraorbital foramen, which lies about 1.5 cm (a finger's breadth) below the inferior orbital margin in line with the pupil. The nerve can also be blocked by an intra-oral approach, injecting above the canine (third) tooth.
- The mental foramen, conveniently, is also in line with the pupil and the *mental* nerve can be blocked in the midpoint of the mandible (although the height of the foramen varies with age, being nearer the alveolar margin in the elderly).
- The superficial branches of the *zygomatic* nerve can be blocked by subcutaneous infiltration or by injection at their sites of emergence from the zygoma.
- The *auriculotemporal* nerve is blocked over the posterior aspect of the zygoma, and the *greater auricular* nerve by infiltration over the mastoid process behind the ear.
- Relatively small volumes of 3–5 ml of local anaesthetic will usually be sufficient to block all these nerves described.

The Sensory Nerve Supply to the Scalp

Commentary

This is really a question of applied anatomy relating to the provision of anaesthesia for awake craniotomy. Other indications for local anaesthesia of the scalp might include excision and grafting of scalp lesions such as basal cell carcinomas in the elderly, but either way it remains something of a niche topic.

Core Information

- A total of seven paired nerves need to be blocked bilaterally to provide adequate anaesthesia over the entire scalp. They need to be targeted with some precision because the potential for local anaesthetic toxicity precludes performing a circumferential block. The rich blood supply results in a more rapid rise in plasma concentrations than in superficial nerve blocks elsewhere in the body.
- Assuming that the nerves are being approached in sequence from the front of the patient they are:
- **Supratrochlear nerve**. This is part of the ophthalmic division of the trigeminal nerve V^1 and supplies the forehead, the anterior scalp and the crown of the head. It is blocked just medial to the supraorbital notch.

- **Supraorbital nerve**. This is also a branch of the ophthalmic division of the trigeminal nerve V^1 and supplies the anterior scalp and the forehead. It is blocked at the supraorbital notch.
- **Zygomaticotemporal nerve**. This is part of the maxillary division of the trigeminal nerve V^2 and supplies a small part of the forehead and temporal area. Despite this small area of innervation, the area of infiltration is quite large, starting at the lateral border of the supraorbital margin and extending as far as the distal part of the zygomatic arch, both deep to and superficial to the temporalis fascia.
- **Auriculotemporal nerve**. This is part of the mandibular division of the trigeminal nerve V^3 and innervates the scalp above the ear and the temporal area. (It also supplies the lower face, lower lip and the ear). The injection point is just above the level of the temporo-mandibular joint and around about 1 cm anterior to the ear (auricle). This block risks inadvertent injection into the superficial temporal artery in relation to which the nerve lies deep.
- **Greater occipital nerve**. This derives from the second and cervical spinal nerves C_2 and C_3 and supplies the skin along the posterior part of the scalp. The nerves are blocked by injection just medial to the occipital arteries which lie about 3–4 cm lateral to the midline (as marked by the external occipital protuberance).
- **Lesser occipital nerve** (C_2, C_3). This derives from the second or sometimes the third cervical spinal nerve, ascending the posterior border of sternocleidomastoid to innervate the lateral part of the scalp behind the auricle. It is blocked by subcutaneous infiltration from the ear lobe to the greater occipital nerve.
- **Greater auricular nerve** (C_2, C_3). This is also derived from the second and third cervical spinal nerves, dividing into anterior and posterior branches to supply the skin over the auricle (as its name suggests), the mastoid process and the parotid. The injection is made at the level of the tragus and some 2 cm posterior to it.

Supplementary and Clinical Information

- The excision of stereotactically identified intracerebral lesions in particularly crucial areas of the brain should be performed ideally with minimal or no damage to eloquent regions. 'Awake' craniotomy helps to achieve this aim. Patients are rarely fully awake throughout; some parts of the procedure are too surgically stimulating to tolerate without the use of short-acting sedatives and/or analgesics. Some anaesthetists prefer to give a controlled general anaesthetic from which the patient is allowed to awaken during surgery so that neurological function can be assessed. Prior to resection or radiofrequency ablation of a lesion, the area is mapped with the specific aim of localizing the speech and motor areas.
- The procedure starts with the insertion of Mayfield pins for the halo, followed by the skin incision, removal of the bone flap and incision of the dura mater. At that point neurocognitive mapping begins with resection of the lesion.
- The heterogeneity of the procedures precludes a single standard technique, and various sedation regimens have been employed, including propofol and remifentanil target-controlled infusions and conventional benzodiazepines.
- Dexmedetomidine, a highly selective α_2-agonist which has been available in the UK since 2014, has several advantages when it is used as a sole agent for this purpose. It provides sedation, anxiolysis and analgesia without causing respiratory depression.

(A typical regimen would be: loading dose of 0.5–1.0 μg kg^{-1} over 15–20 minutes followed by infusion titrated against response, typically up to 0.5–0.7 μg kg hr^{-1}).

- Potential complications: these relate to the duration and nature of the surgery and the patient position. Surgically induced complications include seizures, haemorrhage and venous air embolism. The potential anaesthetic complications are predictable and generic: hypoventilation or apnoea due to over-sedation with potent respiratory depressants, inadequate analgesia, cardiovascular instability, nausea and vomiting, agitation, and restlessness secondary to local anaesthetic toxicity.

The Cervical Plexus

Commentary

This is of particular relevance for carotid endarterectomy (CEA) under local anaesthesia, although cervical plexus blocks have a number of other indications. The question of which of general or local anaesthesia for carotid endarterectomy is the better option was not informed definitively by the GALA trial, not least because lack of funding meant that this was discontinued before the planned 5,000 patients had been recruited and because there was considerable criticism about aspects of its methodology. Clinical practice changed over the years during which patients were recruited, and neither the general anaesthetic nor the regional anaesthetic techniques were standardized. Nonetheless, in conjunction with other evidence it seems clear that in respect of major perioperative outcomes, there is no difference between regional and general anaesthesia, with mortality and stroke rates of around 5% in both groups.

Core Information

- The nerves which supply the lateral aspect of the neck all derive from the ventral rami of the second, third and fourth cervical spinal nerves ($C_{2, 3, 4}$). The first cervical nerve has no sensory distribution to skin.
- **Superficial cervical plexus anatomy:** the cutaneous supply to the anterolateral aspect of the neck is via the anterior primary rami of C_2, C_3 and C_4. These nerves emerge from the posterior border of the sternocleidomastoid muscle midway between the mastoid and the sternum. The accessory nerve is immediately superior at this point. The lesser occipital nerve (the first branch) supplies the skin of the upper and posterior ear, the greater auricular nerve (the second branch) supplies the lower third of the ear and the skin over the angle of the mandible, the anterior cutaneous nerve (the third branch) supplies the skin from the chin down to the suprasternal notch and the supraclavicular nerves (the fourth branch) supply the skin over the lower neck, clavicle and upper chest.
- **Superficial cervical plexus block:** all these nerves can be blocked at the midpoint of the sternocleidomastoid by infiltrating up to 20 ml of local anaesthetic solution between the skin and the muscle. The external jugular vein crosses the muscle at this point and can be a useful landmark.

- **Deep cervical plexus anatomy:** the ventral ramus of the second nerve emerges from between the vertebral arches of the atlas and axis and runs forwards between their transverse processes to exit between longus capitis and levator scapulae. The ventral ramus of the third nerve exits the intervertebral foramen lying in a sulcus in the transverse process, emerging between the longus capitis and scalenus medius muscles. The ventral rami of the fourth and remaining cervical nerves appear between the scalenus anterior and the scalenus medius.
- **Deep cervical plexus block:** deep cervical plexus block in effect is a paravertebral block of C_2, C_3 and C_4. Needles are inserted at each of the three levels, using as landmarks a line between the mastoid process and the prominent tubercle of the sixth cervical vertebra (which is palpable as Chassaignac's tubercle at the level of the cricoid cartilage). The C_2 transverse process is approximately one finger's breadth below the mastoid process along this line with C_3 and C_4 following at similar intervals caudad. After encountering the transverse process, 5–8 ml of local anaesthetic can be injected with due precautions. Because there is little resistance to the spread of solutions through the paravertebral space in the cervical region, adequate anaesthesia can also be obtained using a single needle technique and a larger volume (15–20 ml) at a single level, usually C_3.

Supplementary and Clinical Information

Discussion may include indications for these blocks, and in particular the relative merits of general and local anaesthesia for carotid endarterectomy (CEA). It is inevitable that the answers may be somewhat reciprocal, in that the advantages of one mean that you avoid the disadvantages of the other.

- **Indications for cervical plexus blockade:** these include anaesthesia for carotid surgery under local anaesthesia, clavicular surgery (typically open reduction and internal fixation following trauma) and thyroid surgery.
- **Advantages of CEA under local anaesthesia:** normal cerebration depends on adequate cerebral perfusion, and in the awake patient it is usually obvious whether this is being preserved. In effect the patient acts as their own cerebral function monitor, and signs of cerebral ischaemia are an indication for surgical shunt insertion. Local anaesthesia does not interfere with cerebral autoregulation, and signs of cerebral ischaemia are an indication for surgical shunt insertion. Local anaesthesia does not interfere with cerebral autoregulation, and the requirement for vasoactive drugs is less. Proponents of the technique claimed lower morbidity and mortality rates, but there is no evidence to support that view.
- **Disadvantages of CEA under local anaesthesia:** cerebral oxygen consumption does not fall (the cerebral metabolic rate for oxygen, $CMRO_2$, decreases under general anaesthesia), and a higher pulse and blood pressure during surgery results in higher myocardial oxygen demand than would otherwise be the case. It does also mean, however, that cerebral perfusion pressure is higher. Cooperation can on occasion be a problem; immobility during extended surgery may be very uncomfortable for the patient and, should their cerebration be obtunded by ischaemia, they may become restless and agitated. The nerve blocks may sometimes prove inadequate as surgery proceeds, but local supplementation by the surgeon can circumvent this problem.

- **Advantages of CEA under general anaesthesia:** general anaesthesia allows more control, can be extended indefinitely if necessary and during long procedures is more comfortable for the patient. At concentrations up to 1.0 MAC, sevoflurane decreases cerebral blood flow and $CMRO_2$. Experimental evidence suggests that general anaesthetic agents may confer a degree of neuroprotection, but the data are not robust enough to mandate their use.

- **Disadvantages of CEA under general anaesthesia:** it is clearly more difficult to assess cerebral oxygenation, and, although low concentrations of volatile agents do reduce $CMRO_2$, they may still impair dynamic cerebral autoregulation at MAC levels below 1.0. Monitors of cerebral oxygenation include near-infrared spectroscopy (NIRS), electroencephalography (EEG), somatosensory evoked potentials (SSEPs) and transcranial Doppler. There are in addition the generic complications of general anaesthesia (in which the examiner will have little interest) and those of anaesthesia for head and neck surgery, such as restricted access to the airway.

- **Complications:** superficial cervical plexus block risks mainly what can be described as generic complications of local anaesthesia, namely intravascular injection and systemic toxicity. The complications of deep cervical block are much the same as those associated with interscalene block, which is not surprising given the anatomical similarities, and include injection into the vertebral artery, extension of the block either extradurally or intrathecally, phrenic nerve block and cervical sympathetic block, which will manifest as Horner's syndrome (miosis, ptosis, anhidrosis and enophthalmos). The recurrent laryngeal nerve may also be affected with resultant hoarseness.

- **The GALA trial:** this multicentre trial was conducted over around seven years between 2001 and 2007 and recruited 3.500 of the planned 5,000 patients, who were randomized either to general or regional anaesthesia for carotid endarterectomy. Thereafter, anaesthetists and surgeons were free to follow their routine practice. Primary outcomes were death, stroke or myocardial infarction within 30 days of surgery; secondary outcomes added death at 1 year, length of stay and quality of life. There were essentially no differences between the groups. Criticisms of the trial included the fact that surgical and anaesthetic techniques were very variable; an obvious example being the use or otherwise of shunts, and that both may have changed during the relatively long period during which patients were recruited (GALA Trial [*Lancet* 2008, 372: 2132–42]).

The Larynx

Commentary

You may read in some textbooks that the competent anaesthetist should know as much about the anatomy of the larynx as an ENT surgeon. Examiners do not necessarily make the same assumption, because in reality the clinical applications of such detailed knowledge are quite limited. You will, however, be expected to give a reasonably assured account of the main anatomical features.

Core Information

The Function and Anatomy of the Larynx

- The larynx has a crucial role in protecting the airway from contamination. It does this by invoking what is one of the most powerful physiological reflexes, and one to which every anaesthetist who has managed intractable laryngospasm will attest. The larynx has also evolved into an organ of phonation.
- The larynx extends from the base of the tongue above, to the trachea below, and in the adult male it lies opposite the third to sixth cervical vertebrae. In the adult female and in children it lies higher.
- The larynx comprises a number of articulating cartilages which are joined by ligaments and which are subject to the action of various muscles that move these cartilages in relation to each other.

Cartilaginous Framework

- The cartilaginous framework comprises the thyroid, cricoid and arytenoid cartilages. (The smaller corniculate and cuneiform cartilages contribute little to this structure.)
- The thyroid cartilage comprises two quadrilateral laminae which are fused anteriorly to form the laryngeal prominence. It articulates inferiorly with the cricoid. The thyroid notch lies at the level of C_4.
- The cricoid cartilage is a continuous ring with a narrow anterior arch and a deeper posterior lamina. It articulates on each side with the inferior cornu of the thyroid cartilage and with the base of the arytenoid cartilage.
- Each of the paired arytenoid cartilages is pyramidal in shape. The smooth concave base articulates with the cricoid cartilage. The lateral angle, or muscular process, projects backwards, while the anterior angle, or vocal process, projects forwards. The apex articulates with the corniculate cartilage.
- The two corniculate cartilages are small nodules which are sometimes fused with the arytenoids and which lie in the posterior aryepiglottic folds of mucous membrane. The two cuneiform cartilages lie anterior to the corniculate cartilages, also within the aryepiglottic fold.
- There are a number of intrinsic and extrinsic ligaments. Those of anaesthetic interest include the thyrohyoid membrane, which joins the upper border of the thyroid cartilage to the hyoid bone, and the cricothyroid ligament between the cricoid and thyroid cartilages.
- The vocal cords (also known as the vocal folds) are opalescent folds of mucous membrane which extend from the anterior vocal processes of the arytenoid cartilages as far as the middle of the angle of the thyroid cartilage. The vestibular folds, or false cords, lie lateral to the cords and comprise thicker folds of mucous membrane which also extend from the thyroid cartilage to the arytenoids.

Laryngeal Muscles

- There are a number of extrinsic and intrinsic muscles of the larynx. The extrinsic muscles (the sternothyroid, the thyrohyoid and the inferior constrictor of the pharynx) attach the larynx to adjacent structures. The intrinsic muscles are of more immediate interest to the anaesthetist because they control the opening of the cords during inspiration, the closure of the cords and laryngeal inlet during swallowing, and the tension of the cords during speech.

- **Abduction:** Abduction of the cords is performed by the posterior cricoarytenoid muscles.
- **Adduction:** Adduction of the cords is performed by the lateral cricoarytenoids and the unpaired interarytenoid muscle.
- **Tensors:** the main tensors of the vocal cords are the cricothyroid muscles.
- **Relaxors:** the main relaxors of the vocal cords are the thyroarytenoid muscles.
- **Innervation:** All the muscles of the larynx, with one exception, are innervated by the recurrent laryngeal nerve. The exception is the cricothyroid muscle, which is supplied by the external branch of the superior laryngeal nerve.

Supplementary and Clinical Information

Factors Affecting the Ease of Laryngoscopy

- You will be aware that anaesthetists have long sought a test or a combination of tests that have a high sensitivity and specificity for predicting difficult intubation. None has yet been found. The simplest means of classifying the degree of difficulty is by using the Cormack and Lehane classification. (This describes the best view that is obtained at laryngoscopy: grade I – full view, grade II – posterior part of the glottis only, grade III – epiglottis only, grade IV – soft palate only.)
- The larynx can be seen directly only if there is a single direct plane of view. This means that the three axes of the oral cavity, the pharynx and the larynx must be brought into alignment. In practice this is done by opening the mouth wide, flexing the neck, extending the head at the atlanto-occipital joint and lifting the base of the tongue and epiglottis upwards and forwards.
- Any factor which impedes this alignment will make direct laryngoscopy and intubation more difficult. Such factors include limited (<4 cm) mouth opening, prominent upper incisors, maxillary prognathism and the inability to protrude the lower incisors in front of the upper, limited neck mobility with restricted extension (thyromental distance of <6.5 cm), and a high anterior larynx. Obesity is often cited as a factor, but studies in patients undergoing bariatric surgery have demonstrated no difference in laryngoscopic view between the morbidly obese and those patients of normal body habitus. This is not surprising, as obesity per se, and for that matter pregnancy, do not in themselves impede the ability to obtain a single axis plane of view between the incisors and the glottis. Many other predictors of difficulty have been described, such as the radiological assessment of the atlanto-occipital gap, the C_1–C_2 gap and the anterior-posterior depth of the mandible. These are of limited clinical use, as such radiographs are rarely available (or sought).
- It is important to be able to recognize structures that are seen at laryngoscopy. Beyond the elevated epiglottis are the false and the true vocal cords. Posteriorly are the arytenoid cartilages (together with the bulges of the corniculate and cuneiform cartilages). Between the cords is the laryngeal inlet, or rima glottidis, beyond which may be visible the upper rings of the trachea (Figure 2.4).
- The arytenoids can be dislocated or subluxed during tracheal intubation or laryngeal mask insertion. This will interfere with the function of some of the intrinsic muscles and may compromise the airway. The cricoarytenoid joint may also be affected by

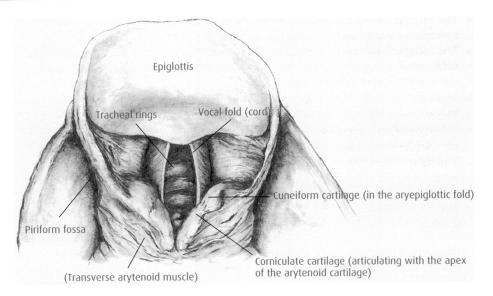

Fig. 2.4 The larynx.

Labels in figure: Epiglottis; Tracheal rings; Vocal fold (cord); Cuneiform cartilage (in the aryepiglottic fold); Piriform fossa; Corniculate cartilage (articulating with the apex of the arytenoid cartilage); (Transverse arytenoid muscle)

systemic inflammatory arthropathies, particularly rheumatoid arthritis and by the tissue changes associated with acromegaly.

- The anatomy of the cricoid cartilage is relevant both for rapid sequence induction of anaesthesia, and also for emergency access to the airway.
- It is also important to be able to recognize the airway signs of injury to the recurrent laryngeal nerve as described in the next section.

The Innervation of the Larynx

Commentary

The innervation of the larynx is another area that is regarded as core anatomy, and it does have immediate relevance for awake fibreoptic intubation. The other traditional question about the laryngeal nerves relates to the consequences of injury, and, although anaesthetists see this very rarely, you may find yourself being questioned as though it were an everyday occurrence.

Core Information

Sensory Innervation

- The sensory innervation of the larynx is via the vagus (tenth cranial nerve), which divides into the superior laryngeal nerve and the recurrent laryngeal nerve. The superior branch divides thereafter into internal and external laryngeal nerves.

- The internal laryngeal nerve innervates the inferior surface of the epiglottis and the supraglottic region as far as the mucous membrane above the vocal folds.
- The recurrent laryngeal nerve provides the sensory supply to the laryngeal mucosa below the vocal cords.

Motor Innervation

- The recurrent laryngeal nerve supplies all the intrinsic muscles of the larynx, with the exception of the cricothyroid muscle. This is supplied from the external branch of the superior laryngeal nerve.
- The right recurrent laryngeal nerve leaves the vagus to loop beneath the subclavian artery, before ascending to the larynx in the groove between the oesophagus and the trachea.
- The left recurrent laryngeal nerve passes beneath the arch of the aorta and similarly ascends in the groove between oesophagus and trachea.

Supplementary and Clinical Information

One obvious clinical area for discussion is the provision of anaesthesia for awake fibreoptic intubation.

Nebulized Lidocaine

- Nebulized local anaesthetic (such as lidocaine 4%) will provide adequate surface anaesthesia of the airway, although the procedure takes some time, and patients may therefore find the mask claustrophobic and uncomfortable. It may not anaesthetize the nasal mucosa adequately.

Topical Anaesthetic

- The nasal mucosa can be anaesthetized with local anaesthetic plus vasoconstrictor to minimize risk of bleeding. Topical cocaine can be used to a maximum dose of 1.5 mg kg^{-1}. If oral intubation is planned, the tongue and posterior pharynx can be anaesthetized using lidocaine 4% or a lidocaine 10% metered pump which delivers 10 mg with each spray.

'Spray as You Go' Technique

- This is another straightforward method of anaesthetising the airway, in which local anaesthetic (usually lidocaine 4%) is introduced under direct vision via the injector channel in the fibreoptic endoscope. In practice this is a simple and almost invariably effective technique. You may nonetheless be asked about supplemental blocks.
- **Glossopharyngeal nerve:** this provides sensory innervation to the oral pharynx, the supraglottic area, the base of the tongue and the vallecula. It can be blocked by submucosal infiltration behind the tonsillar pillars.
- **Superior laryngeal nerve:** this can be anaesthetized by bilateral injections which can be performed either by walking off the greater cornua of the hyoid to penetrate the thyrohyoid membrane, or by walking off the superior alae of the thyroid cartilage.
- **Recurrent laryngeal nerve:** this nerve is usually blocked even if a 'spray as you go' technique has been used to anaesthetize the remainder of the airway. It is blocked via

a transtracheal injection that is made through the cricothyroid membrane during inspiration. The inevitable cough distributes the solution (typically 4 ml of lidocaine 4%) more widely.

Clinical Consequences of Injury to the Laryngeal Nerves

- The external branch of the superior laryngeal nerve supplies the cricothyroid muscle, which tenses the vocal cords. Damage will be followed by hoarseness. If the injury is unilateral, this hoarseness will be temporary, because in time the other cricothyroid muscle will compensate. If it is bilateral the hoarseness will be permanent.
- The recurrent laryngeal nerve supplies all those muscles which control the opening and closing of the laryngeal inlet.
- Partial paralysis affects the abductor muscles more than the adductors, and so with unilateral injury the corresponding vocal cord is paralysed. This also results in hoarseness.
- If both nerves are damaged, then both cords oppose or even overlap each other in the midline. This leads to inspiratory stridor and has the potential to cause total respiratory obstruction.
- If one or both nerves are transected, the vocal cord(s) adopt the cadaveric position in which they lie partially abducted and through which airflow is much less compromised. Phonation may be reduced to a whisper.

The Anatomy of the Trachea and Bronchi

Commentary

Anatomy of these areas is of self-evident importance both in anaesthesia and intensive care. It is possible that you may be given the opportunity to describe every bronchopulmonary segment, but because the terminology is cumbersome with considerable duplication, it is more likely, once you have demonstrated that you know the key points (such as the origin of the right upper lobe bronchus), that the oral will concentrate more on applied clinical aspects.

Core Information

- **Trachea:** the trachea is a tube of cartilage with a membranous lining which is continuous inferiorly with the larynx. The trachea proper is 10–11 cm long, extending downwards from the cricoid cartilage at the level of the sixth cervical vertebra, as far as the sixth thoracic vertebra (in full inspiration). It then divides into left and right main bronchi. Its diameter in the adult is around 20 mm. In the first year of life its diameter is 3 mm or less, and increases thereafter by about 1 mm per year of age until it attains adult dimensions.
  - *Structure*: it comprises 16–20 C-shaped cartilages attached vertically by fibroelastic connective tissue, which helps explain the mobility of the structure. Through most of its course the trachea lies in the midline, although at the bifurcation it is

displaced slightly rightwards by the arch of the aorta. The posterior wall of the trachea is membranous.

— *Anterior relations*: in the upper part of the neck these are confined to skin and fascia, and to the isthmus of the thyroid overlying the second to fourth tracheal rings. In its lower cervical course, the trachea is partly overlain by the sternohyoid and sternothyroid muscles, and by the jugular arch connecting the anterior jugular veins. In its thoracic course the manubrium sterni lies anteriorly, as do the remnants of the thymus, the inferior thyroid veins and the brachiocephalic artery.

— *Posterior relations*: the oesophagus lies posteriorly, and the recurrent laryngeal nerves run in grooves between the trachea and oesophagus.

— *Lateral relations*: in the upper neck, the trachea is related to the lobes of the thyroid and to the carotid sheath. In its lower course, it is related on the right to the lung and pleura, to the brachiocephalic artery and veins, to the azygos vein and to the superior vena cava. On the left, it is related to the arch of the aorta and the left common carotid and subclavian arteries.

- **The right and left main bronchi:** the main bronchi are formed at about the level of T_5. The right is shorter (3 cm long), wider and angled more vertically than the left, which means that foreign bodies and tracheal tubes are more likely to enter its orifice than the left. The left main bronchus is more obliquely placed and is some 5 cm in length. Important relations on the right are the pulmonary artery which lies first below and then anterior to it, with the azygos vein above; on the left side, the main bronchus lies below the arch of the aorta with the descending aorta behind and the left pulmonary artery lying in front. In children, the angles of the bronchi at the carina are equal.

- **Bronchopulmonary segments – right lung:** within about 2.5 cm of the bifurcation, the right main bronchus gives off the right upper lobe bronchus (which divides in turn within 1 cm into apical, anterior and posterior segments). It is this right upper lobe bronchus that is most at risk from inadvertent occlusion by a tracheal tube or a right-sided double-lumen endobronchial tube. The right main then gives off the middle lobe bronchus, which is directed downwards and forwards (before bifurcating into medial and lateral lobes). Just below the origin of the middle lobe bronchus, and opposite to it, is the bronchus of the apical segment of the lower lobe. This directs posteriorly, before dividing into superior, anterior basal and lateral basal segments. The medial, anterior, lateral and posterior basal segments arise in due course from the main stem of the lower lobe bronchus, which continues in its downward direction.

- **Bronchopulmonary segments – left lung:** the longer left main bronchus gives off the left upper lobe bronchus after about 5 cm, and this then divides into a superior division from which arise apical, posterior and anterior segments of the upper lobe, and a lingular bronchus from which arise the superior and inferior lingular segments. The anatomy of the left lower lobe is similar to the right in that the left lower lobe bronchus gives off superior, anterior basal, lateral basal and posterior basal segments. The medial basal bronchopulmonary segment usually arises in common with the anterior basal, however, which means technically there are only four rather than five bronchopulmonary segments on the left (Figure 2.5).

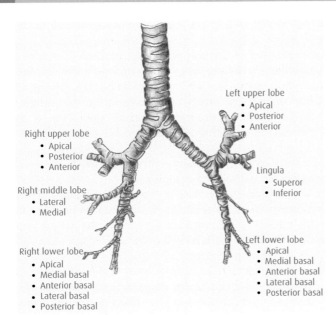

Fig. 2.5 The bronchopulmonary segments.

Supplementary and Clinical Information

- **Pulmonary aspiration of gastric contents:** the anatomy of the lobes and broncho-pulmonary segments influences zonal contamination should pulmonary aspiration occur. If the patient is supine, it is more likely that the apical segments of the lower lobes will be affected because of the direct posterior projection of the bronchus of the apical segment. If the patient is in the lateral position, then aspiration is more likely to affect the upper lobes. If prone, the right middle lobe and lingula will be the site of the problem because of their downward and forward orientation, and if they are sitting, it will be the posterior or lateral basal segments of the lower lobes that are contaminated.

- **Management of aspiration:** the cardinal sign will be otherwise unexplained desaturation. In a patient who has not received neuromuscular blockers this may be preceded by coughing which fails to settle as anaesthesia deepens. In a paralysed patient, aspiration may be silent. Auscultation may reveal rhonchi and/or crepitations. Chest X-ray changes often occur early enough to support the diagnosis of significant aspiration, although they can be delayed for 6 hours or more. Management is essentially expectant. If a patient does not need supplemental oxygen to maintain a normal SpO_2 after 2 hours, then it is unlikely that there will be significant sequelae. (Some anaesthetists prefer to wait 4–6 hours before making that judgement.) Should the patient remain oxygen-dependent, then he or she will need supportive therapy which in severe cases may include intubation and ventilation. There is no evidence of any benefit from the administration of prophylactic antibiotics or steroids.

You may be asked about the main structures that you see at bronchoscopy.

- **Fibreoptic bronchoscopy:** this is essentially a topic which needs visual aids, and so all that you will be required to do is give a brief description of the main structures that you see during bronchoscopy. Examiners will assume that most of your experience of the procedure will have been gained on intensive care, and so your account will start beyond the endotracheal tube in the trachea. You will see first the trachea; the anterior wall, which is composed of complete cartilaginous bands; and the posterior wall, which is membranous. The carina separates the right and left main stem bronchi.

— *Right side view*: the right main bronchus is wider than the left and is shorter at ~3 cm long. It is also angled more vertically than the left. Within ~2.5 cm of the bifurcation can be seen the right upper lobe bronchus. The right main then gives off the middle lobe bronchus, which is directed downwards and forwards. Just below the origin of the middle lobe bronchus and opposite to it is the bronchus of the apical segment of the lower lobe; beyond this the main stem of the lower lobe bronchus continues downwards.

— *Left side view*: the left main bronchus is more obliquely placed and is about 5 cm in length. It gives off the left upper lobe bronchus near its termination at about 5 cm, which then divides into a superior division and a lingular bronchus. The anatomy of the left lower lobe bronchus is similar to the right.

- **Double-lumen endobronchial tubes:** these are used when one lung needs to be isolated so that the other can be collapsed to allow surgery. Such procedures include pulmonary resection, oesophagogastrectomy, surgery of the thoracic aorta, anterior spinal fixation and thoracoscopic sympathectomy. A left-sided tube is almost always favoured because this avoids the risk of inadvertently occluding the origin of the right upper lobe bronchus. Problems with malpositioned tubes are an important cause of mortality and morbidity (see under 'One-Lung Ventilation [One-Lung Anaesthesia]' in Chapter 3). A double-lumen tube is positioned correctly when the upper surface of the bronchial cuff lies immediately distal to the bifurcation of the carina. The position of the tube should be checked endoscopically.

- **Awake fibreoptic intubation:** indications include known difficult intubation, known or suspected difficult intubation in a patient with a full stomach and patients with cervical spine disease or injury. Details of technique vary, but they all involve railroading a tube (oral or, more commonly, nasal) down over the fibrescope and into the airway, which can be anaesthetized using various local anaesthetic techniques.

- **Tracheal damage:** this may be caused by external trauma but has also been reported not infrequently as a complication of tracheal intubation. Clinical features may include alteration of phonation and stridor (if the larynx is involved), hoarseness, subcutaneous emphysema, pain on external palpation and pain on movement of the tongue.

The Surface Anatomy of the Neck (Percutaneous Tracheostomy and Cricothyroidotomy)

Commentary

If these procedures are performed incorrectly the results can be disastrous. The applied anatomy is not complex, but you should be able to give a simple authoritative account of the techniques, particularly in relation to the potentially life-saving manoeuvre of cricothyroidotomy (cricothyrotomy).

Core Information

The surface anatomy of the neck.

- The hyoid bone lies at the level of the third cervical vertebra (C_3). Lying just above and behind is the epiglottis.
- The bifurcation of the common carotid artery is at the level of the fourth cervical vertebra (C_4), slightly above the notch of the thyroid cartilage.
- The larynx lies opposite the fourth, fifth and sixth cervical vertebrae ($C_{4, 5, 6}$).
- The cricoid cartilage is at the level of the sixth cervical vertebra (C_6).
- The trachea extends from the sixth cervical vertebra (C_6) down as far as the fifth or sixth thoracic vertebra ($T_{5, 6}$) at end-inspiration.
- The suprasternal notch is located at the level of the second and third thoracic vertebrae ($T_{2, 3}$).

Anatomy relevant to the two clinical techniques of percutaneous tracheostomy and cricothyroidotomy, which have different indications but broadly similar complications.

- The trachea comprises 16–20 C-shaped cartilages, which lie anteriorly in the neck covered by skin and the superficial and deep fascial layers. The second, third and fourth rings are covered by the isthmus of the thyroid. The great vessels of the neck lie laterally, and so identification of the midline is crucial.
- The cricothyroid membrane spans the inferior border of the thyroid cartilage and the superior border of the cricoid cartilage, and immediately overlies the subglottic region of the larynx. It is covered anteriorly by skin and by superficial and deep fascia. Immediately lateral are the sternocleidomastoid muscle, the sternothyroid and the sternohyoid muscles and the carotid sheath.

Supplementary and Clinical Information

Percutaneous Tracheostomy

- This is an elective, not an emergency procedure, which in the context of intensive care has become a well-established alternative to definitive surgical tracheostomy. Its indications are the same as for formal tracheostomy in the critically ill: typically to simplify airway management in a patient who otherwise would face the problems of long-term tracheal intubation, to allow a reduction in sedation and to facilitate weaning from mechanical ventilation.
- Different techniques have been described (by Ciaglia in 1985, and by Grigg and others). The Fantoni technique is a translaryngeal tracheostomy which is not strictly a percutaneous method and is not widely used. Most are variations on a theme (dilatation over a guidewire), but describe the one with which you are most familiar.
- A typical technique is described as follows.
  — Guided by the surface anatomy a skin incision is made to allow a needle and guidewire to be placed through the fibroelastic tissue that joins the tracheal rings.
  — The isthmus of the thyroid gland covers the second to fourth tracheal rings. A higher approach through the subcricoid membrane or between the first and

second tracheal rings does avoid the thyroid isthmus but is associated with a greater incidence of tracheal stenosis. It is for this reason that many intensivists now prefer a low approach, at the level of the second and third ring.

— The diameter of the hole is enlarged with progressively larger dilators to the point at which it will accept a definitive tracheostomy tube. An alternative is the use of a single tapered dilator.

— A second anaesthetist should monitor this procedure from within the trachea by using a fibreoptic bronchoscope. The posterior wall of the trachea may be so ragged and friable that it can easily be perforated.

Complications

- Haemorrhage (immediate or delayed), the creation of false passage, tracheal or oesophageal perforation, barotrauma, subcutaneous emphysema, failure and accidental decannulation.
- Subglottic stenosis is a cause of serious morbidity; it is more common after cricothyroidotomy than after percutaneous tracheostomy.

Comparison of Percutaneous Tracheostomy with Cricothyroidotomy

- Both techniques bypass the normal translaryngeal route to secure the airway, but the circumstances and urgency of their use differ considerably. Percutaneous tracheostomy is an elective procedure, whereas cricothyroidotomy is an emergency procedure which is usually invoked only when all other attempts to secure a definitive airway have failed and when critical hypoxia is imminent.
- The cricothyroid membrane is used for emergency access because it is readily identifiable and because it is relatively avascular.
- **Difficult Airway Society (DAS) front-of-neck access guidelines**. The 2015 guidelines for the management of unanticipated difficult intubation include the recommendation for emergency front-of-neck access in the 'Can't intubate; can't oxygenate' (CICO) situation. Oxygen should continue to be given via the upper airway (in the absence of complete obstruction and assuming a continued circulation, there will be some apnoeic oxygenation), while the cricothyroid membrane is identified using the so-called laryngeal handshake. (The whole hand is used to palpate the cartilaginous structures of the hyoid, thyroid and cricoid, in much the same way that some anaesthetists check for accurate seating of a laryngeal mask airway). If this proves ineffective and ultrasound is not rapidly available, an 8–10 cm midline incision should be made (caudal to rostral). With the cricothyroid membrane exposed, it should be incised with a transverse stab after which the scalpel blade (number 10) is rotated through 90° with the sharp edge caudad. Without removing the blade, a bougie is passed into the trachea over which a lubricated 6.0 cuffed tracheal tube can be railroaded. (If the cricothyroid membrane is easily identified, the extended midline incision will not be necessary.)
- This procedure is not as straightforward as this description might suggest: the Fourth National Audit Project. (NAP 4) Major complications of airway management in the UK, that was published in 2011 reported that the emergency cricothyrotomy failure rate was 64%. Another review of failed intubation in obstetrics over several decades

reported that of 13 women in whom this procedure was attempted only 6 survived unharmed. A further 6 died, and 1 more suffered hypoxic brain injury (Kinsella *et al. IJOA* 2015, 4: 356–74). The cricothyroid membrane is most accurately located using ultrasound (and is best done before the event).

The Stellate Ganglion

Commentary

Stellate ganglion block is a common procedure in the chronic pain clinic, is simple to perform and has significant potential complications. You may well not have carried out this block yourself, but as one of several procedures in the neck undertaken by anaesthetists (others include interscalene block, deep cervical plexus block and internal jugular cannulation), its anatomy is of some relevance.

Core Information

- The cervical sympathetic chain lies either side of the vertebral column in the fascial space. Posterior lies the fascia over the prevertebral muscles; anterior is the carotid sheath.
- The area where the inferior cervical and the first thoracic ganglia meet, either in close proximity or fusion, is referred to as the stellate ganglion.
- The ganglion extends from the neck of the first rib, where its lower part is covered anteriorly by the dome of the pleura, to the transverse process of C_7, where the vertebral artery lies anterior. By the level of C_6, the vertebral artery has moved posteriorly into the foramen transversarium, pending its ascent into the skull.
- Much of the sympathetic nerve supply to the head and neck as well as to the upper extremity synapses in or near the stellate ganglion. This means that a successful block will be signified by ipsilateral Horner's syndrome (ptosis, miosis, enophthalmos and anhidrosis).
- Sympathetic pre-ganglionic fibres leave the cord from segments as widely separated as T_1–T_6, and, although many converge in or around the stellate ganglion, some may bypass it. For this reason, large volumes of local anaesthetic solution may be needed to fill the space in front of the prevertebral fascia down to T_4, but this will produce reliable sympathetic blockade of the head, neck and upper limb. It is more accurately described as a 'cervicothoracic block'.

Supplementary and Clinical Information

Stellate Ganglion Block

- **Indications:** these include any condition requiring sympathetic block of the head, neck and upper limb. As a generalization, the evidence base for the therapeutic use of stellate ganglion blocks is weak, but the technique has a long tradition of use in the management of chronic pain.

— **Neuropathic pain conditions:** complex regional pain syndromes (CRPS) types I and II, post-herpetic neuralgia of head and neck, shoulder–hand syndrome (following CVA or ischaemia), phantom limb pain and pain associated with upper limb denervation. There is evidence from at least one controlled study which suggests that early stellate ganglion block may prevent the progression of CRPS in some patients.

— **Ischaemic conditions:** thrombosis or microembolism, vasospastic disorders (e.g. Raynaud's disease), scleroderma, frostbite and inadvertent intra-arterial injection in the upper limb.

— **Angina pectoris:** severe refractory chest pain due to coronary ischaemia.

— **Miscellaneous:** hyperhidrosis and treatment of pain associated with Paget's disease of bone.

- **Techniques:** two approaches are described: the anterior (sometimes called the 'paratracheal' anterior) approach and the paratracheal approach. The use of ultrasound guidance allows more precise subfascial placement of the needle, which results in more caudal spread.

  — **Anterior approach:** the trachea and carotid pulse are gently retracted to allow identification of the most prominent cervical transverse process (the Chassaignac tubercle) at C_6, the level of the cricoid cartilage.

  — A lower approach to the ganglion's actual location at C_7 risks both pneumothorax and vertebral artery puncture.

  — The carotid sheath is moved laterally, and the trachea medially, before a 25–30 mm × 23–25G needle is directed perpendicularly down onto the tubercle.

  — Once it has encountered bone, the needle is withdrawn 4–5 mm. If this is not done, there is a higher incidence of upper limb somatic blockade.

  — Local anaesthetic in low concentration and high volume (such as lidocaine 0.5% or bupivacaine 0.125% × 15–20 ml) is injected.

  — **Paratracheal approach:** The needle insertion is two fingerbreadths lateral to the suprasternal notch and two fingerbreadths superior to the clavicle. This identifies the transverse process of C_7, immediately below Chassaignac's tubercle at C_6, at the level of the cricoid cartilage.

  — The sternocleidomastoid and carotid sheath are moved laterally before the needle is directed perpendicularly down onto the transverse process.

  — Once it has encountered bone, the needle is withdrawn 0.5–1.0 cm.

  — Local anaesthetic in low concentration and high volume is injected as described earlier.

  — This lower approach risks pneumothorax as well as vertebral artery puncture.

- **Complications** include local trauma and haematoma (which may compress the airway if severe); recurrent laryngeal nerve block, which causes hoarseness; brachial plexus block, because via the anterior approach only a layer of fascia separates the plexus and the ganglion which is anterior to it; carotid or vertebral arterial puncture and possible intravascular injection (with the paratracheal lower approach); intrathecal injection; pneumothorax (if the approach is too low); and deep cervical plexus block (if the approach is too high).

The Paravertebral Space

Commentary

Thoracic paravertebral blocks can provide ipsilateral analgesia via a technique that is simpler (and probably safer) than a thoracic epidural. First described as long ago as 1905, they have made a resurgence, particularly for procedures such as day case breast surgery. Lumbar paravertebral blocks are less useful and largely have been replaced by transversus abdominis plane (TAP) and rectus sheath blocks.

Core Information

- By definition there are bilateral paravertebral spaces associated with all the vertebrae; the thoracic paravertebral space extends from the level of T1 down to T12.
- The area is triangular (wedge shaped) in all directions.
- The medial wall is formed by the vertebral bodies, intervertebral discs and intervertebral foraminae.
- The anterolateral boundary consists of the parietal pleura and the innermost intercostal membrane.
- The posterior boundary consists of the transverse processes of the thoracic vertebrae, the heads of the thoracic ribs and the superior costotransverse ligament.
- An endothoracic fascial layer divides the space into ventral (anterior) and dorsal (posterior) compartments. This has relevance for the spread of local anaesthetic within the space.
- It contains spinal nerves, as the target for local anaesthetic injection; white and grey rami communicantes; the sympathetic chain; intercostal vessels; lymphatics; and fat.
- It is continuous with a number of areas: the contralateral paravertebral space via the prevertebral fascia, the epidural space immediately medially, and the intercostal space laterally.

Supplementary and Clinical Information

The extent of the thoracic paravertebral space (both thoracic and lumbar) means that unilateral paravertebral block is a versatile analgesic technique that can be used for surgery as diverse as mastectomy and iliac crest bone harvesting.

- **Indications:** paravertebral block can be used to provide analgesia for unilateral surgical operations in the thoracic and upper abdominal region. These include breast, renal and thoracic operations. It can also be used for open cholecystectomy. The block can be used to treat the acute pain of fractured ribs, and may also have a place in the management of chronic pain conditions such as neuropathic pain and the complex regional pain syndrome.
- **Contraindications:** absolute contraindications are typically generic and include patient refusal and local sepsis. Rarely the presence of a tumour in the paravertebral space at the level of injection would also preclude the procedure. Specific relative contraindications to thoracic paravertebral block include respiratory disease involving the diaphragm as a result of which the patient relies on intercostal function.

Coagulopathies, either innate or acquired, are relative contraindications which require a risk-benefit assessment. However, unlike a haematoma in the epidural space, a bleed into the paravertebral space is highly unlikely to lead to spinal cord compression or damage to the spinal nerves themselves.

- **Technique of thoracic paravertebral block:** a number of approaches are described. The following account will be sufficient for the purposes of the oral, but specialist monographs will give much more detail, and in particular describe ultrasound-assisted or ultrasound-guided techniques which are more difficult for a candidate to describe in the context of an oral examination.
- Radiographic studies of local anaesthetic spread have demonstrated that injection into the ventral/anterior compartment is associated with longitudinal spread along several segments, whereas injection into the dorsal/posterior compartment results in much more localized and limited distribution around the level of injection. If injections are made at multiple levels, however, which probably is the more common technique, the needle placement need not be quite as focused.
- **Depth:** the median distance from skin to the thoracic paravertebral space is said to be 5.5 cm, but body habitus, predictably, has an influence on this depth, which can be measured using ultrasound. The space is also shallower in the mid-thoracic region. The key to the efficacy and safety of this block is to limit the advance of the needle to no more than 1.0 cm beyond the superior costotransverse ligament, having walked off the transverse process.
- **In brief:** the block is easiest described by assuming that the patient is awake, but in practice many anaesthetists perform the blocks with the patient anaesthetized with the side to be operated on uppermost.
- The appropriate spinous process is identified in the midline and a point marked 2.5 cm immediately lateral. (Remember that the downward orientation of the thoracic spinous processes means that they lie medial to the transverse process of the vertebra immediately below).
- Following superficial infiltration with local anaesthetic down to the transverse process (in the awake patient), an appropriate needle is advanced perpendicular to skin. An ideal device for this purpose is an 18G paediatric Tuohy needle, which is graduated in 0.5 cm intervals.
- As a safety measure, the operator's forefinger should be placed initially at 35 mm to limit the depth of advancement down onto the transverse process. Should this not be encountered at 35 mm, then the guard distance can be increased in 5 mm increments until it does so.
- Once the needle contacts the transverse process, the forefinger guard is moved 1.0 cm distally and the needle walked off the process caudally (this reduces the risk of inadvertent puncture of the pleura and a likely pneumothorax).
- Advancement of the needle by that 1.0 cm will put the needle tip into the paravertebral space and no further. There is sometimes the sensation of a click as the needle penetrates the superior costotransverse ligament, but this is too subtle for identification by loss of resistance to saline. Loss of resistance to air using an epidural loss-of-resistance device (using a technique analogous to performing a lumbar epidural) can, however, be effective.
- A peripheral nerve stimulator can also be used to aid identification of the space.

- If injections are made at multiple sites, the usual dose would be up to 5.0 ml of local anaesthetic (typically levobupivacaine 0.5%). At a single injection site, 15 ml of solution will give a sensory block over a median of three dermatomes.
- Continuous analgesia can be provided by the insertion of a paravertebral catheter. This should be inserted no deeper than 2.0 cm into the space so as to avoid the risk of catheterizing the epidural space. In adults, a starting infusion rate of 0.1 ml kg hr^{-1} would be appropriate.
- **Levels required for common surgical procedures:** these should be predictable from knowledge of the sensory dermatomes. For example, simple mastectomy, T_3–T_4; mastectomy with axillary clearance, T_1–T_6.
- **Complications:** in addition to generic complications such as vascular puncture and neurapraxia, the complications specific to paravertebral block include pneumothorax (which initially may go unnoticed because injected local anaesthetic will lead to effective intrapleural analgesia), epidural anaesthesia due to medial passage of injectate through the intervertebral foramen, and inadvertent puncture of the dural cuff with intrathecal spread. Paravertebral injections block sensory, motor and autonomic nerves, and so hypotension may also complicate an effective block.
- **Technique of lumbar paravertebral block:** in the lumbar region, there is less continuity between adjacent spaces (nor is there a superior costotransverse ligament), and so multiple injections may be necessary. For inguinal hernia repair, for example, injections will be needed at the levels of T_{12}, L_1 and L_2.

Comparison with Thoracic Epidural Analgesia

- Performing an epidural in the upper thoracic region is a considerably more difficult technique than paravertebral blockade.
- A thoracic epidural cannot reliably provide unilateral analgesia. The catheter may migrate laterally through the intervertebral foramina and into the paravertebral space, at which point of course it become an inadvertent paravertebral block. Otherwise the analgesia provided by the two techniques is comparable.
- This analgesia comes at the expense of predictable consequences of a high bilateral block together with the generic complications of epidural insertion. These are inadvertent dural puncture and subsequent post-dural puncture headache, but with the additional risk of spinal cord damage, failure, unilateral or patchy block, inadvertent subdural block, intravascular injection, epidural haematoma or abscess. The risk of permanent neurological sequelae is small, but in the NAP 3 report on complications of neuraxial blockade, the greatest number of identified problems were associated with peri-operative epidurals. There were 14 epidural abscesses reported, for example, 10 of which were thoracic (Third National Audit Project [NAP3]. National Audit of Major Complications of Central Neuraxial Blockade in the United Kingdom. Royal College of Anaesthetists. 2009).

Effects of Regional Analgesia on Tumour Recurrence

- There is some evidence that effective regional nerve blockade is associated with a lower rate of tumour recurrence. Many, if not most, thoracic paravertebral blocks are performed for surgery for breast malignancy, and so this might be a significant advantage of the technique. The topic is dealt with in more detail under 'Local Anaesthetics – Actions' in Chapter 4.

The Pleura

Commentary

The pleural membranes are important for normal pulmonary function, and their susceptibility to iatrogenic damage heightens their interest for anaesthetists. They lack discrete anatomical features, being essentially a continuous structure, and so are described somewhat arbitrarily according to regions of the thorax as outlined in the following.

Core Information

- The pleura (or strictly speaking the pleurae, as there are two), is the serous membrane that invests the lungs as the visceral pleura, and lines the thoracic cavity as the parietal pleura. They extend from the dome of the pleura superiorly, to the diaphragm inferiorly. The pleural membranes of the left and right lungs do not connect with each other, being separated by the mediastinum.
- **Parietal pleura:** this is continuous but for descriptive purposes is divided into separate parts. These are the cupola (cervical pleura), the costal pleura, the mediastinal pleura and the diaphragmatic pleura.
- **Cupola, or cervical pleura**. This covers the apex of the lung and projects up into the neck above the first rib. It is partly protected in this region by the suprapleural membrane, which is a thickening of the endothoracic fascia. This attaches to the inner margin of the first rib and the transverse process of the seventh cervical vertebra.
- **Costal pleura**. This covers the interior thorax: the inner aspects of the ribs, the costal cartilages and the intercostal muscles. It is separated from these structures and from the sternum by the endothoracic fascia, which in this region is loose connective tissue. Posterior to the dome of the pleura lie the sympathetic trunk and the first thoracic nerve.
- **Mediastinal pleura**. Where the costal pleura turns anteriorly it becomes the mediastinal pleura. The underlying space is the costomediastinal recess. At the root of the lung the mediastinal pleura becomes continuous with the visceral pleura, with a downward projection which is the pulmonary ligament. Medially it is adherent to the pericardium (apart from the area through which the phrenic nerve passes).
- **Diaphragmatic pleura**. This is the most inferior part of the parietal pleura which completely covers the superior thoracic (superior) surface of the diaphragm apart from the central tendon. Beneath it lies the costodiaphragmatic recess. The inferior border of the pleura runs from the xiphersternum down to the level of the 8th rib in the mid-clavicular line, the tenth rib in the mix-axillary line and to the twelfth rib posteriorly.

- **Visceral pleura**. The parietal pleura is reflected onto the lung, at which point it becomes the visceral pleura. It covers the entire surface of the lung, including the fissures which separate the lobes.
- **Pleural space**. This is a potential space between the layers of the visceral and parietal pleura which contains around 10–20 ml of pleural fluid (it has been calculated as being 0.3 ml kg^{-1} body weight). This is produced by the serous membrane and is similar in composition to plasma apart from its much lower protein count. It allows movement between the chest wall and the lung.
- **Innervation:** the visceral pleura receives autonomic innervation via the pulmonary plexus and like the visceral peritoneum is sensitive to stretch but not to pain or temperature. The parietal pleura is innervated by the intercostal nerves and by some branches of the phrenic nerve, which means that pain can be referred to the ipsilateral shoulder.
- **Vascular supply:** the visceral pleurae as well as the parenchyma of the lung are supplied by the internal thoracic arteries. The parietal pleurae are supplied by the intercostal arteries. There is rich lymphatic drainage.

Clinical Applications

- **Pneumothorax**. The pleura is vulnerable to damage from amongst other things trauma, infection and malignancy. There are a number of anaesthetic procedures that can also put it potentially at risk. The topic is described in more detail under 'Pneumothorax' in Chapter 3.
- **Pleural effusion**. The small volume of fluid in the pleural cavity is maintained by the balance of oncotic and hydrostatic pressure and by efficient lymphatic drainage. Increases in the normal volume of pleural fluid are always abnormal, and effusions are classified traditionally as transudative (low protein) and exudative (high protein). **Transudative effusions:** causes include congestive cardiac failure, hyoproteinaemia, cirrhosis of the liver (ascites can cross the diaphragm into the pleural cavity) and the nephrotic syndrome. These are essentially ultrafiltrates produced by alterations in the balance between the oncotic and hydrostatic pressures. Localized collections may occur in the region of a pulmonary embolus due to increased capillary permeability secondary to the cytokines and other inflammatory mediators released by the thrombus.
  Exudative effusions: these are associated with inflammatory pathologies that include infection, primary and secondary malignancy (mesothelioma being the classic tumour of the pleural mesothelial cells) and autoimmune conditions such as rheumatoid arthritis. There may be increased capillary disruption, impaired lymphatic drainage and increased fluid production by the pleural membranes themselves. Exudative effusions can also occur after pulmonary embolism. (As a practical point, it requires the accumulation of 250 ml of fluid before an effusion is apparent on a chest X-ray).
- **Intrapleural catheters**. The injection of local anaesthetic into the intrapleural space, with or without inserting a catheter, can provide effective somatic block of an extensive range of thoracic dermatomes. This makes it a potentially useful intervention for the management of chest and upper abdominal pain from numerous causes. These include rib trauma, surgical pain from thoracotomy and breast surgery, chronic pain syndromes and upper abdominal surgical procedures such as open

cholecystectomy and operations on the kidney. Different techniques for the block have been described using variously loss of resistance and negative intrapleural pressure (during inspiration) to confirm the anatomical location. Ultrasound guidance is increasingly employed for these as for other blocks. The injection is made typically about 10 cm lateral to the posterior midline of the thorax in the seventh or eighth intercostal space. A single shot dose would consist of 20 ml of levobupivacaine 0.5%, and the starting rate for a catheter infusion would usually be 5 ml hr^{-1} of levobupivacaine 0.25%. The main risks of the procedure are pneumothorax (the commonly quoted incidence is 2%) and local anaesthetic toxicity, together with the generic complications of any sharp needle technique. The efficacy of the technique may be limited by uneven spread and by dependent pooling. This does not, however, appear to have a consistently detrimental effect on diaphragmatic function.

The Mediastinum

Commentary

The mediastinum is not a complex area of anatomy to describe, but as it is probably the first part of a chest X-ray that anaesthetists examine it can reveal a substantial amount of relevant pathology.

Core Information

- The mediastinum is the central compartment of the chest and is divided into superior and inferior parts. The inferior part is the larger of the two and is further subdivided into the anterior inferior, the middle inferior and the posterior inferior mediastinum. The separation between superior and inferior is marked by the thoracic plane (of Ludwig), which is an artificial rather than an anatomical plane that extends from the level of the fourth and fifth thoracic vertebrae posteriorly to the sternal angle anteriorly.
- The mediastinum contains the heart and its major vessels, the trachea, the oesophagus, the remnant of the thymus (in adults), the thoracic duct and the phrenic nerves and cardiac nerves, including the vagus. It also contains the lymph nodes that can become massively enlarged in diseases such as lymphomas.
- The relations of the superior mediastinum are superiorly – the thoracic inlet; posteriorly – the vertebral bodies of T_1–T_4; anteriorly – the manubrium; inferiorly – the thoracic plane; laterally – the pleurae.
- The relations of the anterior inferior mediastinum are superiorly – the thoracic plane; posteriorly – the pericardium, aorta and brachiocephalic vessels; anteriorly – the sternum and the costal cartilages and medial parts of the fifth, sixth and seventh ribs; inferiorly – the diaphragm; laterally – the pleurae.
- The middle inferior mediastinum contains the pericardium and the heart. It is therefore bounded anteriorly by the anterior inferior mediastinum and posteriorly by the posterior inferior mediastinum.

- The relations of the posterior inferior mediastinum are superiorly – the thoracic plane; posteriorly – the vertebral bodies of $T_{5/6}$–T_{12}; anteriorly – the pericardium; inferiorly – the diaphragm; laterally – the pleurae.

Supplementary and Clinical information

Various pathological conditions can affect the mediastinum, many of which will be manifest in a standard chest X-ray. (A 'standard' chest X-ray is one taken with the patient upright, in a posterior-anterior (PA) view, in full inspiration, centralized without any rotation, and with adequate penetration that allows the vertebral bodies to be just visible behind the heart. Non-standard X-rays can result in very misleading appearances.)

- **Hilar enlargement**. Massive hilar lymphadenopathy is characteristic of lymphoma, but hilar and paratracheal lymph node enlargement is also typical of sarcoidosis. Enlargement may be due to metastatic disease and also to pulmonary hypertension.
- **Abnormalities of the size, shape and contours of the myocardium**. Numerous conditions can alter the cardiac shadow. These include cardiomegaly due to left and right ventricular hypertrophy or dilated and obstructed cardiomyopathy; left atrial enlargement, secondary, for example, to mitral stenosis, which may manifest as a double right heart border; expansion of the left heart border due to enlargement of the left atrial appendage; and splaying of the carina superiorly, typically by left atrial enlargement, upward displacement of the atrium and mediastinal masses. The cardiac outline is also changed by pericardial effusion. The definition of the heart borders may be lost; if on the left it may be due to consolidation of the lingula, if on the right it may be due to consolidation of the middle lobe of the lung.
- **Abnormalities of the vessels**. This applies particularly to the thoracic aorta, which may be distorted by aneurysmal dilatation and increase the size of the aortic knuckle while also displacing the trachea.
- **Mediastinal widening**. This can be a common artefact, but otherwise can be due to mediastinal masses, particularly paratracheal nodes in the superior mediastinum, and to vascular abnormality.
- **Pneumomediastinum**. This may follow penetrating trauma or perforation of the trachea or oesophagus. It may also occur in patients with chronic lung disease. If the source of the air is pulmonary, then it tracks from ruptured alveoli along the vascular sheaths which accompany the bronchi, and once at the hilum extends proximally into the mediastinum. If air in the mediastinum is under tension it can occasionally compromise cardiac output, but in itself it is usually innocuous and self-limiting. This may not be true of the precipitating cause.
- **Other masses**. These include retrosternal goiters and lesions of the thymus.
- **Mediastinoscopy**. This allows the biopsy of mediastinal masses either for diagnosis or for the staging of disease. The commonest approach is via a relatively small incision in the suprasternal notch. The difficulties faced by the anaesthetist will be influenced largely by the varied nature of the disease. Tracheal compression, for example, may make airway management problematic. Lung cancer is likely to be accompanied by chronic obstructive pulmonary disease and ischaemic heart disease. A thymic mass may be associated with myasthenia gravis. Potential complications

include massive haemorrhage, pneumothorax, air embolism and tracheobronchial injury. However, in many cases mediastinoscopy has been superseded by endobronchial ultrasound-guided fine needle aspiration (EBUS), which is a considerably less invasive technique that spares patients most of the complications outlined here.

Myocardial Blood Supply

Commentary

There is considerable overlap in the arterial supply to areas of the myocardium, and so it is not always possible to diagnose the site of coronary artery occlusion from ECG or echocardiographic changes. After you have been asked about the anatomy, which you may find easier to explain with the help of a simple diagram, the oral may to move on to the physiology of coronary perfusion.

Core Information

You will be asked to describe the arterial supply and venous drainage of the heart.

- **Arterial supply:** the heart is supplied by the right and left coronary arteries; these originate from the ascending aorta (anterior and posterior aortic sinuses, located just above the cusps of the aortic valve) (Figure 2.6).
- **Right coronary artery:** this passes between the pulmonary trunk and the right atrial appendage to descend in the anterior atrioventricular groove.
- It gives off atrial and ventricular short branches to supply those structures.
- At the inferior border of the heart, it effectively divides into the marginal branch which travels along the right ventricle towards the apex and the posterior

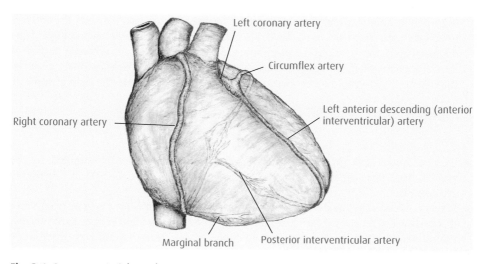

Fig. 2.6 Coronary arterial supply.

interventricular artery which continues in the groove of the same name to anastomose with the circumflex artery (the corresponding branch of the left coronary artery). This anastomosis is variable.

- The right main coronary artery or its branches supply the right ventricle and right atrium, part of the interventricular septum, the sinoatrial node, SAN (in 65%), the bundle of His, the atrioventricular node, AVN (80%) and the conducting system (80%). It also supplies a small diaphragmatic part of the left ventricle.
- **Left coronary artery:** this is larger than the right and, after arising from the posterior aortic sinus, passes between the left atrial appendage and the pulmonary trunk.
- It divides shortly into the anterior interventricular (also known as the left anterior descending, LAD) artery, which passes down the interventricular groove giving off anterior ventricular branches, and into the circumflex artery. This continues in the atrioventricular groove to anastomose with the inferior interventricular artery.
- The left coronary artery or its branches supply the left ventricle and left atrium, part of the interventricular septum, the SAN (in 35%), the AVN (20%) and the conducting system (20%).
- The innermost part of the endocardium receives oxygen directly from the blood within the ventricle.
- **Venous drainage:** as much as a third of cardiac venous blood drains directly into the cardiac chambers via the venae cordis minimae (a network of small veins). The remainder is drained by larger veins which tend to accompany the coronary arteries.
- Most of the remaining venous blood drains into the right atrium via the coronary sinus, which is located to the left of the opening of the inferior vena cava, and which lies in the posterior atrioventricular groove.

This is probably all the information that will be required, but for completeness a fuller account of the venous drainage follows.

- The main veins which drain into the sinus are the *great cardiac vein*, which lies in the anterior interventricular groove (with the LAD); the *middle cardiac vein*, which lies in the inferior interventricular groove containing the anastomosis between the inferior interventricular and the circumflex arteries; the *small cardiac vein* accompanying the marginal branch of the right coronary artery; the *oblique vein* on the posterior surface of the left atrium; and the *anterior cardiac vein*, which lies with the right coronary artery in the anterior atrioventricular groove and which drains directly into the right atrium.

Supplementary and Clinical Information

The Physiology of Coronary Perfusion

- At rest, about 250 ml min^{-1}, or 5%, of the cardiac output is supplied to the myocardium through the coronary arteries. This can increase fivefold during vigorous exercise.
- Flow is governed by the driving pressure. In the presence of a fixed coronary stenosis, this pressure gradient is crucial. In the absence of a stenotic lesion, the main variable that determines flow is the calibre of the blood vessels. Vasodilatation occurs mainly in response to the presence of local metabolites such as hydrogen ions, adenosine,

potassium, phosphate, carbon dioxide and prostaglandins. Autonomic control of vascular tone is present but is a negligible influence in comparison.

- Myocardial tissue has a high oxygen extraction ratio (80%), which limits its capacity for anaerobic metabolism. Increased oxygen demand has to be met by an increase in coronary perfusion.
- During systole, the subendocardial pressure in the left ventricle exceeds that in the outer part of the myocardium, and so, in the main, arterial flow occurs through the arteries only in diastole. There is, however, some flow to the outer areas of the left ventricle throughout the cardiac cycle. In the right side of the heart, which is a lower-pressure system, coronary perfusion persists throughout systole and diastole. At an average heart rate of 72 beats per minute, about 0.3 seconds will be spent in systole and 0.5 in diastole. High heart rates can compromise ventricular perfusion as well as ventricular filling.

Myocardial Oxygen Supply and Demand

- **Supply:** This is dependent on coronary blood flow, O_2 content of blood (dependent on haemoglobin concentration and SpO_2) and the position of the oxygen–haemoglobin dissociation curve.
- **Demand:** This is dependent on systolic arterial pressure (afterload), left ventricular end-diastolic pressure (preload), myocardial contractility and heart rate.

Acute Myocardial Ischaemia

- **Acute coronary syndrome**. This defines any cardiac problem secondary to acutely restricted blood flow to the myocardium, and so includes unstable angina pectoris and myocardial infarction (both NSTEMI and STEMI).
- **STEMI and NSTEMI (ST segment elevation myocardial infarction and non-ST segment elevation myocardial infarction)**. NSTEMI follows partial blockage of a major artery or complete occlusion of one of the minor arteries. Typically, this is with a platelet-rich thrombus or so-called white clot. STEMI accounts for around 65–70% of all cases of myocardial infarction and is due to complete occlusion of one of the major coronary arteries. Typically, this is with a fibrin-rich thrombus or so-called red clot often superimposed on white clot. Clinical presentation is similar, with the typical symptoms of central chest pain, dyspnoea, diaphoresis and nausea. The different ECG changes reflect the degree of myocardial damage, with a STEMI causing full-thickness and an NSTEMI only partial-thickness damage to the ventricular wall. As a result, the biochemical markers of myocardial injury are less elevated. The typical STEMI ECG shows ST segment elevation, q waves in the affected distribution and T-wave inversion. The NSTEMI ECG shows ST segment depression and/or T-wave inversion. If percutaneous coronary intervention (PCI) is not available within 2 hours, then thrombolysis is indicated in STEMI, but it is contra-indicated in NSTEMI because of the risk of reinfarction, which in any event is higher post-hospital discharge (15–25% vs. 5–8%). The platelet-rich core thrombus may have an overlying fibrin cap which partially occludes the vessel but stabilizes the clot. Thrombolyis risks exposing and releasing the platelet core to trigger further thrombus. The differential diagnosis is therefore not academic.

- **NICE guidelines for NSTEMI.** NICE have produced detailed guidelines for the immediate management of NSTEMI. Following diagnosis, it is suggested that aspirin and antithrombin therapy should be 'offered' (as if a patient with crushing central chest pain is going to want to embark on a discussion of the risks and benefits of treatment) and a formal assessment of the risk of future events should be made. (The Global Registry of Adverse Cardiac Events, GRACE, is one such scoring system, which predicts 6-month mortality. See under 'Scoring Systems' in Chapter 5.) The level of predicted risk (low, medium, high) determines further treatment, which can range from conservative management to coronary angiography, PCI and coronary revascularization.
- **Coronary occlusion and the ECG.** Acute thrombotic occlusion of the left anterior descending artery will result in an anterior or anteroseptal myocardial infarction. Occlusion of the posterior interventricular branch of the right coronary artery can result both in inferior and posterior infarction. The right coronary artery supplies the SA and the AV nodes in most individuals, so occlusion will result in conduction abnormalities.
- **Myocardial innervation.** This is likely to form a separate question and also has implications for the transplanted heart as described in the next section.

Myocardial Innervation

Commentary

This sounds straightforward. The oral may include the broad aspects of transplant physiology which are increasingly well recognized given that there are more such patients presenting for non-cardiac surgery; however, just when you think that all is going well, you may be asked about the origin of cardiac pain. This is a deceptively simple question because the neural basis of angina pectoris is more complex than it sounds, and is rarely given much consideration.

Core Information

Innervation
- **Autonomic nervous system:** the innervation of the heart is predominantly auto-nomic. Efferent and afferent fibres originate from the cardiac plexuses, which are aggregations of autonomic nerves and ganglia. The superficial plexus lies below the arch of the aorta in front of the right pulmonary artery, and the deep plexus lies anterior to the bifurcation of the trachea and behind the arch of the aorta.
- **Parasympathetic supply:** this is from branches of the vagus nerves that enter the cardiac plexus. The right vagus innervates the SAN, whereas the left vagus innervates the AVN. There can be some overlap. Vagal efferents supply atrial muscle but innervate the ventricular myocardium only sparsely. Vagal stimulation vasoconstricts the coronary arterial circulation. These effects are mediated via muscarinic receptors.

- **Sympathetic supply:** the sympathetic fibres originate mainly from the upper thoracic spinal cord (segments T_2–T_4) and are distributed through the middle cervical and the stellate (cervicothoracic) ganglia as well as through the first four ganglia of the thoracic sympathetic chain. The fibres pass into the cardiac plexus and thence to the SAN and the cardiac muscle. Ventricular sympathetic innervation is denser than atrial. Sympathetic stimulation dilates coronary arteries via actions on beta-adrenoceptors.

The Physiology of the Transplanted Heart

- **Autonomic denervation:** the transplanted heart loses both sympathetic and parasympathetic efferent and afferent neurons. This leads to a (predictable) alteration in some aspects of cardiac physiology, including the absence of anginal pain.
- **Sympathetic denervation:** despite the lack of a direct neuronal supply, the heart still responds normally to circulating catecholamines. This humoral response is of relatively slow onset and takes some minutes to develop. The response to exogenous catecholamines is similarly delayed.
- **Parasympathetic denervation:** there may be some residual vagal activity associated with the vestigial recipient right atrium which is part of the anastomosis, but this does not extend to the donor atria. Vagal effects are absent, and so drugs which usually have muscarinic actions do not cause bradycardia, and drugs which are vagolytic do not increase the heart rate. In normal individuals, the resting heart rate is governed by vagal tone. In heart transplant patients therefore the rate is higher, commonly around 100 beats per minute.
- **Starling mechanism:** the myocardial response to stress is maintained, with increases in contractility and cardiac output in response to any rise in left ventricular end-diastolic volume (LVEDV). It is important to avoid hypovolaemia in these patients.
- **Other considerations:** a discussion of anaesthetic problems is unlikely to feature at this stage but is summarized briefly here for completeness. Such problems include accelerated graft atherosclerosis owing to chronic rejection; absence of warning symptoms of angina; and immunosuppression by drugs, the commonest of which are corticosteroids (with a wide range of side effects, from myopathy to hyperglycaemia), cyclosporin (with effects on renal and hepatic function) and azathioprine (myelosuppression). Immune reactivity decreases with time, and so dose regimens will be highest in the early months following transplantation.

Supplementary and Clinical Information

Cardiac Pain

- The localization of somatic pain is usually precise, whereas visceral sensations are limited to discomfort (due, for example, to distension) and to pain. There are many fewer visceral sensory fibres than somatic sensory fibres in the dorsal roots, which helps to explain why visceral pain is poorly localized.
- **Origin of cardiac pain:** In a normal heart the oxygen supply can be increased six- to eightfold in response to increased demand, such as during exertion. At the point at which demand exceeds supply there is an accumulation of lactate and other metabolites. Exercise is then limited by fatigue and dyspnoea, but not by cardiac pain. In a patient with coronary artery disease it is common for cardiac pain to precede fatigue.

Why should this be so? A number of substances (which include lactate, potassium, adenosine, prostaglandins and bradykinins) are released from ischaemic areas of the myocardium. It appears that these substances may sensitize sympathetic afferents, in particular those neurons which have a so-called acid-sensing sodium channel. Lactate increases the activity of these channels and enhances their excitability. This increased sensitization is not an acute phenomenon, because systemic lactic acidosis is not associated with chest pain.

- Pain is the only sensation that is evoked from the heart, but it too is more vaguely localized. Sympathetic afferents account for only around 2% of the total number of afferents to the upper thoracic cord. Stimulation of these afferents leads to excitation of spinothalamic tract cells (T_1–T_5) which also receive somatic input from overlying structures. This convergence onto a common pool of spinothalamic tract cells helps account for the classic nature of anginal pain, which is frequently referred to the arm and chest. The convergence is on tracts with afferents from deep (muscle) rather than cutaneous (skin) structures. In addition, vagal afferents transmit nociceptive information to the spinothalamic tract at the level of C_1 and C_2, which explains referred pain in the neck and jaw. This vagal innervation is one of the reasons why not all cases of refractory angina can be treated successfully by sympathetic block.
- Sympathetic afferents from viscera such as the gallbladder and the oesophagus also converge on this pool of spinothalamic tracts; hence the similarity of symptoms that these structures can evoke.
- This discussion is a simplification which does not include other ascending spinal tracts that are involved, and does not entirely account for aspects such as the specific emotional components of cardiac pain. 'Angor animi', for example, which is a profound sense of impending death, is a sensation that is said to be unique to myocardial pain, but one whose neural processing has not been elaborated.

The Intercostal Nerves

Commentary

This area of anatomy was of more direct relevance before thoracic epidural anaesthesia, paravertebral injection and intrapleural catheterization became common analgesic techniques. Intercostal nerve blocks were used to provide analgesia for subcostal surgical incisions and to treat the pain of fractured ribs. The topic, however, continues to be asked, but because the list of indications for intercostal block is shrinking, the oral is likely to focus more on the anatomy and on the distribution of injected drugs than on the (simple) clinical techniques of nerve blockade.

Core Information

- The intercostal nerves are the ventral somatic rami of the spinal nerves from T_1 to T_{11}. T_{12} is a subcostal nerve which is not closely associated with its corresponding rib, and which in addition links with fibres from the first lumbar nerve. T_1, T_2 and, occasionally, T_3 are also atypical, in that some of their fibres join with fibres of the brachial plexus, as well as contributing to the formation of the intercostobrachial nerve.

- The typical intercostal nerve exits the intervertebral foramen to lie initially between the posterior intercostal membrane and the pleura. Thereafter, the nerve lies between the internal and the innermost (intercostalis intimis) intercostal muscles.
- Each nerve lies in the neurovascular bundle comprising the artery, vein and inferiorly the nerve, which runs in a groove beneath each rib. The overhanging external edge of the rib protects this bundle from direct trauma. The groove is also invested in the fascia of the external and internal intercostal muscles.
- The groove is well defined until it reaches the mid-axillary line, at which point the nerve divides.
- Motor filaments supply the intercostal, the transversus thoracis and the serratus posterior muscles. The lower intercostal nerves also supply motor fibres to the abdominal muscles.
- Sensory branches supply the overlying skin as well as supplying the parietal pleura and the costal part of the diaphragm.
- The first sensory branch arises as the posterior cutaneous branch, which supplies the skin and muscles of the paravertebral area.
- The second sensory branch arises as the lateral cutaneous branch after the division of the nerve at around the mid-axillary line. The terminal fibres of this branch supply the skin and subcutaneous tissue of much of the chest and abdominal wall.
- The third and final sensory branch arises as the anterior cutaneous branch which is the continuation of the main intercostal nerve, and which supplies the skin and subcutaneous tissue of the anterior chest and abdominal walls.

Supplementary and Clinical Information

Management of Thoracic Pain and Trauma

- Analgesic options include thoracic epidural anaesthesia (effective, but bilateral in distribution with the generic disadvantages of epidural block), paravertebral block (effective, unilateral, but with potential complications of epidural spread and pneumothorax) and intrapleural block (simple but, according to at least some studies, less effective than the previous two methods). Arguably, intercostal nerve block is also less satisfactory, but none of the other techniques lends themselves as well to a discussion of anatomy.
- **Indications for intercostal nerve block** this can provide effective analgesia for upwards of 12 hours. Historically, it was used for analgesia following subcostal and loin incisions (for gallbladder and renal surgery), after thoracotomy and to provide analgesia for fractured ribs. Only the last indication now applies, and here the technique has been superseded by intrapleural and epidural block. It has been used to alleviate the discomfort of herpes zoster. A block of T_{10}, T_{11} and T_{12} provides effective analgesia following appendicectomy, but it is rarely used for this purpose, possibly because in the UK relatively inexperienced trainees give the majority of anaesthetics for this operation, and because laparoscopic appendicectomy is now routine.

Technique of Intercostal Nerve Blockade

- The intercostal injection is usually made at the angle of the rib, before the nerve divides.
- The skin of the back is tensed gently in a cranial direction before a needle and syringe is advanced to encounter the lower surface of the appropriate rib. The skin tension is then released. This helps the needle to move to its correct position.
- The needle is then carefully walked off the inferior surface, before being directed a further 2–3 mm inwards to pierce the fascia of the innermost intercostal muscle (the posterior intercostal membrane) and enter the subcostal groove.
- Following injection of 3 or 4 ml of solution, for example bupivacaine 0.25–0.5% with adrenaline, the needle is withdrawn to rest on the posterior surface of the rib. The next space can then be located in the same way without risking inadvertent injection in the same space. This can easily happen in individuals even of modest size, and is common in the obese.
- Complications include pneumothorax (incidence of less than 1%), respiratory embarrassment in patients with any diaphragmatic impairment and systemic toxicity if a large number of nerves are blocked. The rich vascular supply to the area means that systemic absorption following intercostal block exceeds that from almost any other site.
- Distribution of local anaesthetic following injection: Contrast studies have confirmed that local anaesthetic spreads not only along the rib but can also track medially as far as the sympathetic chain. It also extends to several dermatomes above and below the site of injection, probably via direct subpleural spread. The intercostal, subpleural and paravertebral spaces are all in anatomical continuity, and so it is not surprising that injection of sufficient volume may lead to spread throughout all three.

The Diaphragm

Commentary

The diaphragm is an important anatomical area for anaesthetists and acts as a radiographic marker for other disease processes. A raised hemidiaphragm, for example, may indicate pulmonary or abdominal pathology, and gas under the diaphragm is pathognomonic of visceral perforation. So even though primary diaphragmatic problems are rare, the examiners will expect you to demonstrate knowledge of the anatomy that allows you to use it as an indicator for these other conditions. The diaphragm is a vital respiratory structure, but its physiological functions are unlikely to figure in any detail in this predominantly anatomical question. However, the oral may be linked to questions about the phrenic nerve. Anatomically, the diaphragm was viewed by the ancient Greeks as a partition between body cavities (it derives from the words for 'across' and 'partition'). Philosophically, however, they believed it to be the organ of thinking, and so also called it the 'phren' (Greek for 'mind'). Hence the derivation of the word 'phrenic'. Here, as elsewhere, this etymological information is probably of more use in a pub quiz than in the final FRCA, but should you get as far as discussing it you will either be doing brilliantly well or will be the victim of a particularly eccentric examiner.

Core Information

The Anatomy of the Diaphragm
- **Diaphragm:** the diaphragm is the dome-shaped muscular and fibrous partition which separates the abdominal from the thoracic viscera.
- **Vertebral part:** this part of the diaphragm originates from the right and left crura, which arise from the front of the vertebral bodies of L_1–L_3 and L_1–L_2, respectively, and from the arcuate ligaments. The median ligament is a fibrous band which links the crura, the medial ligament is a tendinous arch arising as a thickening of the fascia of the psoas major muscle, and the lateral ligament arises as another thickening of fascia, in this case from the quadratus lumborum muscle.
- **Costal part:** this part of the diaphragm arises from the six lowest ribs and their costal cartilages.
- **Sternal part:** this part comprises two small attachments from the xiphisternum.
- **Central tendon:** the muscle fibres converge into the central tendon, which is a tough aponeurosis near the centre of the dome of the diaphragm and which is merged above with the connective tissue of the pericardium.
- **Foramina:** there are three important openings in the diaphragm. Through one foramen at the level of T_8 pass the IVC and some fibres of the right phrenic nerve. Through another aperture at the level of T_{10} pass the oesophagus and vagus nerves. Through the final opening at the level of T_{12} pass the aorta, the thoracic duct and the azygos vein.
- **Motor supply:** motor innervation is supplied solely by the phrenic nerve (mainly derived from C_3, C_4 and C_5) whose long thoracic course reflects the descent of the diaphragm during fetal development.
- **Sensory supply:** the central part of the diaphragm is innervated by the sensory afferents of the phrenic nerve, hence the tendency for subdiaphragmatic pain to be referred to the shoulder tip, which shares the sensory innervation of C_5. The peripheral area of the diaphragm is innervated by the lower intercostal nerves.

The Course of the Phrenic Nerve
- The phrenic nerve arises from the anterior primary ramus, principally of C_4 but with contributions from C_3 and C_5. The nerve is formed from these roots at the upper lateral border of the scalenus anterior muscle, and then descends on the anterior surface of this muscle, behind the prevertebral fascia.
- At the root of the neck it runs in front of the subclavian artery and behind the subclavian vein to enter the thorax. Thereafter, the intrathoracic course of the right and left phrenic nerves is different.
- **Right:** on the right the nerve follows the great veins, passing lateral to the innominate vein, the superior vena cava (SVC), the pericardium overlying the right atrium and the supra-diaphragmatic part of the inferior vena cava (IVC). It penetrates the diaphragm close to the hiatus traversed by the IVC. Some fibres also pass directly through the hiatus.

- **Left:** the course of the left phrenic nerve is longer. After passing between the left subclavian and the left common carotid arteries, the nerve crosses the arch of the aorta, descends anterior to the left hilum of the lung, and continues immediately lateral to the left ventricle before penetrating the diaphragm. On both sides the nerve lies medial to the mediastinal pleura.

Supplementary and Clinical Information

- **Phrenic nerve palsy:** this may be asymptomatic. During quiet breathing, some 75% of respiratory function is diaphragmatic, although when the minute volume is higher, around 60% of the tidal volume is provided by the accessory muscles. It may be found as an incidental finding on a plain chest X-ray which will show a raised hemidiaphragm. (There are other causes, which include pregnancy, ascites, obesity, intra-abdominal malignancy and pulmonary lobar collapse. It may also be iatrogenic.) Fluoroscopy will reveal paradoxical upward movement during inspiration. The phrenic nerve can be paced by stimuli applied where it lies on the scalenus anterior muscle in the neck.
- It is common for the phrenic nerve to be blocked secondarily by local anaesthetic techniques such as interscalene and deep cervical plexus blocks. It may be damaged during surgery, for example, during radical neck dissection, and may also be affected by disease processes, typically metastatic malignant disease of the lung. There are also reports of phrenic nerve palsy complicating long-term central venous catheterization.
- **Spinal cord injury:** cord lesions at the level of C_2 and C_3 cause respiratory tetraplegia. Injuries at C_4 and below permit some phrenic nerve function, but vital capacity is reduced to about 25% of normal. Damage below C_6 allows full diaphragmatic function.
- **Position on chest X-ray:** after forced expiration, the right cupola (which is higher than the left because of the upward pressure of the liver) is level anteriorly with the fourth costal cartilage, and level posteriorly with the eighth rib. During quiet respiration, the diaphragm moves only about 1.5 cm, but this excursion can increase to 10 cm or more with deep inspiration.
- **The cardio-oesophageal sphincter:** the fibres of the crura that surround the cardio-oesophageal junction exert a pinchcock effect on the oesophagus which contributes to the prevention of gastro-oesophageal reflux. Laxity of this oesophageal hiatus is associated with hiatus hernia in which the lower oesophagus and stomach slide into the chest, causing symptoms of dyspepsia and reflux. (This is a sliding hernia; the much less common rolling hernia occurs when the fundus of the stomach rolls up through the hiatus in front of the oesophagus which remains intra-abdominal. Patients have dyspepsia but no reflux.) You should be prepared to detail your management of anaesthesia in a patient with hiatus hernia. This would usually involve a precise clinical history seeking the symptoms and characteristics of oesophageal reflux which, if positive, would mandate rapid sequence induction following administration pre-operatively of agents to reduce gastric acidity.
- **Neuromuscular block:** the diaphragm is amongst the muscles most resistant to muscle relaxants. Postoperative respiration may therefore be adequate even though the patient subjectively may feel profoundly weak.

- **Diaphragmatic hernia:** these may be congenital, occurring in utero (the incidence is 1 in 4,000 live births) and preventing the proper development of the lung, or they may be traumatic. Surgical repair in the neonate requires tertiary paediatric centre expertise, specific details of which you will not be expected to know. Traumatic herniation may be associated with immediate symptoms requiring surgical repair; equally, there are cases in which the abnormality has been diagnosed years after an injury from which the patient has been asymptomatic.

The Liver

Commentary

The liver is an organ of complex metabolic and biosynthetic importance, which means that the clinically orientated parts of the oral could follow one of several routes, examples of which include drug handling, protein synthesis and the anaesthetic implications of impaired liver function. Questions on its basic anatomy are likely to concentrate less on gross anatomy and more on its microstructure. This is not easy. The liver acinus is not a homogenous structure like the glomerulus of the kidney, and the traditional view that was based on the histological appearance of a hepatic lobule has been superseded by the concept of a functional unit. Different parts of the lobule appear to have not only a varied blood supply but also dissimilar metabolic functions. As you are unlikely to have enough time for a coherent discussion of this metabolic zonation, what follows is a simplified account of both the classical and functional anatomy. Because it is complicated it will be enough to describe the basic architecture, particularly if you can also convey that you know this to be an over-simplification. The oral may then move on to the clinical aspects which will be of more interest to you (and the examiner). The following account of liver function is necessarily superficial as it is unlikely to be examined in any depth.

Core Information

The Anatomy of the Liver

- The liver is the largest organ *in* the body, although skin is actually the largest organ *of* the body. Its weight varies with factors such as gender and body habitus, but ranges from 1.0 to 2.5 kg.
- It is divided into right and left lobes, with the right accounting for about 85% of the mass of the whole. It lies directly beneath the diaphragm to fill the right hypochondrium, while its inferior relations include parts of much of the abdominal viscera (including the lesser curve of the stomach, the duodenum, the hepatic flexure of the colon and the right kidney and adrenal gland). It is covered by connective tissue which forms a capsule (Glisson's capsule).
- **Blood supply:** this totals about 1,500 ml min^{-1} (range 1,000–2,000 ml min^{-1} depending on factors such as size) and is derived from two primary sources. These

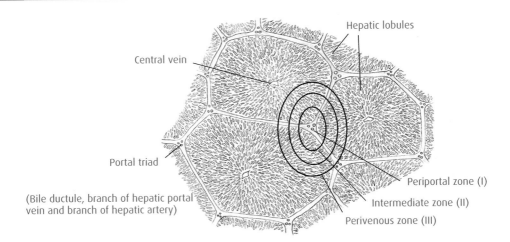

Fig. 2.7 Microscopic anatomy of the liver.

are the **hepatic artery**, which supplies about 30% of the total flow (500 ml min^{-1}), has an oxygen saturation of 98% and accounts for around 50% of total oxygen delivery; and the **portal vein**, which has an oxygen saturation of 60–75% (depending on gastrointestinal metabolic demand), supplies 70% of total flow (1,000 ml min^{-1}) and accounts for the remaining 50% of oxygen delivery.

- **Traditional microscopic architecture (Figure 2.7):** the liver comprises numerous lobules, each approximately 1 mm in diameter and hexagonal in shape. Each lobule contains a central vein, which is a thin-walled venular tributary of the hepatic vein, and from which extend plate-like layers of hepatocytes one cell thick radiating to the borders of the lobule. Between these radiations are sinusoidal blood channels up to 12 μm wide which drain into the central vein and thence via collecting veins to the IVC. At each corner of the lobule is the **portal area** in which lie a branch of the hepatic portal vein, a branch of the hepatic artery, which drains into the sinusoids, and a bile duct (strictly an interlobular bile ductule). These are the **portal triads** (although the portal areas do also contain lymphatics and nerves). The sinusoids are lined by endothelium whose cells include the Kupffer cells, which are mobile phagocytes (although they may have other metabolic functions), and Pitt cells, which are mobile lymphocytes that are active against tumour cells and infective pathogens. Hepatocytes themselves are large polyhedral cells measuring up to 30 × 20 μm.
- **Functional anatomy – Rappaport's acinus (Figure 2.7):** this is a functional unit which consists of more than one lobule and whose central axis is a portal triad. Blood moves from this region towards the centrilobular veins, with a progressive decrease in oxygenation and metabolic activity. This drainage territory is divided into three concentric zones, which are separate functionally, if not anatomically. The **periportal zone (I)** has the highest oxygen saturation. It is also metabolically the most active, containing transaminases which mediate both protein anabolism and catabolism. The **intermediate zone (II)** has similar but diminished functions to those not only of zone I but also of the **perivenous zone (III)**, which has the poorest oxygenation and

which contains perivenous (centrilobular) hepatocytes. These nonetheless have high quantities of cytochromes P450 and are active in drug biotransformation. (You can see that this concept of metabolic zonation is more difficult to encapsulate anatomically, which is why the traditional view is easier to summarize.)

Supplementary and Clinical Information

Liver Functions

- **Drug biotransformation:** the liver metabolizes drugs that reach it via the hepatic and the portal circulations. Phase I reactions, which involve oxidation, reduction and hydrolysis, are catabolic, and, although they render the drug more water-soluble, may create metabolites that are more toxic than the parent compound. Most, but not all phase I reactions involve the P450 mono-oxygenase system (see under 'Cytochrome(s) P450 in Chapter 3) and take place on the smooth endoplasmic reticulum within hepatocytes. Thiopental, for example, is oxidized, while pethidine is metabolized by ester hydrolysis. The P450 system does not degrade ethanol (alcohol), which is metabolized to acetaldehyde by the cytoplasmic enzyme alcohol dehydrogenase. Phase II reactions are anabolic (synthetic) and involve the formation of a conjugate which is more water-soluble than its precursor. A common example is the conjugation of morphine to 3- and 6-glucuronides.
- **Metabolism of nitrogenous compounds:** the liver has a vital role in metabolizing compounds that contain nitrogen, particularly proteins. Proteolysis takes place primarily in the duodenum, and subsequent to hydrolysis small peptides and amino acids by diffusion, facilitated diffusion or active transport, are transferred through enterocytes to the portal circulation. All nitrogen metabolism is based on the recycling of ammonia in its neutral NH_3 or charged ammonium ion NH_4^+ forms. At least 80% of excreted waste nitrogen is in the form of urea produced exclusively in the liver (by the urea cycle). The clinical relevance of this complex metabolic pathway relates to hepatic failure in which detoxification of ammonia is reduced, its peripheral metabolism by skeletal muscle and kidneys (in the glutamine synthetase catalysed formation of glutamine from glutamate) is overwhelmed, and the resultant hyperammonaemia can lead to hepatic encephalopathy. This is defined as a spectrum of neuropsychiatric disturbance secondary to liver dysfunction. Anaesthetists usually encounter these patients in the context of critical care by which point they typically will have grade 3 (somnolence and marked confusion) or grade 4 encephalopathy (coma).
- **Protein synthesis:** the liver produces plasma proteins, amongst the more important of which are albumin, prealbumin and some globulins (α_{1-2}, β but not γ). It synthesizes coagulation factors I (fibrinogen), II (prothrombin), V, VII, IX, X and XI. It also synthesizes antithrombin, protein C and protein S. It produces purine and pyrimidine bases.
- **Carbohydrate metabolism:** the major processes are gluconeogenesis (glucose production from amino acids, lactate and glycerol), glycogenesis (formation of glycogen from glucose) and the converse process of glycogenolysis (formation of glucose from glycogen breakdown).
- **Lipid metabolism:** the liver synthesizes cholesterol as well as high- and low-density lipoproteins. It also produces triglycerides and ketone bodies following partial oxidation of fatty acids.

- **Bile synthesis:** bile emulsifies fats in the gastrointestinal tract and provides a means of eliminating drugs, toxins and other compounds. Hepatic breakdown of haemoglobin produces the bile pigments bilirubin and biliverdin.
- **Storage:** the liver is the major site of storage of a large number of compounds, including vitamins A, B_{12}, D, E and K as well as iron, copper and glycogen.
- **Immunological functions:** Kupffer and Pitt cells are mobile phagocytes that are active against pathogens and tumour cells.
- **Erythropoiesis:** until 32 weeks of gestational age the liver is the primary site of fetal red blood cell production.

You may be asked about the implications of anaesthesia in the jaundiced patient (see under 'Jaundice' in Chapter 3).

- **Implications of jaundice:** these include impaired coagulation; renal failure (hepatorenal syndrome); altered drug metabolism owing to conversion of cytochrome P450 to the inactive P420; hypoproteinaemia may increase the proportion of free active drug; jaundice may be due to an infective disease (hepatitis A, B, C); bradyarrhythmias (owing to high concentrations of bile salts); inaccurate peripheral (and cerebral) oxygen saturation monitoring (the bilirubin absorption coefficient is similar to that of deoxygenated haemoglobin, and so SpO_2 will read artificially low). (See under 'Pulse Oximetry' in Chapter 5).

The Spleen

Commentary
The spleen has a unique anatomical structure and performs a range of functions important enough to make it surprising that humans can survive without it. The clinical aspects of the oral are likely to focus on those functions (much simplified in the following account), the management of splenic injury and the consequences of splenectomy.

Core Information

Gross Anatomy
- The spleen is an irregularly shaped structure around the size of an adult fist which lies mainly in the left hypochondrium. It is sometimes described as being the shape of a shoe but is only around 11–12 cm in craniocaudal length. Its weight in health is around 150 grams. It has a smooth diaphragmatic surface and an irregular and concave visceral surface which contains the hilum.
- The irregular impressions are due to its immediate intimate relations. The superomedial impression is made by the fundus of the stomach, and below it are the impressions made by the upper border of the left kidney, by the tail of the pancreas and inferiorly by the splenic flexure of the colon.
- Posteriorly lies the left hemi-diaphragm, which separates the spleen from the pleura, the left lung and the ninth, tenth and eleventh ribs.

- It is surrounded by peritoneum and is supported by a number of ligaments. The most substantial are the gastro-splenic and the lieno-renal ligaments. The gastro-splenic ligament extends from the hilum to the greater curvature of the stomach and contains the short gastric and the gastro-epiploic vessels, together with sympathetic nerves from the coeliac plexus. The lieno-renal ligament passes from the hilum to the anterior surface of the left kidney and contains the splenic vessels (and the tail of the pancreas).
- **Arterial supply**. It is supplied by the splenic artery (one of the three main branches of the coeliac trunk) through the lieno-renal ligament to the hilum, where it forms numerous terminal branches. Splenic artery aneurysm is uncommon, but occurs more frequently in females, and more than 50% of those that rupture do so either during pregnancy or in parous women.
- **Venous drainage**. The splenic vein forms at the hilum and passes behind the tail of the pancreas to join the superior mesenteric vein and form the portal vein.

Microscopic Anatomy
- Fibroelastic tissue forms the capsule and extends into the body to form trabeculae between which lies the pulp of the spleen. White pulp is formed of lymphatic nodules orientated around an arteriole. Red pulp contains a dense population of mixed cells which include lymphocytes, which readily transform into antibody and immuno-globulin producing plasma cells, together with red blood cells and macrophages. The red pulp contains cords which consist of reticular fibres and fibroblasts but which do not have an endothelium as such, being an open blood system.

Functions of the Spleen
- It is the largest single component of the reticulo-endothelial system with several important functions. **Red cell storage**. Up to 8% are sequestered in the spleen. **Haematopoesis**. This is significant in the fetus but not the adult, except in some cases of myeloid diseases (such as leukaemia and myelosclerosis). **Lymphopoiesis and the immune response**. This function continues through adult life, with transformation of lymphocytes to plasma cells as outlined previously, and the synthesis of opsonins such as properdin (an immunoglobulin that is a component of the alternate complement pathway) and tuftsin (an immunostimulatory tetrapeptide). **Phagocytosis**. In effect the spleen acts as a blood filter, removing ageing red cells (erythrophagocytosis), cells of other types and microorganisms. Platelets are also destroyed in the spleen. The phagocytosis of antigens stimulates cellular and humoral immune responses.

Supplementary and Clinical Information
- **Splenomegaly**. A large number of conditions may give rise to splenomegaly. These include haematological disorders such as idiopathic thrombocytopaenic purpura (ITP), thrombocytopaenic purpura (TTP) and hereditary spherocytosis. In these conditions there is accelerated splenic platelet or erythrocyte consumption. The spleen may enlarge in response to infection (a typical cause in the developed world is infectious mononucleosis; the commonest cause in the developing world is malaria), because of myeloproliferative disorders and lymphomas, and secondary to portal hypertension. An enlarged spleen is more vulnerable to trauma.

- **Hypersplenism**. In this condition the normal functions of the spleen are exaggerated such that it removes normal rather than effete cells. It can sequester temporarily as much as 90% of the circulating platelets and 45% of erythrocytes.
- **Splenectomy**. This is usually indicated in the context of trauma (25% of which is iatrogenic) and for treatment of certain haematological disorders. It may sometimes be necessary because of malignancy in adjacent structures, such as the stomach, whose removal may also involve splenectomy. Splenic trauma is often managed conservatively, but major blunt or penetrating injuries will require surgical intervention. Most elective splenectomies are performed laparoscopically.
- **Sequelae of splenectomy**. Post-procedural sepsis (overwhelming post-splenectomy infection, OPSI) is a potential risk particularly in children, but it can occur at any age. In non-immunised patients, mortality in the first two years is estimated at around 50%. All patients are immunocompromised by splenectomy and should be vaccinated as a minimum against pneumococcal, meningococcal and haemophilus species. This can be done 14 days prior to elective splenectomy or afterwards should it be an emergency. Loss of splenic function (so-called autosplenectomy) can occur in association with a number of diseases, including ulcerative colitis, coeliac disease and sickle cell anaemia.
- **Management of splenic injury**. Treatment ranges from the conservative, through radiographic embolization of splenic vessels, to open splenectomy. The anaesthetic management of a haemodynamically unstable patient is largely generic, and as for any trauma patient with uncontrolled blood loss. One point of which to be aware is the possible tamponade of splenic haemorrhage. This may be relieved when the abdomen is open with further sudden blood loss and instability.

The Blood Supply to the Abdominal Viscera (the Splanchnic Circulation)

Commentary

The splanchnic circulation supplies the abdominal viscera: the small and large gut, the liver, spleen, stomach and pancreas. Clinically, it is the blood supply to the small and large intestine that is of most interest because of the potentially disastrous sequelae of arterial occlusion, ischaemia that is not due to occlusion and reperfusion injury.

Core Information

Arterial Supply to the Viscera
The splanchnic circulation arises from three main branches of the aorta.

- **Coeliac artery**. This is a very short (1.25 cm) vessel which almost immediately branches to form the common hepatic artery, the left gastric artery and splenic artery. These supply the liver, stomach, pancreas, spleen and the upper part of the duodenum.

- **Superior mesenteric artery**. The superior mesenteric artery leaves the aorta 1–2 cm lower than the coeliac, at the level of L_1, and divides almost immediately into five major arteries which supply the lower part of the duodenum, the remainder of the small gut, the ascending colon and the first two-thirds of the transverse colon. (For completeness the branches are the pancreaticoduodenal, the intestinal, the ileocolic, the right and the middle colic arteries.)
- **Inferior mesenteric artery**. The inferior mesenteric artery leaves the abdominal aorta at the level of L_3 to supply the remainder of the colon and the rectum via the left colic artery, the sigmoid branches and the superior rectal artery.

Physiological Characteristics

- The arterial supply is able to adapt to changing requirements by a number of regulatory mechanisms. Under neutral resting conditions it requires around 25% of the cardiac output, but this rises substantially in response to eating. Equally, the arterial supply can more than halve in circumstances in which blood is diverted to other vascular beds or if there is a significant fall in cardiac output with associated hypoperfusion.
- **Regulatory control**. The vascular bed autoregulates so as to maintain splanchnic blood flow and does so both by metabolic and myogenic mechanisms. As in other regional circulations, local accumulated metabolites (including H^+ ions, K^+ and CO_2) are vasodilatory. Vascular smooth muscle will also relax in response to a decrease in transmural tension and will contract if wall tension is high. As elsewhere in the circulation the final mediator of this response is a change in intracellular calcium.
- **Humoral regulators**. Increased blood supply is necessary for digestion, and enhanced mucosal activity results in the production of local vasodilatory metabolites (H^+ ions and CO_2, as described, plus adenosine). Systemic peptide hormones whose levels increase after ingestion of food also have splanchnic vasodilatory actions. These hormones include gastrin, secretin, cholecystokinin and vasoactive intestinal polypeptide (VIP).
- **Autonomic influences**. The sympathetic supply to the gut originates from the coeliac ganglion, the superior mesenteric ganglion and the inferior mesenteric ganglion, and the post-ganglionic fibres tend to accompany the arteries of the same name. Noradrenaline-mediated vasoconstriction allows effective diversion of blood away from the viscera to ensure perfusion of more critical organs such as the brain, heart and kidney in response to trauma, blood loss or sepsis. The parasympathetic supply originates from vagal and pelvic nerves which synapse in the gut wall. Stimulation increases the vegetative functions of the gut with an increase in gastrointestinal secretions and motility. An increase in mucosal blood flow follows vascular smooth muscle relaxation mediated by nitric oxide (NO) which is released after stimulation of endothelial muscarinic receptors.

Supplementary and Clinical Information

- **Gut barrier function**. The most catastrophic manifestation of splanchnic hypoperfusion is infarction of the bowel secondary to acute occlusion by arterial embolus or thrombus. The presentation is rapid and dramatic, with all the features of septic shock, and the prognosis is very poor unless treated with extreme urgency. Otherwise translocation of bacteria following compromise of the gut's natural barrier function is implicated in the systemic inflammatory response syndrome (SIRS) and its potential evolution into the multi-organ dysfunction syndrome (MODS). This can happen following hypoperfusion and ischaemia from causes which include hypovolaemia (blood loss or dehydration) and circulatory failure secondary to low cardiac output states. Restoration of adequate splanchnic blood supply is also associated with a reperfusion syndrome which results in an increase in the permeability of the endothelium and release of inflammatory mediators into the circulation (see under 'Sepsis' in Chapter 3). These mediators may enter the systemic circulation via a route that includes lymphatics in the mesentery which lead to the thoracic duct, the subclavian vein and thence to the lungs. To an extent therefore the liver is bypassed.

- **Abdominal compartment syndrome**. The normal intra-abdominal pressure is between 5–7 mmHg (higher in the obese and in pregnancy), and abnormal elevations may compromise splanchnic blood flow. These may occur as the primary result of intra-abdominal pathology or less commonly may be secondary to extra-abdominal injury. End-stage ascites accumulation may also lead to excess pressures. Luminal collapse and vascular compromise results in bacterial translocation and multi-organ dysfunction. This, in combination with the severity of the predisposing cause, is responsible for the high mortality associated with the condition.

- **Influence of anaesthesia on splanchnic blood flow**. General anaesthetic agents have predominantly vasodilatory effects, but the specific effects on the blood supply to the gut have not clearly been elaborated. Much the same applies to neuraxial anaesthesia in which the likely benefits of sympathetic block may be offset by a fall in mean arterial pressure and splanchnic perfusion. This may better be corrected by vasopressor rather than fluid administration, particularly in the context of major anastomotic bowel surgery. Receptor effects include α_1 vasoconstriction, β_2 vasodilatation and dopamine DA_1 and DA_2 vasodilatation. Therefore, α_1 agonists reduce splanchnic blood flow locally, although they may increase it via their systemic pressor actions. This does not appear to apply to noradrenaline whose effects in this context are minimal. Intermittent positive pressure ventilation (IPPV), particularly with high airway and end-expiratory pressures, reduces venous return and cardiac output, and has both indirect and direct effects on splanchnic perfusion. This may fall both as a result of diminished cardiac output and because of an increase in vascular resistance in the mesenteric and portal circulations. Moderate hypercapnia may result in an increase in perfusion as it does in other vascular beds.

The Coeliac Plexus

Commentary

You will have had little, if any, direct experience of coeliac plexus block. It is no longer a procedure that can be undertaken blind without imaging, and its indications are limited to severe, intractable pain. This question, however, remains a perennial favourite despite the fact that most examiners expect only theoretical knowledge. You will nonetheless need to know the anatomy reasonably well, because even the most sympathetic examiner has no choice but to pursue the topic. There is nowhere else to go, and the 7 or 8 minutes otherwise will seem interminable.

Core Information

- The coeliac plexus is the largest sympathetic plexus and lies anterior to the abdominal aorta where, as a dense network of nerve fibres, it surrounds the root of the coeliac artery at the level of L_1.
- It is a bilateral structure. There are two ganglia, right and left, which are closely related to the crura of the diaphragm.
- The plexus receives the greater splanchnic nerve (fibres from T_5 to T_9 or $_{10}$) and the lesser splanchnic nerve (fibres from $T_{9/10}$ or $T_{10/11}$).
- The plexus also receives some filaments bilaterally both from the vagus and the phrenic nerves.
- Superiorly lie the crura of the diaphragm; posteriorly is the abdominal aorta; laterally are the adrenal glands in the superior poles of left and right kidneys. The important anterior relation is the pancreas.

Supplementary and Clinical Information

Coeliac Plexus Block

- **Diagnostic:** coeliac plexus block using local anaesthetic alone can be used for diagnostic purposes, and for attempting to break a sympathetically mediated acute pain cycle.
- **Therapeutic:** the plexus can be blocked in conjunction with intercostal nerves to provide analgesia for intra-abdominal surgery. This technique does not have many enthusiasts. More commonly it is used for the relief of malignant visceral pain, typically that due to carcinoma of the pancreas. Neurolytic blocks give good analgesia in up to 90% of patients, although the effect may only last for a number of months.
- **Non-malignant pain:** the commonest such condition is chronic pancreatitis. Many clinicians are reluctant to use coeliac plexus block in such patients both because of the risks of paraplegia (1–2 per 1,000 owing to acute ischaemia at the watershed area of the cord) and because its effective duration is limited. Coeliac plexus block for non-malignant visceral pain is also generally less successful, with only around 60–70% of patients reporting good pain relief.

Technique of Coeliac Plexus Block

Your and even the examiner's knowledge may be largely theoretical, and your collective experience may be limited. You are unlikely to be picked up on small details as long as your overall account is plausible and safe. If your examiner does happen to work in chronic pain management they should not allow their specialist knowledge to influence the standard that is expected of you.

- The patient lies prone. The procedure should be done under X-ray control.
- The spinous process of T_{12} forms the apex of a flattened triangle whose base is a line joining the twelfth ribs, and which ends 7–8 cm from the midline.

- A 10–15 cm 20G needle (depending on the size of the patient) is directed medially and rostrally along the lines of this triangle, and towards the lateral border of the body of the first lumbar vertebra.
- When the needle encounters the vertebral body it is withdrawn almost to skin before redirection so that it can be walked off the anterolateral side of the vertebra to advance a further 2–3 cm.
- The diffuse nature of the para-aortic plexus means that 20–25 ml of local anaesthetic will be required on each side. Neurolytic agents should be injected only under X-ray control, after needle placement has been confirmed by contrast media.
- All neurolytic drugs lead to indiscriminate neural destruction. Alcohol (50–100%) is usually preferred to phenol (5–8%) for coeliac plexus block. It can be very painful on injection, but does not cause the vascular injury that is associated with phenol (which is a potential problem for a block such as this, which is para-aortic). Transient intoxication may occur in the elderly.
- The duration of effective action may be limited to 1–6 months. The neuritis that can accompany the regeneration of nerves may be as severe as the original symptoms.
- **Complications:** these include hypotension (it is a sympathetic block); anterior spinal artery syndrome (see under 'The Blood Suppply to the Spinal Cord'); subarachnoid, epidural and intrapsoas injection; intravascular injection (the aorta is very accessible on the left, the inferior vena cava is less vulnerable on the right); retroperitoneal haemorrhage; and visceral puncture. The kidney is the organ that is most vulnerable. The neurolytic agent may also spread unpredictably, causing paresis, paralysis and dysaesthesia.

The Blood Supply to the Spinal Cord

Commentary
The main clinical relevance lies in the potential for catastrophic neurological damage secondary to ischaemia. For most anaesthetists, happily, this is theoretical, but it is of obvious importance for those involved in surgery of the thoracic aorta. Otherwise the required knowledge may perhaps allow you some day to astound colleagues as you alone correctly diagnose an anterior spinal artery syndrome.

Core Information
- The spinal cord is supplied by paired posterior arteries and a single anterior artery, together with a series of smaller feeder radicular arteries.
- The two posterior arteries arise from the posterior inferior cerebellar arteries. These descend to the posterior nerve roots, to which they lie medially, and give off penetrating vessels to the posterior white columns and the rest of the posterior grey columns.
- The anterior spinal artery is a single midline artery, which is formed between the pyramids of the medulla oblongata from terminal branches of the vertebral arteries.

It descends the cord in the midline in the anterior median fissure, giving off numerous circumferential vessels. The central branches of the artery supply up to two-thirds of the cross-sectional area of the cord.

- The anterior and two posterior arteries are fed by a variable number of smaller radicular arteries which approach the spinal cord along both ventral and dorsal nerve roots. These arteries, whose number may vary from about 25 to 40, arise from the spinal branches of the subclavian artery, the aorta and the iliac arteries inferiorly.
- In the cervical and upper thoracic regions, the anterior spinal artery begins with contributions from the vertebrals and then receives feeders from the subclavian, the thyrocostal and the costocervical arteries. From the level of T_4 down to T_9 the feeding branches of the intercostal arteries are relatively small.
- The three main arteries are also supplied by a few of the spinal branches of the vertebral, deep cervical, ascending cervical, posterior intercostal, lumbar and lateral sacral arteries. Only about six or seven of these make any significant contribution to the anterior artery, and a similar number supply the posterior arteries (but not at the same level). These feeding arteries terminate in a series of short lengths which anastomose across the midline from posterior to anterior. The posterior radicular arteries are larger than the anterior.
- The largest of the feeder arteries is the radicularis magna, or anterior radicular artery of Adamkiewicz. This originates from the aorta at a variable level and supplies the low thoracic and lumbar regions of the cord. It enters on the left in 80% of subjects, through any one of the intervertebral foramina between T_8 and L_3. In a small number of patients (around 15%), the artery of Adamkiewicz originates high on the aorta, at the level of T_5, in which event the contribution of iliac tributaries to the lumbar cord enlarges. This renders the conus medullaris vulnerable should there be subsequent damage to this iliac supply, for example, by ligation during pelvic surgery.
- This anatomical arrangement ensures an adequate blood supply across three large and discrete areas of the cord: the cervical, the upper thoracic and the thoracolumbar. There is, however, a much poorer vertical anastomosis between the cervical, thoracic and lumbar areas, and at these watershed zones, particularly at T_4/T_5, the spinal cord is acutely vulnerable to ischaemia.

Supplementary and Clinical Information

Clinical Situations in Which Cord Damage May Arise
- This may occur following profound hypotension from any cause, including subarachnoid and extradural anaesthesia. Spinal cord ischaemic damage has also been associated specifically with hypotension secondary to coeliac plexus block.
- Injury may result from aortic surgery, particularly for repair of aneurysms of the thoracic aorta, although the incidence in elective procedures is now quoted as less than 5%. Risk factors, predictably, are those which worsen ischaemia – in particular, the duration of aortic cross-clamp time, as well as the pre-morbid state of the patient's circulation, the patient's age and the difficulty of the surgical procedure.

Attenuation of Risks to the Cord during Aneurysm Surgery
- Spinal cord function can be monitored using somatosensory evoked potentials (SSEPs) (see under 'Evoked Potentials' in Chapter 5).

- Non-pharmacological methods include hypothermia, the use of shunts and oxygenated bypass circuits and cerebrospinal fluid (CSF) drainage. By analogy with cerebral perfusion pressure (CPP), the mean spinal arterial pressure (MAP) can be increased if CSF pressure is reduced. (CPP = MAP – [CVP + ICP], where CVP is central venous pressure and ICP is intracranial pressure.) Some surgeons have advocated reattachment of intercostal vessels, although others contend that the routine reimplantation of segmental vessels is not supported by evidence.
- Pharmacological interventions include intrathecal vasodilators such as papaverine, systemic calcium channel blockers and the use of oxygen-derived free radical scavengers such as mannitol and n-acetyl cysteine.

Anterior Spinal Artery Syndrome

- This describes the situation in which critical ischaemia of the anterior part of the spinal cord leads to loss of the corticospinal and vestibulospinal tracts, which are motor, and the spinothalamic tracts, which subserve deep touch and pressure sensation. This results in a lesion that is primarily motor below the level of cord damage. Vibration sense, light touch and proprioception are mediated via the posterior columns and these remain undamaged.

The Lumbar Sympathetic Chain

Commentary

The anatomy of this area is not detailed, and so the oral is likely to move on quite quickly to clinical aspects of the subject. Lumbar sympathectomy is a procedure which is undertaken mainly by chronic pain specialists, and you may well not have seen it done. The same may apply to lumbar plexus (psoas compartment) block, which may also arise in discussion. If you are struggling for facts then do not guess; instead, fall back on the anatomy. If you are able to show that you could work out a safe theoretical approach by virtue of your anatomical knowledge, then you are likely to pass the question, even though the practical details may be incomplete.

Core Information

The Anatomy of the Lumbar Sympathetic Chain

- The sympathetic outflow originates in the hypothalamus, medulla and spinal cord as pre-ganglionic myelinated efferents. These exit the cord with the ventral nerve roots of the first thoracic nerve down to the second, third and, in some subjects, the fourth lumbar spinal nerves (T_1–L_{2-4}). These efferents pass via the white rami communicantes to synapse in the sympathetic ganglia of the paravertebral sympathetic trunk, which is closely related to the spinal column throughout its length.
- The lumbar part of the sympathetic trunk lies in a fascial plane on the anterolateral aspect of the vertebral bodies. Posterolaterally is the fascia of the sheath of psoas

major, and anterolaterally is peritoneum. On the left side the anterior relation is the aorta, and on the right it is the inferior vena cava (IVC).

Lumbar Sympathectomy

- **Indications:** the block is performed to improve impaired circulation of the lower limb, the commonest cause of which is peripheral vascular disease. It is also used to treat syndromes in which sympathetically maintained pain is a feature, such as the complex regional pain syndrome, and for phantom limb and other neuropathic pain. It has been used to alleviate renal colic, and to manage chronic urogenital pain.

Supplementary and Clinical Information

Techniques of Lumbar Sympathetic Block

- **Technique:** several techniques have been described. Choose the one with which you are familiar, but if you have never seen this procedure performed then you can cite the account which follows as the 'traditional approach'. The block should always be undertaken with the help of an image intensifier. With the patient in the lateral position and after infiltration of the skin, a 120-mm needle is inserted 8–10 cm from the midline at the lateral margin of the erector spinae muscle and at the level of the L_2 spinous process (the procedure is repeated at L_3 and L_4). The needle is then directed inward and medially at an angle of $45°$ towards the vertebral body. As soon as the needle encounters bone it is partly withdrawn prior to reinsertion at a steeper angle, which will allow the needle (with the bevel facing towards the vertebra) to slide past the vertebral body and through the psoas fascia to lie close to the sympathetic chain. After aspiration checks for blood (the aorta is on the left, the IVC on the right), a small volume of contrast medium is injected. Correct placement is indicated by localized linear spread along the vertebral column. If the needle is lying within the psoas compartment, then the contrast will track away from the vertebral body. Local anaesthetic is then injected, or, if a permanent block is sought, either absolute alcohol or a dilute solution of phenol (5%) can be used.
- **Complications:** these include puncture of the aorta or IVC, inadvertent subarachnoid injection, profound hypotension, genitofemoral nerve neuritis (occurring in 5–10% of patients and presenting as pain in the groin), injury to somatic nerves (1%) and perforation of the intervertebral disc. Some of these complications are associated with mechanical damage caused by the advancing needle, others by the substance that is injected. L_1 genitofemoral neuralgia, for example, is much more common after alcohol has been used. Ureteric strictures have also been reported following the use of alcohol and phenol.

Lumbar Sympathetic Block Contrasted with Lumbar Plexus Block

- The lumbar plexus is formed from the anterior primary rami of the first four lumbar nerves, together with a small contribution from the twelfth thoracic nerve. After emerging from the intervertebral foramina, the nerves lie just within the substance of the psoas major muscle (and within its sheath). The nerves formed by the plexus include the femoral, obturator, iliohypogastric, ilioinguinal, genitofemoral and the lateral cutaneous nerve of the thigh. All except the obturator nerve emerge laterally in the plane between the psoas and quadratus lumborum. The obturator nerve issues medially before descending beneath the iliac vessels.

- **Lumbar plexus block:** this block (sometimes called psoas compartment block) can provide effective analgesia (as well as motor block) to much of the groin and upper leg. It should therefore offer a useful alternative to field block for inguinal herniorrhaphy, and to '3-in-1' blocks for proximal hip surgery (cannulated and dynamic hip screws). The analgesia afforded by the block is rarely dense enough to allow surgery without general anaesthesia, and nerves such as the femoral and obturator can as readily be blocked at more distal sites.

- **Technique:** various approaches have been described. With the patient in the lateral position with the side to be blocked uppermost, a needle is directed perpendicular to the skin to encounter the transverse process of L3. This site is chosen because the process is longer and wider than those of the other lumbar vertebrae. The needle is then walked off superiorly, penetrating first the fascia of quadratus lumborum and then that of the psoas sheath. Some anaesthetists use a nerve stimulator, although because the fibres of the plexus are separated and embedded within the body of the muscle this technique may not always succeed. An alternative is to use a Tuohy epidural needle with a loss-of-resistance device attached. The loss of resistance as the needle penetrates the sheath is not dissimilar to that which occurs when the epidural space is entered. The advantage of this approach is that an epidural catheter can be inserted to provide continuous analgesia. It also allows verification of placement, because an injection of contrast medium will outline the borders of the psoas compartment should the catheter be in the correct place. (Various catheter-over-needle sets are now available.) A single bolus injection may require 20–40 ml of local anaesthetic to achieve a satisfactory block.

The Anterior Abdominal Wall

Commentary
The apparent waning enthusiasm in some units for epidurals for analgesia following abdominal surgery has been matched by increasing enthusiasm for techniques such as rectus sheath and transversus abdominis plane (TAP) blocks. There is overlap with the anatomy and innervation of the inguinal region.

Core Information
- The anterior abdominal wall is not a strictly defined anatomical area, but in effect it is bounded superiorly by the xiphoid process of the sternum and the inferior costal margins, laterally by the mid-axillary line and inferiorly by the inguinal ligaments and the pubic symphysis.
- The three muscle layers of the abdominal wall are the external oblique, the internal oblique and the transversus abdominis. Each is contained within a fascial sheath. Either side of the midline is the muscle layer formed by the paired rectus abdominis muscles (the 'recti').

- The external oblique muscle originates from the middle and lower ribs, and its fibres, as the name suggests, slope obliquely down to the iliac crest. Below that level they form an aponeurosis.
- The internal oblique muscle originates from the iliac crests and from the inguinal ligaments (outer two-thirds) and slopes obliquely upwards towards the midline.
- The transversus abdominis is the innermost muscle of the three with its fibres crossing transversely.
- In the midline are the paired rectus abdominis muscles, separated by the linea alba. The muscles are vertical in orientation, they thicken as they move inferiorly, and are enclosed for the most part within the rectus sheath. Over the lower quarter to one-third of the muscles the posterior layer of the sheath is deficient. The arcuate line at this site is the point at which the posterior aponeurosis of the internal oblique and that of the transversus abdominis merge into part of the rectus sheath anteriorly. Posteriorly the sheath is covered only by the thin transversalis fascia. As an anatomical landmark the arcuate line is located one-third of the way down a line joining the umbilicus and the pubic crest.
- The nerve supply to the abdominal wall consists of the anterior primary rami of the six lower thoracic nerves from T_7 to T_{12} and that of the first lumbar nerve L_1, which supplies skin as well as muscle and the parietal peritoneum. These nerves run in the plane between the internal oblique and the transversus abdominis muscles to pierce the posterior wall of the rectus sheath as anterior cutaneous branches. They supply only the abdominal wall and not the viscera.
- The dermatomal levels are familiar: T_7 innervates skin just inferior to the xiphisternum, and T_{10} supplies the umbilicus. Skin below the umbilicus is innervated by T_{11}, T_{12} and by the ilioinguinal and iliohypogastric nerves, which both originate from L_1.

Supplementary and Clinical Information

Nerve Blocks of the Anterior Abdominal Wall
Transversus Abdominis Plane Block (TAP block)

- The TAP block anaesthetizes the sensory nerves that supply the abdominal wall before they enter the musculature. As the nerves lie within the spacious fascial plane between transversus and internal oblique, the block requires a large volume of local anaesthetic, typically 20 ml.
- The original landmark technique involved identifying the triangle of Petit, which is the area bounded inferiorly by the iliac crest, posteriorly by the latissimus dorsi and anteriorly by the external oblique muscle.
- Having identified the triangle (which is not always easy even in only moderately overweight patients), a short-bevelled block needle (which allows better appreciation of passage through the fascial layers) is advanced perpendicularly to the skin and through the fascia of the external oblique. A second click or pop should be felt as the needle penetrates the fascia of the internal oblique to enter the transversus abdominis plane.
- If bilateral blocks are indicated, care must be taken not to exceed recommended total doses of local anaesthetic.
- The use of ultrasound to perform TAP blocks is becoming routine, and, given the difficulty in reliably identifying the triangle of Petit is the better way of locating the

plane. A probe placed transversely between the iliac crest and the twelfth rib will usually give a view that is accurate enough to allow an in-plane approach.

- **Efficacy**. TAP blocks do not provide analgesia that is as dense or as effective as that provided by thoracic epidurals, but they decrease opioid consumption after abdominal procedures, including caesarean section.
- **Complications**. These are predictable from the anatomical location and include inadvertent intra-peritoneal injection with the risk of visceral puncture. Otherwise the complications are largely generic: intravascular injection, local anaesthetic toxicity and failure.

Rectus Sheath Block

- These blocks can provide useful post-operative analgesia following surgery with midline incisions, by blocking the cutaneous branches of T_9, T_{10} and T_{11} which run in the transversus/internal oblique plane to pierce the posterior wall of rectus abdominis.
- Here too ultrasound has superseded the blind anatomical landmark techniques, not least because in up to 30% of individuals the anterior cutaneous branches of the nerves do not penetrate the posterior rectus sheath; instead, they form proximally to it.
- Standard technique: the entry point of the needle (either a short-bevelled 5 cm needle or a paediatric or 18g Tuohy needle) is inserted about 3 cm from the midline and slightly cephalad of the umbilicus (this may vary according to body habitus). The approach is a right angle to the skin, and the needle is advanced through the anterior rectus sheath and through the muscle as far as the posterior wall. Penetration of the fascial plane should normally be appreciated as a definite click or pop. A bolus technique will usually require the injection of 15–20 ml of local anaesthetic, but there is increasing interest in using catheter techniques which allow continuous post-operative infusion. With bilateral catheters, a typical dosing regimen would be 15 ml h^{-1} of levobupivacaine 0.125% increasing to 20 ml hr^{-1} according to response.
- Complications include intra-peritoneal injection with failure of the block; potential injury to bowel; potential trauma to blood vessels, particularly the inferior epigastric vessels; local anaesthetic toxicity due to the large volumes necessary to fill the posterior compartments.

Ilioinguinal and Iliohypogastric Nerve Blocks

- These are described under 'The Innervation of the Inguinal Region'.

The Innervation of the Inguinal Region

Commentary

This in essence is a straightforward question about field block for inguinal hernia repair based on anatomical knowledge. (If you provide reasonably comprehensive anatomical details it should prevent the oral moving too far away from the core topic).

Core Information

The Nerve Supply to the Inguinal Region

- **Supply:** the skin over the lower abdomen is supplied by the first and second nerves of the lumbar plexus, L_1 and L_2, together with a contribution from the subcostal nerve, T_{12}.
- **Iliohypogastric nerve:** this arises from L_1, emerges from the lateral border of the psoas muscle and passes obliquely behind the kidney to perforate the posterior part of the transversus abdominis muscle above the iliac crest. It lies then between transversus and the internal oblique where it divides. Its anterior cutaneous branch runs forwards between those muscles before passing through the internal oblique about 2 cm medial to the anterior superior iliac spine. It pierces the aponeurosis of the external oblique muscle about 3 cm above the external inguinal ring and supplies sensation to suprapubic skin.
- **Ilioinguinal nerve:** this also arises from L_1, emerging from the lateral border of the psoas muscle and passing below the larger iliohypogastric nerve to perforate the posterior part of the transversus abdominis muscle near the anterior iliac crest. It lies below the internal oblique, before piercing it to traverse the inguinal canal accompanied by the spermatic cord. It exits the external inguinal ring to supply the skin of the upper thigh, the skin over the root of the penis or the mons pubis and the skin of the scrotum or labia.
- **Genitofemoral nerve:** this arises from L_1 and L_2, emerging on the abdominal surface of the psoas muscle opposite the third or fourth lumbar vertebra. It runs down on the body of the psoas muscle, retroperitoneally, and divides above the inguinal ligament into genital and femoral branches. The genital branch enters the inguinal canal via the deep inguinal ring to supply the cremaster muscle and to send some fine terminal branches to innervate scrotal skin. In women, it accompanies the broad ligament and contributes to cutaneous sensation of the mons and labia. The femoral branch passes behind the inguinal ligament to enter the femoral sheath, lateral to the artery, before perforating the sheath and fascia lata anteriorly to supply the skin over the upper femoral triangle.

Supplementary and Clinical Information

Various techniques of local anaesthetic 'field block' for inguinal herniorrhaphy have been described. It is increasingly common for ultrasound guidance to be used, but as always an appreciation of the landmark anatomy will be required.

- Reliable anaesthesia for inguinal hernia repair is not always easy to achieve, and if the operation is done with the patient awake it is common for surgeons to infiltrate considerable volumes of supplemental local anaesthetic. Field block, however, is useful for postoperative analgesia.
- All three nerves need to be blocked, and subsequent infiltration may also be required over the skin incision itself, depending on its extent, and at the internal ring.
- A short-bevelled needle is advanced via a point approximately 2 cm medial and 2 cm caudal to the anterior superior iliac spine. This blunter needle will better appreciate the resistance offered by the external oblique aponeurosis, which is penetrated often

with a definite click. Injection of around 5 ml of local anaesthetic should be sufficient to block the iliohypogastric nerve at this point. If the needle is then advanced through the internal oblique muscle for about 1–2 cm the same volume should block the ilioinguinal nerve which at this point lies below the muscle. The genitofemoral nerve is approached via an injection made from the pubic tubercle and extending fanwise from the midline to the external inguinal ring.

- Alternative techniques include the fanwise injection of large-volume low-concentration solutions in and between the oblique muscles (plus genitofemoral nerve block as described), lumbar plexus, lumbar paravertebral and transverse abdominis plane (TAP) blocks. The latter technique has become increasingly popular.

The Brachial Plexus

Commentary

An understanding of the anatomy of the brachial plexus is the key to successful regional anaesthesia of the upper limb. The anatomy is detailed but is not so complex that it cannot be incorporated into a 7- or 8-minute oral question. It is a clinically important area of anatomy and is asked frequently. It is worth learning a schematic diagram of the plexus because it makes it much easier to explain it to the examiners. As it is a core topic of obvious clinical relevance, it is likely that the pure anatomy part of the question will precede discussion of its clinical aspects.

Core Information

The Brachial Plexus (Figure 2.8)

- The plexus forms in the neck from the anterior primary rami of C_5, C_6, C_7, C_8 and T_1.
- These five roots merge in the posterior triangle of the neck to form three trunks.
- C_5 and C_6 form the upper trunk, C_7 the middle trunk (above the subclavian artery) and C_8 and T_1 form the lower trunk (posterior to the subclavian artery).
- At the lateral border of the first rib the three trunks each divide into anterior and posterior divisions.
- The three posterior divisions form the posterior cord (described according to its relationship with the axillary artery), from which derives the radial nerve (also the axillary, thoracodorsal and upper and lower subscapular nerves).
- The anterior divisions of the upper and middle trunks form the lateral cord, from which derive the median nerve (lateral head) and the musculocutaneous nerve (also the lateral pectoral nerve).
- There are several cutaneous nerves of the upper limb: intercostobrachial (T_2); upper lateral cutaneous of the arm ($C_{5,\,6}$); posterior cutaneous of arm ($C_{5,\,6,\,7,\,8}$); medial cutaneous of arm (C_8, T_1); posterior cutaneous of forearm ($C_{5,\,6,\,7,\,8}$); medial cutaneous of forearm (C_8, T_1); lateral cutaneous of forearm ($C_{5,\,6}$).

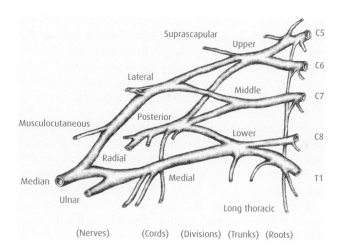

Fig. 2.8 The brachial plexus.

(Nerves)   (Cords)   (Divisions) (Trunks) (Roots)

- The anterior division of the lower trunk continues as the medial cord, from which derive the ulnar nerve and the median nerve (medial head) (also the medial cutaneous nerves of arm and forearm and the medial pectoral nerve).

Supplementary and Clinical Information

Brachial Plexus Block
There are several different approaches. If offered a choice, describe the one with which you are most familiar.

- **Interscalene block**
  - Interscalene local anaesthesia blocks the anterior primary rami of the nerves of C_5–C_8 and T_1 before they merge in the posterior triangle to form the trunks of the brachial plexus.
  - The cervical nerves leave the intervertebral foramina, and pass caudad and laterally between the scalenus anterior and the scalenus medius muscles. The nerves are enclosed within a fascial compartment which comprises the posterior fascia of the anterior scalene muscle and the anterior fascia of the middle scalene muscle.
  - The patient should lie supine with the head turned slightly away from the side of injection and with the arm by the side (gently pulled down if necessary to depress the shoulder).
  - What follows is a description of the landmark technique which for many is becoming obsolete, as ultrasound guidance becomes the norm. As with other techniques to which that applies, however, ultrasound does not absolve the anaesthetist of the need to be familiar with the relevant detailed anatomy.
  - After standard aseptic preparation, the interscalene groove between scalenus anterior and medius should be identified at the level of the cricoid cartilage (C_6).
  - If the awake patient is asked to lift the head off the pillow (which tenses the sternocleidomastoid muscles) or to give a sniff, the groove becomes more evident. In the anaesthetized patient, identification is helped by the fact that in more than 90% of subjects, the external jugular vein overlies the groove at this level.

— The groove and the roots beyond are superficial, and in most cases a stimulating needle no longer than 30 mm is needed. The needle should be held perpendicular to the skin in all planes as it is directed medially, posteriorly and caudally (inwards, backwards and downwards) towards the transverse process of C_6 (Chassaignac's tubercle). This is the approach as described by Winnie. An alternative is Meier's approach, in which the needle is directed caudad down the interscalene groove towards the subclavian artery.

— Once muscle stimulation is apparent in the required distribution (usually shoulder or biceps movements mediated by $C_{5, 6}$), 20 ml of solution may be injected after aspiration and with all due precautions. In common with most plexus blocks into fascial compartments, large volumes of appropriately dilute solutions may be needed to obtain adequate analgesia of all the nerves involved. Typically, an interscalene block will last for 12–16 hours. The addition of dexamethasone to the local anaesthetic solution will prolong the duration of analgesia, but the same applies if the drug is given intravenously. This may be a better option in view of the fact that dexamethasone is neurotoxic.

— Historically, the plexus was identified using a peripheral nerve stimulator alone, but ultrasound-guided location is now commonplace, if not essential.

— Using ultrasound, the needle can be advanced out-of-plane using the approach as described earlier. This may seem contrary to the abiding principle of ultrasound-assisted nerve blockade, which is the ability to see exactly the position of the needle tip, but it has two advantages. One is the fact that the plexus is very superficial at this point and is frequently located at less than a centimetre from the skin. The second is that it removes the risk of damage to the dorsal scapular (from C_5) and long thoracic nerves ($C_{5, 6, 7}$) which are potentially vulnerable using the in-plane approach and which can be hard to identify on ultrasound. Damage to one or other of these nerves can lead to disabling motor weakness and a winged scapula. This problem can be avoided by using a nerve stimulator with the current set at 0.2–0.3 mA. This will be enough to stimulate movement of the scapula should the needle be too close to one or other of those nerves.

— Interscalene block is indicated particularly for shoulder surgery. It can be used to provide analgesia for more distal structures in the upper limb, but it does not provide reliable block of C_8 and T_1, and so ulnar sparing is frequent (some reports quote 30–40%). It does not block the C_4, nerve root and so if lower port sites are used for arthroscopic work then analgesia may not be sufficient. The acromioclavicular joint and the clavicle also have innervation from C_4, and so superficial cervical block and/or supplemental infiltration will be necessary.

— Successful analgesia is almost invariably associated with block of the phrenic nerve which lies on scalenus anterior. The block therefore should be used cautiously in patients with respiratory disease because it may reduce the functional residual capacity by up to 30%. The accompanying diaphragmatic palsy is usually asymptomatic, but the occasional patient may complain of chest discomfort (rather than dyspnea) as a result. Given the potential respiratory embarrassment, bilateral blocks should not be performed.

— **Complications:** these include intravascular injection (particularly into the vertebral artery; central spread via inadvertent dural puncture leading to a total spinal;

phrenic nerve palsy [90%]; Horner's syndrome [cervical sympathetic block, which is usually innocuous (20%)]; vagal and recurrent laryngeal nerve block, which may cause hoarseness [15%] but is usually benign; and pneumothorax [rare]). (There are also the generic complications such as systemic toxicity and neurapraxia.)

- **Supraclavicular block**
  - This block provides analgesia for most of the upper limb, and has been described as the 'spinal' of the arm. It can also be used for shoulder surgery, although the interscalene approach is usually preferred.
  - The three trunks lie on the first rib, between the insertion of the scalenus anterior and scalenus medius muscles, and immediately posterior to the subclavian artery (the pulsations of which can provide a landmark).
  - The trunks cross the rib at about the midpoint of the clavicle before separating into anterior and posterior divisions.
  - The use of ultrasound has superseded the various landmark techniques (most of which directed the needle down on to the first rib to contact the brachial plexus where it lies cephaloposterior to the subclavian artery). The in-plane approach allows clear identification of the first rib, the underlying pleura and lung, the subclavian artery and the adjacent divisions of the plexus which typically lie superolateral to the vessel.
  - With accurate localization, 20 ml of appropriate local anaesthetic solution (such as levobupivacaine 0.25–0.5%) may be injected after aspiration and with the usual precautions.
  - **Complications:** these include pneumothorax with the landmark technique (the incidence may be 0.5–1.0% even in experienced hands, and may take up to 24 hours to develop), although the use of ultrasound is likely, although not yet proven, to reduce this figure; intravascular injection or puncture (subclavian artery or vein), phrenic nerve palsy (in 40–60%); Horner's syndrome in 70–90% (cervical sympathetic block); and neuritis (plus generic complications as discussed previously).
- **Subclavian perivascular or vertical infraclavicular block** (Several variations have been described.)
  - In effect this is an approach to the axillary sheath from a proximal direction, although the block provides analgesia similar to that offered by the supraclavicular approach. The subclavian perivascular block is actually made through a needle inserted above the clavicle. The brachial plexus at this level is deeper, the angle of approach is steeper, and needle repositioning is usually required to ensure that the local anaesthetic surrounds the axillary artery.
- **Axillary block**
  - This has fewer complications than other approaches, is generally effective and remains a popular technique with some anaesthetists.
  - The block provides good analgesia for surgery below the elbow. The musculocutaneous nerve may leave the axillary sheath proximal to the site of injection, in which event supplemental analgesia may be needed by blocking the nerve between brachioradialis and the lateral epicondyle at the elbow. This nerve innervates a substantial part of the radial side of the forearm, and so local anaesthetic sparing of this area is not purely academic.

— The arm is abducted to 90° (hyperabduction may abolish the arterial pulsation). The advancing needle is directed at an angle of about 45° to the skin as far proximally as possible. In practice, this often means injecting at the lateral border of pectoralis major.

— Axillary block is now usually performed with ultrasound guidance, with or without the use of a peripheral nerve stimulator. It takes just over 40 ml of solution to fill the axillary sheath as far as the coracoid process in adults, and, in theory, complete block of all three cords will follow circumferential spread round the sheath. Some anaesthetists prefer to identify the major nerves of the upper limb separately, and block each one in turn. This reduces the total dose of local anaesthetic.

— Historically, an alternative approach used axillary arterial puncture as an end point. Following transfixion of the vessel, the needle was either advanced or withdrawn until aspiration is negative. This technique is obsolete where ultrasound and nerve stimulation are available.

— Axillary brachial plexus block does not provide dense analgesia of the upper arm and does not block the intercostobrachial nerve (which arises from T_2 and T_3 and supplies the skin of the posterior upper arm). Patients may therefore be unable to tolerate the arterial tourniquet.

— Cadaver studies have suggested that the connective tissue of the sheath can form septae between the parts of the plexus, effectively forming a fascial compartment for each nerve and thus limiting the circumferential, but not the longitudinal, spread of injected local anaesthetic. This may explain patchy and incomplete blocks (while providing a useful excuse for their failure).

The Ulnar Nerve

Commentary

You may well not get a full question on this single nerve; indications for isolated ulnar block are restricted (for example to dermofasciectomy of the fifth finger), and so it might be linked to a discussion of the radial and median nerves. Other clinical aspects could include its vulnerability to damage during general anaesthesia and the clinical features of injury.

Core Information

• The ulnar nerve arises from the brachial plexus. The anterior division of the lower trunk continues as the medial cord, from which derives the ulnar nerve. Its fibres originate mainly from C_8 and T_1, although it may also receive a contribution from C_7.

• It passes through the extensor compartment of the upper arm, lying medial to the axillary and brachial arteries. It then continues medially on the anterior aspect of the medial head of triceps to pass beneath the medial epicondyle of the humerus, where it lies in the ulnar groove.

- It enters the forearm between the two heads of flexor carpi ulnaris. In the upper part of the forearm, it lies deep to this muscle and separated from the ulnar artery. In the distal forearm, it lies lateral to flexor carpi ulnaris and near to the medial side of the artery.
- About 5 cm above the wrist, it gives off a dorsal branch before continuing into the hand lateral to the pisiform bone and above the flexor retinaculum.
- The ulnar nerve provides the motor supply to flexor carpi ulnaris, to the medial part of flexor digitorum profundus and to the hypothenar muscles. It also supplies all the small muscles of the hand apart from the lateral two lumbricals and the three muscles of the thenar eminence (abductor pollicis brevis, opponens pollicis and part of flexor pollicis brevis). It innervates the deep head of flexor pollicis.
- It supplies sensation to the elbow joint but gives off no branches in the upper arm. It supplies the skin over the hypothenar eminence and over the fifth finger as well as over the medial part of the fourth finger.

Supplementary and Clinical Information

Indications for Ulnar Nerve Block

- Ulnar nerve block provides analgesia for procedures on the medial (ulnar) side of the hand and forearm. The nerve supplies sensation to a relatively small area. Digital nerve blocks ('ring' blocks) are an easy and reliable method of providing anaesthesia for finger surgery, and so ulnar block is usually reserved for more proximal operations such as palmar fasciectomy. It would be used in isolation only for disease that was restricted to the fifth finger and so is commonly performed jointly with blocks of the other major nerves of the arm.

Ulnar Nerve Blockade

- **At the brachial plexus (for example by supraclavicular or axillary block).**
- **At mid-humeral level:** a line is drawn between the upper border of pectoralis major in the axilla and the mid-point of the flexor crease of the elbow. A parallel line is drawn along the middle of the humerus about 1 cm medial to it, and, via a single injection point at this mid-point, all three major nerves of the forearm can be reached with a 50-mm stimulator needle. The ulnar nerve is below and medial to the brachial artery and superficial to the triceps muscle.
- **At the elbow:** the nerve can be blocked with about 5 ml of solution injected 2–3 cm proximal to the ulnar groove. Injection into the actual fibrous sheath at the elbow is associated with a higher incidence of residual neuritis.
- **In the mid-forearm:** using ultrasound guidance the nerve can be blocked with about 5 ml of solution injected immediately medial to the ulnar artery. More proximally the artery and nerve are more widely separated.
- **At the wrist:** the nerve lies beneath the tendon of flexor carpi ulnaris, proximal to the pisiform bone and medial and deep to the ulnar artery. An approach from the ulnar side of the tendon (3–5 ml of solution injected at a depth of around 1.5 cm) is less likely to encounter the artery, and will also block the cutaneous branches.

Ulnar Nerve Damage and Its Clinical Signs

- **Damage:** even when the arm is lying in the neutral position by the side of the anaesthetized patient, it is vulnerable to pressure, either from arm supports or from the table. It has become routine practice to protect the elbow with padding, and it has also become routine to blame anaesthesia for any ulnar nerve damage. This is despite the fact that ulnar nerve palsy has been reported even when every precaution has been taken. The nerve is also vulnerable to stretch, and so the upper arm should not be displaced posteriorly, nor abducted to greater than 90°.

- **Symptoms and signs of injury:** apart from the sensory loss and paraesthesia of which the patient will complain, ulnar nerve injury is associated with the classic 'main en griffe', or 'claw hand'. This is because the extensors of the fingers and the long flexors of the hand act unopposed. If the nerve is transected at the elbow the clawing is less marked. This so-called ulnar paradox occurs because the flexor digitorum profundus is also paralyzed.

The Radial Nerve

Commentary

The radial nerve is another of the three main nerves of the upper limb, and comprises another well-defined area of anatomy. Upper limb surgery and surgery following trauma is common, and radial nerve block is a reliable means of producing useful analgesia. The nerve has a relatively large number of terminal branches whose detailed anatomy should be beyond the scope of this oral, but you will need to know the effects of blocking the radial nerve proximal to its main divisions. Again, you may find that the questioning incorporates the other two main nerves of the upper limb.

Core Information

The Anatomy of the Radial Nerve

- The radial nerve arises from the brachial plexus. The posterior divisions from each of the three trunks form the posterior cord (described according to its relationship with the axillary artery), from which derives the radial nerve. Its fibres therefore originate from C_5, C_6, C_7, C_8 and T_1, and it is the largest branch of the brachial plexus.
- The radial nerve descends beneath the axillary artery and passes between the long and medial heads of the triceps muscle into the posterior compartment of the arm. It then passes obliquely behind the humerus where it lies in a shallow spiral groove.
- In the lower third of the humerus, the radial nerve enters the anterior compartment of the upper arm, descending into the forearm between brachialis medially and brachioradialis laterally. At the lateral epicondyle of the humerus, it divides into its terminal deep and superficial branches.
- It is motor in the upper arm to triceps and in the lower arm to brachialis, brachioradialis and to the extensor muscles of the wrist and hand.

- The area of sensory innervation that is of particular anaesthetic relevance includes much of the dorsum of the hand and part of the radial side of the forearm. (The ulnar nerve supplies the skin over the distal phalanges, the fifth finger and medial side of the fourth finger, and over the fifth and fourth metacarpals.) The radial nerve also supplies cutaneous sensation to the posterior aspect of the forearm and to the skin over the dorsal base of the thumb. (The musculocutaneous nerve supplies much of the radial surface of the forearm.)

Indications for Radial Nerve Blockade

- Its main use is in conjunction with other blocks to provide analgesia for procedures on the lateral, radial side of the hand and forearm. Digital nerve blocks provide reliable anaesthesia for finger surgery, but radial block can be used for procedures on the base of the thumb and, in combination with musculocutaneous block, to allow the creation of forearm arteriovenous fistulas for dialysis.

Supplementary and Clinical Information

Radial Nerve Blockade

- **At the brachial plexus: (for example by supraclavicular or axillary block).**
- **At mid-humeral level:** via the single injection point at this mid-point the nerve can be located below and medial to the brachial artery where it lies on the posterior surface of the humerus in the spiral groove.
- **At the elbow:** the nerve can be blocked as it traverses the anterior aspect of the lateral epicondyle of the humerus. The needle is inserted some 2 cm lateral to the biceps tendon and directed towards the bone. Up to 10 ml of solution can be injected in a fanwise direction as the needle is withdrawn. The musculocutaneous nerve can also be blocked at the elbow between the biceps and brachioradialis muscles.
- **At the wrist:** nerve block at the wrist is effectively a superficial field block of the terminal sensory branches. Local anaesthetic solution can be injected along the lateral border of the radial artery, extending dorsally to include the area delineated by the extensor tendons of the thumb.

Radial Nerve Damage and Its Clinical Signs

- **Damage:** the radial nerve is subject to various types of injury and may be damaged by compression against the upper humerus, as in the so-called Saturday night or crutch palsy. The pressure exerted by an arterial tourniquet can also damage the nerve by the same mechanism. Its close relation to the humerus makes it vulnerable to damage in mid-humeral fractures, and the posterior interosseous branch may be traumatized in injuries to the head of the radius.
- **Symptoms and signs of injury:** overlap of innervation means that sensory loss and paraesthesia may be confined to a relatively small area on the dorsum of the hand. Otherwise radial nerve injury is typically associated with wrist drop due to paralysis of the extensor muscles. If the damage to the nerve has occurred below the elbow, then the functional preservation of extensor carpi radialis longus will minimize this effect.

The Median Nerve

Commentary

This is the third of the main nerves of the upper limb, and is another well-defined area of anatomy. As with the questions on the ulnar and radial nerves, you will be expected to outline the anatomy and to discuss the relevant local anaesthetic blocks. The oral is likely to include questions on the other nerves of the upper limb.

Core Information

The Anatomy of the Median Nerve

- The median nerve arises from the brachial plexus. The anterior divisions of the upper and middle trunks form the lateral cord, from which derives the lateral head of the median nerve.
- The anterior division of the lower trunk continues as the medial cord, from which derives the medial head of the median nerve. Its fibres originate therefore from C_5, C_6, C_7, C_8 and T_1.
- The nerve passes into the arm lying lateral to the brachial artery, which it then crosses to descend on its medial side to the antecubital fossa, where it is protected by the bicipital aponeurosis.
- It passes down into the forearm between the bellies of the deep and superficial flexors of the fingers (flexor digitorum profundus and superficialis) and at the wrist lies lateral to or just beneath the tendon of palmaris longus, and medial to flexor carpi radialis.
- It enters the hand beneath the flexor retinaculum before dividing into a leash of terminal branches.
- It is motor in the forearm to several of the superficial flexors (excluding flexor carpi ulnaris) and in the hand to muscles of the thenar eminence: abductor pollicis brevis, part of flexor pollicis brevis and the opponens pollicis. Its anterior interosseous branch also supplies flexor pollicis longus, pronator quadratus and part of flexor digitorum profundus.
- The cutaneous innervation extends to the radial aspect of the palm, and the palmar surface of the radial 3½ digits, together with their dorsal tips as far as the first interphalangeal joint.

Indications for Median Nerve Blockade

- Its main use is the provision of analgesia for procedures on the radial palm. The fingers and distal thumb can readily be anaesthetized using digital nerve blocks, but median nerve block is useful for procedures such as carpal tunnel release and palmar fasciectomy.

Supplementary and Clinical Information

Median Nerve Blockade

- **At the brachial plexus: (for example by supraclavicular or axillary block).**

- **At mid-humeral level:** Via the single injection point at the mid-point, the nerve lies above the brachial artery with which it runs parallel.
- **At the elbow:** the nerve can be blocked immediately medial to the brachial artery as it crosses the intercondylar line. The needle is directed perpendicularly and should find the nerve within 1–2 cm.
- **In the mid-forearm:** using ultrasound guidance, the nerve can be traced upwards from its position on the volar surface of the wrist. It lies between flexor digitorum profundus and flexor digitorum superficialis and is usually medial and deep to the radial artery from which it is 1–2 cm distant.
- **At the wrist:** the nerve lies in the midline on the radial border of the palmaris longus tendon. The needle is directed perpendicularly some 2 cm proximal to the distal flexor crease of the wrist. The nerve is superficial and lies beneath the deep fascia at a depth of 1 cm or less.

Median Nerve Damage and Its Clinical Signs
- **Damage:** the median nerve is most vulnerable to trauma at the wrist, although it can be injured in supracondylar humeral fractures and following injury to the distal radius. The commonest lesion occurs as a result of compression of the nerve in the carpal tunnel.
- **Symptoms and signs of injury:** trauma at the wrist will paralyze the thenar muscles and cause significant sensory loss. More proximal injury leads to weak wrist flexion, loss of pronation, and loss of flexion of the thumb, index and middle finger. Atrophic changes and wasting of the thenar eminence flatten the contours of the hand.

The Antecubital Fossa

Commentary
In common with the femoral triangle, the anatomy of the antecubital fossa is straight-forward, and it too lends itself readily to simple diagrams which are worth practising. Alternatively, you may find yourself automatically demonstrating on your own arm. This can be an effective technique which may make the anatomy easier to learn. Questioning may extend to practical clinical matters such as inadvertent intra-arterial injection, nerve blocks at the elbow and the insertion of long lines. Non-medical personnel who undergo training in venepuncture and cannulation are required to learn the detailed anatomy of this area, and so the FRCA examiners will expect at least as much.

Core Information

The anatomy (Figure 2.9).
- The antecubital, or cubital, fossa is a triangular intermuscular depression on the anterior surface of the elbow joint.
- The base of the triangle is formed by the line which joins the medial and lateral epicondyles of the humerus.

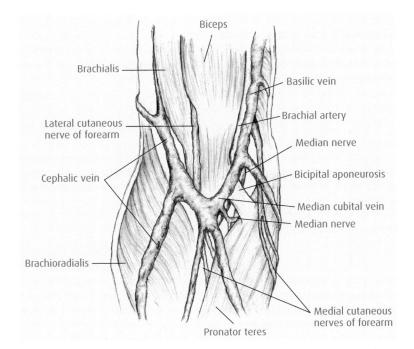

Fig. 2.9 The antecubital fossa.

- The lateral side of the triangle is formed by the medial edge of the brachioradialis muscle, while the medial side is formed by the lateral border of the pronator teres.
- The floor consists of the brachialis and supinator muscles.
- The roof (from above down) comprises skin, subcutaneous tissue and the deep fascia, which includes the bicipital aponeurosis.
- Within the fossa lie the tendon of the biceps muscle and the terminal part of the brachial artery, which lies in the centre of the fossa prior to its division into the radial and ulnar arteries opposite the neck of the radius. It also contains the associated veins and the median and radial nerves.
- The anatomy of the superficial veins varies greatly, but that of a typical subject can be described as follows.
  — **Cephalic vein:** this drains the radial side of the forearm, and ascends over the lateral side of the fossa to lie in a groove along the lateral edge of the biceps. At the lower border of pectoralis major it moves deeper to lie between pectoralis major and deltoid before penetrating the clavipectoral fascia to join the axillary vein.
  — **Basilic vein:** this drains the ulnar side of the forearm and rises along the medial border of biceps to pierce the deep fascia in the middle upper arm before going on to form the axillary vein.
  — **Median cubital vein:** this originates from the cephalic vein distal to the lateral epicondyle, and then runs upwards and medially across the antecubital fossa to join the basilic vein above the elbow.

Supplementary and Clinical Information

- The antecubital fossa is the commonest site for venepuncture as well as being a site for venous cannulation. One potential hazard is inadvertent puncture or injection into the brachial artery. The danger of this happening is lessened by the presence of the bicipital aponeurosis, which is an extension of the medial lower border of the muscle and tendon of biceps. It passes downwards and medially to merge with the deep fascia at the origin of the forearm flexor muscles, separating as it does so the brachial artery from the median cubital vein. (This is the reason why historically it was known as the 'grâce à Dieu' – 'by the grace of God' – fascia.)
- The lateral cutaneous nerve of the forearm crosses the fascia of the roof of the fossa and, although it lies deep to the cephalic vein, may still be vulnerable to damage from a needle or cannula.
- Long lines can be inserted via the antecubital veins, which offer a safer route to the central veins. Although cannulation at the elbow may be simple, the acute curve at the clavipectoral fascia may prevent a long venous catheter from gaining access to the central venous circulation. The length of the catheter precludes the rapid infusion of fluid.
- Inadvertent intra-arterial injection is detailed in the next section. An anomalous ulnar artery which lies superficially just below the median cubital vein is present in 2% of the population, and so it is not only accidental injection into the brachial artery of which anaesthetists must be aware.
- Nerve blocks at the elbow are described in the previous accounts of the ulnar, median and radial nerves.

The Arterial Supply of the Hand

Commentary

This is a straightforward area of anatomy. The topic is not large and so you may exhaust it quickly. The questioning may include topics such as the modified Allen test, the indications for direct intra-arterial blood pressure monitoring and problems associated with intra-arterial injection and their management.

Core Information

Basic anatomy of the arterial supply: the hand is supplied by the radial and ulnar arteries.

- **Radial artery:** in the distal forearm the radial artery lies between the flexor carpi radialis and brachioradialis. The tendons of these muscles comprise the landmarks between which the artery is palpated at the wrist.
  - Beyond the radial pulse the artery supplies a branch which contributes to the superficial palmar arch.
  - The main arterial branch continues over the scaphoid and beneath the extensor and abductor tendons of the thumb (extensor pollicis longus and brevis, and

abductor pollicis longus), and passes between the first and second metacarpal bones to contribute to the deep palmar arch.

- **Ulnar artery:** in the distal forearm the ulnar artery lies superficially between the tendons of flexor carpi ulnaris and flexor digitorum superficialis.
  — It crosses beneath the flexor retinaculum to complete the superficial palmar arch. The ulnar arterial component is much more significant than the radial.
  — The deep branch enters the palm where it forms an anastomosis with the radial artery to complete the deep palmar arch.
  — The superficial palmar arch then gives off further branches including dorsal metacarpal and dorsal digital arteries. The deep palmar arch similarly branches to form palmar metacarpal and palmar digital arteries.

Indications for Direct Intra-Arterial Monitoring

- **Indications:** intra-arterial monitoring gives beat-to-beat information about the blood pressure, which is particularly useful in patients with actual or potential cardiovascular instability. Many anaesthetists would also regard its use as mandatory whenever intravenous vasoactive drugs, particularly hypotensive agents, are used to manipulate the blood pressure. It is useful in patients in whom regular arterial blood gas analysis is indicated, and it is used routinely in the critically ill and the critically hypovolaemic. It may also be indicated in patients in whom anatomical factors such as morbid obesity make it impossible to measure blood pressure by any other means.

Clinical Tests for Arterial Patency

- **Modified Allen test:** both the radial and ulnar arteries can be cannulated to allow direct intra-arterial measurement of blood pressure, but anaesthetists prefer reassurance that the circulation of the hand will not be jeopardized. The traditional method for assessing the adequacy of radial or ulnar arterial flow is the modified Allen test. After compression of both arteries at the wrist, the patient is asked to blanch the palm by clenching and then opening the hand. On releasing the compression of one or other of the arteries, depending on which is chosen as the site of cannulation, the palm should reperfuse, demonstrating thereby the adequacy of flow. Seven seconds or less is considered normal; longer than 15 seconds is abnormal. Although the test continues to be used widely, it has a poor predictive value. Ischaemic complications have been reported following a normal Allen test and vice versa.

Supplementary and Clinical Information

- **Intra-arterial injection:** this may occur when an intra-arterial catheter is mistaken for a venous cannula, when there is anomalous vascular anatomy such as an aberrant radial artery that can be mistaken for the cephalic vein at the wrist or when the arterial pulsation is so feeble in a hypotensive patient that the vessel is thought to be a vein. Drugs that have been so injected include phenytoin, benzodiazepines, anaesthetic induction agents and antibiotics. In the awake patient, severe pain in the hand is a cardinal feature. In the anaesthetized or sedated patient, there may be ischaemic colour changes in the distal limb which, because of arterial spasm, may be pale, mottled or cyanosed. Thrombosis may follow. The degree of damage depends on the substance injected. Thiopental causes substantial damage because at body pH it precipitates into crystals which occlude small arterial vessels and provoke intense vasospasm mediated via local noradrenaline release. In contrast, propofol does not cause the same problems and is relatively innocuous in comparison. Any such injection, however, should be treated as for the worst-case scenario, because clinical experience of intra-arterial injection of many drugs is limited.

- **Management:** arterial thrombosis and extremity ischaemia puts tissue at risk of necrosis, and so anti-coagulation is an important priority. Intravenous heparin 500–1,000 units would be a typical initial dose, following which warm NaCl 0.9% can be infused in an attempt to dilute whatever substance has been injected into the artery. Arterial spasm can be treated with papaverine 40–80 mg, prostacyclin at a rate of 1 μg min^{-1}, tolazoline (which is a noradrenaline antagonist) and phenoxybenzamine (which is an α_1-antagonist). Thromboxane inhibitors, of which aspirin is the simplest example, have also been used. Sound though the recommendation may be, these drugs might well not be immediately available, and this advice may be impractical. Dexamethasone 8 mg given immediately may reduce arterial oedema. Perfusion can be enhanced by sympatholysis, either by a stellate ganglion block (which is quick to perform) or via a brachial plexus block using a catheter technique to provide continuous analgesia. Maintenance anticoagulation is recommended for up to 14 days, and hyperbaric oxygen has also been suggested as a means of minimizing final ischaemic damage.
- **Direct intra-arterial monitoring:** see under 'Intra-Arterial Blood Pressure Measurement' in Chapter 5.

Anatomy Relevant to Subarachnoid (Spinal) Anaesthesia

Commentary

Every candidate for this exam will have performed spinal anaesthesia. It is the default technique for obstetric anaesthesia and is widely used in orthopaedic surgery, both in hip fracture fixation and as part of an enhanced recovery protocol for lower limb joint arthroplasty. Together with epidural analgesia it is a central area of anaesthetic practice. Ignorance of its main aspects can potentially put patients at grave harm, and so you will be expected to demonstrate that your knowledge is sound.

Core Information

Anatomy of the subarachnoid space

Just as with the epidural space, this is an area of such obvious clinical importance that the examiner will not feel the need to introduce it in any other way.

- The **subarachnoid space** is defined by its relation to the arachnoid mater, which is one of the three meningeal layers.
- **Meningeal layers:** there is continuity between the cranial and spinal meninges. The spinal subarachnoid space communicates freely with the ventricular system of the brain.
- **Dura mater:** this is the strongest of the meningeal coverings and consists of fibroelastic connective tissue. The cranial dura has two layers: an outer endosteal layer which lines the skull, and a meningeal layer which invests the brain. These two layers are closely applied, except where they separate to accommodate the large venous sinuses. At the spinal level, the endosteal layer continues down the vertebral canal as a lining of periosteum. The inner layer continues downwards as the spinal dura. The width of the dura varies with the spinal level; in the lumbar region it is said to be between 0.3 and 0.5 mm thick (the data are largely historical and based on small numbers of cadaver studies), and it becomes progressively thicker towards the cervical region. The dura thickens with age. The spinal dura also provides a cuff for nerve roots, which thins as each nerve approaches the intervertebral foramen. In some subjects this cuff is a more substantial structure, containing cerebrospinal fluid (CSF) which does not communicate with intrathecal CSF. These structures are known as Tarlov's cysts and may (rarely) explain the apparently impeccable spinal which then completely fails to work. It is usually not possible to inject into these structures.
- **Arachnoid mater:** this is a fine non-vascular membrane, which is closely applied to the dura. The subdural space between these two layers is a potential capillary space, containing a small amount of lubricant serous fluid. It is widest in the cervical region and, laterally, adjacent to the nerve roots themselves.
- **Pia mater:** this is a fine vascular membrane which invests the spinal cord. Its lateral projections form the denticulate ligament, which attaches to the dura and supports the cord. The filum terminale is the terminal extension of the pia mater which runs from the end of the spinal cord to attach to coccygeal periosteum. It is not purely vestigial; it stabilizes and anchors the cord within the CSF and tethers the dura within the lower part of the epidural space. The filum contains neither neural tissue nor CSF.
- **Subarachnoid space:** this contains CSF, and the anterior and posterior roots of the 31 pairs of spinal nerves. The subarachnoid space extends laterally as far as the dorsal root ganglion.
- **CSF:** cerebrospinal fluid is an ultrafiltrate of plasma, which is found in the spinal and cranial subarachnoid spaces and within the cerebral ventricles. It is formed by secretion and ultrafiltration from the choroid arterial plexus in the lateral third ventricles and the fourth ventricle. Its rate of production is constant at around 0.4 ml min^{-1} (575 ml per day). Its specific gravity at body temperature ranges from 1.003 to 1.009 (mean 1.006). The total volume in adults is between 120 and 150 ml, around 25–35 ml of which is found in the spinal subarachnoid space and most of which is distal to the cord in the area of the cauda equina. The PCO_2 is higher than that of blood, and the pH of CSF is slightly below arterial pH at 7.32. Electrolyte concentrations are similar (but not identical) to plasma. The protein concentration is less, but levels are not uniform and demonstrate a gradient between the ventricles,

where the concentration is low, and the lumbar region, where they are highest. The mean protein concentration is 23–28 mg dl^{-1}.

- **Thoracic kyphosis and lumbar lordosis:** the adult spine has a number of natural curves, the high points of which (in the supine position) are the fifth cervical (C_5) and the second or third lumbar ($L_{2/3}$) vertebrae, and the low points of which are the fifth and sixth thoracic ($T_{5/6}$) and the second sacral (S_2) vertebrae. This has relevance for the spread of intrathecal hyperbaric solutions.

Supplementary and Clinical Information

Surface Landmarks for Identifying Vertebral Levels

- The spinal cord in the adult ends at the level of the intervertebral disc at L_1/L_2. There is some variation, and in up to 10% of subjects the cord may end as high as T_{12}/L_1 or as low as L_2/L_3. (In the neonate the cord ends at the lower border of L_3.) It is of obvious importance to identify the vertebral level as accurately as possible.
- A line drawn between the highest points of the iliac crests (the intercristal or Tuffier's line) passes across either the spinous process of L_4 or the L_4/L_5 interspace. (Some textbooks say L_3/L_4, but examination of any plain PA X-ray will show this in most cases to be wrong.) This is the technique that is most commonly used by anaesthetists, but various studies have compared palpation with MR imaging to demonstrate that its accuracy is limited. This among other reasons is why neurosurgeons operating on the back always identify the level radiologically prior to operation. Anaesthetists must be aware of this potential for inaccuracy, because a spinal needle which is advanced too high or without due care risks penetrating the conus medullaris with permanent neurological deficit, particularly if any solution is injected into the spinal cord itself. The use of ultrasound to identify the vertebral level more accurately is likely to become more common.
- The lowest rib (which is palpable only in very thin subjects) is at the level of T_{12}.
- The first spinous process which is clearly palpable is C_7, which is the vertebra prominens (although the spinous process of T_1 below it is actually more prominent still).
- The inferior angle of the scapula in the neutral position is at the level of T_7 or T_8.

Factors That Influence Intrathecal Spread

- **Drug dose:** one prime determinant of spread is the mass of drug. The greater the amount of drug, the higher and more prolonged the block. The volume is of minimal importance: it has been demonstrated in obstetric anaesthesia, for example, that the injection of bupivacaine 15 mg in 15 ml (0.1%) will achieve a block of similar height to that obtained after injection of bupivacaine 15 mg in 3 ml (0.5%).
- **Level of injection:** in the supine patient with a normal spine the maximum height of the lumbar lordosis is at L_2/L_3. Less local anaesthetic will move rostrally if the injection is made below that level. In practice the final block height is similar, but it may take longer to achieve.
- **Baricity of drug:** this is another important determinant. Plain solutions of local anaesthetic are approximately isobaric relative to CSF at room temperature (mean CSF specific density is 1.006). At body temperature they become slightly hypobaric. Hyperbaric ('heavy') solutions are made so by the addition of glucose. 'Heavy'

bupivacaine contains glucose 8% (which is much more than the 0.8% which would render the solution hyperbaric). In the supine patient with a normal spine, hyperbaric solutions tend to pool in the thoracic kyphosis at $T_{5/6}$, and produce blocks which are generally higher but which are claimed to be more predictable than those produced by isobaric solutions. Solutions which pool in the lumbosacral area may have a relatively enhanced effect because the nerves of the cauda equina have a large surface area and only a thin layer of pia mater. This appears to increase their sensitivity to local anaesthetic.

- **Patient position:** this is linked to baricity. If the patient is in the decubitus position, the curves of the spine have no influence. Trendelenberg positioning will clearly increase the rostral spread of a hyperbaric solution.
- **Patient height:** there may be reduced cephalad spread in taller subject; the relationship is not reliable enough to allow accurate prediction.
- **Patient age:** there may be increased cephalad spread with advancing age, although again the block height cannot reliably be predicted.
- **Pregnancy:** term pregnancy is said to be associated with greater block height, which is made higher still with multiple pregnancy. The mechanism may relate to the relatively smaller volume of the dural sheath because of encroachment in the epidural space by the engorged venous plexus. In clinical practice this is not reliably true.
- **Speed and direction of injection:** forceful injection shortens the onset time but does not usually influence the final height of block. There are some data to suggest that if the side hole of a pencil point needle is directed rostrally, then block height may be increased.
- **Barbotage, weight of patient, gender of patient, adjuvant drugs, vasoconstrictors:** none of these factors has any significant effect on block height.

Failure of Subarachnoid Anaesthesia

One of the early pioneers of regional anaesthesia was Gaston Labat who in 1922 wrote that 'two conditions are . . . absolutely necessary to produce spinal anesthesia: puncture of the dura mater and subarachnoid injection of an anesthetic agent', which from a twenty-first century perspective seems somewhat self-evident. But Labat's precept has too often been used to explain all failures of spinal anaesthesia; if a block does not work it is claimed to be either because the needle has been wrongly placed or the incorrect solution has been injected. Those may certainly explain some failures, but the reality is more complex.

- **Needle misplacement:** pencil-point needles have side ports of varying dimensions, and there are some in which these can be 1.0 mm in length. It is theoretically possible therefore to puncture the dura and to obtain CSF but to straddle the dura (which is around 0.3 mm thick) with the side port and inject some of the solution proximally into the epidural space. Slower injection will increase the volume which escapes proximally.
- **Incorrect injectate:** this is a possibility – typically, although not that commonly, with the substitution of bupivacaine with the lidocaine used for infiltration anaesthesia. Suboptimal anaesthesia is sometimes blamed on the intrathecal drug itself, with the claim that it may be part of a faulty batch. In most instances this is unlikely: of

562 product defect notifications to Astra Zeneca between 2001–2007, no faulty samples were identified.

- **Lumbar CSF volume:** extracranial CSF volume as measured using MRI has been reported as ranging from 10 to 81 ml, and at least one (small) study has found that volume does correlate with the extent of sensory block. Nonetheless, individuals at the extremes of this reported range must be rare, because spinal anaesthesia in most cases is consistent and reliable.

- **Intrathecal septae:** the same applies to the possibility of intrathecal septae, whose existence has been confirmed both in cadaveric studies and by spinaloscopy. However, maldistribution of local anaesthetic is a well-recognized phenomenon in the literature and may explain a block of uneven density or one that is restricted to the sacral routes.

- **Innate resistance to local anaesthetics:** some, if not many authorities discount this possibility, and the term 'rachi-resistance', which was coined by a Belgian surgeon named Joseph Sebrechts in the 1930s to describe patients who were resistant to local anaesthetic action, has long since disappeared from the textbooks. There are, however, case reports, supported by most clinicians' empirical experience, to suggest that there clearly are very occasional patients in whom local anaesthesia is at least partly ineffective, and it seems logical to attribute this to some form of mutation of the sodium channel. However, although numerous mutations of the voltage-gated sodium channel have been described in other contexts and which can have profound effects on function, no such mutation has yet been identified for the local anaesthetic binding site (which is on domain D-IV, subunit S6). It is sometimes said that in patients with Ehlers-Danlos syndrome and other connective tissue disorders, local anaesthetic may be ineffective. This may apply to infiltration anaesthesia but is not true of plexus or neuraxial anaesthesia.

- **Acquired resistance to local anaesthetics:** for completeness, it is of interest that scorpion and other envenomation can be associated with local anaesthetic resistance. Such venoms block ionic channels and are highly antigenic. In individuals who have been stung there may be an increase in latency or an anaesthetic block that is inadequately dense. The mechanism by which this occurs is thought to be competitive inhibition by antibody/antigen complexes at sodium channel receptor sites.

Influence on Mortality

- **General or spinal anaesthesia for hip fracture fixation:** this is an issue of perennial debate, but the data tend to disappoint proponents of each technique. One large recent observational study in the UK of 30,130 patients receiving general anaesthesia and 22,999 given spinals showed no difference in mortality at either 5 or 30 days (White *et al. Anaesthesia* 2014, 69: 224–30). It may be, however, that more sophisticated subgroup analysis is needed, because a large American series reported improved survival in patients undergoing fixation of intertrochanteric fractures under neuraxial block. In respect of femoral neck fractures there was no difference (Neuman *et al. Anesthesiology* 2012,117: 72–92). So the standard mantra remains: there is no overwhelming evidence to support one or other of the techniques, but it is more important to ensure cardiovascular stability throughout. Intraoperative hypotension is associated with worse outcomes.

The Extradural (Epidural) Space

Commentary

This is another key subject for anaesthetists. The popularity of epidural analgesia for surgery appears to have subsided, despite its benefits (see the following), and it now has a more restricted range of indications. For labour, however, epidural analgesia remains a standard technique on UK delivery suites with an overall rate of 22% (the reported range is from 4–38%). Detailed knowledge will be expected: you will be required to demonstrate a good three-dimensional grasp of the anatomy as well as being aware of all the material complications and their management. This applies both to lumbar and to thoracic epidurals.

Core Information

Basic Anatomy

- The extradural (epidural) space is sometimes referred to as a 'potential' space. This is inaccurate. A potential space is one in which two structures are closely opposed but which can be separated, for example by fluid or by air. Such potential spaces include that between the parietal and visceral pleura and that between the dura and arachnoid maters. The epidural space posteriorly is an actual space whose posterior dimensions can be seen easily on any coronal CT or MR scan of the vertebral column.
- This actual space is the area surrounding the dural sheath as it lies within the vertebral canal.
- It extends from the foramen magnum superiorly (where the dura is fused to the skull) to the sacral hiatus inferiorly. (This means that extradural local anaesthetic cannot under normal circumstances spread intracranially. So, in contrast to a 'total spinal', a patient with a high cervical epidural block may stop breathing but will not be unconscious. There may be some intracranial diffusion of local anaesthetic, but this is unlikely to be significant.)
- The space is traversed by the dural sheath, whose thickness in the lumbar region is about 0.3–0.5 mm, and which comprises the membranes of the dura and arachnoid maters, the subarachnoid space containing CSF, the spinal nerves of the cauda equina and the filum terminale. The filum terminale is an extension of the pia mater, which runs from the conus medullaris to the coccyx, effectively acting to stabilize the cord. It contains neither neural tissue nor CSF.
- Anteriorly, the epidural space is bounded by the bodies of the vertebrae and by the intervertebral discs, over which lies the posterior longitudinal ligament. The anterior dura mater and the posterior longitudinal ligament are closely apposed, and so anteriorly the epidural space is 'potential'.
- Laterally, the epidural space is bounded by the pedicles and the intervertebral foramina.
- Posteriorly, it is bounded by the laminae of the neural arches.

- **Ligamenta flava:** these are not continuous but are metameric; that is, they form a series of ligaments with a structure that is fundamentally similar. At each level, there are two ligaments which meet in the midline and which connect the laminae of adjacent vertebrae. Each ligament extends from the lower part of the anterior surface of the lamina above to the posterior surface of, and upper margin of, the lamina below. Their fibres run in a perpendicular direction, but when viewed in the sagittal plane the ligaments are triangular in shape, with the apex of the triangle formed at the upper lamina. This explains why the ligamenta flava in different (or even the same) patients can appear to vary in thickness. This will depend on whether the advancing needle penetrates the wider base of the triangle or the thinner apex. The ligaments contain yellow elastic connective tissue: hence the name ('flavus' is Latin for 'yellow').
- At the level of a typical lumbar vertebra, for example L_3, the space contains the spinal nerves, each of which is invested with a cuff of dura, with loosely packed fat, areolar connective tissue, lymphatics and blood vessels. These vessels include the rich valveless vertebral venous plexus of Batson. (The lack of valves means that they will engorge as intra-abdominal pressure increases, for example during a contraction in labour.)
- The depth of the posterior epidural space (between the ligamenta flava and the dura) varies with the vertebral level. In the mid-cervical region it is only 1.0–1.5 mm wide, and at T_6 it is deeper, at around 2.5–3.0 mm. The greatest depth is at the L_2 interspace in men, in whom this is 5.0–6.0 mm.

Supplementary and Clinical Information

Complications Associated with the Procedure
- These include inadvertent dural puncture and subsequent post-dural puncture head-ache (PDPH) (incidence of 0.5%); failure (1%); unilateral or patchy block (5–10%); inadvertent subdural block (0.1%); intravascular injection; retention of a fragment of needle or catheter; epidural haematoma. The risk of permanent neurological sequelae is very small. The incidence is quoted at 1 in 10–15,000 epidurals but many of these complications are relatively minor, comprising, for example, little more than a patch of residual numbness, and even this figure is likely to be too high because childbirth itself may cause permanent neurological deficit (1 in 2,000). In the NAP 3 report on complications of central neuraxial blockade in the UK (2009), the incidence of permanent harm, considering the 'pessimistic' interpretation, was 1 in 161,550. There is finally no evidence, despite much debate fueled by the lay press, that routine epidurals lead to chronic back pain.

Complications Associated with Drugs That Are Injected
- These include hypotension owing to sympathetic block; high spinal block; evidence of systemic toxicity of local anaesthetic; urinary retention; pruritus, nausea and vomiting (usually associated with extradural opiate); respiratory depression. A total spinal may follow inadvertent intrathecal injection, depending on the epidural dose. There are many case reports of accidental injection of the wrong solution. Numerous substances have been administered in this way, including various antibiotics; solutions of total parenteral nutrition (which apparently provided good quality analgesia); chlorhexidine, with catastrophic sequelae; and thiopental. Obstetric

epidurals do not have any influence on caesarean section rates but do increase the likelihood of instrumental delivery by up to 14%.

Following are diagnosis and management of some of the more common and more complex complications.

Post-Dural Puncture Headache (PDPH)

- **Diagnosis:** the incidence of inadvertent dural puncture should not exceed 0.5%, and the incidence is usually quoted at between 0.5% and 1.0%. The incidence of PDPH is highest in obstetric patients, more than 80% of whom will develop symptoms. These are probably caused by traction on intracranial pain-sensitive structures such as the tentorium and blood vessel, and by adenosine-mediated reflex intracerebral vasodilatation. The low-pressure headache results from the failure of the choroid plexus to produce sufficient CSF to compensate for the loss through the breach in the dura. The onset is variable, with the headache commonly starting after about 12–24 hours. It can occur earlier or later. The headache may be frontal or occipital rather than global, but typically it is postural and relieved by recumbency or abdominal pressure. It may also be associated with photophobia, visual disturbance, neck and shoulder stiffness, and tinnitus. If the patient also complains of anorexia, nausea and vomiting, this is an indication that there is significant sagging of intracranial contents, with pressure on the brain stem at the foramen magnum. The patient may feel systemically unwell. The presentation is not always typical. Differential diagnosis of significant post-partum headache includes migraine, pre-eclampsia (which can present post-delivery), intracranial haemorrhage (associated with severe hypertension), meningitis and cortical vein thrombosis.
- **Management of severe PDPH:** assuming the failure of initial conservative treatment, advising recumbence when headache supervenes and simple analgesia, management may move on to other treatments. Cerebral vasoconstrictors such as caffeine and sumatriptan may improve symptoms, but they will not address the cause. Patients are instructed frequently to overhydrate. This has no influence on CSF production. The only agents which may increase it are corticosteroids, and accordingly there is some evidence to support the administration of ACTH analogues such as tetracosactrin (Synacthen), which stimulate glucocorticoid release. Epidural morphine reduces PDPH, as does the technique of prophylactically injecting autologous blood down the epidural catheter. As is the case with any relatively rare complication, however, the numbers in these supportive studies are small. The only technique that is likely to provide immediate relief is an extradural blood patch (EBP). This will abolish symptoms in almost all patients, but in at least 30% of mothers the procedure will need to be repeated. EBP has been associated with the development of chronic low back pain, and this risk must be weighed against those of persistent long-term headache or of neurological disaster (such as subdural haemorrhage), of which there are numerous reports in the literature. In many such reports, a common theme is PDPH that has been neglected.

Inadvertent Subdural Block

- A catheter or needle may deposit solution in the subdural space between the dura and arachnoid mater. Radiologists maintain that during myelography there is a 1%

incidence of subdural injection. It is much less commonly diagnosed in clinical anaesthesia. Some authorities cite an incidence of 1 in 1,000.

- Subdural block is often patchy; it may be extensive and unilateral, may extend very high (the subdural space extends into the cranium) and it often spares the sacral roots. The dura and arachnoid are more densely adherent to each other anteriorly, and so there may be a relative sparing of motor fibres. Sympathetic block may be minimal, and analgesia may be delayed. Horner's syndrome may be apparent.
- The use of a multi-holed catheter may further confuse the picture, because it is theoretically possible for the catheter to lie partly within the epidural and partly within the subdural space. Slow injection will favour emergence of the solution from the proximal epidural holes; more vigorous injection will favour dispersal through the distal subdural hole.

High Block or Total Spinal

- A high block or developing total spinal is characterized by the development of paraesthesia and weakness of the upper limbs, respiratory embarrassment owing to intercostal paralysis, a weak voice and cough, and sensory loss over the skin of the neck and eventually the jaw. If the block is a total spinal then apnoea and unconsciousness will supervene. Pupils dilate. It is usually asserted that a high sympathetic block will lead to hypotension and bradycardia because of local anaesthetic effects on the cardiac accelerator fibres (T_1–T_4). In practice, the cardiovascular changes are by no means always so predictable. High blocks regress quickly, whereas it might be some hours before a total spinal has worn off to the point at which comfortable respiration will be possible. Until this happens, anaesthesia must be maintained to prevent awareness.

Thoracic Epidural Analgesia

- **Techniques of insertion**. The technique of thoracic epidural block is similar to that used for lumbar catheter placement, although the different anatomy makes it appreciably more difficult. The spinous processes of the thoracic spine are significantly angled downwards and overlap such that the process of one thoracic vertebra is opposite the transverse process of the one below. This means that if a midline approach to the epidural space is used, the advancing needle will have to be at an angle of at least $45°$ to the spinal column, depending on which interspace is being used. For this reason, many anaesthetists prefer the paramedian approach.
- **Indications**. A thoracic epidural can provide effective analgesia following thoracic and major abdominal surgery, can attenuate the stress response to surgery and decreases adverse peri-operative cardiac events. The conclusions of a systematic review and meta-analysis of 125 trials comparing epidural with systemic opioid analgesia and published in 2014 were unequivocal. The authors asserted epidural analgesia decreased the risks of death, of atrial fibrillation and other supraventricular tachycardias, of deep venous thrombosis, respiratory depression, atelectasis and pneumonia, and post-operative nausea and vomiting. It also decreased ileus and accelerated the recovery of bowel function. Predictably the technique increased the

risk of arterial hypotension, pruritus, urinary retention and motor block, but these complications, some of which are readily manageable, would not seem to outweigh the substantial advantages (D.M. Popping *et al. Ann Surg* 2014, 259: 1056–67). Crucial to the success of epidural analgesia, however, is post-operative management, because if, for example, episodes of hypotension are always attributed to the epidural and are always treated with fluid boluses, then the benefits may be negated.

The Sacrum

Commentary

Caudal (sacral extradural) anaesthesia is a popular technique, particularly in children, in whom it can provide analgesia similar to that provided by a low lumbar epidural. In contrast to other neuraxial blocks, it requires no equipment other than a needle, syringe and/or intravenous cannula, and is simple to perform. This is a core area of anatomy applied to anaesthetic practice.

Core Information

The Basic Anatomy

(You will not be asked the origin of the name, but its etymological origins do add a certain poetry to the bare anatomical facts.)

- The sacrum was believed by the ancients to be the site of the soul, the bone which was the last to decompose, and thus the one around which the new body would form. Less fancifully it was believed to be the part of the animal that was offered in various sacrificial rituals. Hence it was called the 'sacred bone'. The original Greek word for 'sacred' or 'holy' is the same as that for 'big' or 'strong'. Galen used the word to describe the sacrum, and so more prosaically it may just represent a mistranslation from Greek to Latin.
- It is a large triangular-shaped bone that articulates superiorly with the fifth lumbar vertebra, inferiorly with the coccyx and laterally with the ilia.
- The dorsal roof comprises the fused laminae of the five sacral vertebrae and is convex dorsally (the curve is variable between sexes and races).
- In the midline there is a median crest, which represents the sacral spinous processes.
- Lateral to this is the intermediate sacral crest with a row of four tubercles, which represent the articular processes. The S_5 processes are remnants only and form the cornua, which are the main landmarks for identifying the sacral hiatus.
- At S_5 this failure of development of the spinous processes and laminae results in a hiatus in the roof of the canal. It is this sacral hiatus which allows access to the extradural space. It is covered by the sacrococcygeal membrane.
- Along the lateral border are anterior and posterior foramina which are the sacral equivalent of intervertebral foramina of higher levels, and through which the sacral nerve roots pass.

- In addition to the dura superiorly, the canal contains areolar connective tissue, fat, the sacral nerves, lymphatics, the filum terminale (which is an extension of the pia mater originating from the conus medullaris at the end of the spinal cord and which extends to the coccyx) and a rich venous plexus.

Supplementary and Clinical Information

Sacral Extradural (Caudal) Anaesthesia

- Access to the canal is via the sacral hiatus at the level of the fifth sacral vertebra through the sacrococcygeal membrane. In up to 7% of subjects, fusion has taken place and so access is impossible. (Some authorities believe this to be an overestimate.)
- **Identification:** there are several ways of identifying the hiatus.
  - The sacral hiatus is at the apex of an equilateral triangle completed by the posterior superior iliac spines.
  - If the tip of the index finger palpates the coccyx, the midpoint of the middle interphalangeal joint of the finger identifies the hiatus (in an 'average' adult).
  - With the hips flexed at 90°, a line extended along the midpoint of the thigh will end at the hiatus.
  - Palpation of the midline sacral crest caudally until the cornua are identified is useful only in lean subjects in whom the anatomy is not obscured by a sacral fat pad.
- **Drug doses:** in adults, a typical dose would be levobupivacaine 0.5% × 20 ml. In children, various formulae have been elaborated to achieve blocks of adequate height. A commonly used regimen is that described by Armitage in 1979: 0.5 ml kg^{-1} of (levo)bupivacaine 0.25% for sacral block (circumcision, hypospadias, anal procedures), 1.0 ml kg^{-1} for low thoracic block (for inguinal herniotomy) and 1.25 ml kg^{-1} for higher thoracic block up to T_8 (for orchidopexy). (E.N. Armitage. *Anaesthesia*, 1979, 34: 396.) The addition of clonidine 2.0 μg kg^{-1} will double the duration of effective analgesia, while ketamine 0.5 mg kg^{-1} (preservative free) has been shown to increase it by four times. However, concern about the effects of ketamine on the developing nervous system have led many anaesthetists to abandon this practice. Ketamine is highly lipid-soluble, and both CSF and plasma concentrations rise rapidly after caudal injection. Given the well-recognized association between ketamine and accelerated neuronal apoptosis in young animals, the potential risks would seem to far outweigh the benefits of any increased duration of analgesia.
- The 'whoosh' and 'swoosh' tests have been described as methods of verifying accurate needle placement. In the 'whoosh' test a small volume of air (2 ml) is injected while the anaesthetist listens with a stethoscope over the lumbar spine. Some first deposit a small volume of fluid in the space; correct needle placement is confirmed by definite crepitus. The injection of air into the extradural space has well-recognized disadvantages; the subsequent block may be patchy, and venous air embolism has been reported. The 'swoosh' test is similar in principle, except that auscultation is performed as the local anaesthetic itself is being injected.
- **Differences between adults and children:** the dura mater usually ends at the level of S_2 in adults (although it can descend to within about 5 cm of the hiatus in some subjects). At birth the dura is as low as S_4, but by around 2 years of age it ascends to

adult levels. The sacral hiatus is easier to locate in children because it is not overlain by the sacral fat pad that later develops in adults.

- **Spread of solution:** in the sacral extradural space this is influenced in adults by total volume, speed of injection and posture (one study has reported that higher levels are reached if the patient is 15° head up).
- There is good correlation in children between spread of a given dose and age. There is poor correlation between spread and weight and/or height.
- The sacral extradural space in children offers lower resistance to longitudinal spread than the adult. Epidural fat in children has a loose and wide-meshed texture, whereas in adults it becomes more densely packed and fibrous. There is less fibrous connective tissue in the sacral epidural space than in adults, and this combination of factors means that local anaesthetic spread is greater.
- In children it is possible to direct a 20G 51-mm cannula rostrally to escape the sacral space altogether and allow what is in effect a lower lumbar epidural block. Generous volumes can be employed therefore if a high block is required. High blocks are much more difficult to achieve in adults. Hypodermic needles should not be used to perform caudal blocks in children; a cannula sized 20G or smaller should be used to minimize the risk of unrecognized vascular or dural puncture.
- Complications such as intrathecal injection are more likely in children less than 2 years of age. Otherwise the incidence both of intrathecal and intravascular injection does not differ from that seen in adults. If too large an aspirating pressure is applied to a syringe used to check that the needle is not intravascular, this may collapse the vessel and give a false negative. For that reason, the syringe should be removed from the needle or cannula, which should be allowed to drain freely.
- **Sympathetic effects:** children up to and beyond the age of 6 years show cardiovascular stability in the face of blocks that would cause sympathetic blockade and hypotension in adults. This is probably due to delay in the maturation of the autonomic nervous system.
- **Complications:** these include failure; intravascular injection (false negative aspiration may occur in 10% or more of cases, as negative pressure collapses the vein); intraosseous injection in young children; bowel perforation; dural and subdural puncture (which is characterized by an extensive, patchy block of slow onset). In obstetric practice the fetal head is vulnerable to an inaccurately placed needle. There are also the potential complications associated with the particular drugs injected (local anaesthetics, opiates, clonidine, ketamine).

The Blood Supply to the Lower Limb

Commentary

Long (and dispiriting) lower limb revascularization procedures provide a ready opportunity to contemplate the arterial supply of the lower limb, although the details are not really essential to the practice even of vascular anaesthesia. The blood supply of the lower limb may appear as a topic for the anatomy oral with clinical aspects focusing on the acutely ischaemic limb, anaesthesia for revascularization and venous thromboembolism.

Core Information

Arterial Supply of the Lower Limb

- The arterial supply to the lower limb arises from the external iliac artery which is a terminal branch of the abdominal aorta.
- The upper part of the limb is supplied by the obturator artery. This is a branch of the internal iliac artery which passes into the thigh via the obturator canal. It then divides into the anterior branch which supplies the adductor muscles plus pectineus and gracilis, and the posterior branch which primarily supplies the gluteal muscles.
- At the level of the inguinal ligament it continues as the common femoral artery to enter the femoral triangle.
- Posterolaterally the femoral artery gives off the profunda femoris (the 'deep' femoral artery) with its three main branches: the perforating arteries which perforate adductor magnus and contribute part of the supply to the medial and posterior muscles of the thigh, the lateral circumflex artery which passes round the antero-lateral aspect of the femur to supply the lateral thigh muscles, and the medial circumflex which wraps around the posterior femur to supply the femoral neck and head.
- The femoral artery (at this point described as the superficial femoral artery) enters the adductor canal in the anteromedial aspect of the thigh, supplying as it does so the anterior thigh muscles, and exits the canal at the adductor hiatus.
- As it moves into the posterior compartment of the thigh it becomes the popliteal artery, which in turn divides into the anterior tibial artery and the tibioperoneal trunk.
- The anterior tibial artery passes through the interosseous membrane to reach the anterior compartment of the leg and then continues to the dorsum of the foot as the dorsalis pedis artery.
- The tibioperoneal trunk divides into the posterior tibial artery and the peroneal artery. The posterior tibial passes downwards and backwards behind the medial malleolus (in conjunction with the tibial nerve) to divide into the medial and lateral plantar arteries (plantar arches). The peroneal artery terminates at the ankle, having run down the posterior interosseous membrane in close proximity to the fibula.
- The plantar arch gives off the metatarsal arteries and the plantar digital arteries to supply the extremities.

Venous Drainage of the Lower Limb

- The deep veins in general travel with, and have the same name as, the major arteries. Within vascular sheaths the two are closely enough opposed to allow arterial pulsation to assist venous return.
- Thus, the medial and lateral plantar veins of the foot combine to form the posterior tibial vein, which accompanies the posterior tibial artery and the fibular vein. This

unites with the anterior and posterior tibial veins to form the popliteal vein which passes up into the thigh through the adductor canal.

- Once in the thigh the popliteal vein becomes the femoral vein which travels in close apposition to the femoral artery.
- The profunda femoris ('deep' femoral) vein drains the thigh muscle via a series of perforating veins.
- There are two significant superficial veins. First, the long saphenous (also known as the great saphenous vein) is formed from the dorsal venous arch of the foot and the dorsal vein of the hallux. This passes up the medial side of the lower leg, lying anterior to the medial malleolus, where it is a suitable site for cannulation (and historically for venous cut down). It enters the thigh posterior to the medial condyle of the knee and drains into the femoral vein at around the level of the inguinal ligament. The superficial long course and size of the vessel makes it suitable for use in coronary revascularization surgery. Second is the small (short) saphenous vein, which is also formed from the dorsal venous arch of the foot with a contribution from the dorsal vein of the fifth toe. It passes into the lower leg posterior to the lateral malleolus, between the two heads of gastrocnemius, and drains into the popliteal vein in the popliteal fossa.

Supplementary and Clinical Information

- **Acute lower limb ischaemia**. This is a vascular emergency due to occlusion of part of the arterial circulation of the lower limb by thrombus. It may be secondary to a prothrombotic state or to conditions such as atrial fibrillation and cardiac failure. Other causes include trauma and inadvertent arterial injection of thrombogenic substances by intravenous drug users. The typical clinical presentation will be of a patient with a white, pulseless and painful limb, often with paresis or paralysis and a global loss of normal sensation. The restoration of vascular patency is vital if the limb is to be salvaged, and there are various surgical and radiological approaches to the problem. These include arterial embolectomy, usually under local anaesthesia; thrombolysis; and therapeutic anti-coagulation with heparin. The more prolonged the period of complete ischaemia the more likely is the patient to develop compartment syndrome. This equally will threaten the viability of the limb and mandates emergency fasciotomy. Following successful embolectomy, patients may require angioplasty, endovascular stenting or bypass revascularization procedures.
- **Reperfusion injury**. Reperfusion of previously ischaemic tissue is associated with an inflammatory response that is both local and systemic. The cellular effects of hypoxia are complex in their detail, but in simplified summary the failure of oxidative phosphorylation secondary to the depletion of substrate (oxygen) diminishes the resynthesis of substances such as ATP and phosphocreatine. This in turn affects the function of ATP-dependent ionic pumps, with the accumulation of intracellular sodium, calcium and water. Intracellular catabolism also leads to the production of molecules such as hypoxanthine from ATP degradation, which when perfusion is restored react with molecular oxygen to form toxic oxygen radicals. These reactive species cause direct damage to the cell membrane by lipid peroxidation. Ischaemia also 'primes' the endothelium which produces a number of proinflammatory species such as cytokines, endothelin and thromboxane A_2, while inhibiting protective

molecules including nitric oxide synthase and prostacyclin. Leucocyte activation is another significant process that is involved. Polymorphonuclear leucocytes migrate from the intravascular space to the insterstitium (partly mediated by interleukin-8 which is released from hypoxic tissues), and once there release a number of highly deleterious factors including reactive oxygen species, together with elastase and protease enzymes. At its most severe this cascade of events (amplified by complement activation) leads to an increase in the permeability of the vascular endothelium, thrombotic occlusion, oedema and cell death. Systemically this may result in the systemic inflammatory response syndrome (SIRS) and even to multiple organ dysfunction syndrome (MODS). Leucocyte adherence and platelet aggregation may also explain the so-called 'no reflow' phenomenon, whereby tissue blood flow remains reduced even after relief of the thrombotic or surgical occlusion. (To add to the complexity, these leucocytes can also mediate a protective response that can enhance the barrier represented by the vascular endothelium, but a discussion of these paradoxical effects will be beyond the scope of the oral.)

- **Patients presenting for lower limb revascularization procedures**. These patients are high risk, usually presenting with multiple comorbidity. Thirty-day mortality for elective procedures is as high as 8% and is higher still following emergency surgery. Mortality at 1 year is quoted at around 35%. In contrast, patients with abdominal aortic aneurysms, who are commonly perceived to be at even higher risk, have a much lower 1-year mortality of 10–15%. The high mortality of patients with peripheral vascular disease is associated with age, multi-system atherosclerosis (more than 60% have severe coronary artery disease and the overall incidence approaches 90%), attendant hypertension, type 2 diabetes mellitus and renovascular disease. Most of the patients are smokers, or ex-smokers with the resultant complications. Pre-operative assessment of these patients is essentially generic, as are the available anaesthetic techniques. Regional anaesthesia has the usual indications and contraindications, and although it confers the theoretical advantage of sympathetic block with vasodilatation of the affected limbs, there is no evidence of longer limb or patient survival when compared with general anaesthesia.
- **Venous thromboembolism**. See under 'Drugs Affecting Coagulation' in Chapter 4.

The Femoral Triangle

Commentary

The anatomy of the femoral triangle is straightforward. It lends itself readily to simple diagrams: the first being the triangle itself, the second a transverse view to demonstrate that you realize the femoral nerve lies in a fascial compartment quite separate from the femoral sheath. The question may then move on to the structures of significance to the anaesthetist, namely the femoral nerve, the femoral vein and the femoral artery. There is not a large amount of detail to cover.

Core Information

- The triangle is bounded superiorly by the inguinal ligament (which curves from the anterior superior iliac spine to the pubic tubercle).
- Its lateral border is formed by the sartorius. (This is the 'tailor's muscle' which runs across the thigh from its origin at the anterior superior iliac spine to the medial side of the upper tibia, and is the longest muscle in the body.)
- Its medial border is formed by the adductor longus muscle (whose insertion is at the superior ramus of the pubis and which has a linear attachment to the linea aspera on the posterior aspect of the femur).
- Its roof is formed by areolar tissue, fascia lata, subcutaneous tissue and skin.
- Its floor is a trough composed of the iliacus, psoas and pectineus muscles.
- Within the triangle lie the femoral canal, containing lymphatics, and immediately lateral to it, the femoral sheath, containing the femoral vein (medial) and femoral artery (lateral).
- Outside the femoral sheath and lying lateral to it is the femoral nerve. The nerve is invested in the fascia of the iliacus muscle (fascia iliaca), which separates it from the femoral sheath. Above this is the fascia of the tensor fascia lata muscle. The distance by which it is separated is variable. It may bear a close relation to the pulsation of the femoral artery or may be 1–2 cm or more lateral to it. It can also be separated from the femoral sheath by a small part of the psoas muscle.

Supplementary and Clinical Information

- **Femoral vein:** this is useful for central venous access (if other sites are unsuitable) and for siting large-bore cannulae for haemodiafiltration. It is the central vein of choice in infants and young children. It is also the site of access for insertion of vena caval filters. Access to the femoral vein is not always easy; it is commonly overlaid by the superficial femoral artery and its anatomy can be variable. The route is used commonly in children but is more of a last resort in adults in whom the subclavian veins are usually a better alternative.
- **Femoral artery:** this is used for arterial sampling and monitoring (again if other sites are unsuitable). The artery also provides access for angiography and for the insertion of intra-aortic balloon pump catheters.
- **Femoral nerve:** this can readily be blocked in this site (Figure 2.10).
- **Indications:** these include analgesia for fractured shaft of femur, perioperative analgesia for knee surgery and perioperative analgesia for hip surgery (usually as part of a 3-in-1 block). **Technique:** see next section.

The Femoral Nerve

Commentary

The applied anatomy of the femoral nerve is not entirely straightforward because the course of the nerve in the groin can be variable. Femoral nerve block is still performed

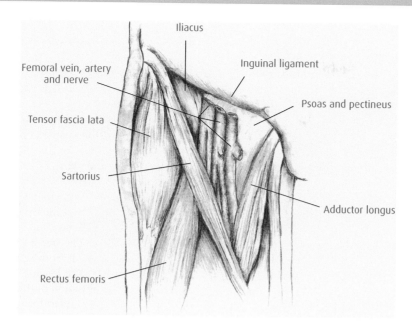

Fig. 2.10 The femoral triangle.

blind in many Accident and Emergency departments, but ultrasound guidance is becoming routine in anaesthetic practice. The increasing emphasis on enhanced recovery after surgery (ERAS) means that femoral nerve block is used less than once it was for surgery on the knee, including arthroplasty.

Core Information

- The femoral nerve originates from the anterior primary rami of L_2, L_3 and L_4 and enters the anterior thigh beneath the inguinal ligament (which runs from the anterior superior iliac spine to the pubic tubercle).
- The femoral sheath is formed from an extension of the extraperitoneal fascia and contains the femoral vein (medially) and artery (laterally). It does not contain the femoral nerve.
- The nerve is invested in the fascia of the iliacus muscle (fascia iliaca), which separates it from the femoral sheath. Above this is the fascia lata (see Figure 2.11).
- The distance by which it is separated from the vessel is variable. It may bear a close relation to the pulsation of the femoral artery or may be 1–2 cm or even more lateral to it. It can be separated from the femoral sheath by a part of the psoas muscle, and can also lie posterior to the artery.
- The nerve usually starts to divide into its terminal branches at the base of the femoral triangle. In some subjects this division can start above the inguinal ligament.
- It divides into a leash of nerves which supply the muscles of the thigh. One of the main divisions continues as the saphenous nerve, which passes medially across the knee to provide sensory innervation as far as the medial aspect of the ankle and rear foot.

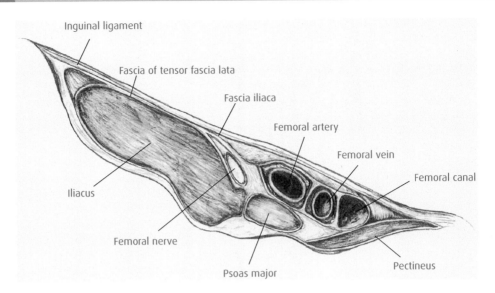

Inguinal ligament

Fascia of tensor fascia lata

Fascia iliaca

Femoral artery

Femoral vein

Femoral canal

Iliacus

Femoral nerve

Pectineus

Psoas major

Fig. 2.11 The femoral nerve.

Supplementary and Clinical Information

Femoral Nerve, 3-in-1 and Fascia Iliaca blocks

- It is common for anaesthetists and others to assume that it is straightforward to perform a femoral nerve block and that the 3-in-1 block provides useful analgesia for hip surgery. Neither is necessarily true; the anatomy of the femoral nerve is variable and the benefits of 3-in-1 block are inconsistent.
- **Supply:** the nerve supplies the shaft of the femur, the muscles and skin of the anterior thigh as far as the knee, and via the saphenous nerve, the medial side of the lower leg as far as an area surrounding the medial malleolus.
- **Indications:** these include the provision of analgesia for fractured shaft of femur (which is usually very effective, particularly if an indwelling catheter technique is used), perioperative analgesia for knee surgery, and perioperative analgesia for hip surgery (usually as part of a 3-in-1 block).
- **3-in-1 block:** this describes a single injection, which aims to block the **femoral** nerve, the **obturator** nerve and the **lateral cutaneous** nerve of the thigh. A larger volume of local anaesthetic is used, and during injection firm distal pressure is applied. In theory, this spreads the local anaesthetic rostrally back up into the psoas compartment so that all three nerves are blocked. The obturator nerve supplies the adductor muscles of the hip, part of the hip joint, skin on the medial side of the thigh and part of the knee joint. The lateral cutaneous nerve supplies skin over the anterolateral thigh as far as the knee, and the over the lateral thigh from the greater trochanter down to the level of the mid-thigh. These nerves can also be blocked within the psoas compartment itself.
- **Efficacy:** 3-in-1 block can be effective for cannulated hip screws and sometimes for dynamic hip screws, but, as its anatomy demonstrates, in many cases it will not

provide reliable analgesia for cutaneous sensation above the level of the greater trochanter, which is the site of incision for much hip surgery. It has been described, not entirely unfairly, as 'a nerve block in search of an operation'.

- **Fascia iliaca block:** this is an alternative to the standard 3-in-1 block, and which also blocks the femoral, lateral cutaneous and obturator nerves. Local anaesthetic is injected behind the fascia iliaca at the junction of the lateral with the two medial thirds of the inguinal ligament, and is directed upwards by the application of distal pressure. A short-bevelled needle allows identification of the two fascial layers (producing 'clicks' as it passes through tensor fascia lata and fascia iliaca), and it is not necessary to seek a motor response using a nerve stimulator. The fascial layers of the iliacus muscle form a potential space in which are found the three nerves. Some studies have claimed that fascia iliaca block provides better analgesia than either femoral or 3-in-1 blocks, but, given the anatomy, it is hard to see why this should be so. In essence, it is a different mode of detection rather than a different nerve block.

- **Technique of femoral and 3-in-1 nerve block:** the success of these blocks is increased substantially by the use of ultrasound with or without a peripheral nerve stimulator (see under 'Peripheral Nerve Stimulators' in Chapter 5). A plexus or block needle is inserted at an angle of about 45° and directed rostrally just below the inguinal ligament and lateral to the pulsation of the femoral artery. Movement of the patella (quadriceps femoris) is the best indicator of correct placement (at around 0.5 mA). The mass of drug injected will depend on whether other nerves, such as the sciatic and obturator, are being blocked at the same time, but the general dose range is 15–20 ml of 0.5% levobupivacaine for a femoral nerve block, and 30 ml or more for a 3-in-1 block.

- **Adductor canal block:** traditional combined sciatic-femoral nerve block militates against the early mobilization after knee surgery which is now the norm, but knee arthroplasty especially can be particularly painful in the immediate post-operative period. The adductor canal block can provide analgesia comparable to that of a formal femoral nerve block but is relatively motor sparing and so does not delay immediate post-operative rehabilitation. The saphenous nerve is the terminal sensory branch of the femoral nerve and can be blocked in the adductor canal which is the space formed by the sartorius (superiorly), vastus medialis (laterally) and adductor longus and magnus (medially). The space contains the neurovascular bundle, and it is the femoral artery that provides the key anatomical landmark, as the nerve itself is not always clearly seen on ultrasound. Lower volume and lower concentration local anaesthetic is sufficient to provide analgesia without the risk of motor block to vastus medialis; a typical dose would be 10–20 ml of levobupivacaine 0.25%.

- **SPANK block:** the knee joint is supplied by what are termed the genicular nerves, which are essentially the articular branches of the major nerves of the lower limb: the tibial, the common peroneal, the saphenous, the femoral and the obturator. These branches are described according to their anatomical positions (superior lateral, superior medial, etc.), but it is sufficient to note that in effect they form a plexus that supplies the entire posterior capsule of the knee. SPANK is an acronym for **Sensory Posterior Articular Nerves of the Knee.** (As one review in an American journal put it – 'Yes, they really did call it that.') Traditionally the nerves have been approached using three separate injection sites, but a more recent technique describes a single large-volume injection which anaesthetizes the posterior capsule of the knee while sparing the motor components of the tibial and the common peroneal nerves. Cadaver studies have demonstrated a deep tissue plane that is superficial to the periosteum of the posterior femur, and 20 ml of solution (e.g. levobupivacaine 0.25%) will spread to block the genicular nerves. A 100-mm block needle or 22G spinal needle is inserted just behind the medial epicondyle and then advanced until it encounters the shaft of femur. The needle is then withdrawn sufficiently to avoid the periosteum and then advanced to the posterior border before injection. There is a variation in the form of the **iPACK** block (injection into the **i**nterspace between the **P**opliteal **A**rtery and the posterior **C**apsule of the **K**nee). This is a modified superior genicular nerve block with the same point of injection as for the SPANK block. The needle is advanced until it is lateral to the popliteal artery and then solution is injected continuously during gradual withdrawal.

The Sciatic Nerve

Commentary
The sciatic nerve is the largest peripheral nerve in the body, and it is accessible from a number of sites. Sciatic nerve block provides good analgesia for much lower limb surgery, and the variety of possible approaches provides an appropriate test of applied anatomy. As always with questions which include practical procedures, it will help the credibility of your answer if you can convince the examiner that you have done some of these blocks. You will not, however, be expected to be familiar with every approach.

Core Information
- The sciatic nerve arises from the sacral plexus, which is formed by the union of the L_4, L_5, S_1, S_2 and S_3 nerve roots, and which lies separated from the anterior sacrum by the piriformis muscle.
- The nerve, which is the largest in the body, is about 2 cm in diameter as it exits the pelvis posteriorly via the greater sciatic notch.
- It continues its descent into the thigh between the ischial tuberosity and the greater trochanter, and then lies behind the femur before dividing in the popliteal fossa into the common peroneal and the posterior tibial nerves.
- The sciatic nerve provides a sensory supply to much of the lower leg via its main terminal branches (the tibial and common peroneal).
- It supplies the knee joint (via articular branches) and almost all of the structures below the knee.
- It does not supply a variable, but extensive, cutaneous area over the medial side of the knee, lower leg and ankle, and medial side of the foot around the medial malleolus. This area is supplied by the saphenous nerve (from the femoral).
- Sciatic nerve block alone will provide reliable analgesia for surgical procedures which involve the forefoot, the sole of the foot and the lateral side of the foot and ankle.

In conjunction with femoral and obturator nerve block, it provides good analgesia for major knee surgery (although it is less popular than previously because the motor block and temporary loss of proprioception will delay early mobilization).

- Sciatic nerve irritation can result from lumbar disc prolapse, leading to classic symptoms of sciatica in the distribution of the root that is affected. Impingement of the nerve can also occur in the pelvis where it crosses beneath or, in 15% of subjects, through the piriformis muscle leading to the so-called piriformis syndrome. The nerve can be damaged by direct trauma, including surgical trauma, as well as by ill-directed intramuscular injections in the buttock. One of its peripheral branches, the common peroneal nerve, is particularly vulnerable as it winds round the fibular head.

Supplementary and Clinical Information

Sciatic Nerve Block

A number of approaches have been described. As with other peripheral nerve and plexus blocks, ultrasound guidance is now routine.

- **Posterior approach**
  - The patient lies in the supine position with the upper leg flexed to 90° at the hip and knee.
  - A line is drawn from the greater trochanter to the ischial tuberosity. The nerve can be located just medial to the midpoint of this line at a depth of around 6 cm. The depth clearly varies with the size of the patient.
  - The needle is inserted at right angles to the skin, attached to a nerve stimulator. A twitch in the lower limb (usually dorsiflexion of the foot) elicited at about 0.5 mA is a sign of accurate placement, and 20 ml levobupivacaine 0.5% is injected.
  - The stimulator technique and drug dose apply to the other proximal approaches to the sciatic nerve.
- **Posterior (classic approach of Labat)**
  - The patient lies in the decubitus position with the upper leg flexed to 90°at hip and knee.
  - A line is drawn from the greater trochanter to the posterior superior iliac spine. From the midpoint of this line a perpendicular is dropped 3–5 cm.
  - The needle is inserted vertically to the skin, and the nerve is sought at around 6–8 cm. Alternatively, a line can be drawn from the greater trochanter to the sacral hiatus and the injection made at its midpoint.
- **Anterior approach**
  - The nerve emerges from the greater sciatic foramen and lies between the ischial tuberosity and the greater trochanter of the femur. Before it passes down behind the bone it is accessible medial to the femur and just below the lesser trochanter.
  - The patient lies supine and a line is drawn from the anterior superior iliac spine to the pubic tubercle. A line parallel to it is drawn from the greater trochanter. At the junction of the medial third and lateral two-thirds of the upper line, a perpendicular is dropped to meet the lower.
  - At this junction, a long (150-mm) needle is inserted vertical to the skin until it contacts the medial shaft of femur. It is then redirected medially to slide off the

femur before advancing another 5 cm or so to encounter the nerve in the region of the lesser trochanter.

— It is worth noting that in around 15% of patients the sciatic nerve lies immediately posterior to the femur at this point and so is inaccessible to the anterior approach.

- **Lateral approach**
  — The patient lies supine.
  — A long needle is inserted 3 cm distal to the most prominent part of the greater trochanter and seeks the nerve as it descends behind the femur. It is not as easy as it sounds, and this approach is not commonly used in the UK.

- **Popliteal fossa block**
  — The sciatic nerve can be blocked in the popliteal fossa before it divides into its tibial and common peroneal branches. This is a particularly useful block for providing analgesia for forefoot surgery.
  — The patient lies lateral or prone, and the proximal flexor skin crease of the knee is identified.
  — A line is drawn vertically for about 7 cm from the midpoint of the skin crease, and the injection is made about 1 cm lateral to this point.
  — If dorsiflexion is elicited it may be the common peroneal nerve alone that is being stimulated, and the sciatic nerve may have already branched. Plantar flexion or inversion of the foot indicates successful location of the posterior tibial nerve. Ultrasound allows much more precise identification of the level at which the nerve divides.
  — Drug dose: 10–20 ml levobupivacaine 0.5%.

The Sensory Innervation of the Foot

Commentary

This is a predictable question about applied anatomy. There are several ways to provide analgesia for forefoot surgery and, although an ankle block does not necessarily provide the best analgesia, its applied anatomy has always made it a good topic for anatomical discussion. Five separate nerves need to be identified. Give yourself an advantage by observing or performing some ankle blocks so that you will have recent practical experience on which to draw.

Core Information

Basic anatomy and Peripheral Nerve Blocks

Ankle block can provide effective and prolonged analgesia for the forefoot. Five nerves need to be blocked before local anaesthesia is complete. Concentrations may need to be reduced if the patient is frail or if the procedure is bilateral.

— **Saphenous nerve:** this supplies a variable portion of the medial border of the foot and ankle. It is a terminal branch of the femoral nerve and is anaesthetized immediately anterior to the medial malleolus where it is superficial, close to the saphenous vein. It is blocked with subcutaneous local anaesthetic, for example, levobupivacaine 0.5% × 5 ml.

— **Posterior tibial nerve:** this supplies the plantar surface of the foot. It is a branch of the sciatic nerve (which divides into tibial and common peroneal branches in the popliteal fossa) and is blocked behind the medial malleolus where it lies posterior to the posterior tibial artery. The needle is gently directed perpendicular to the skin until it encounters bone, and is then withdrawn 1–2 mm prior to injection of 3–5 ml levobupivacaine 0.5% on either side of the artery. This nerve can also reliably be blocked in the popliteal fossa.

— **Deep peroneal nerve:** this supplies only a small area of skin on the dorsum of the foot between the first and second toes. It passes beneath the extensor retinaculum at the front of the ankle joint and is most readily blocked between the tendons of extensor hallucis longus and extensor digitorum longus where it lies lateral to the dorsalis pedis artery. It is blocked with a total of 3–5 ml levobupivacaine 0.5% placed on either side of the artery and deep to the fascia.

— **Sural nerve:** this supplies sensation to the fifth toe and the lateral border of the foot. It is a branch of the tibial nerve; at the level of the ankle it lies superficially behind the lateral malleolus. Subcutaneous infiltration of levobupivacaine 0.5% × 5 ml between the lateral malleolus and the tendo Achilles usually provides effective analgesia.

— **Superficial peroneal nerve:** this supplies much of the dorsum of the foot (excepting the small area supplied by the deep peroneal nerve, and the lateral foot which is supplied by the sural nerve). It is a branch of the common peroneal nerve, which divides further into terminal branches at the level of the malleoli. It is blocked with a ring of superficial infiltration of levobupivacaine 0.5% × 10 ml between the anterior tibia and the lateral malleolus.

Supplementary and Clinical Information

Foot surgery can be disproportionately painful and there are other methods of providing anaesthesia and analgesia.

- **Possible local anaesthetic techniques:** these include subarachnoid (spinal) block, lumbar extradural (epidural) block, sacral extradural (caudal) block, sciatic nerve block at the hip, sciatic nerve block in the popliteal fossa, intraosseous nerve block between the metatarsals (for procedures in the distal foot which cannot be performed under digital nerve [ring] block), intravenous regional anaesthesia (Bier's block, which needs high compression pressures and high volumes to obtain satisfactory analgesia), and local infiltration (this is unlikely to be satisfactory for awake surgery but is included for completeness).

- **Indications:** these include all forefoot surgery, such as metatarsal osteotomy for hallux valgus, excision of neuromata and foreign body removal.

- **Complications:** these are largely generic and include failure and partial failure, local anaesthetic toxicity (you may need to modify the concentrations quoted above to reduce the total dose), nerve and vessel damage, intravascular and intraneural injection, and complications related to the lower limb arterial tourniquet (see under 'The Arterial Tourniquet' in Chapter 3)

Cross-Sectional Areas of Interest (Eye, Neck, Lower Thoracic and Lumbar Regions)

Commentary

You may be asked to draw a cross-sectional diagram of anatomical interest, or you may be shown a CT or MR image in the coronal plane, which will then be followed by a discussion of an aspect of clinical relevance. Such typical areas are the eye, the neck at the level of the sixth cervical vertebra and the lumbar spine. (If you practise talking as you draw, and if you can include more anatomical detail than is strictly necessary, then you may be able to limit the examiner's opportunity for further questioning.) The following descriptions are deliberately constructed in this way to try and reflect the way in which people might sketch the diagrams.

Core Information

The Eye (Figure 2.12)

- The anterior structures of the globe are more complex than the posterior, and so the question is likely to include reference to the drainage of aqueous humour. The probable discussion about narrow angle glaucoma may extend to the pharmacological management of glaucoma and to determinants of intraocular pressure (see under 'Intraocular Pressure' in Chapter 3).
- **Outer layers:** the three layers of the eyeball consist of the outer fibrous *sclera*, the middle vascular *choroid* and the inner layer of the *retina*. The sclera is continuous posteriorly with the dural cuff that surrounds the optic nerve, and is continuous anteriorly with the cornea.

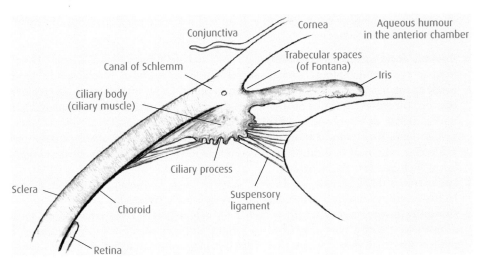

Fig. 2.12 The eye.

- **Contents of the globe:** the posterior part contains *vitreous humour*, which is a colourless transparent gel and which constitutes about 80% of the total contents. Anteriorly, the vitreous body is bounded by the capsule of the *lens* and its suspensory ligaments. These ligaments extend to the *ciliary body*, which is a direct anterior continuation of the choroid and comprises the muscle involved in accommodation of the lens. The ciliary body also secretes *aqueous humour* into the anterior chamber, where it circulates before draining via spaces in the trabecular meshwork through the *canal of Schlemm*. The anterior chamber of the eye contains the *iris*, which itself is a forward continuation of the choroid via the ciliary body.

The Neck at the Level of C_6 (Figure 2.13)

- You may be asked to sketch a cross-sectional diagram of the neck at the level of C_6. This allows the examiner the choice of a number of follow-up questions which include central venous cannulation, the larynx, the phrenic nerve and the vagus nerve
- C_6 is the level of the *cricoid cartilage* whose lower border marks the beginning of the *trachea*. Immediately posterior is the *oesophagus*, which is separated from the body of the sixth cervical vertebra only by the *pretracheal fascia*. Immediately anterior is the isthmus of the *thyroid*. Posterolaterally is the *carotid sheath*, which encloses the common carotid artery, the internal jugular vein and the vagus nerve. Behind the sheath lies part of the *sympathetic chain*. Immediately lateral to the vertebral body are the *vertebral artery* and *vein*, beyond which are the *scalene* muscles. Between these lie the trunks of the *brachial plexus*.

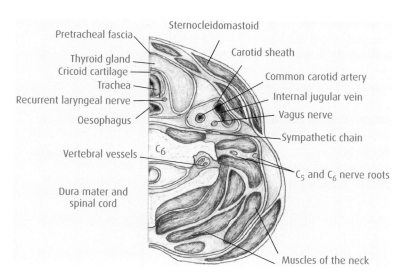

Fig. 2.13 Transverse section of the neck (right side) at the level of C_6.

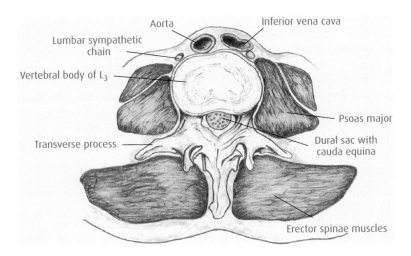

Fig. 2.14 Cross-sectional view at the level of the third lumbar vertebra.

The Lumbar Region at the Level of L₃ (Figure 2.14)

- You may be asked to draw a cross-section of the lumbar area at the level of L_3. Questioning thereafter could include spinal anaesthesia, epidural anaesthesia, lumbar sympathectomy or psoas compartment (lumbar plexus) block.
- Immediately anterior to the *vertebral body* are the *aorta* (on the left) and the *inferior vena cava* (on the right). On the lateral surface on each side lies the *sympathetic trunk*. Immediately lateral to the vertebral body at this level lies the *psoas major* muscle. Further lateral are the lower poles of the *kidney*. Posterior to the vertebral body is the *vertebral canal*, which, at the level of L_3, contains the *theca* (comprising the dura and arachnoid maters), within which are *CSF* and the *cauda equina*. The theca is surrounded by the *epidural space*. This is minimal anteriorly because the dura is closely apposed to the vertebral body. The vertebral arch is completed by the *pedicles, transverse processes, laminae* and *spinous processes*.

The Lower Thoracic Region at the Level of T₁₀ (Figure 2.15)

- You may be shown a CT or MR scan taken through the level of T_{10} and asked to identify the structures.
- Remember that you are effectively looking up at the image, and so the left side of the patient is on the right as you view it. The structures are as identified on the CT image reproduced in Figure 2.15 and show the liver, stomach, spleen and blood vessels.

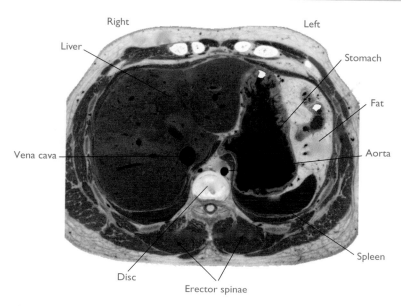

Fig. 2.15 The lower thoracic region at the level of T_{10}.

3

Physiology

Pneumothorax

Commentary

Pneumothorax is an important complication in anaesthesia, trauma and medicine. This oral will concentrate both on the precise mechanisms by which pneumothoraces occur and on details of recognition and treatment. A pneumothorax can develop rapidly into a life-threatening emergency, and so you must ensure that your management is competent.

Core Information

- By definition, a pneumothorax exists when there is air in the pleural space. This is a potential space in the area between the parietal and the visceral layers of the pleura which are usually in close apposition and separated only by a small amount of serous fluid.
- At the end of expiration there is no pressure differential between intra-alveolar and atmospheric pressure. However, the intrapleural, or transpulmonary, pressure is subatmospheric, and the slight negative pressure of around 4–6 cm H_2O (caused by the opposing elastic recoil of the lung and the chest wall) keeps the lungs expanded. This pressure differential also opposes the tendency of the thoracic wall to move outwards.
- When air gains access to the intrapleural space, the negative transpulmonary pressure is lost and the stretched lung collapses while the chest wall moves outwards.
- Air can enter the intrapleural space via a breach in the parietal or visceral pleura (or both), or via the mediastinal pleura as a consequence of intrapulmonary alveolar rupture. Gas insufflated into the abdomen under pressure may also enter the interpleural space via the mediastinal pleura.
- The size of a pneumothorax will increase if the patient is ventilated with positive pressure, or if nitrous oxide is given. (Paramedics routinely carry Entonox to provide

131

analgesia for accident victims.) It will also increase if there is a significant reduction in atmospheric pressure, which has obvious implications for the air evacuation of trauma patients.

Causes of Pleural Breach (Parietal and Visceral)

- **Traumatic:** pneumothorax can follow penetrating injury, rib fracture or blast injury.
- **Iatrogenic (surgical):** it may occur during procedures such as nephrectomy, in spinal surgery, during tracheostomy (especially in children), laparoscopy or as a consequence of oesophageal or mediastinal perforation.
- **Iatrogenic (anaesthetic):** pneumothorax may result from attempted central venous puncture and various nerve blocks. These include supraclavicular, interscalene, intercostal and paravertebral blocks. It may be caused by barotrauma due to mechanical ventilation and from gas injector systems.
- **Miscellaneous:** it may occur if the alveolar septa are weakened, as described in the following, and is associated with many pulmonary diseases, including asthma. There are some bizarre and unusual causes; recurring catamenial pneumothorax, for example, is a spontaneous pneumothorax, usually right-sided, which occurs in phase with the menstrual cycle.

Intrapulmonary Alveolar Rupture

- Gas escapes from the alveolus, dissects towards the hilum and ruptures the mediastinal pleura. Causes include barotrauma from mechanical ventilation (caused by excessive pressures in the context of reduced lung compliance) or high-pressure gas delivery systems (injectors). Patients with chronic obstructive pulmonary disease (COPD) with bullous emphysema are also at risk. It is also caused by blast injury and may occur in asthmatics and in patients in whom the alveolar septa are weakened or distorted by infection, collagen vascular disease or connective tissue disorders, such as Ehlers–Danlos and Marfan's syndromes. Severe hypovolaemia has been implicated as a risk factor for the same reason.

Supplementary Information and Clinical Considerations

Diagnosis of Pneumothorax in the Awake Patient

- Typical features (which are not invariable and which will depend on the size of the pneumothorax and whether it is expanding) include chest pain, referred shoulder tip pain, cough, dyspnoea, tachypnoea and tachycardia. There may be reduced movement of the affected hemithorax, hyperresonance on percussion, diminished breath sounds and decreased vocal fremitus. The coin test (*bruit d'airain* – 'noise of bronze') may be positive, as may Hamman's sign (auscultation reveals a 'crunching' sound of air in the mediastinum which occurs in time with the heartbeat). In the coin test, the tapping of one coin against another placed flat on the chest wall can be heard on auscultation as a ringing sound. These signs are less definitive than chest X-ray which will confirm the clinical diagnosis. If a patient is relatively symptom-free and is managed conservatively, the rate of reabsorption of air from a pneumothorax cavity is slow at up to 2% of the volume of the hemithorax in 24 hours.

- If the pneumothorax is expanding under tension, the clinical features are more dramatic because mediastinal compression by the expanding mass decreases venous return, impairs ventricular function and reduces cardiac output. Patients will complain of dyspnoea; signs include tachypnoea and eventual cyanosis. Cardiovascular compromise will manifest as tachycardia, hypotension and, ultimately, cardiac arrest. There may be tracheal deviation (which is not always easy to identify) and subcutaneous emphysema. Tension pneumothorax can be bilateral. The diagnosis of a tension pneumothorax should never await chest X-ray confirmation.

Diagnosis of Pneumothorax in the Anaesthetized Patient

- Initial signs may be non-specific, with hypotension and tachycardia; others include diminished unilateral chest movement, wheeze, hyperresonance, decreased breath sounds and increased airway pressure. There may be tracheal deviation and elevated central venous pressure (if it is being monitored). Cyanosis, arrhythmias and circulatory collapse may supervene. If the diagnosis is suspected, treatment must not be delayed pending chest X-ray. Ultrasound provides effective diagnosis in experienced hands. The critical care patient with acute respiratory distress syndrome (ARDS) may have a pneumothorax but with little evidence of pulmonary collapse. This is because the non-compliant lung loses the elasticity which would otherwise allow it to collapse away from the chest wall. Pneumothoraces in patients with chronic lung disease may be loculated.

Management of Pneumothorax

- **Management:** discontinue nitrous oxide (in the anaesthetized patient) and give 100% oxygen. Immediate management is decompression via needle thoracocentesis followed rapidly by insertion of a definitive chest drain (intravenous cannulae are too small to provide continued effective decompression). The traditional recommended site is the fourth intercostal space in the mid-axillary line. The British Thoracic Society (BTS) suggests that the drain should be inserted in the so-called safe triangle, which is the area bordered by the lateral border of the pectoralis major muscle, by the anterior border of the latissimus dorsi and by a line superior to the horizontal level of the nipple. Its apex is just below the axilla. The BTS recommend small-size drains for simple pneumothorax (8–14 F), there being no evidence of benefit from larger diameter tubes; however, larger sizes (24–28 F) are recommended for drainage of blood or fluid.
- **Underwater seal drain:** air from the pneumothorax drains under water via a submerged tube in a sealed bottle and is then vented to the atmosphere. The depth of water is important: if it is too shallow, air may be entrained back into the drainage tube; if it is too deep, the pressure may be too great to blow off the pneumothorax gas. The typical depth is 3–5 cm. Clamping a chest drain risks converting a simple pneumothorax to one that is under tension.

Other Air Leaks

- Pneumothorax is the commonest leak from an air-filled space that is seen in anaesthetic practice. Others include subcutaneous emphysema which is formed by air that tracks along tissue planes. It can be seen on X-ray but simple palpation will elicit the characteristic crepitus. The condition can be dramatic, extending up into the tissues of the neck or, in males, down into the scrotum but usually presents no undue threat to the patient. This is also true of pneumomediastinum itself, but not of its underlying causes, which include pharyngeal, oesophageal and gastrointestinal tract perforation. Pneumopericardium in contrast may be associated with cardiac tamponade and the need for immediate pericardiocentesis.

Control of Breathing

Commentary

This question has many potential complexities, but there will be insufficient time to cover these in any detail. The oral is likely to include disorders of respiration, most of which are straightforward.

Core Information

- **Overview:** the control of breathing is coordinated by centres within the central nervous system by receptors in respiratory muscles and the lung, and by specialized chemoreceptors such as the carotid bodies.
- **Respiratory centre:** a brain stem 'respiratory centre' mediates automatic rhythmic breathing, which is influenced by physical and chemical reflexes. Breathing is a complex activity, which can be interrupted by coughing, vomiting, sneezing, hiccoughing and swallowing. It is also subject to voluntary control from the cerebral cortex to allow activities such as singing, reading (during which the cortex computes the appropriate size of breath for the proposed segment), speech and vigorous exercise, during which expiration may be almost entirely an active process.
- **Inputs:** the 'centre' is in the medulla, where the respiratory pattern is generated and where the voluntary and involuntary impulses are coordinated. It contains receptors for excitatory neurotransmitters such as glutamate (whose activity is inhibited by opioids) and inhibitory neurotransmitters such as gamma-aminobutyric acid (GABA) and glycine. The centre receives a large number of afferents from the cortex, the vagus, the hypothalamus and the pons. An area in the upper pons, the pontine respiratory group (formerly known as the pneumotaxic centre), contributes to fine control of respiratory rhythm by influencing the medullary neurons, which comprise two main groups.
- **Dorsal respiratory neurons:** these are primarily inspiratory and are responsible for the basic ventilatory rhythm.
- **Ventral neurons:** these are predominantly expiratory.
- **Reciprocal innervation:** as activity increases in one or other of these groups of neurons, so inhibitory impulses are relayed from the other, resulting eventually in the reversal of the respiratory phase.
- **Central chemoreceptors:** these lie on the anterolateral surface of the medulla, and are acutely sensitive to alterations in H^+ ion concentration. A rise in $PaCO_2$ increases

CSF PCO_2, cerebral tissue PCO_2 and jugular venous PCO_2 (which all exceed $PaCO_2$ by about 1.3 kPa or 10 mmHg). This rise in CSF PCO_2 decreases CSF pH. The acidosis stimulates chemosensitive areas by a mechanism not yet fully explained. Respiratory acidosis stimulates greater ventilatory change than metabolic acidosis despite the same blood–pH, because the blood/brain barrier is permeable to CO_2 but not to H^+ ions. Over a period of hours this CSF acidosis is corrected by the bicarbonate shift.

- **Peripheral chemoreceptors:** these are located in the carotid bodies, which are small structures with a volume of only around 6 mm^3, which are found close to the bifurcation of the common carotid artery and in the aortic bodies along the aortic arch. Afferents from the carotid bodies travel via the glossopharyngeal nerve, and those from the aortic bodies travel via the vagus. These are sensitive primarily to hypoxia but, as sensors of arterial gas partial pressures, are less sensitive to a decline in oxygen content. This means that they mediate minimal respiratory stimulation in patients who are anaemic, or when there is carboxyhaemoglobinaemia. Their response time is of the order of 1–3 seconds. They are stimulated minimally by an increased CO_2. Acidaemia stimulates respiration, regardless of whether its cause is metabolic or respiratory. This rapid response is mediated via the peripheral chemo-receptors. Pyrexia is another stimulus mediated via the peripheral chemoreceptors, and which also enhances the responses to hypercapnia and hypoxia. Hypoperfusion is also a stimulant, presumably due to 'stagnant' hypoxia. Peripheral chemoreceptor stimulation may also mediate increases in bronchiolar tone, adrenal secretion, hypertension and bradycardia. Aortic body stimulation has a proportionately greater effect on the circulation. (The nerves to the carotid bodies may be lost during carotid endarterectomy. The subsequent loss of hypoxic ventilatory drive is not usually significant.)
- **Mechanoreceptors:** mechanical as well as chemical stimulation of pulmonary receptors leads to afferent input to the respiratory centre by the vagus nerve. Their importance remains contentious, as patients with denervated transplanted lungs or with (experimental) bilateral vagal block demonstrate normal ventilatory patterns. The inflation reflex comprises the inhibition of inspiration in response to an increased transmural pressure gradient with sustained inflation. In the deflation reflex, inspiration is augmented via a reflex excitatory effect in response to the decrease in lung volume.

Supplementary and Clinical Information

Disorders of Respiration Seen in Anaesthesia and Critical Care

- **Apnoea and hypoventilation:** common primary causes include anaesthetic drugs such as opioids, neuromuscular blockers and inhalational agents. Hypocapnia will suppress respiratory drive, as will profound hypercapnia. It may follow hypoxic or traumatic brain injury and occurs in patients with type 2 respiratory failure who rely on hypoxaemic drive for respiration and who have been given supplemental oxygen (>24%). Primary alveolar hypoventilation syndrome (Ondine's curse) is a rare disorder that is characterized by the loss of automatic respiration. Breathing becomes a voluntary activity and ceases when patients either stop concentrating or fall asleep.

- **Hyperventilation:** in the anaesthetized patient this may reflect inadequate anaesthesia or analgesia. It will occur in response to a rising CO_2 due to rebreathing. Rare causes include malignant hyperpyrexia, of which hyperventilation is a cardinal sign, and pontine haemorrhage. In the non-anaesthetized patient it may be due to pain or anxiety. Kussmaul respiration ('air hunger') is a form of hyperventilation characterized by increased tidal volume and reduced respiratory frequency. Typically it accompanies severe metabolic acidosis.

- **Abnormal respiratory patterns:** Cheyne–Stokes respiration (periodic breathing) is characterized by sequential increases and decreases in tidal volume interspersed with periods of apnoea. It is associated with conditions such as stroke, hypoxia, cardiac failure and altitude sickness, and appears to be caused by the failure of the respiratory centre to compensate rapidly enough for changes in PaO_2 and $PaCO_2$. Kussmaul respiration is described previously under Hyperventilation. 'Fish-mouth' breathing occurs typically when a patient with chronic obstructive airways disease breathes out through pursed lips, thereby generating enough positive-end expiratory pressure (PEEP) to keep alveoli open. 'Grunting' respiration in neonates is another example of the same phenomenon.

- **Obstructive sleep apnoea (OSA):** obstructive sleep apnoea is not strictly a state of apnoea, which is defined strictly as the 'suspension of respiration without movement of respiratory muscles', but the terminology is too well established to challenge. There are a number of different predisposing conditions (including adenotonsillar hypertrophy in children), but the classic patient is an obese and sedentary middle-aged male with a neck circumference greater than 40 cm (which is a better indicator than raised body mass index alone). 'STOP-BANG' is both a mnemonic and a questionnaire which predicts risk. Three of more of the following predict a high risk of OSA: (**S** – snoring; **T** – daytime somnolence (tired); **O** – obstructive episodes observed; **P** – raised blood pressure; **B** – body mass index >35 kg m^{-2}; **A** – age >50 years; **N** – neck circumference >40 cm; **G** – male gender. Directly associated morbidity includes ischaemic heart disease, cerebrovascular events and venous thromboembolism. Also well-recognized are cognitive impairment secondary to irreversible changes in intracerebral grey matter, and disordered endocrine function. This includes impaired glucose metabolism and a disruption of the normal circadian activity of the hypothalamic-pituitary-adrenal axis. Such patients presenting for elective surgery are therefore at risk of predictable complications and are particularly sensitive to the sedative effects of anaesthetic and analgesic drugs. Wherever possible, surgery should be deferred until a combination of controlled weight loss and nocturnal airway support (CPAP) improves symptoms. Patients who require emergency surgery should be managed with regional anaesthetic techniques or local anaesthetic supplementation where this is practicable, and if general anaesthesia is unavoidable, with the use of short-acting agents. This may not always be possible because clearly patients cannot be denied analgesia after surgery, and so they should be cared for in a high-dependency area with the continued use of CPAP.

Ventilation Response Curves Following Changes in $PaCO_2$ and PaO_2

- **$PaCO_2$/ventilation response curve** (Figure 3.1). In response to an increase in $PaCO_2$ there is an increase in respiratory rate and depth. This response is linear over the range of usual clinical values, although the slope varies. There is inter-individual variation, and the slope is also altered by disease, drugs and hormonal changes. The minute volume for a given increase in $PaCO_2$ is influenced by the PaO_2, so that a lower PaO_2 shifts the line up and to the left, leading to a greater increase in minute ventilation.

- **PaO_2/ventilation response curve** (Figure 3.2). This curve is a rectangular hyperbola, asymptotic to the ventilation at high PaO_2 (when there is zero hypoxic drive) and to the PaO_2 at which theoretically ventilation becomes infinite at around 4.3 kPa. (The response is easier to gauge if it is linear, and a graph of ventilation plotted against oxygen saturation is linear down to about 70%.)

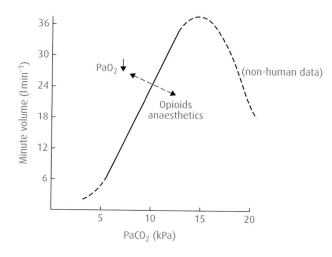

Fig. 3.1 $PaCO_2$/ventilation response curve.

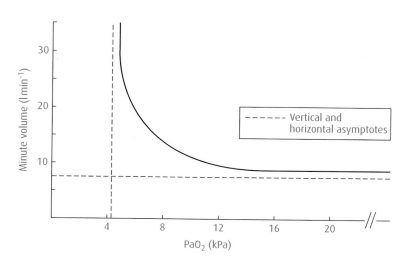

Fig. 3.2 PaO_2/ventilation response curve.

The Influence of Anaesthesia on These Mechanisms

- **Anaesthetics:** all anaesthetic agents have a depressant effect on the initial ventilatory response to hypoxia by the peripheral chemoreceptors. They also depress the response to increases in $PaCO_2$ (shifting the line of the CO_2 response curve down and to the right).
- **Hypoxia:** hypoxia has a direct depressant effect on the respiratory centre. Should the medulla be subjected to severe ischaemic or hypoxic hypoxia, then apnoea will result.
- **Opioids:** these exert a powerful central respiratory depressant action at the medulla.
- **Respiratory stimulants:** drugs such as **doxapram** and **almitrine** act at peripheral carotid chemoreceptors. The exact mechanism of action remains unclear, but doxapram is thought to inhibit potassium channels (subfamilies 3 and 9). **Progesterone** is also a potent respiratory stimulant and acts on nuclear receptors in the carotid body and in brainstem respiratory nuclei. (It was once quite commonly used in critical care, but has long since lost its popularity in this context.)

Apnoea and Hypoventilation

Commentary

Questions about breathing and gas exchange can come from different angles, and so you may be asked what happens during apnoea (either obstructed or non-obstructed) and about the consequences of hypoventilation. Neither of these patterns of respiration is uncommon in anaesthetic practice, and so you will be expected to explain them with some clarity.

Core Information

Arterial blood gases during apnoea.

PaO$_2$

- **Obstructed apnoea:** the basal requirement for oxygen is around 250 ml min^{-1}. The functional residual capacity (FRC) in an adult is about 2,000–2,500 ml (21% of which is oxygen). Under normal circumstances therefore, if a patient obstructs when breathing air, the oxygen reserves will be exhausted in about 2 minutes, and the partial pressure will fall from the normal 13 kPa down to about 5 kPa. The lung volume also falls, by the difference between the O_2 uptake and CO_2 output (which ceases). Pre-oxygenation increases the reserves substantially, which is the rationale behind this routine anaesthetic technique.
- **Non-obstructed apnoea:** if the airway is patent, the lung volume does not fall because ambient gas is drawn into the lungs by mass movement down the trachea. If the ambient gas is room air, then hypoxia will occur almost as swiftly as it does in obstructed apnoea. If, however, the ambient gas is 100% oxygen then it can be calculated (according to the eminent anaesthetic respiratory physiologist Professor J.F. Nunn) that in theory it will take 100 minutes before hypoxia will supervene.

(This assumes that the patient has effectively been pre-oxygenated by breathing 100% oxygen prior to becoming apnoeic.)

- **Rate of oxygen desaturation:** this depends on the alveolar oxygen (P_AO_2), the FRC and the oxygen consumption.
  — **Oxygen reserves:** these are mainly in the alveoli. The circulating oxygen is sufficient to maintain metabolism for only 2–3 minutes, and there is no real 'storage' capacity. Efficient pre-oxygenation (either for 3–5 minutes or with three vital capacity breaths) will replace alveolar air with 100% oxygen. If nitrogen washout has been completed, then 8–10 minutes may elapse before desaturation starts to take place.
  — **Lung volume:** the volume of the FRC decreases in pregnancy, in the obese and with some forms of pulmonary disease. FRC is decreased or is exceeded by closing capacity in children up to the age of 6 years and adults (in the supine position) over the age of 44 years.
  — **Oxygen consumption:** this is increased by any rise in metabolic rate such as is seen in children, in pregnancy, thyroid disease, sepsis and pyrexia. It is decreased by hypothermia, myxoedema and a range of drugs, including anaesthetic agents.

PaCO$_2$

- **PaCO$_2$:** during apnoea, CO_2 elimination stops and arterial CO_2 rises at a rate of between 0.4 and 0.8 kPa min^{-1}. (In patients in whom the metabolic rate may be low, as in a patient undergoing tests for brain stem death, this rate of rise may be much slower.) The body stores of CO_2 total around 120 litres (compared with 1.5 litres of oxygen). In non-obstructed apnoea the CO_2 still rises, because elimination via convection or diffusion is opposed by the mass inward movement of ambient gas.
- This rise in PaCO$_2$ is inevitable and, should it reach too high a level, will lead to a respiratory acidosis and start to exert negative inotropic effects on the myocardium (at around 9–10 kPa). It also influences cerebral blood flow, which increases in a linear fashion by around 7.5 ml 100g^{-1} min^{-1} for each 1 kPa rise from baseline, to maximal at 10.5 kPa, above which no further vasodilatation is possible (see Figure 3.11). Carbon dioxide narcosis will occur at a PaCO$_2$ of around 12 kPa in nonhabituated individuals.
- **Effect on oxygenation:** as the PaCO$_2$ and P_ACO_2 rise, the P_AO_2 falls by an amount that can be quantified by the alveolar gas equation, which states that the $P_AO_2 = P_IO_2 - P_ACO_2/RQ$ where RQ is the respiratory quotient. (The P_IO_2 is obtained by multiplying the inspired oxygen fraction [F_IO_2] by the atmospheric pressure [BPatm] and subtracting the saturated vapour pressure of water [SVP H_2O], 47 mmHg or 6.3 kPa [$P_IO_2 = F_IO_2 \times BPatm - SVP\ H_2O$.]) This means that if a patient who is breathing room air has a P_ACO_2 of 12 kPa, their P_AO_2 will fall to only 5 kPa.

Supplementary Information and Clinical Considerations

- **Apnoeic oxygenation:** this technique is used during the apnoea test for brain stem death testing, when PaCO$_2$ must rise to 6.6 kPa or above. Oxygenation can be achieved by simple insufflation. It can also be used during airway endoscopy and at critical points of complex upper airway surgery.

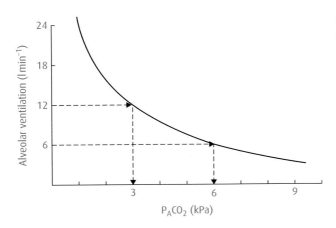

Fig. 3.3 Relationship of alveolar ventilation to P_ACO_2.

Hypoventilation

- The relations of alveolar gas tensions to alveolar ventilation are described by rect-angular hyperbolas (concave upwards for eliminated gases such as CO_2 and concave downwards for gases that are taken up by the lung, such as O_2).
- In the case of the P_ACO_2 this relationship (which is given by the equation $P_ACO_2 = CO_2$ output/alveolar ventilation) means that if the alveolar ventilation halves the P_ACO_2 will double (Figure 3.3). The alveolar air equation makes it inevitable that a hypoventilating patient who is breathing air will become hypoxic. Oxygen enrich-ment to 30% will increase the P_AO_2 by almost 9 kPa, thereby restoring it almost to normal (while having no effect on the P_ACO_2). This can mask ventilatory failure because supplemental oxygen will ensure that oxygen saturations remain high even in the presence of a high P_ACO_2.

Post-Operative Apnoea

- Potential causes of postoperative apnoea are straightforward and include persistent narcosis secondary to opioid administration, residual neuromuscular blockade, hypo-capnia and severe hypercapnia with CO_2 narcosis. Causes that you would never want to encounter are cardiac arrest and an intracerebral catastrophe such as acute haemorrhage.

Compliance

Commentary

Compliance is an important concept with obvious implications for ventilatory management of patients, and this particular oral should divide quite evenly between the basic science and its clinical application. It will probably be linked with a discussion of management of a patient with deteriorating respiratory function (see under 'The Failing Lung'). It will help if you are able to draw a typical pressure–volume curve (see Figure 3.4).

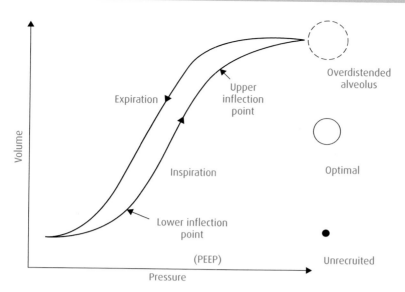

Fig. 3.4 Pulmonary pressure–volume curve.

Core Information

- **Definition:** compliance is defined by the change in lung volume per unit change in pressure. It has two components: the compliance of the lung itself and the compliance of the chest wall. Lung compliance is determined both by the elastic properties of pulmonary connective tissue and by the surface tension at the fluid–air interface within alveoli. Both normal lung compliance and normal chest wall compliance are 1.5–$2.0\,l\,kPa^{-1}$ (150–200 ml cmH_2O^{-1}). Total compliance is about $1.0\,l\,kPa^{-1}$ (100 ml cmH_2O^{-1}), and is determined from the sum of the reciprocals of the two values.
- **Static compliance:** a pressure–volume curve is obtained by applying distending pressures to the lung and measuring the increase in lung volume. The measurements are made when there is no gas flow. (The patient expires in measured increments and the intrapleural pressure at each step is estimated via oesophageal pressure.)
- **Dynamic compliance:** a pressure–volume curve is plotted continuously throughout the respiratory cycle.
- **P–V curves:** pressure–volume curves are useful, but they may oversimplify what is happening in the lung. In particular, accurate dynamic compliance curves can be difficult to generate in diseased lungs. The final curve also represents the total rather than the separate lung units, whose individual compliance may be very different. In ARDS about a third of the lung may remain normal. The curve can be used to set PEEP and to control ventilation.
- **Hysteresis:** the inspiratory and expiratory pressure–volume curves are not identical, which gives rise to a hysteresis loop. Hysteresis describes the process in which a measurement (or electrical signal) differs according to whether the value is rising or falling. It usually implies absorption of energy, for example due to friction, as in this case. The area of the hysteresis loop represents the energy lost as elastic tissues stretch and then recoil (viscous losses) and as airway resistance is overcome (frictional losses).

- **Specific compliance:** compliance is related to lung volume, and this potential distortion can be removed by using specific compliance, which is defined as compliance divided by the FRC. This correction for different lung volumes demonstrates, for instance, that the lungs of a healthy neonate have the same specific compliance as those of a healthy adult.
- **Factors which alter compliance:** ARDS and pulmonary oedema decrease respiratory compliance by reducing lung compliance. Restrictive conditions such as ankylosing spondylitis or circumferential thoracic burns reduce it by decreasing the compliance of the chest wall. Compliance is also decreased if the FRC is either higher or lower than normal. At high lung volumes, tissues are stretched to near their elastic limit, whereas at low volumes greater pressures are required to recruit alveoli. In acute asthma, therefore, patients are ventilating at a high FRC, at which the compliance is lower and the work of breathing correspondingly greater. Compliance is also affected by posture, being maximal in the standing position. Obesity may reduce compliance both via a reduction in FRC and a decrease in chest wall compliance due to the cuirass of adipose tissue. Age has no influence.

Supplementary Information and Clinical Considerations

Intermittent positive pressure ventilation (IPPV) and decreased compliance.

- **Constant-pressure generators:** these ventilators generate an increase in airway pressure which produces inspiratory flow whose rate depends on the compliance and resistance of the whole system (patient and breathing circuit). The sudden initial mouth–alveoli pressure gradient produces high flow into the lungs, which then decreases exponentially as the lungs fill and the gradient narrows. In lungs with low compliance, the alveolar pressure increases much more rapidly, the pressure differential reduces and inspiratory flow declines.
- **Constant-flow generators:** these ventilators produce an incremental increase in flow rate to generate a tidal volume that is a product of the flow rate and the inspiratory time. The pressure of the driving source is much greater than that in the airways, and so flow into the lungs is not affected by sudden decreases in pulmonary compliance or increases in airway resistance. The delivery of an unchanged tidal volume in the face of decreased compliance will be associated with a more rapid increase in alveolar pressure and a higher airways pressure.
- **Acute lung injury:** anaesthetic interest in compliance relates particularly to the ventilatory management of patients with acute lung disease, particularly with severely reduced compliance as seen typically in ARDS.

The Failing Lung

Commentary

This is a question about the underlying theory of what has now become the routine management of patients whose respiratory function is deteriorating because of acute lung injury (ALI) and ARDS. There has been considerable research effort aimed at providing an evidence base for lung-protective strategies, and what follows is an abbreviated synthesis. It should nonetheless allow you to give a convincing overview of the main principles. The ARDS network has probably produced the most influential studies, but the structure of the oral is unlikely to allow a detailed discussion of this research (some aspects of which have been criticized, as described in the following).

Core Information

Principles of Ventilation in the Critically Ill

- **Conventional ventilation:** traditional methods of ventilating patients with ALI maximized oxygenation by using normal tidal volumes (10–12 ml kg^{-1}), which in non-compliant lungs were associated with very high peak and plateau airways pressures. The ventilatory mode was usually volume-controlled with synchronized intermittent mandatory ventilation (SIMV). A major concern was barotrauma. It has more recently become apparent that barotrauma is much less of a problem than *volutrauma* (caused by over distension of the lung), *atelectrauma* (owing to cyclical shearing forces generated by alveoli closing and reopening), and *biotrauma* (so-called because of surfactant reduction and cytokine release in response to this repetitive injury).
- **'Lung-protective' ventilation:** it has now become standard practice to try to minimize ventilator-associated lung injury (VALI) by using 'lung-protective' ventilation in which plateau airways pressures are limited to 30 cmH$_2$O by means of much reduced tidal volumes, typically of 6 ml kg^{-1}. There are two consequences of this technique: the minute ventilation may be insufficient for adequate removal of CO$_2$, and low tidal volumes will predispose to closure of alveoli and gas trapping. The first problem is dealt with by allowing the PaCO$_2$ to rise: this is 'permissive hypercapnia'. The second is addressed by adding PEEP to maximize the recruitment of alveoli.
- **Permissive hypercapnia:** this is a key part of current ventilatory strategies, and there are experimental data to suggest that it is safe (up to a PaCO$_2$ of ~9.0 kPa and pH of ~7.2) and that it might confer some protection in the context of lung injury and associated systemic organ damage. Hypercapnic acidosis (as opposed to metabolic acidosis) appears to attenuate VALI, particularly that associated with volutrauma rather than atelectrauma. It also has some myocardial protective effects, and although a PaCO$_2$ of >10 kPa does depress myocardial contractility, cardiac output can still increase as a result of a decrease in systemic vascular resistance. In other tissues, hypercapnic acidosis attenuates reperfusion brain injury and delays hepatocyte cell death. In addition, it appears to modify some key components of the inflammatory response (such as TNFα and IL-1). It reduces lung neutrophil recruitment as well as free radical production and oxidant tissue injury. In particular, hypercapnic acidosis attenuates damage mediated by xanthine oxidase, a complex enzyme system whose production is increased during periods of tissue injury and which is a potent source of free radicals in the lung. However, its anti-inflammatory properties may also limit the host response to live bacterial pathogens, because free radical production is also central to the bactericidal activity of neutrophils and macrophages. This may be problematic with ongoing bacterial sepsis.

- **Positive end-expiratory pressure (PEEP):** although PEEP increases airways pressures and may contribute to a fall in cardiac output, most clinicians consider it essential for alveolar recruitment and prevention of atelectrauma. It does not appear that outcomes are influenced by the use of 'high' (~13 cmH$_2$O) rather than 'low' PEEP (~8 cmH$_2$O). Typically PEEP is set at 5–10 cmH$_2$O, but ideally this should be done with reference to the static pressure–volume curve (Figure 3.4). The upper inflection point represents probable encroachment on total lung capacity, and so the distending pressure should be kept below this point to avoid overexpansion. The lower inflection point is where small airways and alveoli open (and is effectively the closing volume), and the inflation pressure should be just above this point to avoid de-recruitment of alveoli. Pressure-controlled ventilation on the steep linear part of the curve midway between the two points reduces the peak airway pressure for a given mean airway pressure and minimizes intrinsic PEEP. In practice, however, although modern ventilators will produce pressure–volume curves, the inflection points are often difficult to identify.

Supplementary Information and Clinical Considerations

Other strategies to improve gas exchange in the critically ill.

- **High frequency ventilation:** ventilation at very high rates with low tidal volumes is theoretically 'lung-protective'. High frequency jet ventilation (HFJV) uses rates of between 60 and 300 min^{-1}, while high frequency oscillation (HFO) uses still higher rates of 300–1800 min^{-1}. HFJV is used for the management of ARDS in some units and can be useful in differential lung ventilation (via a double-lumen tube) and in patients with bronchopleural fistulae. HFO, in which there is considerable experience in children, is probably used more widely. HFO applies a constant mean airway pressure which prevents alveolar de-recruitment and minimizes peak pressures. The OSCILLATE trial, however, terminated early because of higher mortality in the group receiving high frequency oscillatory ventilation (47% v 35%). (This was a multicentre trial which randomized 548 patients with ARDS to conventional or oscillatory ventilation.) (*NEMJ* 2013, 368: 795–805.) That HFOV conferred no benefit was also suggested by the OSCAR trial (HF **Osc**illation in **AR**DS) which randomized 795 patients to the same two treatments and which found no differences between them (*NEJM* 2013, 368: 806–13). Proponents of HFOV still maintain that it may be of benefit if used early and in some subsets of patients; further studies are necessary to confirm whether such arguments are valid.
- **Prone ventilation:** the practice waxes and wanes in popularity, but meta-analyses of the numerous trials that have been performed suggest that in patients with severe ARDS, it confers a survival benefit of around 10%, and that in most, although not all patients, the PaO$_2$ will improve. Any positive response is usually observed within the first hour. Prone ventilation reduces shunt and improves oxygenation by mechanisms which are thought to include better distribution of ventilation to previously dependent areas of lung, perfusion of less oedematous areas of lung, a rise in end-expiratory volume and an increase in diaphragmatic excursion. These improvements, however, are not explained by the traditional gravitational theories of improved perfusion of dependent areas and are thought to relate more to the geometry of

the pulmonary airways and vasculature. This is discussed in more detail under 'The Prone Position in Anaesthesia'.

- **Inverse ratio ventilation:** changing the I:E ratio from 1:2 to 2:1 or even 3:1 will increase the inspiratory time sufficiently to allow ventilation of lung units with prolonged time constants. In effect, this may just be a way of increasing PEEP.
- **Airway Pressure Release Ventilation (APRV):** This is a technique that provides continuous positive airway pressure (CPAP) with a brief release of minimal duration. In effect it is inverse ratio, pressure controlled, intermittent mandatory ventilation throughout which the patient is able to breathe spontaneously. It is a means of providing 'open lung' ventilation. Two levels of PEEP, high and low, are set, with the time spent in high PEEP set, for example, at around 4.5–6.0 seconds and in low PEEP at a brief 0.5–0.8 seconds. The airway pressure release time is usually set at around 1 time constant (the time that it takes to empty 63% of the lung volume). As complete emptying requires 4 time constants, this short release time results in a degree of auto PEEP which further reduces alveolar collapse. The technique recruits alveoli and improves oxygenation while allowing spontaneous ventilation, but this may be at the expense of increased transpulmonary pressure, elevated work of breathing and the risk of dynamic hyperinflation. Although APRV improves oxygenation, there is no evidence to show that it improves mortality in ARDS because there have been no defined standard settings, not least because the time constants referred to previously will vary substantially according to the degree of acute lung injury.
- **Nitric oxide (NO):** inhaled NO is delivered to better-recruited alveoli where it dilates the associated pulmonary vessels and reduces shunt fraction. It improves oxygenation, but no study has established that this is mirrored by better outcomes.
- **Miscellaneous:** these include nebulized prostacyclin PGI_2 (less effective than NO in improving oxygenation), artificial recombinant protein C-based surfactant (evidence is awaited of its benefit in adult patients), partial liquid ventilation with perfluorocarbons which preferentially fill and recruit dependent atelectatic areas of lung (there is no evidence as yet of improved outcomes), and interventional lung assist membrane ventilator devices (such as the Novalung).
- **Extracorporeal membrane oxygenation (ECMO):** the indications for ECMO have widened from its use in neonates with respiratory distress syndrome to adults who require respiratory support and to those who need cardiorespiratory support after, for example, acute myocardial infarction. Evidence suggests that ECMO for respiratory support is safe, but its efficacy has not been established. It was hoped that the CESAR trial would do so (*Lancet* 2009, 374: 1351–630), but because ECMO was carried out in a single centre after referral from hospitals which in contrast had very heterogeneous management strategies, the interpretation of the results was equivocal. There are, however, data from the Extracorporeal Life Support Organization registry which indicate that the recent survival rate for patients with ARDS and treated with ECMO is 60–70%. The technique is relatively straightforward. Venovenous ECMO is appropriate for patients who do not need cardiac assistance, and involves passing desaturated blood from the vena cava through a membrane oxygenator across which gas exchange can take place. Venoarterial ECMO is used if myocardial support is also necessary.

Bronchomotor Tone (Asthma)

Commentary

This is another topic that is central to anaesthesia but with a basic science component that is relatively well circumscribed. Much of the oral therefore should feel clinically relevant.

Core Information

Changes in bronchial smooth muscle tone are mediated via the autonomic nervous system.

- **Parasympathetic:** this is dominant in the control of airway smooth muscle tone. Vagal stimulation of muscarinic cholinergic receptors causes bronchoconstriction, mucus secretion and vasodilatation of bronchial vessels. Increases in bronchial smooth muscle tone are mediated via the second messenger cyclic GMP under parasympathetic control.
- **Sympathetic:** sympathetic efferent nerves may control vasomotor tone, but there is no direct sympathetic innervation of bronchial smooth muscle, despite the fact that β_2-adrenoceptors are abundantly expressed on human airway smooth muscle and their stimulation leads to bronchodilatation. Smooth muscle fibre relaxation occurs via the production of cyclic AMP and the activation of myosin light chain kinase.
- **Non-adrenergic non-cholinergic (NANC) nerves:** the only neural bronchodilator pathways may be those of the inhibitory NANC nerves which contain nitric oxide and vasoactive intestinal polypeptide. In addition, there are excitatory NANC nerves which cause bronchoconstriction, vasodilatation, mucus secretion and vascular hyperpermeability.
- **Drugs:** β_2-agonists such as salbutamol, terbutaline and adrenaline cause bronchodilatation by increasing cAMP formation. Phosphodiesterase (PDE) inhibitors such as theophyllines do not inhibit intracellular PDE at therapeutic doses, and their mechanisms of action remain speculative. Antimuscarinic drugs such as ipratropium antagonize cholinergic receptors. (This is non-specific antagonism of M_1–M_5 receptors.)

Supplementary Information and Clinical Considerations

Assessment of Acute Severe Asthma

- **Criteria for ventilatory support:** in essence this is a clinical decision rather than one based on numerical criteria such as measurements of peak expiratory flow rate (PEFR) and arterial blood gases. These are particularly useful in quantifying the response to treatment but should not represent the main criteria for ventilation.
- **Clinical features:** the patient with severe acute asthma is unable to talk in sentences and uses all the accessory muscles of ventilation. Their respiratory rate will be high (>25 min^{-1}), as will the heart rate (>100 min^{-1}). Oxygenation is usually maintained and the $PaCO_2$ is low. A normal $PaCO_2$ is ominous. The PEFR may be between 33% and 50% either of predicted or of the patient's recent best effort. Pulsus paradoxus

(in which the arterial pressure changes in response to the large intrathoracic pressure swings) is no longer regarded as a useful sign. Life-threatening asthma is characterized by exhaustion, failing respiratory effort, a silent chest and sometimes confusion. Patients may be bradycardic, hypotensive and mentally obtunded. PEFR is below 33% of predicted, SpO_2 is less than 92% and the $PaCO_2$ is elevated. At SpO_2 above 92% patients are unlikely to be hypercapnic.

Management

The most recent national clinical guideline from the British Thoracic Society and the Scottish Intercollegiate Guideline Group (BTS/SIGN) was published in September 2016. Interestingly, the document stressed that it should be seen to represent a standard of care, and included the comment that 'guideline recommendations . . . should not be construed as including all proper methods of care or excluding other methods of care aimed at the same result'. With that caveat in mind, their recommendations for the management of acute asthma do encompass some of the following.

- **Treatment of bronchoconstriction:** this consists of humidified oxygen at flow rates to maintain an oxygen saturation of 94% or greater, nebulized salbutamol 5.0 mg or terbutaline 2.5 mg, and ipratropium 0.5 mg (both via an oxygen-driven device). Nebulized adrenaline is not superior to salbutamol or terbutaline. A single dose of magnesium sulphate 1.2–2.0 g infused over 20 minutes may improve lung function in the acute short term, but the BTS is cautious about recommending its routine use, both because of the absence of robust evidence and because of concerns about toxicity. Hydrocortisone 100 mg or other corticosteroids will also have been given. The use of aminophylline is contentious; there is no firm evidence of additional benefit, although a 5 mg kg^{-1} loading dose and infusion of around 0.5 mg kg^{-1} h^{-1} may improve symptoms in a subgroup of patients whose response to other therapies has been poor. The use of heliox (helium/oxygen mixtures in ratios of 80:20 or 70:30) is also not recommended, although the guideline acknowledges that in patients with severe obstruction there is the possibility of benefit. Similarly, it acknowledges that while ketamine is a potent bronchodilator, prospective trials are needed to confirm its value in the context of acute severe asthma. Critical care physicians are usually a bit less timorous, and ketamine is frequently administered to patients with refractory asthma (0.5–2.0 mg kg^{-1} hr^{-1}). The value of intravenous leukotriene receptor antagonists also awaits further studies according to BTS/SIGN, and there is no parenteral preparation available in the British National Formulary. Nonetheless, their mechanism of action suggests that they might be of benefit. Volatile anaesthetics are also sometimes used in difficult cases in which other treatment options have been exhausted.
- **Treatment of respiratory failure:** non-invasive ventilation has not yet established a place in management, and there is insufficient evidence to support the use of helium–oxygen mixtures. Patients will need general anaesthesia, administered cautiously because of the sudden loss of adrenergic stimulation. Traditional teaching has always held that these patients are dehydrated and need fluid resuscitation. The risk may have been exaggerated; there is some evidence, in children at least, that acute asthma attacks are accompanied by ADH release, and so hypovolaemia may be less of a danger. Ventilation can be problematic. Airways resistance is high, and lung

compliance is reduced by over distension. High inflation pressures are almost inevitable and may lead to barotrauma. The distribution of ventilation in asthmatics is uneven, and high inflation pressures may be directed preferentially to relatively unobstructed bronchi. It is important to maximize expiration, if necessary by adjusting the ventilatory pattern, including the I:E ratio, so as to prevent further distension. It may be impossible to ensure minute ventilation that will clear CO_2, and so permissive hypercapnia may be necessary. It may even be desirable, because hyperventilation to reduce $PaCO_2$ can be associated with a substantial acute reduction in cardiac output.

- **Wheeze:** the classic auscultatory sounds of asthma, rhonchi, are musical but they are not actually generated by simple airway narrowing as is usually assumed. The noise is actually generated by the apposition of the bronchial walls, which vibrate together in response to airflow and act in effect like the reed of a wind instrument. It is the multiple different dimensions of the bronchi and bronchioles that make the sounds polyphonic. This is of clinical relevance because it suggests that any persistent wheeze means that the calibre of at least some of the airways has narrowed substantially to the point at which the airway transiently is almost closed.

Smoking and Anaesthesia

Commentary

The numbers of users of tobacco products in the UK has fallen, but some 20% of adults in the UK still smoke regularly and therefore put themselves at increased risk of a long list of conditions that may require surgery. These include pulmonary, bladder and gastrointestinal malignancy as well as peripheral vascular and coronary heart disease. Smoking also increases postoperative morbidity and worsens surgical outcomes. Anaesthetists are unlikely to influence those factors significantly, but they do need to be aware of the chronic and acute effects, and to mitigate these where possible.

Core Information

- **Diseases associated with smoking:** the chronic problems are well known and include obstructive pulmonary disease, coronary heart disease, hypertension, cerebrovascular disease and an increased risk of malignancies in several systems. Its only benefits appear to be a reduction in the risk of pre-eclampsia in pregnancy and a lower incidence in smokers of postoperative nausea and vomiting.
- **Nicotine:** this is a potent toxin with an LD_{50} in adults as low as 30–60 mg (one cigarette contains as much as 10 mg, but much of this is destroyed in combustion). It acts directly on receptors at ganglia, indirectly on chromaffin cells via catecholamine release and on excitatory nicotinic receptors within the central nervous systems. Dopaminergic stimulation inputs the 'reward' centre in the hypothalamus, elevates mood and establishes a cycle of dependence. (There is some evidence that smoking alters the cytochrome P450 CYP2A6 gene and can lead to inherited dependence to

nicotine.) The immediate physical effects are familiar: sympathetic stimulation leads to tachycardia and hypertension, decreased cutaneous blood flow and coronary arterial vasoconstriction. At a cellular level, nicotine increases the formation of reactive oxygen species with lipid peroxidation, and accelerates neuronal apoptosis. It reaches the brain within 10–20 seconds of inhalation and has a half-life of 1–2 hours. One of its metabolites, cotinine, is pharmacologically active and has a much longer half-life of 20 hours.

- **Carbon monoxide (CO):** cigarette smokers can have carbon monoxide (CO) concentrations of 10% and sometimes higher (in non-smokers <1.5%) at which level the physiological effects are significant. CO affinity for haemoglobin is 250 times that of oxygen, and it also shifts the oxygen–haemoglobin dissociation curve to the left with direct implications for oxygen delivery to the tissues. It inhibits cytochrome oxidase (required for mitochondrial ATP synthesis) and also forms carboxymyoglobin to the detriment of myocardial performance. It is also a cellular toxin, which appears to inhibit cellular respiration via cytochrome A_3, as well as impairing the function of neutrophils.

- **Hydrocarbons and toxic metabolites:** cigarette smoke contains at least 4,000 compounds, including polycyclic aromatic hydrocarbons, aldehydes, nitrogen oxides, metals and hydrogen cyanide. This diverse chemical array acts as a potent inducer of the enzyme cytochrome P450 CYP1A2 which also metabolizes many commonly prescribed drugs. It is this enzyme induction that is believed to confer some protection against postoperative nausea and vomiting in smokers.

- **Pathophysiology of chronic smoking:** the list of smoking-related health complications is a familiar one. Patients are at greater risk of numerous forms of malignancy, including lung (more women in the USA die from lung cancer than from breast cancer), larynx, oropharynx, oesophagus, bladder and cervix. Coronary artery disease, peripheral vascular disease and cerebrovascular disease occur much more commonly (fourfold), and some degree of chronic obstructive pulmonary disease (COPD) is almost invariably present. More severe forms of COPD with bullous emphysema denote significant destruction of pulmonary tissue and condemn a patient to a dyspnoeic, hypoxic and premature death. Cutaneous hypoperfusion gives rise to the typical smoker's facies in around 10% of individuals.

Supplementary Information and Clinical Considerations

- **Smoking cessation in the immediate pre-operative period:** this allows greater clearance of carbon monoxide, but it may be at the expense of increased anxiety and agitation, which in its most extreme form may even manifest as a postoperative nicotine withdrawal syndrome. A patient who has just had a cigarette may have a CO concentration of 10% with all the adverse physiological effects outlined previously. At rest, the elimination half-life of CO is 4–6 hours, which is reduced to around an hour if breathing 100% oxygen. This suggests that even 12–24 hours of abstinence is of benefit.

- **Longer-term cessation:** If a patient gives up smoking 6 months prior to surgery their postoperative respiratory complication rate falls to that seen in non-smokers, although at 1–2 months pulmonary complications increase. This may be due to a reactive bronchorrhoea which occurs before ciliary function has returned to normal.

The hyper-reactivity of the smoker's airway starts to reduce within about 48 hours of cessation, but it may take 10–14 days before it disappears completely.

- **Anaesthetic implications:** These are straightforward. Superimposed on smoking-related co-morbidity are the problems of an over-reactive airway which may respond to inhaled and potentially irritant volatile agents with coughing, breath-holding, laryngospasm and bronchoconstriction. The increased FiO_2 of normal general anaesthesia is likely to correct any reduction otherwise in oxygen delivery. Regional anaesthesia is a suitable alternative, although there are some procedures, such as trans-urethral and intra-ocular surgery during which persistent coughing may seriously compromise the surgery. Nicotine addiction does have the one benefit of promoting early mobilization as some patients are desperate to have a first post-operative cigarette. Specific postoperative problems are predominantly respiratory, but smokers may have complications related to any of their chronic conditions.

Non-Respiratory Functions of the Lung

Commentary

Gas exchange remains the most complex and interesting of the functions of the lung, and is the prime focus of most anaesthetists. But even if you have not given the non-respiratory functions much consideration, there are sufficient to provide material for an oral question, and you do not want to be taken by surprise.

Core Information

- **Metabolic functions:** the best-known metabolic function of the lung is probably the enzymatic conversion of angiotensin I to angiotensin II by angiotensin converting enzyme (ACE). (Angiotensin I is an inert decapeptide from which two residues are removed to form the active angiotensin II which subsequently passes through the lung without any further metabolic change.) ACE also catalyzes the degradation of bradykinin, which is another short peptide (9 residues). The persistence of bradykinin in patients receiving ACE inhibitors is responsible for the cough that can be a problematic side effect of the treatment. Otherwise the lung also metabolizes some amines: noradrenaline (by monoamine oxidase, MAO and by catechol-O-methyl-transferase, COMT) and 5-hydroxytrytamine (by MAO). Adrenaline, dopamine and histamine are unaffected. Such selective metabolism is also seen with prostaglandins; PGE, PGE_2 and $PGF_{2\alpha}$ are degraded, whereas PGA_2 and PGI_2 remain unchanged. Purines such as adenosine mono-, di- and tri-phosphate (AMP, ADP, ATP) are metabolized to adenosine. Atrial natriuretic peptide is also inactivated.
- **Neuroendocrine functions:** in addition to its metabolic functions the lung also secretes a number of substances (some of which it also degrades). These include 5-hydroxytryptamine, histamine, substance P, heparin, bradykinins and prostaglandins. Type II alveolar cells produce surfactant, which is essential for healthy lung function.

- **Drug metabolism:** some drugs in the systemic circulation, such as local anaesthetics, are sequestered in the lung and thereby may protect the systemic circulation from excessively high concentrations. Prilocaine is the exception in that it is actually metabolized in the lung (although not exclusively in this site). Many inhaled drugs and other substances are metabolized by pulmonary cytochrome P450 isoforms. Some of the inhaled steroids are pro-drugs. An example is beclomethasone, which is converted by pulmonary esterases to its active 17-monopropionate form. Some drugs can compete for pulmonary binding sites, and so their combination may increase plasma concentrations (this can happen with β-adrenoceptor blockers and some anti-depressants), whereas others may accumulate locally. Amiodarone is one such drug, which accumulates in several tissues, including lung, where it can give rise to an acute or subacute pneumonitis.

- **Pulmonary sequestration:** the extravascular pH of lung is lower than that of plasma, and so this can lead to ion trapping and the sequestration of some drugs. This can be important in the attenuation of potential drug toxicity, such as that which follows high doses of local anaesthetics.

- **Barrier function:** the upper airways provide the first barrier to inhaled noxious substances and toxins, which strictly speaking is a 'respiratory function' albeit not one that is involved directly in gas exchange. The muco-ciliary escalator consists of a double-layered system in which a layer of high viscosity mucopolysaccharide is carried proximally on an underlying layer of low-viscosity serous bronchial secretion. This extends from the respiratory bronchioles upwards. Beating cilia move the viscous layer towards the pharynx at a frequency of around 10–15 beats per second and at a rate of up to 20 mm min^{-1} in the trachea. This surface layer traps particles of diameter 5 μm and above.

- **Filtration:** the lung is very efficient at filtering embolic matter of all types, including thrombus, fat and air. The system clearly has a limit to its capacity and can be overwhelmed, for instance by a massive pulmonary embolus. This will result in at best a substantial shunt and at worst, circulatory collapse. Microemboli may stimulate the release of local inflammatory mediators which can precipitate in due course the clinical features of acute lung injury. Pulmonary endothelium can produce both anticoagulant (heparin and fibrinolysin) and procoagulant substances (thromboplastin) and so has a role in regulating the balance between these two processes.

- **Immune functions:** inhaled particles that are smaller than 5 μm in diameter pass into the distal airways. Those between 2 and 5 μm are deposited on the airway walls with the smaller particles reaching the alveoli. Only around 20% of these stay within the alveolus; the remainder are exhaled. Particles less than 0.3 μm in diameter remain as aerosols. Pulmonary macrophages are effective against bacteria, and they also phagocytose other particles. Epithelial cells secrete various non-specific substances such as lysozyme and nitric oxide, which are active against pathogens. As with most other tissues they can also generate a similar range of inflammatory mediators at the site of injury. These include as interleukins, cytokines, tumour necrosis factor and oxygen radicals. IgA is the most abundant immunoglobulin and is found mainly in bronchial secretions.

- **Vascular reserve:** the pulmonary vessels essentially accommodate the cardiac output in a low-pressure, elastic circulation which at rest is not fully perfused but which will distend as cardiac output increases. The potential increase in blood volume can be as high as 1,000 ml, but this is not an effective vascular reserve that can be utilized in hypovolaemic states because under such circumstances cardiac output will increase to maximize oxygen delivery to tissues.

One-Lung Ventilation (One-Lung Anaesthesia)

Commentary
The physiological changes of one-lung ventilation (OLV) are of particular anaesthetic relevance, which make it an attractive science-based clinical topic. The examiners will not expect you necessarily to have had much direct experience, but as this is a standard and predictable question, you will have to show that you understand the basic principles.

Core Information

Indications for One-Lung Anaesthesia
- The indications for single-lung anaesthesia (during which one lung is deliberately collapsed to facilitate surgical exposure) include pulmonary, oesophageal and spinal surgery. It may be necessary during surgery on the thoracic aorta, and it is also used for relatively minor procedures such as transthoracic cervical sympathectomy and pleurodesis. It may be indicated to prevent contamination of the contralateral lung by empyema or significant endobronchial haemorrhage. Lung isolation or protection is also necessary in cases of bronchopleural fistula.

Physiological Changes Associated with One-Lung Ventilation
- For the duration of anaesthesia the surgical side is uppermost, and the non-ventilated upper lung is usually described as the non-dependent lung.
- When ventilation is interrupted, the remaining blood flow takes no part in gas exchange, creating ventilation–perfusion mismatch and a shunt, which contributes to hypoxia.
- The shunt is partly reduced because gravity favours flow to the dependent lung, and because surgical compression and retraction may further decrease blood flow to the non-ventilated lung.
- The shunt will further reduce if non-dependent blood vessels are ligated surgically, and will largely disappear if, for example, the pulmonary artery is clamped prior to pneumonectomy.
- Hypoxic pulmonary vasoconstriction (HPV) decreases the flow to the non-dependent lung by around 50%, and may reduce the shunt from 50% down to 30% (which is nonetheless still significant).
- The dependent lung loses volume because of compression, but hypoxic vasoconstriction, should it occur, may compensate partially by diverting some blood to the non-dependent lung.

- Secretions may pool in the dependent lung, but suction removal via a double-lumen tube may be very difficult.

Adjustment of Ventilator Settings during OLV

- The ventilator settings are similar to those used for double-lung ventilation with tidal volumes of around 10–12 ml kg^{-1}. Higher volumes increase both mean airways (P_{aw}) and vascular resistance, with the result that more blood may flow to the non-ventilated lung and increase shunt. Lower tidal volumes are likely to lead to pulmonary atelectasis.
- Although shunt is not substantially improved by supplemental oxygen, many anaesthetists routinely increase the FiO$_2$ to 0.8–1.0.
- The respiratory rate is adjusted to keep the end-tidal carbon dioxide (ETCO$_2$) at around 5–6% or 40 mmHg.

Supplementary Information

Management of an Unexpected Episode of Hypoxia

- Pre-existing disease, either pulmonary or cardiac, may be an important contributory factor.
- Check the FiO$_2$ and increase it if necessary. This may not help if significant shunt is the problem, but it is probably the swiftest intervention available.
- Check the tidal volume and other ventilator indices. Again, these are interventions that can be made rapidly. The ETCO$_2$ should be maintained at 5–6% because hypocapnia may decrease hypoxic pulmonary vasoconstriction, although small increases in tidal volume can help oxygenation.
- The double-lumen tube position should then be checked with a fibreoptic bronchoscope. Displacement to a suboptimal position is very common, particularly if the patient has been moved.
- If oxygenation still does not improve, then CPAP of around 5 cmH$_2$O can be added to the upper lung, but the surgeon will have to be warned that the lung may partially re-expand. Alternatively, oxygen can be insufflated in the upper lung, but many anaesthetists do this routinely from the start of surgery.
- PEEP (~5 cmH$_2$O) can be added to the lower lung, which may increase volume in potentially atelectatic areas. This manoeuvre may, however, increase vascular resistance and divert blood to the non-ventilated upper lung.
- Both CPAP and PEEP can be increased in small increments.
- If none of these interventions is successful, intermittent inflation can be tried, or it may finally be necessary to revert to full double-lung ventilation (with lung retraction which will allow surgery to continue).

Problems Associated with Double-Lumen Tubes

- Difficulties with double-lumen tubes are probably the most important cause of mortality and morbidity associated with one-lung anaesthesia. In the 1998 National Confidential Enquiry into Peri-Operative Deaths (NCEPOD), which looked at oesophagogastrectomy, problems with double-lumen tubes were implicated in 30% of perioperative deaths. Studies have confirmed that critical malpositioning occurs in more than 25% of cases, and general misplacements complicate more than 80% of uses.

- This is not surprising. The anatomy may be distorted by tumour or effusion, and the tubes are bulky and more complex to insert than single-lumen tubes, requiring rotation within the airway of between 90° and 180°.
- Complications include failure to achieve adequate lung separation and one-lung ventilation, prolonged surgical retraction and associated pulmonary trauma, occlusion of a major bronchus with lobar collapse and secondary infection, contamination of the dependent lung by infected secretions from the upper lung and trauma during insertion.
- A double-lumen tube is positioned correctly when the upper surface of the bronchial cuff lies immediately distal to the bifurcation of the carina. This tube position can be assessed clinically, but this may be unreliable. The average depth of insertion for a patient of height 170 cm is 29 cm, and the distance alters by 1 cm for every 10 cm change in height. This distance from the incisors can be used as an approximate guide. Auscultation of the lung fields during clamping and release can be performed, although findings may be equivocal if access to the chest wall is limited because surgery has begun. Oximetry and capnography will not give specific enough information about where the tube is sited. The tube position should therefore be checked using a fibreoptic bronchoscope.

Pulmonary Oedema

Commentary

Pulmonary oedema is common in critical care, if less so in anaesthesia. This question explores your understanding of the various forces that allow its development as well as your ability to apply that knowledge to its rational management.

Core Information

Pulmonary oedema is defined by the presence of fluid in the alveoli. It is formed by movement of that fluid across capillary membranes to which a number of factors contribute.

- Fluid flux across the capillary into the interstitium and thence into the alveolus is governed by Starling's hypothesis for capillary fluid exchanges.
- **Starling equation:** fluid flux $= k\,(p_{cap} - p_{is}) - \sum(\pi_{cap} - \pi_{is})$
  - k: this is the capillary filtration coefficient, a proportionality constant which is a measure of the ease with which fluid traverses the endothelial boundary. It is the product of the area of capillary wall and its permeability to water. 'Leaky' capillaries have a high filtration coefficient.
  - p_{cap} and p_{is}: these are the capillary and interstitial hydrostatic pressures, respectively.

— $\sum$ (also written sometimes as σ or δ): this is the reflection (or reflectance) coefficient, which is an indication of the permeability of the capillary barrier (acting as a semi-permeable membrane) to solute. A coefficient of 1 indicates total 'reflection', with no solute passing into the interstitium. A coefficient of zero indicates that the capillary wall allows free passage of solute.

— π_{cap} and π_{is}: these are the capillary and interstitial oncotic pressures, respectively.

— The net sum of the four forces is usually outwards, with the extravasated fluid being cleared by the lymphatics. This is despite the lower hydrostatic pressures in the pulmonary circulation. The normal clearance rate of 10–20 ml h^{-1} (in the lungs) can increase to 200 ml h^{-1} before the system is overwhelmed.

— The oncotic pressure is the contribution made to total osmolality by colloids. (Hence the alternative term 'colloid osmotic pressure'.) The plasma oncotic pressure, at 25–28 mmHg, is only about 0.5% that of total plasma osmotic pressure, but is significant because, from the Starling equation, it can be seen that it is the only force whose effect is to retain fluid within the pulmonary capillary.

From the equation, it can be seen that pulmonary oedema may arise from a number of different mechanisms.

- **Increased capillary hydrostatic pressure (p_{cap}):** this is common and explains the formation of pulmonary oedema as a consequence of left ventricular failure, fluid overload, mitral stenosis and any other condition that may cause pulmonary venous hypertension. Hydrostatic pressure is clearly greater in the dependent parts of the lung. Neurogenic pulmonary oedema (such as that associated with subarachnoid haemorrhage) may be caused by a sudden increase in hydrostatic pressure in response to a massive catecholamine surge.
- **Decreased interstitial pressure (p_{is}):** if interstitial pressure becomes acutely negative, pulmonary oedema may develop as the lymphatics are overwhelmed. This can occur with upper airway obstruction during which very high negative intrathoracic pressures may be generated, creating a gradient which favours transudation.
- **Decreased capillary oncotic pressure (π_{cap}):** this commonly worsens oedema that has another primary cause. Hypoproteinaemia, hypoalbuminaemia, haemodilution, liver failure and the nephrotic syndrome are all conditions which will decrease the gradient between the oncotic pressure and the pulmonary capillary occlusion (or 'wedge') pressure (PCWP). If this gradient does not exceed 4 mmHg, then oedema formation is inevitable. Albumin makes a substantial contribution to colloid oncotic pressure, and if the plasma albumin concentration × 0.57 does not exceed PCWP, then pulmonary oedema will supervene.
- **Decreased reflection coefficient ($\sum$):** capillary endothelial damage may reduce $\sum$ to zero, so that protein will diffuse freely across the wall such that no effective oncotic pressure can be exerted. This form of capillary leak characterizes ARDS. Capillary injury will also increase permeability to water, with a rise in the filtration coefficient, k.
- **Decreased lymphatic clearance:** this is uncommon, but will accompany any disease process which obliterates lymphatic vessels. Examples include severe fibrosing lung disease, silicosis and lymphangitis carcinomatosis (lymphangitis obliterans).
- **Idiopathic:** other causes of pulmonary oedema include ascent to altitude and rapid lung re-expansion after collapse. The mechanisms are uncertain.

Supplementary Information and Clinical Considerations

These principles can be applied to the rational management of pulmonary oedema.

- Hydrostatic pulmonary oedema is treated by reducing left atrial pressure. This can be achieved by offloading the left ventricle using nitrates or ACE inhibitors to improve myocardial function. The emergency treatment of acute left ventricular failure commonly involves intravenous diamorphine and diuretic. These probably alleviate symptoms by the same mechanism. Myocardial contractility can be enhanced using positive inotropes.
- Decreased capillary oncotic pressure is usually contributory rather than primary. In theory, the restoration of the capillary oncotic pressure by giving albumin should be beneficial, but this is rarely done. Plasma albumin concentrations in the critically ill can be maintained only if the patient's condition begins to improve.
- Increased alveolar pressure: PEEP is now believed to increase the capacity of the interstitium to hold fluid. (The pulmonary interstitium can accommodate 500 ml with an increase in pressure of only 1.5 mmHg.) It is a useful therapy following negative pressure pulmonary oedema secondary to airway obstruction. PEEP also increases alveolar recruitment.

Pulmonary Hypertension

Commentary

Pulmonary hypertension has numerous causes, but for most general anaesthetists it is a theoretical rather than a practical problem. It is, however, of particular importance to anaesthetists who deal regularly with both children and adults with congenital cardiac disease. The subject allows some discussion of pulmonary pathophysiology and its clinical implications. It may be linked to a question about hypoxic pulmonary vasoconstriction.

Core Information

Pulmonary Hypertension: Diagnosis and Causes

- **Diagnosis:** definitive diagnosis requires determination of pulmonary arterial pressures (PAP). The normal mean PAP is 12–16 mmHg; pulmonary hypertension is defined by mean pressures at rest of >25 mmHg or >30 mmHg with exercise.
- **'Arterial hypertension'.** It can be caused by excessive pulmonary blood flow. This 'arterial' hypertension is associated with conditions such as congenital cardiac anomalies involving left-to-right shunts, and with collagen vascular disease. It may also be a problem in later life for elite endurance athletes such as marathon runners and professional cyclists who during the course of many years of high-intensity training will have subjected their pulmonary circulations to very high right ventricular output.
- **'Venous hypertension'.** It can also result from increased resistance to pulmonary venous drainage. This 'venous' hypertension occurs typically as a result of chronic left ventricular failure and mitral valve disease. The rise in left atrial pressure is transmitted retrogradely through the pulmonary circulation.

- **'Hypoxic hypertension'.** Pulmonary hypertension occurs commonly in response to alveolar hypoxia with obliteration of part of the capillary bed. Causes of this 'hypoxic' hypertension include chronic obstructive pulmonary disease (COPD), obstructive sleep apnoea syndrome (OSAS) and interstitial lung disease.
- **'Thrombotic hypertension'.** This is associated with thrombotic disease. 'Thrombotic' hypertension may develop as a consequence of chronic proximal embolic disease or as a result of obstruction of distal vessels by thrombus. (These vessels can also become occluded by parasites, such as schistosomes, or by foreign material, as can happen in intravenous drug abusers.) Acute proximal obstruction owing to pulmonary emboli leads to only moderate rises in pulmonary artery pressure, because without chronic adaptation the right ventricle can generate a systolic pressure no greater than about 50 mmHg. The right ventricle may therefore fail acutely in the presence of massive pulmonary thromboembolism.
- **'Drug-induced hypertension'.** It may follow the use of appetite suppressants such as fenfluramine (definite link), amphetamines and L-tryptophan (probable link) and cocaine (possible link).
- **'Idiopathic hypertension'.** Pulmonary hypertension can occur without obvious cause or in association with infective or inflammatory conditions such as HIV and schistosomiasis and sarcoidosis.

Supplementary Information and Clinical Considerations

- **Anaesthetic implications:** cardiac output from the right ventricle is crucially dependent on right ventricle filling pressure and on PAP. It is thus compromised by any decrease in venous return or any increase in pulmonary vascular resistance. The aims of any anaesthetic technique therefore should be to avoid tachycardia which may reduce ventricular filling, to maintain sinus rhythm and to optimize preload. A reduction in afterload is acceptable as long as the pulmonary hypertension is not secondary to a left-to-right shunt which has the potential to reverse (Eisenmenger syndrome).
- **Increase in pulmonary vascular resistance (PVR):** PVR rises with hypoxia, hypercapnia, acidosis, the use of nitrous oxide (only in the presence of pre-existing pulmonary hypertension), catecholamines and exogenous pressors which increase systemic vascular resistance.
- **Falls in PVR:** agents that can reduce PVR include oxygen, calcium-channel blockers, prostacyclin, nitric oxide and phosphodiesterase-5 inhibitors such as sildenafil. Specific endothelin receptor antagonists such as bosentan both reduce PVR and improve exercise capacity. (Endothelin is a potent vasoconstricting peptide.)

Hypoxic Pulmonary Vasoconstriction (HPV)

Commentary

Hypoxic pulmonary vasoconstriction is one of several factors that influence ventilation–perfusion relationships in the lung, and anaesthetists rarely intervene directly to exploit the mechanism. In that sense it is theoretical, but the mechanism is influenced by anaesthetic drugs and does have relevance for special situations such as one-lung anaesthesia.

Core Information

- **Definition:** HPV is a mechanism that diverts blood flow away from areas of the lung where the alveolar oxygen tension is low, shunting it to better ventilated zones and improving the ventilation–perfusion ratio. (Elsewhere in the circulatory system, hypoxia always results in the vasodilatation of vascular beds.)
- **Significance:** HPV is of little importance in health, but it is more significant in disease. It explains, for example, the upper lobe diversion characteristic of left ventricular failure, as blood in the congested and hypoxaemic lower parts of the lung is diverted away. It is significant during one-lung anaesthesia.
- **Response:** this occurs via the constriction of small arterioles; it is not neurally mediated. It is seen, for example, in denervated lungs (following transplantation). Nor is it mediated by humoral vasoconstrictors but rather by pulmonary mixed venous oxygenation and, more importantly, by alveolar oxygenation. Larger blood vessels may be affected globally, as in the fetal pulmonary circulation in which the low PaO_2 reduces pulmonary blood flow to about 15% of the cardiac output.
- **Onset:** this is within seconds of the decrease in PaO_2, and lobar blood flow may halve within minutes from its value during normoxia. The phenomenon is biphasic, with the vascular resistance returning almost to baseline before the onset of a second phase of slower and sustained vasoconstriction that reaches a plateau at 40 minutes.
- **Mediators:** the mechanisms have not been fully identified. The pulmonary vasculature is maintained in a state of active vasodilatation to which nitric oxide may contribute, and so suppression of endothelial nitric oxide production will lead to vasoconstriction. In addition, hypoxia stimulates production of the peptide endothelin, which is the most potent vasoconstrictor yet identified in humans. It is also known that pulmonary blood vessels have oxygen-sensitive potassium channels such that the membrane potential alters in response to hypoxia, with opening of calcium channels and smooth muscle contraction. This phenomenon is not seen in the systemic vasculature.
- **Influences:** acidosis and hypercarbia potentiate HPV, while alkalosis either attenuates or abolishes it and causes pulmonary vasodilatation.

Clinical Applications

The Influence of Anaesthesia on HPV

- **Anaesthesia:** all inhalational anaesthetics inhibit HPV. The effect is dose-dependent and is similar for all the agents apart from nitrous oxide, whose action is less potent. The dose–response curve is of typical sigmoid shape; the ED_{50} is just under 2 MAC, and the ED_{90} is around 3 MAC. At 1.3 MAC, HPV is diminished by around 30%. Intravenous induction agents have little effect.
- **Oxygen:** a high FiO_2 may inhibit HPV by maintaining higher PaO_2 even in underventilated alveoli.

- **Cardiac output:** any factor which depresses cardiac output will reduce mixed venous PO_2 and so may enhance HPV.
- **Drug effects:** drugs such as calcium-channel blockers, sodium nitroprusside, glyceryl trinitrate, bronchodilators, nitric oxide and dobutamine all attenuate HPV. It is potentiated by cyclo-oxygenase inhibitors, propranolol and by the respiratory stimulant almitrine. (Although not used in the UK, it acts by stimulating carotid body chemoreceptors. It also enhances the effect of HPV in situations in which it is deficient.)

The Oxygen–Haemoglobin Dissociation Curve

Commentary

This is a standard and predictable question (which like some others in this chapter may seem more appropriate for the Primary FRCA examination). However, it is seen as core knowledge that is basic to an understanding of respiratory physiology and monitoring. You will be expected to answer it with some facility. Ensure that you can readily draw the curve; it will reinforce the impression of your familiarity with the subject.

Core Information

- **The oxygen–haemoglobin dissociation curve (OHDC)** (Figure 3.5. This defines the relationship between the partial pressure of oxygen and the percentage saturation of

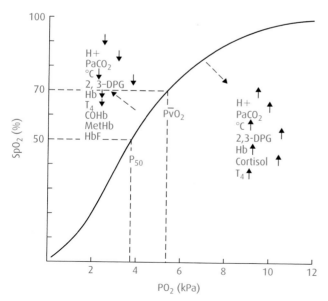

Fig. 3.5 Oxygen–haemoglobin dissociation curve. COHb, Carboxyhaemoglobin; MetHb, methaemoglobin; T_4, thyroxine.

oxygen. In solutions of blood substitutes, such as perfluorocarbons, this curve is linear, with saturation being directly proportional to partial pressure. In solutions containing haemoglobin, however, the curve is sigmoid-shaped. This is because as haemoglobin binds each of its four molecules of oxygen, its affinity for the next increases. Haemoglobin exists in two forms, an 'R' or 'relaxed' state in which the affinity for oxygen is high, and a 'T' or 'tense' state in which affinity for oxygen is low. As haemoglobin takes up oxygen this effects an allosteric change in the structure of the molecule, which increases affinity and enhances uptake with each of the combination steps.

- **Shifts in the OHDC:** the curve can be displaced in either direction along the x axis; movement that is usually quantified in terms of the P_{50}, which is the partial pressure of oxygen at which haemoglobin is 50% saturated. This is normally 3.5 kPa. The P_{50} is decreased (leftward shift) by alkalosis, by reduced $PaCO_2$, by hypothermia, and by reduced concentrations of 2,3-diphosphoglycerate (2,3-DPG). The curve for fetal haemoglobin (HbF) lies to the left of that for adult haemoglobin (HbA). A shift to the right is associated with acidosis, by increased $PaCO_2$, by pyrexia, by anaemia and by increases in 2,3-DPG. In most instances, a shift to the right is accompanied by increased tissue oxygenation. A better reflection of this is the venous PO_2, which can be determined from the curve, assuming an arteriovenous saturation difference of 25%. At low PaO_2 levels, however (on the steep part of the curve), hypoxia may outweigh the benefits of decreased affinity and increased tissue off-loading. Under these circumstances, a rightward shift is actually deleterious for tissue oxygenation. At high altitude, with the critical reduction in arterial PO_2, the curve shifts to the left.

- **Haldane effect:** the deoxygenation of blood increases its ability to transport CO_2. In the pulmonary capillaries, oxygenation increases CO_2 release, and in peripheral blood deoxygenation increases uptake.

- **The double Haldane effect:** this applies in the uteroplacental circulation, in which maternal CO_2 uptake increases while fetal CO_2 affinity decreases, thereby enhancing the transfer of CO_2 from fetal to maternal blood.

- **Bohr effect:** this describes the change in the affinity of oxygen for haemoglobin which is associated with changes in pH. In perfused tissues, CO_2 enters the red cells to form carbonic acid and hydrogen ions ($CO_2 + H_2O \leftrightarrow H_2CO_3 \leftrightarrow H^+ + HCO_3^-$). The increase in H^+ shifts the curve to the right, decreases the affinity of oxygen and increases oxygen delivery to the tissues. In the pulmonary capillaries the process is reversed, with the leftward shift of the curve enhancing oxygen uptake.

- **The double Bohr effect:** this is a mechanism which increases fetal oxygenation. Maternal uptake of fetal CO_2 shifts the maternal curve to the right and the fetal curve to the left. The simultaneous and reverse changes in pH move the curves in opposite directions and enhance fetal oxygenation.

- **Carboxyhaemoglobin and methaemoglobin:** other ligands can combine with the iron in haemoglobin, the most important of which is carbon monoxide. Its affinity for haemoglobin is 300 times that of oxygen, and not only does it reduce the percentage saturation of oxygen proportionately, it also shifts the curve to the left. In methaemoglobinaemia, the iron is oxidized from the ferrous (Fe^{2+}) to the ferric (Fe^{3+}) form, in which state it is unable to combine with oxygen. This happens when haemoglobin acts as a natural scavenger of nitric oxide (NO), when a subject inhales NO or when they receive certain drugs, including prilocaine and nitrates.

- **2,3-DPG:** this is an organic phosphate which exerts a conformational change on the beta chain of the haemoglobin molecule and decreases oxygen affinity. Deoxyhaemoglobin bonds specifically with 2,3-DPG to maintain the 'T' (low affinity) state. Changes in 2,3-DPG levels do alter the P_{50}, but the clinical significance of this seems to be small. It is true that concentrations of 2,3-DPG in stored blood are depleted (and are reduced to zero after 2 weeks) and that it can take up to 48 hours before pre-transfusion levels are restored. There is, however, little evidence that massive transfusion is associated with severe tissue hypoxia, and this is borne out by clinical experience with such patients.

- **Abnormal haemoglobins:** fetal haemoglobin is abnormal only if it persists into adult life, as in thalassaemia. (It consists of two α-and two γ- or δ-chains, forming HbA_2 or HbF, respectively, rather than the two α- and two β-chains in the normal adult.) Haemoglobin S, which is found in sickle cell disease, is formed by the simple substitution of valine for glutamic acid in position six on the β-chains. The P_{50} is lower than normal and the 'standard' OHDC for HbS is shifted leftwards. The anaemia that is associated with the condition then shifts the curve to the right. There are other haemoglobinopathies, including HbC and HbD (mild haemolytic anaemia without sickling), HbE, Hb Chesapeake and Hb Kansas. You will not be expected to know about these in any detail; they are rare conditions which most anaesthetists would need to look up in a textbook of uncommon diseases should they encounter a case in clinical practice.

Hyperbaric Oxygen

Commentary

This topic is clinically orientated, but in fact it also allows an exploration of some basic respiratory physiology. During the discussion you will have to make clear, for example, that you appreciate the difference between oxygen saturation, oxygen partial pressure and oxygen content. Be prepared to cite some figures to demonstrate that you understand the principles.

Core Information

The principles underlying hyperbaric oxygen therapy and the rationale for its use.

- **Predicted PaO_2 from FiO_2:** there is a useful formula that predicts the partial pressure of oxygen in arterial blood (PaO_2) by multiplying the inspired oxygen percentage by 0.66. A young adult in good health and breathing room air therefore will have a PaO_2 of $20.93 \times 0.66 = 13.3$ kPa (100 mmHg). Vigorous hyperventilation can increase this to around 16 kPa (from the alveolar gas equation, the fall in $PaCO_2$ allowing a rise in PaO_2), but further rises are possible only by enriching the inspired oxygen concentration. From the empirical formula here it can be seen that the maximum PaO_2 that can be achieved by breathing 100% oxygen is around 66 kPa. (In practice it may be slightly higher.)

- **Saturation, partial pressure and content:** at a partial pressure of oxygen of 13.3 kPa, haemoglobin is almost 100% saturated. Further increases in inspired oxygen (FiO_2) can therefore increase the oxygen saturation (SpO_2) only marginally, although the PaO_2 will rise substantially. The sigmoid shape of the OHDC, moreover, means that oxygen will start to be released to the tissues only when the PaO_2 is around 13.3 kPa. It is also important to note that, although the increase in PaO_2 is very high, the rise in oxygen content is relatively modest. If a subject changes from breathing room air to breathing 100% oxygen at barometric pressure, the arterial oxygen content rises from around 19 ml dl^{-1} to only 21 ml dl^{-1}. In practice, the venous oxygen content is probably more significant because this reflects more reliably the minimum tissue PO_2. In this situation, the venous arterial content rises from about 14 to 16 ml dl^{-1}. This is the same as the arterial rise, because the arteriovenous O_2 difference remains constant.

- **Hyperbaric oxygenation:** this is an example of an application of Henry's Law, which states that the number of molecules (in this case oxygen) which dissolve in the solvent (plasma) is directly proportional to the partial pressure of the gas at the surface of the liquid. It is the only means whereby very high arterial PaO_2 values (greater than 80 kPa) can be obtained. Thus, at 2 atmospheres the PaO_2 will be 175 kPa. Even at these levels, however, the venous content will only be of the order of 18 ml dl^{-1}, and it is not until the blood is exposed to oxygen at 3 atmospheres of pressure, at which the arterial content is 25.5 ml dl^{-1} and the venous content 20.5 ml dl^{-1}, that all the tissue requirements can be met by dissolved oxygen. Content is determined by the product of the [Hb] × [% saturation] × [1.31] (O_2-carrying capacity of Hb) plus dissolved oxygen. Dissolved oxygen (0.003 ml dl^{-1} $mmHg^{-1}$) is small and is usually ignored, except under these hyperbaric conditions when it assumes great importance.

Supplementary Information and Clinical Applications

In respect of indications for hyperbaric oxygen therapy (HBOT) many claims of benefit have been made; few have been supported by evidence.

- **Decompression sickness:** recreational divers use compressed air mixtures which they breathe at hyperbaric pressures; each 10 metres of descent increases the pressure by 1 atmosphere. At depth, the tissues become supersaturated with nitrogen. If the diver ascends too rapidly, the partial pressure of nitrogen in tissues exceeds the ambient pressure, and so the gas forms bubbles in the circulation and elsewhere. Most remains in the venous side of the circulation to be filtered out by the lung, but some may gain access to the arterial (and hence the cerebral) circulations via hitherto innocuous shunts. Hyperbaric treatment mimics controlled ascent from depth, and this allows the nitrogen to wash out exponentially without causing symptoms.

- **Infection:** the evidence supports the use of hyperbaric oxygen therapy as part of the management of patients with bacterial infections. The main indications are for anaerobic bacterial infections, particularly with clostridia, osteomyelitis and necro-tizing soft tissue infections. Oxygen-derived free radicals are bactericidal.

- **Carbon monoxide (CO) poisoning:** the half-life of CO while breathing 100% oxygen is reduced to an hour. This is reduced further to about 20 minutes in a hyperbaric chamber, but, unless the chamber is on site, the transfer time alone will make this benefit negligible. CO is, however, a cellular toxin, which appears to inhibit cellular respiration via cytochrome A_3, as well as impairing the function of neutrophils. The rationale for hyperbaric treatment rests on the presumption, as yet unproven, that it attenuates these toxic effects.
- **Delayed wound healing:** hyperbaric oxygen therapy may be of benefit to patients in whom wound healing is delayed by ischaemia. Its theoretical role in the treatment of thermal injury has not been supported by recent studies. Angiogenesis is, however, stimulated at hyperbaric pressure by a mechanism that is unclear.
- **Anaemic hypoxia:** Jehovah's witnesses who have lost blood but whose religious beliefs prohibit transfusion, and others in whom very low haemoglobin concentrations have compromised oxygen delivery to tissues, have been managed successfully using hyperbaric oxygen.
- **Ischaemia and reperfusion injury:** HBOT confers some protection against oxygen free radicals, but it is most effective if given early following reperfusion. This is rarely practical in the UK but is more commonly done in the USA to improve graft and free-flap survival after reconstructive surgery.
- **Soft tissue injuries:** early treatment has been used in elite athletes to treat soft tissue injuries and some fractures. There is no good evidence for benefit.
- **Multiple sclerosis:** hyperbaric therapy for this disease still has its enthusiasts, despite the many controlled trials that have shown no benefit.
- **Fibromyalgia:** this is a chronic pain condition which primarily affects women (90%). Its aetiology is mysterious (and in common with conditions such as chronic fatigue and irritable bowel syndromes is disputed as an entity by some), but part of the symptomatology is related to central pain afferent processing. It is claimed that by enhancing cerebral oxygenation HBOT facilitates repair of some of the abnormal neurons that may be responsible. There is some weak trial evidence to support the claim, but a much larger randomized control trial would be needed to confirm the finding.
- **Summary:** the Mayo Clinic in the USA (which is an institution of global renown) lists on their website the indications for which there is evidence of benefit following HBOT: severe anaemia, cerebral abscess, arterial gas embolism, burns, decompression sickness, CO poisoning, crush injury, sudden hearing loss, gangrene, severe tissue infection, non-healing wounds (particularly in diabetics), radiation damage, compromised skin graft or flap, sudden painless loss of vision. The list of conditions for which there is no evidence that HBOT offers benefit is much longer: AIDS, allergies, Alzheimer's disease, arthritides, asthma, autism, Bell's palsy, cerebral injury, cerebral tumours, malignancy in general, cerebral palsy, chronic fatigue syndrome, cirrhosis of the liver, depression, fibromyalgia, peptic ulceration, cardiac disease, heatstroke, hepatitis, migraine, multiple sclerosis, Parkinson's disease, spinal cord injury, sports injuries, cerebrovascular accidents (stroke).
- **Potential complications:** the main problem relates to oxygen toxicity (discussed in the next section.)

Oxygen Toxicity

Commentary

One of the most basic principles of anaesthesia and intensive care is the maintenance of oxygenation, and so it is paradoxical that a molecule which is essential to life can, under certain circumstances, be lethal. It is important that anaesthetists realize that oxygen is potentially toxic, and the oral is testing your recognition of that reality.

Core Information

The conditions under which oxygen may become toxic and possible underlying mechanisms.

Adverse Effects at Atmospheric Pressure

- **Pulmonary pathology:** oxygen causes pathological changes which begin with tracheobronchitis, neutrophil recruitment and the release of inflammatory mediators. Surfactant production is impaired, pulmonary interstitial oedema appears, followed, after around 1 week of exposure, by the development of pulmonary fibrosis. Toxicity also accelerates lung injury in the critically ill. In patients receiving certain cytotoxic drugs, particularly bleomycin and mitomycin C, ARDS and respiratory failure may supervene after 'normal' doses of oxygen (see under 'Chemotherapeutic (Cytotoxic) Drugs' in Chapter 4.)
- **Mechanism of toxicity:** this is complex and not fully elucidated. Although oxygen is a stable molecule, it is readily transformed into substances that are potentially toxic. In various normal metabolic pathways and enzymatic reactions, oxygen becomes partially reduced to a superoxide anion (O_2^-). At normoxia this leads to the formation of hydrogen peroxide (H_2O_2) and water in a reaction catalyzed by superoxide dismutase. Both H_2O_2 and O_2^- are potentially toxic and in higher concentrations interact to produce highly reactive species of which the hydroxyl free radical is the most dangerous. These oxidant toxins appear particularly to affect enzyme systems which contain sulphydryl groups as well as nucleotides and lipid membranes (which undergo lipid peroxidation).
- **Oxygen toxicity:** the major problem is dose-related direct toxicity. Dose–time curves have been constructed to allow the recommendation that 100% should be administered for no longer than 12 hours at atmospheric pressure, 80% for no longer than 24 hours and 60% for no longer than 36 hours. An FiO_2 of 0.5 can be maintained indefinitely.
- **Defence mechanisms:** up to a partial pressure of oxygen of about 60 kPa, a number of endogenous antioxidant enzymes are effective. These include catalase, superoxide dismutase and glutathione peroxidase.

Supplementary Information and Clinical Considerations

Clinical features of oxygen toxicity.

- These are most marked in conscious patients who are breathing oxygen under hyperbaric conditions.

- Initial symptoms include retrosternal discomfort, carinal irritation and coughing. This becomes more severe with time, with a burning pain that is accompanied by the urge to breathe deeply and to cough. As exposure continues, symptoms progress to severe dyspnoea with paroxysmal coughing.
- CNS symptoms may supervene, with nausea, facial twitching and numbness as well as disturbances of taste and smell. Convulsions may occur, preceded by a premonitory aura.
- In long-term ventilated patients in whom high inspired oxygen concentrations tend to be the norm, the non-specific clinical signs will be those of progressively impaired gas exchange with decreased pulmonary compliance.

Adverse Effects in Obstetrics

- Conventional wisdom has always held that pregnant women undergoing operative delivery under regional anaesthesia benefit from supplemental oxygen, it being argued that this optimizes fetal oxygenation. This may not in reality be best practice. An FiO_2 as high as 0.6 is associated with only a small increase in umbilical venous oxygenation. However, what do rise are markers of oxygen free radical activity in both mother and baby. These radicals deplete intrinsic antioxidant systems. The placenta also increases its release of inflammatory mediators. Neonatal hyperoxia is known, moreover, to mediate tissue damage in conditions as diverse as retinopathy of prematurity, necrotizing enterocolitis, bronchopulmonary dysplasia and intracranial haemorrhage. Maternal cardiac function is also affected. In response to an FiO_2 of 0.4, the cardiac index falls and systemic vascular resistance rises, hyperoxia appearing to exert direct vasopressor effects.

Toxic Effects under Hyperbaric Conditions

- This toxicity presents the major limitation of hyperbaric oxygen therapy. It is dose-dependent and affects not only the lung but also the CNS, the visual system and probably the myocardium, liver and renal tract.
- **Pulmonary toxicity:** oxygen at 2 atmospheres produces symptoms in healthy volunteers at 8–10 hours, together with a quantifiable decrease in vital capacity which starts as early as 4 hours. This persists after exposure ceases.
- **CNS:** oxygen at 2 atmospheres is associated with nausea, facial twitching and numbness, olfactory and gustatory disturbance. Tonic–clonic seizures may then supervene without any prodrome, although some subjects report a premonitory aura.
- **Eyes:** hyperoxia may be associated in adults with narrowing of the visual fields and myopia.

Adverse Effects in Other Circumstances

- **Paediatrics:** neonates and infants of post-conceptual age less than 44 weeks may develop retrolental fibroplasia if they are allowed to maintain a PaO_2 greater than 10.6 kPa (80 mmHg) for longer than 3 hours. In practice, this means keeping the oxygen saturation (SpO_2) in these babies at around 90%. The condition, however, is almost certainly multifactorial and not related to oxygen toxicity alone.
- **Absorption atelectasis:** this is a predictable adverse effect of therapy.

- **Hypoventilation:** oxygen concentrations higher than 24% may suppress respiration in patients who are reliant on hypoxaemic ventilatory drive. This is another adverse effect of therapy. (It is a phenomenon that seems to worry physicians more than anaesthetists, most of whom have seen it only rarely and who generally believe its importance to be overstated.)

Pre-Operative Assessment of Cardiac Function

Commentary

Cardiac complications are a major cause of perioperative morbidity and mortality, and so there is much interest in methods of identifying, evaluating and protecting those patients who are at greatest risk. Such science as you will be asked in this oral will be largely descriptive (and is of sufficient clinical relevance to keep most anaesthetists interested).

Core Information

Clinical predictors of perioperative cardiac risk.

- **Cardiac risk:** this is usually defined as myocardial infarction, heart failure or death, and its incidence in adults undergoing non-cardiac surgery is quoted as being in the order of 0.5–1% (which is higher than in most anaesthetists' experience).
- **Clinical predictors: Minor** predictors include advanced age, any abnormalities in the ECG, any rhythm other than sinus, reduced FRC, past history of cerebrovascular accident and uncontrolled systemic hypertension. **Intermediate** predictors include a history of prior myocardial infarction, mild angina pectoris, diabetes mellitus, compensated cardiac failure and renal impairment. **Major** predictors of risk include unstable coronary syndrome, decompensated heart failure, any potentially malignant cardiac arrhythmia and severe valvular disease.
- **Risk classifications:** the Goldman index, which was first described in 1977, identified nine independent variables amongst which were recent myocardial infarction and heart failure. It was modified by Detsky but still remained cumbersome to apply. An index of risk that has since been validated in several studies is that described by Lee *et al.* in 1999. This is a further simplification of Goldman which identifies six independent predictors of adverse cardiac outcome. In outline summary, these are (1) high-risk surgery, (2) ischaemic heart disease, (3) heart failure, (4) cerebrovascular disease, (5) type 1 diabetes mellitus and (6) chronic renal impairment. (In patients with none of these factors the cardiac risk is 0.5%. In patients with three or more the risk is 9%.) (It is of interest that in none of these scoring systems does hypertension feature as a material risk factor.) The **P**hysiological and **O**perative **S**everity **S**core for the en**u**meration of **M**ortality and **M**orbidity (POSSuM) is a more complex scoring system that uses variable weighting for factors known to be associated with worse outcomes (see under 'Scoring Systems' in Chapter 5.) (T.H. Lee *et al. Circulation* 1999, **100**: 1043–9).
- **Surgery-specific risk: high-risk surgery** (>5% cardiac risk): includes all emergency major operations (especially in the elderly), prolonged procedures involving large

fluid shifts or blood loss, major vascular and peripheral vascular surgery. Of **intermediate-risk** (1–5%) are intraperitoneal and intrathoracic surgery, orthopaedic and prostatic surgery, carotid endarterectomy and other head and neck surgery. **Low-risk** procedures (<1%) include breast surgery, cataract surgery and endoscopic procedures.

Evaluation and Investigation of Patients Identified as Being at Risk

- **Clinical assessment:** in addition to history and examination, the patient's functional capacity can be quantified by the metabolic equivalent of task level (MET). One MET represents the oxygen consumption of a resting adult (3.5 ml kg^{-1} min^{-1}), with four METs representing normal daily activities such as light housework or climbing a flight of stairs. Cardiac risks are increased in patients unable to meet a four-MET demand. Symptoms can be classified according to the New York Heart Association (NYHA) functional classification for patients with cardiac disease. In simplified outline:
  — Class I – ordinary physical activity causes no symptoms.
  — Class II – slight symptomatic limitation of physical activity.
  — Class III – marked limitation of physical activity.
  — Class IV – symptoms on minimal exertion; may have symptoms at rest.

- **Electrocardiography:** this is a routine investigation which may reveal ischaemic, hypertrophic and conduction abnormalities. A normal ECG, however, does not exclude cardiac pathology; hence the value of exercise ECG stress testing which may unmask ischaemic heart disease and establish thresholds at which symptoms appear.

- **Echocardiography:** this identifies impaired left ventricular function, determines the ejection fraction (EF), gives information about ventricular wall and septal motion abnormalities, and detects valvular heart disease. The EF as determined by echocardiography is not a good predictor of adverse perioperative cardiac events, and in fact the retrospective analysis of a large cohort of patients (40,000) who underwent resting echocardiography as part of pre-operative assessment prior to non-cardiac surgery demonstrated that there were no outcome differences between this group and controls (R.M. Pearse *et al. British Medical Journal J*, 2011, 343: 734–9).

- **Dobutamine stress echocardiography:** this is useful in patients in whom treadmill exercise testing is not possible and gives more information than the investigation performed at rest. Dobutamine increases cardiac output and myocardial oxygen demand, and a stress echocardiogram can identify regional wall motion abnormalities which may develop as the myocardium develops areas of focal ischaemia.

- **Dipyridamole–thallium scintigraphy scanning:** dipyridamole prevents the cellular uptake of adenosine and so potentiates its powerful vasodilatory effects on the small resistance vessels of the coronary circulation. In patients without coronary artery disease, blood flow can increase fivefold, but if there is a significant coronary stenosis the distal vessels are already maximally dilated. Infusion of dipyridamole creates regional heterogeneity of blood flow, with the diseased areas being underperfused. Thallium allows this heterogeneity of flow to be imaged using a gamma camera.

- **Coronary angiography:** although invasive, this investigation gives definitive information about the myocardial arterial supply in patients who are at such high potential risk that coronary revascularization should be considered.

- **Cardiopulmonary exercise testing (CPET):** in CPET patients are exposed to incremental increases in workload on a cycle ergometer (some centres have arm ergometers for patients with peripheral vascular disease in whom lower limb claudication pain may end testing prematurely). Inspired and expired gas analysis allows estimation of maximal oxygen consumption, or VO_2 max, which is a guide to the patient's functional capacity. To achieve 4 METs, which is a very modest level of activity, a subject needs a VO_2 max of 15 ml O_2 kg min^{-1}. Postoperative physiological stress imposes a lower demand of around 5.0 ml O_2 kg min^{-1}, but this is sustained over a much longer period, and so patients who cannot achieve 15 ml O_2 kg min^{-1} are at risk of cardiac insufficiency after surgery. This is because most subjects are unable to sustain oxygen consumption at any more than 40% of VO_2 max for any prolonged period. (By way of comparison and at the other end of the physiological spectrum are endurance athletes, such as professional cyclists and cross-country skiers, in some of whom maximal oxygen consumption levels have been measured at more than 90 ml O_2 kg min^{-1}. These athletes are also able to function for sustained periods at around 85% of these levels). CPET also identifies the anaerobic threshold (AT), which is the point at which the oxygen consumption of exercising muscle outstrips aerobic supply and metabolism switches to anaerobic glycolysis with the production of lactic acid. An AT of less than 11 ml kg^{-1} min^{-1} is associated with higher mortality rates, particularly if signs of myocardial ischaemia accompany the ergonomic test. A low AT indicates poor ventricular function and an inability to increase oxygen supply in response to the physiological stress of major surgery.
- **Biological markers:** in response to myocardial ischaemia or to abnormal stretch of the ventricular wall, cardiac myocytes release natriuretic peptides (NP). Elevated NP concentrations are powerful and consistent predictors of postoperative cardiac events. Troponins are a marker of myocardial injury and do not predict pre-operative risk, although peak troponin levels following surgery do correlate with postoperative mortality at 30 days.

Reduction of risks of an adverse cardiac outcome.

- **Risk reduction:** the strategy may need to be tailored to the particular patient, but it could include pre-optimization, perioperative β-adrenoceptor blockade and limiting the duration of surgery by staging procedures where appropriate. Important generic measures include maintaining normothermia, avoiding anaemia, delivering post-operative oxygen therapy and ensuring good postoperative analgesia. Coordination of high quality care is also of self-evident importance.

Mitral Valve Disease

Commentary

Valvular pathology is of clinical interest because of the risk that anaesthesia and surgery will cause perioperative decompensation. Mitral valve disease is a popular topic because it allows discussion of physiology and pharmacology applied to a fixed cardiac output state.

Core Information

Mitral Stenosis

- Mitral stenosis is almost always due to untreated rheumatic fever, usually following streptococcal infection. It is increasingly rare to see this in the UK.
- **Pathophysiology:**
  - The pressure gradient across the narrowed valve is less reliable than estimations of valvular area, which is the key factor determining flow. The cross-sectional area of a normal mitral valve area is 4–6 cm^2. Stenosis may be graded as mild (1.6–2.5 cm^2), moderate (1.1–1.5 cm^2) and severe (<1 cm^2). Between 2.5 and 4.0 cm^2 the narrowing is not clinically significant.
  - As the stenosis worsens, the left atrium dilates and hypertrophies, and the contribution of atrial contraction to left ventricular filling becomes progressively more important, increasing from 15% up to 40%. Compensatory bradycardia allows sufficient time for diastolic flow across the stenosis. These factors explain why the onset of atrial fibrillation (AF) with the loss of this crucial contribution to left ventricular filling can be calamitous. In time, the increased left atrial pressure (LAP) is reflected in pulmonary hypertension and right ventricular overload.
  - As pulmonary venous pressure increases, symptoms will include dyspnoea on exertion, orthopnoea and paroxysmal nocturnal dyspnoea. Impaired exercise tolerance is a good guide to disease severity. Pulmonary sequelae of mitral stenosis may encompass reduced lung compliance and a rise in airway resistance, both of which increase the work of breathing. Gas exchange worsens with a widening of the alveolar–arterial oxygen difference (A–aDO$_2$).

Anaesthetic Implications of Mitral Stenosis

- Mitral stenosis can lead to a fixed output state. Anaesthesia must minimize interference with compensatory mechanisms, because attempts to manipulate the cardiac output by the use of fluids or vasoactive drugs may prove fruitless.
- **Heart rate and rhythm:** bradycardia may allow increased stroke volume but at the expense of cardiac output; tachycardia will reduce stroke volume and also reduce cardiac output.
- **Maintenance of cardiac rhythm:** sudden onset of AF must be treated aggressively, with DC cardioversion if necessary, otherwise pulmonary oedema may develop. If AF is already present, the ventricular response rate must be controlled.
- **Circulating volume:** normovolaemia is important. If LAP drops because of reduced venous return, then cardiac output will fall as flow across the stenotic valve decreases. Patients may also be very sensitive to increases in venous return; in severe stenosis cardiac output cannot change, and pulmonary oedema may supervene.
- **Contractility:** effective myocardial contraction is important and depression must be minimized.

- **Systemic vascular resistance (SVR):** normal SVR ensures adequate coronary perfusion during diastole.
- **Pulmonary vascular resistance (PVR):** hypercapnia, hypoxia and acidosis will all increase PVR. Nitrous oxide further increases PVR in the presence of pre-existing pulmonary hypertension and so should be avoided.
- **Infective bacterial endocarditis:** see under 'Mitral Incompetence' in the next section.
- **Anticoagulation:** patients may be taking oral anticoagulants which may need to be changed to parenteral heparin during the perioperative period, depending on the surgery to be undertaken.

Mitral Incompetence

- Mitral incompetence is commoner than stenosis. It is rheumatic in origin in around 50% of cases. Other causes include disruption of the chordae tendinae and papillary muscle supporting structures (this can follow myocardial infarction), and dilatation of the valve ring itself.
- **Pathophysiology**
  — During systolic left ventricular contraction there is regurgitant flow back into the left atrium in addition to forward flow through the aorta. This can be quantified by measuring the regurgitant fraction: up to 0.3 is classified as mild; a fraction of 0.6 or greater is severe.
  — This regurgitant flow leads to volume overload of left atrium and left ventricle. Although left ventricular end-diastolic volume (LVEDV) may increase fourfold, the function of the ventricle is usually well preserved because the larger volume of blood can be unloaded both through the aorta and the mitral valve, and so systolic ventricular wall tension is not high. In time, however, this process leads to an irreversible decline in contractile function.
  — The left atrium dilates, and AF may supervene, but this does not cause the critical decompensation in cardiac function that may be seen in mitral stenosis. Mitral incompetence does not in general impose large costs in terms of myocardial oxygen demand (owing to ventricular wall tension, contractility and heart rate). This allows some compensation by a relatively rapid heart rate, which reduces the time for further ventricular overload. The prolonged filling time associated with a bradycardia increases ventricular volume, may cause further functional dilatation of the annulus and with it a rise in the regurgitant fraction. The left ventricle also dilates, with an increase in LVEDV and pressure. Forward flow of blood into the systemic circulation depends on the relative impedances of the two parallel paths, and so is enhanced by low PVR.

Anaesthetic Implications of Mitral Incompetence

- **Heart rate:** relative tachycardia is preferable to bradycardia because it reduces left ventricular overload. Bradycardia may increase ventricular filling and further dilate the valve ring.
- **Circulating volume:** patients may be sensitive to large rises in preload, because this will further distend the left atrium and predispose to pulmonary oedema.

- **Contractility:** myocardial depression should be avoided.
- **SVR:** the forward flow of blood is dependent on low peripheral resistance. Vasoconstrictors should be used with caution.
- **Infective bacterial endocarditis:** up until a decade ago, empirical antibiotic prophylaxis was routine for any patient undergoing surgery. Following the recommendations of various specialist working parties, this has changed completely in what the National Institute for Health and Clinical Excellence (NICE) themselves described in 2008 as a 'paradigm shift'. Their most recent guidelines (2015 and 2016) reiterate that although patients with acquired valvular disease should be considered to be at increased risk of developing infective endocarditis, they should not be given routine prophylactic antibiotics. In essence this conclusion was drawn from the lack of any supporting evidence, together with more mundane examples to suggest that prophylaxis is redundant when it is known, for example, that the fact of simple tooth brushing is associated with a transient bacteraemia comparable to that produced by surgical trauma.

Aortic Valve Disease

Commentary

As with other cardiac valvular conditions, anaesthetic interest in aortic valve disease centres on the need to avoid perioperative decompensation. Like mitral pathology, it is a popular exam topic because it allows discussion of applied physiology and pharmacology.

Core Information

Aortic Stenosis

- Aortic stenosis may be caused by rheumatic heart disease, degeneration and calcification of the valve, either as a result of ageing, or in a congenitally abnormal (usually bicuspid) valve. The distinction between a 'stenotic' and a 'sclerotic' valve is artificial. Sclerosis does stenose the valve but rarely to a critical degree. Severe aortic stenosis is said to affect 2% of those aged greater than 65 years in the developed world, with that figure doubling to 4% in the over-85-year-old group.
- **Pathophysiology**
  - Determination of the peak pressure gradient across the valve is less reliable than estimations of valvular area, but the quoted values for grading severity are: Normal <10 (mmHg); Mild <40; Moderate 40–65; Severe >65. The cross-sectional area of a normal aortic valve is 2.5–3.5 cm^2. An area <1.0 cm^2 is usually an indication for urgent surgical valve replacement. At areas of <0.7 cm^2 ('critical' stenosis), any demand for increased cardiac output, such as occurs during advancing pregnancy or during exercise, is likely to be associated with angina pectoris, syncope and sudden death. Asymptomatic but severe aortic

stenosis carries a risk of sudden death of around 1%. Once symptoms supervene, then life expectancy shrinks to 2 years with a 50% probability of sudden death. Clinical signs of the disease include narrowed pulse pressure (a value of <30 mmHg suggests severe disease), and a coarse systolic murmur in the aortic area. Systolic blood pressure may be lower than expected because of the reduced cardiac output. The gradient may be misleadingly low in a patient whose failing left ventricle is unable to generate high systolic intraventricular pressures.

— As narrowing progresses there is increased pressure loading on the left ventricle, which undergoes concentric hypertrophy. The hypertrophic left ventricle is less compliant, thus myocardial oxygen demand increases while supply falls. Systole through the stenosed valve is prolonged, and so diastolic time during the cardiac cycle is proportionately reduced. The high intraventricular pressures almost completely abolish systolic coronary flow. Diastolic subendocardial perfusion also decreases unless perfusion pressures remain high.

— The decrease in ventricular compliance and the loss of ventricular filling by passive elastic recoil means that the atrial contribution to filling becomes more important. It may in some cases be responsible for up to 50% of LVEDV. Atrial fibrillation may lead to cardiac decompensation.

Anaesthetic Implications of Aortic Stenosis

- Aortic stenosis leads to a fixed output state, which is maintained by compensatory mechanisms that may be disrupted by anaesthesia. Decompensated mitral stenosis manifests as heart failure; decompensated aortic stenosis may manifest as death. It is particularly important to maintain coronary perfusion during diastole.
- **Contractility:** effective contraction maintains cardiac output in aortic stenosis (as in all valvular lesions), and undue myocardial depression should be avoided. Increasing myocardial drive, however, does increase myocardial work and oxygen demand, and may precipitate subendocardial ischaemia.
- **Maintenance of systemic vascular resistance (SVR) and diastolic blood pressure:** if SVR falls, then coronary diastolic perfusion may fail, with potentially disastrous consequences. Vasodilatation must be avoided and preload maintained to ensure flow across the stenotic valve. This has obvious implications for the use of the many anaesthetic agents which decrease SVR, including local anaesthetics used in neuraxial block. Cardiopulmonary resuscitation in the presence of aortic stenosis and left ventricular hypertrophy is rarely successful.
- **Heart rate and rhythm:** bradycardia will decrease cardiac output, but tachycardia is more detrimental because it limits the time for diastolic coronary perfusion. The optimal heart rate in sinus rhythm is 60–80 beats per minute. Arrhythmias, including AF, require urgent treatment, but myocardial depressants such as β-adrenoceptor blockers are better avoided.
- **Infective bacterial endocarditis:** the 2015 update from the National Institute for Health and Care Excellence (NICE), (whose name changed from 'Clinical' Excellence to 'Care' Excellence in 2012), recommended that individuals with acquired valvular heart disease should be considered to be at increased risk of infective endocarditis, but that such patients should not be given prophylactic antibiotics as routine.

- Patients with severe aortic stenosis can be difficult to manage. Cases presenting for non-emergency surgery should be referred to a specialist centre for consideration of aortic valve replacement. Otherwise anaesthesia should include invasive monitoring of intra-arterial and central venous pressure, and it may be necessary to run a continuous infusion of vasopressor (such as noradrenaline) to ensure that SVR is maintained.

Aortic Incompetence

- Aortic incompetence has numerous causes, most of them quite rare. The overall prevalence in the general population is quoted as around 1%. There are infectious causes (bacterial endocarditis, syphilis, rheumatic fever), congenital abnormalities (bicuspid valve), degenerative and connective tissue disorders (Marfan's syndrome, Ehlers–Danlos) and inflammatory conditions (rheumatoid arthritis, systemic lupus erythematosus). Abnormal dilatation of the ascending aorta itself may cause regurgitation in the absence of pathology affecting the valve itself.
- **Pathophysiology**
  — The condition is usually chronic, although acute aortic regurgitation can occur with dissection or as the result of destruction of the valve by bacterial endocarditis.
  — The regurgitation during diastole of part of the left ventricular stroke volume decreases forward blood flow through the aorta. This results in continuous volume overload of the left ventricle, which initially dilates to accommodate this extra volume. On the ascending part of the Frank–Starling pressure–volume curve, the increase in myofibril length improves the efficiency of contraction. With increasing dilatation, the heart moves on to the descending part of the curve, at which point acute cardiac failure may supervene. In acute aortic incompetence, the left ventricle is unable to dilate, and there is an increase in left ventricular diastolic pressure and pulmonary venous pressure with the potential for pulmonary oedema.
  — Compensatory mechanisms act to reduce the volume of regurgitant blood. As with mitral incompetence, a regurgitant fraction of 0.6 or greater denotes severe disease. There is an increase in left ventricular size with eccentric hypertrophy. There is also an increase in ventricular compliance, which allows an increase in volume at the same pressure. This means that end-diastolic pressure is reduced, and with it ventricular wall tension which is an important determinant of myocardial oxygen demand. The left ventricular ejection fraction is maintained, since the stroke volume and LVEDV increase together.
  — A rapid heart rate is advantageous, because it reduces the time for diastolic filling. LVEDV is decreased, and so there is less ventricular over distension.
  — Lower SVR offloads the myocardium and ensures forward flow.

Anaesthetic Implications of Aortic Incompetence

- **Preload:** normovolaemia should be maintained to ensure that the dilated ventricle remains well filled.
- **SVR:** this should be kept low so as not to increase the impedance to outflow with an increase in the regurgitant fraction.

- **Heart rate:** bradycardia increases the time for ventricular over distension. A relative tachycardia will reduce the regurgitant fraction.
- **Contractility:** it is obvious that undue myocardial depression should be avoided.
- **Infective bacterial endocarditis:** as with other valvular lesions the 2015 update from NICE recommended that individuals with acquired valvular heart disease should not be given prophylactic antibiotics as routine, although they should be considered as being at increased risk.

Oxygen Delivery

Commentary

An organism survives by means of effective oxygen delivery to mitochondria. There is perennial interest in the concept of optimizing oxygen flux both in critically ill patients and in those undergoing major surgery. An understanding of the underlying principles may be linked to the continuing debate about goal-directed therapy (see under 'Sepsis' in the next section.)

Core Information

Factors that determine oxygen delivery.

- Oxygen is required for energy generation in mitochondria via the process of oxidative phosphorylation.
- Oxygen delivery (oxygen flux) to the tissues is governed by cardiac output (heart rate [HR] × stroke volume [SV]) and arterial oxygen content. Content is determined by:

$$[\text{Haemoglobin concentration}] \times [\%\text{saturation}] \times [1:31]$$

1.31 is the O_2-carrying capacity of haemoglobin. The theoretical figure of 1.39, which was based on a more exact determination of the molecular weight of haemoglobin, has been superseded by this figure of 1.306 ml g^{-1}, derived from direct measurements of oxygen capacity and haemoglobin concentration. Dissolved oxygen (0.003 ml dl^{-1} $mmHg^{-1}$) is small and can be ignored unless hyperbaric therapy is contemplated.

- The formal equation relates delivery to cardiac index (cardiac output/body surface area [BSA]) and so is given by:

$$O_2 \text{ flux} = \left[HR \times SV \left(l \min^{-1}\right)/BSA \times SaO_2(SpO_2)\% \right] / \left[100 \times Hb \left(g\,l^{-1}\right) \times 1.31 \right]$$

Supplementary Information

Optimization of Oxygen Flux

- There are only four variables that can be manipulated: heart rate (HR), stroke volume (SV), haemoglobin concentration (Hb) and oxygen saturation (SpO_2).

- **Cardiac output:** HR and SV are affected by various factors, including venous return and myocardial contractility. Ventricular preload can be improved by optimizing volaemic status, and contractility can be augmented by inotropes.
- **Measurement:** cardiac output determination is discussed under 'Measurement of Cardiac Ouput' in Chapter 5.
- **Oxygen saturation:** this may be improved by enhancing cardiac performance as discussed previously. It will also be influenced by primary pulmonary factors affecting gas exchange, some of which may be amenable to treatment. Conditions that can be improved include chest infections, atelectasis and bronchoconstriction. Supplemental oxygen will increase PaO_2, although intra-pulmonary shunting will diminish the effectiveness of increasing the FiO_2.
- **Haemoglobin concentration:** the oxygen delivery equation confirms the importance of haemoglobin: given a cardiac output of 5 l min^{-1} and an SpO_2 of 100%, O_2 delivery at a [Hb] of 100 g l^{-1} is 670 ml min^{-1}; at 150 g l^{-1} it rises to 1,005 ml min^{-1}. It is therefore clear that oxygen flux can be improved significantly if a low haemoglobin is increased by transfusion. 'Low' in the context of anaesthesia and intensive therapy does not of course mean 100 g l^{-1}. An oxygen delivery of 670 ml min^{-1} is more than adequate, and few intensivists would wish to transfuse such a patient.
- **Dissolved oxygen:** at atmospheric pressure breathing air, the O_2 solubility coefficient (0.003 ml dl^{-1} $mmHg^{-1}$) means that dissolved O_2 content is around 0.26 ml dl^{-1}. If a subject breathes 100% oxygen, this increases to 1.7 ml dl^{-1} and, at 3 atmospheres in a hyperbaric chamber, it reaches 5.6 ml dl^{-1}. At this level, dissolved oxygen can make a significant contribution to delivery to the tissues.

Sepsis

Commentary

The profile of sepsis recognition and management has been increased greatly by the Surviving Sepsis Campaign and the introduction of care bundles, particularly the so-called Sepsis Six. These bundles are simple, unlike the underlying pathological processes, which can be complex. In addition, the terminology of sepsis can be somewhat confusing. Research papers which deal with the subject include as keywords 'sepsis', 'septic shock', 'sepsis syndrome' and 'systemic inflammatory response syndrome'. The most recent NICE guidelines (2016) suggest restricting the terminology to 'sepsis' and 'septic shock'. The pathophysiology of sepsis is very detailed, and so a relatively superficial overview of some of the important mediators should be adequate. The clinical aspects are likely to concentrate on initial and critical care management, and you should be familiar with the broad principles.

Core Information

- **Definitions:** *sepsis* is defined as infection (suspected or proven) together with a systemic inflammatory response syndrome (SIRS). Sepsis plus organ dysfunction is described as *severe sepsis*, and, if this is accompanied by hypotension unrelieved by fluid resuscitation, it is known as *septic shock*. (This nomenclature has mainly been useful in designing randomized controlled trials [RCTs]). In the oral it will be acceptable to discuss 'sepsis' as a single entity.)

- **SIRS:** this comprises features of the inflammatory response in the absence of an identifiable pathogen, end-organ damage or the need for circulatory support. It is therefore distinct from sepsis and its variants. Once a pathogen has been isolated, then the working diagnosis in a patient shifts from SIRS to sepsis, severe sepsis or septic shock. Once end-organ damage supervenes the diagnosis becomes that of early multiple organ dysfunction syndrome (MODS). SIRS is defined by the presence of two or more of the following: temperature $>38\,^{\circ}C$ or $<36\,^{\circ}C$; tachycardia >90 beats min^{-1}; tachypnoea >20 breaths min^{-1} (or $PaCO_2 <4.3$ kPa); white cell count $>12 \times 10^3$ mm^{-3} or $<4 \times 10^3$ mm^{-3}.

- **The 'Sepsis Six':** this is a simple care bundle (a bundle being defined as a group of interventions that together have a greater effect on beneficial outcome than when the individual interventions are given in a disparate manner) that should be implemented as soon as the diagnosis of sepsis is suspected. If initiated within the first hour associated mortality is substantially reduced (up to 50%). The elements consist of (1) Oxygen at high flows to maintain SpO_2 $>94\%$, (2) Blood cultures, (3) Antibiotics, broad spectrum, given intravenously, (4) Fluid resuscitation (e.g. 20 ml.kg^{-1} initially), (5) Lactate measurement: a level >4 mmol l^{-1} is consistent with severe sepsis and (6) Urine output monitoring (hourly). (This shouldn't be too difficult to remember, but if your mind goes blank the acronym 'OBAFLU' may act as a mnemonic.)

- **NICE guidelines (2016):** these stressed early recognition, the non-specific nature of presentation, the identification of high-risk groups (including those who are immunocompromised, patients taking corticosteroids, diabetics, the elderly, intravenous drug users, those who have recently undergone surgery or have given birth) and initial management broadly in line with the 'Sepsis Six'. In addition to blood lactate determination, NICE recommended that laboratory investigations should include full blood count, electrolytes, coagulation, C-reactive protein, creatinine and venous blood gases. Senior involvement is required early, as is timely referral to critical care.

- **The inflammatory response:** this is systemic rather than localized and is part of an exaggerated or uncontrolled host response to a pathological insult. It is highly complex, comprising a sequence of reactions which involves not only the secretion of key signalling molecules such as the cytokines (protein immunoregulators that include interleukins IL-1, 5, 6, 8, 11 and 15, tumour necrosis factor, colony-stimulating factors, interferons and platelet-activating factor) but also the activation of complement. Other inflammatory mediators such as kinins and histamine lead to vasodilatation and increased capillary permeability, while leukotrienes stimulate inward granulocyte migration. In addition, there is an increase in acute phase proteins such as haptoglobin, fibrinogen and C-reactive protein (CRP). CRP activates monocytes, increases cytokine production and can activate the complement cascade. Other aspects of immune function, such as cell-mediated and humoral immunity, may also be mobilized.

- **Procoagulant–anticoagulant balance:** sepsis alters this balance in favour of procoagulant factors. Endothelial cells appear to upregulate tissue factor and thereby activate coagulation and the formation of microvascular thrombus. The anticoagulant factors suppress coagulation and enhance fibrinolysis. They include protein C, its co-factor protein S, antithrombin III and tissue factor-pathway inhibitor. All are decreased by sepsis.
- **Causes and clinical features:** the final common pathway to the inflammatory response can be triggered by numerous insults such as trauma, major surgery and challenges to the immune system by various antigens, including infective agents and the transfusion of blood and blood products. The major infective sources are respiratory (30–50%), urinary tract (10–20%) and abdominal (20–25%). Consistent with the diagnostic criteria described earlier, patients typically exhibit tachycardia, disturbed temperature regulation, tachypnoea, a narrowed pulse pressure secondary to the reduced effective circulating volume and oliguria. The hypoperfusion is responsible for the lactic acidosis that is a typical feature of the condition (see under 'Massive Haemorrhage: Compensatory Responses and Management'). These clinical signs are relatively non-specific.

Supplementary Information and Clinical Considerations

- **Early goal-directed therapy (EGDT):** This is discussed later in this section.
- **Ventilation:** acute lung injury with capillary leak frequently complicates sepsis. Lung-protective ventilation reduces mortality (see under 'The Failing Lung').
- **Antibiotics:** empirical broad-spectrum antibiotics are usually necessary until a pathogen has been identified. Expert microbiological advice is helpful, particularly in respect of factors such as local patterns of antibiotic usage and bacterial susceptibility.
- **Glycaemic control:** sepsis is associated with insulin resistance and hyperglycaemia, whose adverse effects in critical illness are well established. It is procoagulant, induces apoptosis, impairs neutrophil function and delays wound healing. Insulin counteracts all these effects. Tight glycaemic control which maintains blood glucose levels at between 4.4 and 6.1 mmol l^{-1} reduces mortality rates in critically ill surgical patients. The same benefit has not been demonstrated in critically ill medical patients.
- **Vasopressin:** vasopressin deficiency and receptor downregulation occur commonly in sepsis, and vasopressin infusion improves haemodynamic indices and reduces concomitant inotrope requirements. This is at the expense in some patients of decreased cardiac output and gastrointestinal ischaemia. Hazards increase at infusion rates greater than 0.04 units min^{-1}.
- **Transfusion:** data are equivocal, but although severely anaemic patients should be transfused with red cells, the threshold appears to be low, with haemoglobin levels of between 70 and 90 g l^{-1} being acceptable.
- **Renal replacement therapy (RRT):** there is little evidence that early RRT alters outcomes, but it clearly cannot be withheld from patients with acute renal dysfunction and deranged biochemistry.
- **Other drugs**
  - **Corticosteroids:** RCTs of high-dose early glucocorticoids have shown no improvement in survival.

— **Nitric oxide synthetase inhibitors:** excess production of nitric oxide (NO) may be associated with the early vasodilatation and myocardial depression that is seen in septic shock, but NO synthetase inhibitors such as arginine derivatives increase mortality rates.

— **Monoclonal antibodies:** there is no evidence of benefit from the use of monoclonal antibodies such as anti-TNF.

— **Selenium:** there is some evidence that adjuvant treatment with high-dose selenium is associated with a reduction in 28-day mortality rates. Selenium is an important antioxidant whose levels fall in sepsis. It has a relatively narrow therapeutic index.

— **Activated protein C (APC):** the PROWESS trial of APC in severe sepsis (published in 2001) was halted early because of the significant improvement in mortality that was demonstrated in the treatment group. Doubts about the methodology of the study brought these results into question, however, and subsequent trials failed to show the same benefits. The drug was withdrawn from the market in 2011, perhaps prematurely, because further studies might have identified a group of patients in whom it would have reduced mortality. The agent had powerful disease-modulating properties which included the inactivation of clotting factors Va and VIIIa, enhanced fibrinolysis, decreased cytokine production and reduced leucocyte activation.

Goal-Directed and Early Goal-Directed Therapy

- **Goal-directed therapy (GDT)** is a term used to describe the use of specific indices to guide intravenous fluid, oxygen and inotrope therapy. Its origins lie in studies published in the 1980s (by, amongst others, Bland and Shoemaker), which suggested that survival in high-risk surgical patients was higher in those in whom supranormal levels of oxygen delivery (DO_2) were achieved. (Shoemaker *et al.* Chest 1988, 94: 1176–86).

- The strategy involves the manipulation of cardiac preload and myocardial contractility to optimize systemic oxygen delivery. Typical 'goals' include supra-normal DO_2 of >600 ml min^{-1}, central venous pressure (CVP) of 8–12 mmHg, mixed venous oxygen saturation (SvO_2) $>70\%$, mean arterial pressure >65 mmHg, urine output >0.5 ml kg^{-1} h^{-1}, oxygen saturation (SpO_2) $>93\%$ and haematocrit $>30\%$. The state of tissue perfusion is assessed best by measuring SvO_2, blood lactate concentration, base deficit and intramucosal gastric pH (pHi). (Normal oxygen utilization is around 110 ml min^{-1} m^{-2}. This rises to over 170 ml min^{-1} m^{-2} following major surgery, which in patients of normal size is still well below the DO_2 that has been advocated.)

- The aim of sustaining a supranormal DO_2 may be an oversimplification. High global oxygen delivery does not exclude regional perfusion deficiencies. This is especially true of the splanchnic circulation, which is the first to falter and the last to recover. Any drop in cardiac output appears to be accompanied by a disproportionately large fall in splanchnic perfusion, which can lead to disruption of the enteric mucosal barrier, bacterial translocation and endotoxic triggering of the inflammatory cytokine pathways.

- A number of trials and meta-analyses supported the benefits of the approach which was extended to the management of patients with sepsis, and one particularly influential study suggested that EGDT improved survival in the critically ill

(E. Rivers *et al. N Engl J Med* 2001, 345: 1368–77). EGDT emphasizes intensive fluid therapy within 6 hours of onset, titrated against standard physiological variables. If it was delayed, then EGDT was shown either to make no difference or to worsen outcome. In due course, however, the methodology of this study was challenged, and several subsequent large studies, the most recent of which was the ProMISe (proto-colised management of sepsis) trial which enrolled 1,260 patients in the UK, have suggested that following appropriate fluid resuscitation and intravenous antibiotics in patients with septic shock, the manipulation of haemodynamic indices according to strict EGDT protocols makes no difference to outcome (P.R. Mouncey *et al. N Engl J Med* 2015, 372: 1301–11). Two other influential studies were the ProCESS trial (protocolized care for early septic shock) and the ARISE trial (Australasian resuscitation in sepsis evaluation), both of which failed to show any outcome benefit from EGDT.

Central Venous Pressure and Cannulation

Commentary

Central venous catheters (CVCs) are used widely in critical care and in major anaesthetic cases, and so although the underpinning principles are not complex, questions on the topic reappear. An understanding will be expected of how to interpret measurements and the normal waveform, insertion of the devices and familiarity with most of the very long list of potential complications. The topic may form part of an anatomy-based question on the internal jugular vein (see under 'The Internal Jugular Vein' in Chapter 2).

Core Information

Central Venous Pressure (CVP): The Waveform

- This comprises three upstrokes (the 'a', 'c' and 'v' waves) and two descents (the 'x' and 'y') that relate to the cardiac cycle.
- **'a' wave:** this occurs at the end of diastole and is caused by increased **a**trial pressure as the atrium contracts (occurs at end-diastole).
- **'x' (or 'x") descent:** this reflects the fall in atrial pressure as the atrium relaxes.
- **'c' wave:** this supervenes before full atrial relaxation, and is caused by the bulging of the **c**losed tricuspid valve into the atrium at the start of isovolumetric right ventricular **c**ontraction.
- **'x' descent:** this is a continuation of the 'x" descent (interrupted by the 'c' wave) and represents the pressure drop as the ventricle and valve 'screw' downwards at the end of systole.
- **'v' wave:** this is the increase in right atrial pressure as it is filled by the venous return against a closed tricuspid valve.
- **'y' descent:** this reflects the drop in pressure as the right ventricle relaxes, the tricuspid valve opens and the atrium empties into the ventricle.

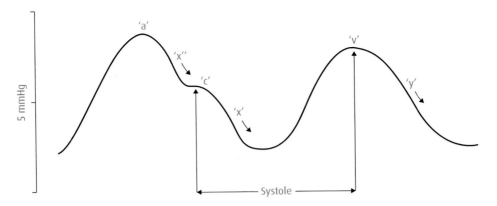

Fig. 3.6 Central venous pressure waveform.

- Any event that alters the normal relationship between these events will alter the shape of the waveform. For example, in atrial fibrillation the 'a' wave is lost; in tricuspid incompetence, a giant 'v' wave replaces the 'c' wave, the 'x' descent and the 'v' wave. 'Cannon' waves are seen when there is atrial contraction against a closed tricuspid valve (as occurs at a regular interval if there is a junctional rhythm, or at an irregular interval if there is complete atrioventricular conduction block).

Indications for Central Venous Catheterization

- **Indications:** CVC catheters are used for the monitoring of central venous pressures, for the insertion of pulmonary artery catheters and to provide access for haemofiltration and transvenous cardiac pacing. Central venous lines also allow the administration of drugs that cannot be given peripherally, such as inotropes and cytotoxic agents, and the infusion of total parenteral nutrition. It is suggested that they can be used to aspirate air from the right side of the heart after massive air embolism, although very few anaesthetists have ever used them for this purpose.
- **Function of CVP monitoring – intravascular volume:** the CVP is the hydrostatic pressure generated by the blood within the right atrium (RA) or the great veins of the thorax. It provides an indication of volaemic status because the capacitance system, including all the large veins of the thorax, abdomen and proximal extremities, forms a large compliant reservoir for around two-thirds of the total blood volume. Hypovolaemia may be actual or effective, caused, for example, by subarachnoid block or sepsis, in which loss of venoconstrictor tone or venodilatation decreases venous return and reduces CVP. A single reading may be unhelpful, whereas trends are more useful, particularly when combined with fluid challenges.

- **Function of CVP monitoring – right ventricular function:** CVP measurements also provide an indication of right ventricular (RV) function. Any impairment of RV function will be reflected by the higher filling pressures that are needed to maintain the same stroke volume (SV).
- **Normal values:** the normal range is 0–8 mmHg, measured at the level of the tricuspid valve. The tip of the catheter should lie just above the RA in the superior vena cava.
- **CVP decreases:** if the blood volume is unchanged, then the CVP will alter with changes in cardiac output (CO). It will fall as the CO rises because the rate at which blood is removed from the venous reservoir also increases. This reflects the essentially passive volume–pressure characteristics of the venous vascular system. The major cause of a fall in CVP is depletion of effective intravascular volume. (Raising the transducer will lead to an apparent fall in CVP.)
- **CVP increases:** potential causes for an increase in CVP include a fall in CO (the converse of the effect described previously). Ventilatory modes may also cause the increase which is seen with IPPV, PEEP and CPAP. The CVP also rises in response to volume overload, if there is RV failure, pulmonary embolus, cardiac tamponade or tension pneumothorax. Rarer causes include obstruction of the superior vena cava (assuming that the catheter tip lies proximally) and portal hypertension leading to inferior vena caval backpressure. (Moving the reference point and lowering the transducer will also lead to an apparent increase.)
- **Complications of insertion:** these are numerous and include arterial puncture (carotid and subclavian), haemorrhage, air embolism, cardiac arrhythmias, pneumothorax, haemothorax, chylothorax, neurapraxia, cardiac tamponade and thoracic duct injury. Anatomically proximate structures such as the oesophagus and trachea can also be damaged. Parts of catheters or entire guidewires can embolise into the circulation. Ultrasound guidance can reduce complications associated with catheter insertion. Endocarditis and cardiac rupture have been reported. Venous thrombosis is common, but the risk may be reduced by the use of heparin-bonded catheters. Infection is a problem, and occurs in up to 12% of placements. Its risk is reduced by full aseptic precautions, by the use of antiseptic- and antibiotic-coated catheters (in high-risk patients) and by using the subclavian approach. There is no definite evidence of benefit for tunnelling, for prophylactic line changes or for the use of prophylactic antibiotics. These complications can be fatal: the confidential maternal mortality reports alone have documented three deaths caused by central catheterization.

Supplementary Information

CVP measurements are sometimes recorded as negative values.

- If the CVP is measured from the accurate reference point of the tricuspid valve, then a sustained negative intravascular pressure is impossible. Certainly, the negative intrathoracic pressure during inspiration will be transmitted to the central veins, and if there is respiratory obstruction this negative pressure will be high. It will, however, be transient. If a mean CVP reading is consistently negative it can only be because the transducer has been placed above the level of the right atrium.

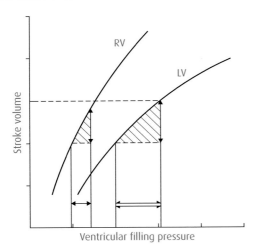

Fig. 3.7 Ventricular function curves. In response to a fluid challenge there is a differential rise in ventricular filling pressures, although the increase in stroke volume is the same. RV, right ventricle; LV, left ventricle.

CVP measurement and left ventricular function.

- The right atrial pressure reflects the right ventricular end-diastolic pressure (RVEDP), and it is frequently assumed that this also reflects the left ventricular end-diastolic pressure (LVEDP). This is not strictly true even in health, because the right ventricle ejects into a low-pressure system, and so the normal RV function curve (in which SV is plotted against filling pressure) is steeper than the LV curve (Figure 3.7). This means that, for a given fluid load, the increase in SV of each ventricle is identical, but the rise in filling pressure in the left ventricle exceeds that in the right. This discrepancy is accentuated by LV dysfunction, and under these circumstances accurate diagnostic information has to be obtained by other means.

Fluid Therapy

Commentary

The optimum choice of fluids for many different clinical circumstances remains confusing and contentious, and you will not be expected to resolve the various controversies. Volume restoration, however, is such an important part of anaesthetic practice that you will be expected to demonstrate both an understanding of the fluid compartments of the body and a logical appreciation of the characteristics of the different replacement fluids.

Core Information

- **Normal body fluid compartments:** of the total body weight in men, 60% is water. In women, who have a higher proportion of body fat, it is 50–55%. These proportions change with age; total body water (TBW) as a percentage of body weight may be 80%

in the neonate and 50% in the elderly. Two-thirds of TBW is intracellular water (ICW); the remaining third is extracellular fluid (ECF), which can be divided further into interstitial fluid (ISF) and the intravascular volume. There is a small volume of residual transcellular fluid, which has been secreted, but which remains separated from plasma, for example as cerebrospinal or intraocular fluid.

Fluid Loss from Body Compartments

- **Blood loss:** this is straightforward. Intravascular volume may be depleted directly by trauma or during surgery. It may occur pre-operatively, for example following the rupture of a varicose venous ulcer or an arterial aneurysm, or postoperatively.
- **Pure dehydration:** this implies a loss of water alone, without electrolytes. This may be caused by prolonged lack of fluid intake, protracted pre-operative fasting and as a result of any condition that may prevent swallowing. Dehydration depletes all the fluid compartments and is corrected by a solution that equilibrates across all three, namely glucose 5%. Even in these situations there are always some electrolyte losses.
- **Dehydration:** in the context of clinical medicine, most water deficits are also accompanied by electrolyte losses. The causes are numerous and include inappropriate diuretic therapy, diarrhoea and vomiting, intestinal obstruction, pre-operative bowel preparation, diabetes mellitus (and insipidus) and pyrexia. Insensible losses in a healthy individual in a temperate climate are of the order of 0.5 ml kg^{-1} h^{-1}.
- **Perioperative fluid losses:** these include the fluid deficits accrued as a result of pre-operative fasting, pre-operative pathology, intraoperative haemorrhage and what are termed 'third space' losses. This refers to fluid that is sequestered at the site of injury. Losses are variable, but, during the course of a long laparotomy through a large abdominal incision, fluid replacement may be needed by a balanced salt solution at a rate of up to 15 ml kg^{-1} h^{-1}.

Restoration of volaemic status.

- **Crystalloids**
  — A crystalloid solution is defined chemically as one containing a water-soluble crystalline substance capable of diffusion through a semi-permeable membrane.
  — Crystalloids can be infused rapidly in large volumes, are readily available and are cheap. Disadvantages include their short duration in the circulation, with only about 50% of the infused volume remaining in the intravascular compartment at 20 minutes. This increases the potential for overinfusion, circulatory overload and pulmonary oedema. Crystalloids have no oxygen-carrying capacity.
  — **Normal saline (NaCl 0.9%):** this contains 154 mmol l^{-1} each of sodium and chloride ions and is isotonic. The excess of chloride ions means that if large volumes are infused, a hyperchloraemic acidosis may supervene. This can be a particular problem in children.
  — **Hartmann's (compound sodium lactate):** this is a balanced salt solution whose composition approximates that of ECF. The lactate in Hartmann's is gluconeogenic, and so it has been recommended that the solution should not be used in diabetics. Given that basal lactate production is around 1,300 mmol 24^{-1} (0.8 mmol kg^{-1} hr^{-1}), however, it seems unlikely that the 29 mmol of lactate in a litre

of Hartmann's solution is going to make a substantial difference to any diabetic's glycaemic status, and so this is a prohibition that many anaesthetists are happy to ignore, viewing the infusion of normal saline as the greater problem.

— **Glucose 5%:** this is effectively a means of giving free water. Isotonic glucose solutions are appropriate for resuscitation of the intracellular compartment, but will have minimal impact on intravascular volumes because they will equilibrate throughout the 42 litres of water in the body's fluid compartments. Fluids which contain glucose have no place in acute fluid resuscitation.

- **Colloids**
  — A colloid is defined chemically as a dispersion, or suspension, of finely divided particles in a continuous medium. It is not therefore a solution. A butterfly's wing is a colloid, as are, more prosaically, foam rubber and fog.
  — Colloids are theoretically more effective than crystalloids in resuscitation, but the evidence to support their superiority is equivocal. All contain NaCl 0.9%, and Haemaccel contains small amounts of potassium and calcium. Blood is also a colloid, but by convention it is treated separately.
  — **Gelatins:** gelatins (Gelofusine and Haemaccel) contain modified gelatin of molecular weight between 30,000 and 35,000 Da, and have an effective half-life within the circulation of 3 hours. However, if the endothelial glycocalyx is impaired, as it is in sepsis, this circulatory half-life becomes no longer than that of crystalloid solutions. Their use in severe sepsis is also associated with a higher incidence of kidney injury, and they carry the additional risk of allergic reactions (quoted as 1 in 25,000). The CRISTAL trial randomized critically ill patients to fluid resuscitation with any colloid or any crystalloid and found no difference in mortality at 28 days (*JAMA* 2013, 310: 1809–17).
  — **Human albumin solution (HAS):** this was previously supplied as plasma protein fraction (PPF) and has an intravascular half-life of 24 hours. It is derived from pooled human plasma but is sterile. There remains uncertainty about prion diseases, vanishingly small though the risk may be, and there is controversy about its role in resuscitation. Some argue that if albumin crosses damaged cerebral and pulmonary capillary membranes, its use will only worsen outcome (by increasing interstitial fluid because of the osmotic pressure that it exerts). In general, however, albumin is not the 'killer fluid' identified by a (notoriously weak) systematic review but rather is a useful volume expander that has been shown in other studies to improve survival.
  — **Starches:** these, however, did turn out to be the killer fluid that human albumin never was. A number of randomized controlled trials together with meta-analyses have identified greater risks of kidney injury associated with the use of starches, and a higher mortality in the critically ill. Accordingly, in 2013 the Medicines and Healthcare Products Regulatory Agency (MHRA) announced the withdrawal of all hydroxyl ethyl starch products in the UK. (For information, as the Food and Drug Administration in the USA [US FDA] have not yet banned starches, they consist of amylopectin that is etherified with hydroxyethyl groups. They comprise a wide range of molecular weights and remain within the circulation for much longer than gelatins, with an effective intravascular half-life of 24 hours. Smaller

molecular weight particles [less than 50,000] are excreted renally, but the average molecular weight of hetastarch is 450,000 Da, so much of it remains in the body after partial degradation by α-amylase. Some of the starch molecules are taken up by the reticuloendothelial system and may persist there for over a year. Intractable pruritus has been reported as a complication of their use. Tetrastarches were newer preparations of lower molecular weight [130,000; degree of substitution 0.4]. Overall these preparations were associated with renal damage, a higher mortality in sepsis and other critical illness, and an increase in bleeding tendency.)

— **Dextrans:** these polysaccharides are classified according to their molecular weight: 40, 70 and 110×10^3. They also remain within the circulation for longer than crystalloids, with an effective half-life of 3 hours and upwards, but they have enjoyed only fitful popularity in the UK. They can also precipitate allergic reactions, may interfere with blood cross-matching (Dextran 70) and can cause renal problems (Dextran 40).

- **Blood:** blood is also a colloid, but it is convenient to discuss it separately. In acute blood loss, fresh whole blood is arguably the ideal replacement; it has oxygen-carrying capacity and expands the intravascular volume. Red cell concentrates, such as SAG-M, supply oxygen carriage but are not ideal intravascular expanders when given alone, as each unit only has a volume of around 300 ml. Blood is the most physiological solution, but homologous transfusion has numerous potential disadvantages which must be set against the urgency of optimal intravascular resuscitation (see under 'Complications of Blood Transfusion'.) Autologous transfusion is ideal but may be impractical in unexpected major blood loss. Blood is also an expensive commodity.

Alternative solutions of potential clinical value.

- **Perfluorocarbons:** these are inert, halogenated compounds which have the capacity to carry oxygen in solution, according to Henry's Law (the amount of gas that is dissolved in a liquid at a given temperature is proportional to the partial pressure in the gas in equilibrium with the solution). Older preparations, such as Fluosol DA20, had limited usefulness because of the requirement for high inspired oxygen concentrations, their relative inefficiency of oxygen carriage and the potential for adverse reactions. Newer compounds, such as perfluoro-octobromide, allow the carriage of oxygen equivalent to a haemoglobin concentration of up to 70 g l^{-1} and show more clinical promise.

- **Stroma-free haemoglobin solutions:** free haemoglobin is able to carry and deliver oxygen molecules, but to minimize the risk of toxicity it must be stroma-free (with no residual red cell debris). It has a higher affinity for oxygen than red cell haemoglobin (the P_{50} is 1.6 kPa compared to 3.6 kPa for red cell haemoglobin), and this marked leftward shift of the oxygen–haemoglobin dissociation curve reduces oxygen delivery to tissues. The molecules are also rapidly degraded in the body, may impair the immune response and can cause renal failure.

- **Micro-encapsulated haemoglobin:** haemoglobin can be enclosed within artificial microspheres of diameter around 1 μm and which retain 2,3-DPG inside the membrane. Such solutions are experimental.

Massive Haemorrhage: Compensatory Responses and Management

Commentary

This is a standard question, and so you need to be confident about your handling of any of the clinical scenarios with which you may be presented. In addition, it must be clear that your management is rational, based both on an understanding of the homeostatic mechanisms involved and on familiarity with the characteristics of the fluids that you may give.

Core Information

The normal compensatory responses to the loss of intravascular volume.

- The function of the circulation is to distribute the cardiac output to tissues sufficient to meet their metabolic demands. Any progressive loss of circulating volume is accompanied by a redistribution of flow aimed to ensure that the brain and myocardium continue to receive oxygenated blood.
- As blood loss continues, the decreases in venous return, right atrial pressure and cardiac output activate baroreceptor reflexes (mediated by stretch-sensitive receptors in the carotid sinus and aortic arch). This is an immediate response. The decreased afferent input to the medullary cardiovascular centres inhibits parasympathetic and enhances sympathetic activity.
- There follows an increase in cardiac output together with alterations in the resistance of vascular beds in an attempt to maintain tissue perfusion. These changes are mediated via direct sympathetic innervation, by circulating humoral vasopressors such as adrenaline, angiotensin, noradrenaline and vasopressin, and by local tissue mediators, including hydrogen ions, potassium, adenosine and nitric oxide. (The renal vasculature is especially sensitive.) Hypovolaemia encourages movement of fluid into capillaries, the decreased capillary hydrostatic pressure favouring absorption of interstitial fluid with a resultant increase in plasma volume and restoration of arterial pressure towards normal (Starling forces). These mechanisms are particularly efficient in situations in which blood loss is slow and progressive.
- The hypothalamo–pituitary–adrenal response is also important, although it is slower. Reduced renal blood flow stimulates intrarenal baroreceptors which mediate renin release from the juxta-glomerular apparatus. Renin converts circulating angiotensinogen to angiotensin I, from which angiotensin II (AT II) is formed in the lung. AT II is a potent arteriolar vasoconstrictor that stimulates aldosterone release from the adrenal cortex and arginine vasopressin (ADH) release from the posterior pituitary. ADH release is also stimulated by atrial receptors, which respond to the decrease in extracellular volume. These changes enhance sodium and water reabsorption at the distal renal tubule as the body attempts to conserve fluid. Sympathetic stimulation also mediates secretion of catecholamines and cortisol.
- **Inflammatory response.** It is also clear that there is a significant inflammatory response to major haemorrhage. Hypoperfused and hypoxic endothelium releases

the familiar inflammatory mediators, oxidants and cytokines as is seen in sepsis and reperfusion injuries, and these may similarly mediate coagulopathy and a systemic inflammatory response syndrome (SIRS). This phenomenon emphasizes the importance of flow rather than pressure. Endogenous catecholamines and exogenous vasopressors may increase arterial pressure, but at the level of the microcirculation, pre-capillary arteriolar constriction will simply decrease flow through the capillary bed, compromise tissue perfusion further and accelerate the inflammatory response.

- **Acute Trauma Coagulopathy (ACT).** Major trauma is associated with the development of coagulopathy that is proportional to the severity of the injury and which is now specifically described as 'acute trauma coagulopathy'. Its mechanisms have not fully been elucidated, but it is likely that critically underperfused vascular endothelium accelerates activation of the coagulation cycle with consumption particularly of Factor V and fibrinogen (Factor I). The effectiveness of coagulation is also compromised by hypothermia and acidaemia, both of which may frequently complicate severe trauma.

The Metabolic Acidosis Associated with Blood Loss

- **Lactic acidosis:** decreased tissue perfusion causes a progressive decline in aerobic metabolism, which is accompanied by a compensatory increase in anaerobic metabolism. This shift to anaerobic metabolism results in a decrease in energy production and the development of a metabolic acidosis. In the aerobic tricarboxylic acid (TCA) cycle, the hydrogen ions which are produced are carried by NADH and $NADH_2$ to the electron transport chain in which the final acceptor is molecular oxygen, which is then converted to water. In the absence of molecular oxygen, the final acceptor is missing and so NADH accumulates. The lack of NAD^+ effectively blocks the TCA cycle, and so pyruvate (CH_3-C = O-COOH) also accumulates (at the 'entrance' to the cycle). NADH and pyruvate react to form lactate (CH_3-HCOH-COOH) and NAD^+. The lactate then diffuses out of the cell to accumulate as lactic acid; NAD^+ meanwhile allows anaerobic glycolysis to proceed.

- **Summary of clinical features:** redistribution of blood flow is responsible for the typical pallor, cold peripheries, peripheral cyanosis and oliguria. Sympathetic stimulation explains the tachycardia and the increase in respiratory rate. Carotid chemoreceptors also stimulate ventilation in response to changes in PaO_2, $PaCO_2$ and pH. Systolic blood pressure is a relatively crude index which may show little change until substantial volumes have been lost, particularly in young patients. The pulse pressure may be more useful; as blood loss continues, it narrows, and the mean arterial pressure may increase. This occurs because diastolic blood pressure is under the influence of catecholamines which rise in response to haemorrhage. Capillary refill time is a simple and effective measure. A delay of more than 2 seconds is abnormal, and trends can be used to gauge the effectiveness of fluid resuscitation. Confusion or other changes in mental state indicate cerebral hypoxaemia and hypoperfusion.

Massive Haemorrhage: Principles of Management

- The management of the patient with massive haemorrhage continues to evolve, particularly in the light of military trauma management. Airway and Breathing remain important components of the ABCDE assessment and management mantra, but C for Circulation is now less obvious. Controlling the bleeding at source is the key priority, whether it be due to trauma, post-partum haemorrhage or a ruptured aortic aneurysm. In some situations, particularly following trauma, this will be damage-control resuscitation prior to definitive surgical repair.

In addition to rapid surgical control of haemorrhage, the anaesthetist needs to ensure adequate tissue perfusion, and although from the anaesthetic perspective it may seem counter-intuitive, it can be deleterious to resuscitate the patient to euvolaemia and normotension. This may contribute a dilutional element to the coagulopathy, and may reduce the oxygen-carrying capacity of the circulation while jeopardizing flow through the capillary bed, as described earlier. Current practice is to aim for 'permissive hypotension' with a systolic blood pressure of around 80 mmHg and the more cautious titration of fluids against response. In the acute phase, moreover, it is clear that the optimal resuscitation fluids are blood, coagulation factors (in fresh frozen plasma and cryoprecipitate) and platelets. Military studies support initial transfusion of fresh frozen plasma (FFP) and packed red blood cells (PRC) in a 1:1 ratio, with platelets and cryoprecipitate given ideally in response to point of care coagulation tests, with tranexamic acid given as routine. Civilian protocols tend to vary, with FFP and PRC sometimes given in a 1:2 ratio. Although it may seem formulaic, it is clearly associated with better outcomes than the previous practice of transfusing red cells and then giving coagulation factors after a sometimes lengthy wait for a clotting profile, which in a dynamic situation may be inaccurate by the time that that is measured. (For general complications of blood transfusion, including those associated with rapid infusion, see under 'Complications of Blood Transfusion'.)

- **Fluids used in resuscitation:** see under 'Fluid Therapy'.

Blood Groups

Commentary
The subject of blood groups might appear alone, linked to a clinical question about acute haemolytic reactions; alternatively, it may arise as part of a general discussion of the complications of blood transfusion. The importance of the topic is self-evident, and so examiners could well assume that your knowledge of the clinical aspects is secure and will concentrate more on the science of the ABO blood group typing system. After the relatively straightforward concepts of the major types, the subject becomes too complex to explore in a short oral, and the questioning is likely to revert to clinical aspects.

Core Information

The Major Blood Groups
- The red cell membrane contains various blood group antigens, or agglutinogens. These are complex oligosaccharides which vary in their terminal sugar molecule (*N*-acetylgalactosamine in group A, and galactose in group B).

- The most important of many variants are the A and the B antigens. These are inherited as Mendelian dominants which allows separation of individuals into one of four main types: group A, which have the A antigen; B, which have the B antigen; AB, which carry both antigens; and group O, which carry neither. Red blood cells of all types carry an H antigen which also differs in the terminal sugar residues.
- Antibodies against these red cell agglutinogens are known as red cell agglutinins, and these are formed early in life. Individuals do not necessarily require exposure to blood; antigens that are related to A and B are found in gut bacteria and even in some foods, and so neonates develop early antibody responses. Type A individuals develop anti-B antibodies, type B develop anti-A antibodies, type AB develop neither, while type O develop both. Type O blood will therefore agglutinate (clump) blood of all other types, while group AB will agglutinate none. Thus, AB (rhesus negative) is the universal recipient and O (rhesus negative) the universal donor. Around 45% of individuals in the UK have the blood group O; 40% group A; 10% group B; and 5% group AB.
- **Other agglutinogens:** there are a large number of systems of which the rhesus is the most significant. (Others, amongst many, include the Lutheran, the Kidd and the Kell systems.) The rhesus factor comprises C, D and E antigens, of which D is the most important, being by far the most antigenic. Eighty-five per cent of the Caucasian population and 99% of the non-Caucasian population are D-rhesus-positive. In contrast to ABO antigens, individuals do require exposure to the D antigen in blood to develop antibodies, and this happens either by transfusion or by exposure of the maternal circulation to small amounts of fetal D-positive blood. This is significant for subsequent pregnancies should a mother be rhesus-negative but carrying a rhesus-positive fetus. Maternal antibodies will cross the placenta to cause haemolytic disease of the newborn. Hence the importance of administering rhesus immune globulin in the postpartum period to prevent the mother forming active antibodies.

Supplementary and Clinical Information

Suspected Transfusion Reactions and Immediate Management

- The acute antigen–antibody reaction can be triggered by transfusion of only very small volumes of blood. The donor cells are destroyed by antibodies in the recipient plasma, with haemolysis; this leads in some cases to intravascular fibrin deposition, disseminated intravascular coagulation and renal failure. If the patient is conscious then the relatively non-specific symptoms include dyspnoea, loin and chest pain, headache, nausea and vomiting. The patient may become pyrexial, may have rigors, can develop an urticarial rash and usually becomes hypotensive. In the anaesthetized patient, most of these features are lost apart from the possible urticaria and hypotension. As the reaction continues the patient may develop haemoglobinuria and a coagulopathy.
- **Management:** after stopping the transfusion, management is directed mainly towards standard cardiorespiratory support with airway intervention, fluids and inotropes as indicated. It is important to maximize renal perfusion because the risk of acute renal failure is high. Acute haemolytic reactions due to ABO or rhesus incompatibility are very rare (the Serious Hazards of Transfusion [SHOT] report of

2015 reported one death due to ABO incompatibility and six due to haemolysis) and occur usually as a result of human error.

- **Reducing the requirement for banked blood** (some of this would also be relevant to a question about the management of a Jehovah's Witness These individuals refuse blood on religious grounds, and although there is a spectrum of attitudes, the most committed believers will not accept blood, blood products or even autologous blood unless it remains in continuity with the circulation. This may therefore be the focus for a brief consideration of ethical issues).

- **Ethical concerns:** the situation is problematic for doctors, but legally there is no ambiguity: an individual with capacity has the absolute right to refuse treatment even should that decision lead to his or her death. The health professional's duty of care otherwise remains unchanged, difficult though it may be to have to withhold an intervention that would be life-saving. In children, the situation is more complicated, and made more so by the concept of 'Gillick competence', which holds that children under the age of 16 years can be judged to be legally competent if they have 'sufficient understanding and maturity to understand what is being proposed'. If a 'competent' child wishes to have treatment, then this decision cannot be overridden; if, however, he or she wishes to refuse treatment, then those with parental responsibility can give consent and override that wish. In the case of much younger children and in situations where the medical professionals feel that blood transfusion may be necessary, it is possible to apply to the High Court for a 'specific issue order'. If time is too restricted for such an application then blood can be given, if indicated.

- **Pre-operative optimization:** this would include haematinics, intravenous iron (if total body iron is depleted, this limits haematopoiesis) and the use of erythropoietin (EPO). (see under 'Anaemia'). Because these are patients who are healthy, are not anaemic and are not losing blood the response to EPO is not blunted. As an approximate guide, and depending on the dosing regimen, EPO can potentially increase the haemoglobin concentration by up to 10 g l^{-1} in a week.

- **Autologous donation:** patients donate 450 ml (1 unit) of blood up to twice a week, but more commonly weekly, up to 72 hours before surgery. Iron supplementation is routine. The production of endogenous erythropoietin is enhanced during twice-weekly donation, but is more modest if donation is less frequent. The procedure is useful for patients undergoing surgery with anticipated major blood loss. Units stored should be matched against likely usage, but wastage is high (around 50%).

- **Surgical and anaesthetic technique:** this applies to all situations, as clearly no surgical team ever wants to lose more blood than necessary. Typical strategies would include discontinuation of any anti-platelet or anticoagulant medication (where clinically appropriate), scrupulous surgical haemostasis, the use of red cell salvage, efforts to minimize any venous congestion which would encourage oozing, judicious hypotensive anaesthesia, the use of regional and neuraxial blocks where appropriate and the routine administration of tranexamic acid.

- **Acute normovolaemic haemodilution:** whole blood is removed from the patient and replaced with crystalloid and/or colloid solutions prior to the anticipated blood loss. Blood is then reinfused as appropriate, but in the reverse order of collection, because the first unit collected has the highest haematocrit and the greatest concentrations of platelets and clotting factors. The technique is conceptually attractive, but mathematical modeling demonstrates that the actual volumes of saved blood are relatively small (amounting to the equivalent of 1 unit of packed cells). For example, it has been calculated that a patient from whom 3 units totalling 1,350 ml are withdrawn prior to a blood loss of 2,600 ml will require only about 215 ml less allogeneic blood than otherwise would be the case. It also poses obvious logistical difficulties.

- **Acute hypervolaemic haemodilution:** the patient is rendered hypervolaemic with crystalloid and/or non-blood colloid. This is a simpler technique, although it runs the risk of precipitating circulatory overload. Mathematical modeling suggests that it is superior to normovolaemic haemodilution, at least for blood losses up to 40% of total blood volume.

- **Perioperative autologous blood recovery:** intraoperative cell-saver devices can be very efficient, saving the equivalent of up to 10 units hourly should massive transfusion be necessary. Its cost-effectiveness is disputed, and some prospective trials in major vascular patients have demonstrated that it does not reduce the requirement to give allogeneic blood. Its economic benefits have, however, been confirmed in obstetric practice. In obstetrics it may also ensure the avoidance of allogeneic blood transfusion which may be of particular importance to young women of childbearing age. Reinfused blood may contain sufficient red cells to stimulate an antibody response in a mother who is rhesus negative. If the baby is rhesus D-positive or rhesus status unknown, the mother should therefore receive a minimum of 1,500 i.u. of anti-D immunoglobulin.

Cell salvage also has the advantage of providing blood relatively rapidly, although the collection and washing processes are not swift. (Postoperative reinfusion of blood collected from drains has been used after orthopaedic surgery, but the blood so salvaged has a low haematocrit of around 0.20, is partly haemolysed and may be rich in cytokines. Its benefits are debated and the practice is no longer widespread.)

- **Transfusion triggers:** evidence that outcomes were favourable in patients in critical care whose haemoglobin concentrations were maintained at between 70–90 g l^{-1} rather than being transfused to levels above 100 g l^{-1} led to a re-evaluation of transfusion thresholds. It is now well recognized that healthy individuals can tolerate very low haemoglobin levels and that efficient aerobic metabolism continues until concentrations fall below 50 g l^{-1}. In other surgical populations, mortality shows no increase as long as the haemoglobin concentration remains greater than 80 g l^{-1}. This includes patients with cardiorespiratory disease.

Complications of Blood Transfusion

Commentary

The 2015 Serious Hazards of Transfusion (SHOT) Report identified 1,858 incidents and 26 deaths (2 definitely associated, 9 probably associated, and 15 possibly associated with transfusion). This was out of a total of almost 2.6 million blood components that were issued by the Blood Transfusion Service. A possible mortality rate of 0.001% is low, but it is almost three times that associated with anaesthesia, and so it is important that anaesthetists should be familiar with the complications of transfusion of blood and blood products.

Core Information

Complications of Blood Transfusion

- **Acute haemolytic reactions:** an acute antigen–antibody reaction is initiated by ABO or rhesus incompatibility (see under 'Blood Groups'.]) Donor cells are destroyed by antibodies in the recipient plasma, with the resultant haemolysis leading in some cases to intravascular fibrin deposition, disseminated intravascular coagulation and renal failure. In the 2015 SHOT report, there was one death attributed to ABO incompatibility and five more due to haemolytic reactions. Cumulative SHOT data suggest that around a third of ABO-incompatible transfusions result in death or serious harm.

- **Transfusion-related acute lung injury (TRALI):** there were four deaths attributed to TRALI in the 2015 report, which makes it a significant complication. TRALI presents with an acute respiratory distress syndrome either immediately or within 6 hours of transfusion. The plasma of donor blood can contain leucocyte antibodies which target recipient neutrophils. Within the pulmonary microvasculature there is destruction of capillary endothelium by oxygen free radicals and proteolytic enzymes, with resultant exudation of fluid and proteinaceous material into the alveoli and the development of pulmonary oedema. The same phenomenon can occur in the absence of measurable leucocyte antibodies but in the presence of some other trigger in donor plasma. This is referred to as non-immune TRALI (mortality is lower). TRALI is more likely in response to blood products with a high plasma component such as fresh frozen plasma (FFP), platelets and cryoprecipitate, and especially if the donor is female. (Human leucocyte antigen antibodies are commoner in multiparous women.) The risk is reduced by leucocyte depletion and by the use of male donors.

- **Transfusion-associated circulatory overload (TACO):** this was the most frequent cause of death and major morbidity in the 2015 report, being associated with seven deaths and 35 cases, respectively. It is a clinical diagnosis made when a patient develops four out of the five following symptoms within 6 hours of transfusion: acute respiratory distress, tachycardia, hypertension, pulmonary oedema and positive fluid balance. Confirmation of the diagnosis is assisted if the patient responds to conventional treatments for pulmonary oedema. The SHOT report acknowledges that these diagnostic criteria lack specificity, and so they are currently under revision, and may include for example, measurements of brain-natriuretic peptide (BNP) as an indicator of myocardial stress.

- **Non-haemolytic (febrile) reactions:** these are common and are mediated by donor leucocyte antigens which react with recipient antibodies to form a complex that binds complement and releases pyrogenic inflammatory mediators such as IL-1 and IL-6 and TNFα. Cytokines can also be introduced directly into the circulation by contaminated residual leucocytes in platelet concentrates. Leucodepletion attenuates the risk.

- **Allergic and anaphylactic reactions:** allergic reactions to proteins in donor plasma are relatively common, are usually mild and present with typical features of pruritus and urticaria. Anaphylactic reactions are rare.
- **Complications of massive transfusion:** the replacement of a patient's total blood volume within 24 hours (which is one simple definition of a massive transfusion) can affect their temperature, their biochemistry and their coagulation.
  - **Temperature:** blood infused directly from storage will be at around 4 °C. One litre of unwarmed blood can lower core temperature by 0.5 °C. The effects of peri-operative hypothermia are well known and include reduced oxygen delivery (because of the leftward shift of the oxygen–haemoglobin dissociation curve), impaired wound healing, abnormalities of coagulation and increased infection rates. Hypothermia also slows enzymatic reactions so that metabolism of the citrate and lactate in stored blood is reduced.
  - **Biochemistry:** hyperkalaemia is rarely a problem because although the potassium in stored blood can be many times higher than normal, once within the circulation intracellular re-uptake is rapid. Potassium may nonetheless rise if large volumes of blood are infused within a short time, such as in the resuscitation of patients with major trauma. However, if cold blood is infused quickly through a central venous cannula (in error) it will be cardioplegic. Stored blood contains citrate as an anticoagulant, which, when metabolized to bicarbonate in large amounts, can contribute to a metabolic alkalosis (which further impairs enzyme function). Citrate also chelates calcium, and so hypocalcaemia can be associated with the rapid infusion of large volumes of stored blood.
  - **Coagulation:** plasma-reduced blood contains minimal coagulation factors which rapidly become depleted during massive transfusion. This dilutional coagulopathy may be complicated by the onset of disseminated intravascular coagulation associated with persistent haemorrhage.
- **Immunomodulation:** the immunosuppressive effect of homologous blood was exploited deliberately in early renal transplantation to reduce rejection rates. It is now evident that transfusion suppresses IL-2 production, killer cell activity and macrophage function. It also lowers the CD4/CD8 cell count ratio (which is the ratio of T lymphocytes that express the C4 antigen to those that express the C8 antigen, and is an indicator of the overall level of immune suppression). This immunomodulation is associated with increased rates of metastasis and tumour recurrence following surgery for colonic and other cancers, with a heightened risk of postoperative infection, and with the activation of latent chronic viral infection (such as herpes simplex).
- **Transmission of infection:** bacterial contamination of blood and blood products is possible, and, because transfusion will ensure a large intravenous inoculum of pathogen, such contamination can result in fulminant septicaemia. (Gram-negative species thrive at the blood storage temperature of 4 °C.) Viral contamination may be more insidious, and there are many recipients who are now suffering the consequences of receiving blood that at the time was unknowingly contaminated with the hepatitis B and C viruses, and with HIV. Although blood is now screened for these

viruses as well as T cell lymphotrophic virus, syphilis and cytomegalovirus, there remains a transmission window during which the donor may be infected but still seronegative. Prion diseases (such as variant Creutzfeld–Jacob disease) are more insidious still; the latent period may be very long and there are no diagnostic tests. (There was one such transfusion-transmitted death reported in 2015.)

- **Graft-versus-host disease:** this is a very rare complication which can occur in recipients who are immunocompromised. Donor immune cells, particularly T lymphocytes, attack host tissue, which includes bone marrow stem cells. Ninety per cent of cases are fatal.

Anaemia

Commentary

Anaemia is important for anaesthetists, both in the context of surgery, obstetric anaesthesia and in critical care. More than a quarter of the world's population is anaemic, with iron deficiency accounting for more than half of the cases. This is clearly a much greater problem in the developing than the developed world. This oral may include some medicine (causes of chronic anaemia), pathology (abnormal erythrocyte morphology), pharmacology (treatment with intravenous iron), and clinical anaesthesia.

Core Information

- **Definition:** anaemia is defined as a reduction of red cell mass, but typically is described in terms of the haemoglobin concentration, whose normal range in adult males is quoted as between 130–180 g l^{-1}, and in adult females 115–160 g l^{-1}. These reference data do vary between laboratories but encompass the 95% of adults who are within two standard deviations of the mean.
- **Causes:** there are only three ways in which red cell mass will decrease: through blood loss; because of red cell destruction, usually by haemolysis; and by failure of red cell production. Within these three broad categories, however, there lie a myriad of causes.
- **Red cell loss:** Obvious causes include surgical, civilian and military trauma, ruptured aneurysms (typically abdominal aortic), ruptured spleen, burns, ruptured ectopic pregnancy, and antepartum and postpartum haemorrhage (placental abruption, placenta praevia, uterine atony).
- **Red cell destruction:** there are both congenital and acquired causes of haemolysis. Congenital causes include hereditary spheroctytosis, haemoglobinopathies such as sickle cell disease, and erythrocytic metabolic disorders such as glucose-6-phosphate dehydrogenase deficiency. (This is the commonest enzyme deficiency in humans. Haemolysis can be precipitated following consumption of some foods, particularly the broad bean, *Vicia fava*, which is why it is also called favism). Amongst the

numerous acquired causes are infection (such as mycoplasma, malaria, clostridia); autoimmiune conditions such as autoimmune haemolytic anaemia itself, rheumatoid arthritis and systemic lupus erythematosus; paroxysmal nocturnal haemoglobinuria in which haemolysis is secondary to complement activation; and HELLP syndrome in pregnancy (haemolysis, elevated liver enzymes and low platelets).

- **Failure of red cell production:** common nutritional causes include lack of dietary iron, generalized malnutrition, and vitamin B12 and folate deficiency. Erythropoiesis is suppressed by the uraemia of chronic renal impairment and is reduced, partially or even completely in some myelodysplastic and myeloproliferative disorders.

- **Erythropoiesis:** red cell precursors from pluripotent stem cells are produced in the bone marrow and are released into the circulation as reticulocytes (so named because they contain a reticular matrix of rRNA). Within 24–48 hours these mature into erythrocytes and then remain viable for about 120 days. Red cell production is under the influence of erythropoietin (EPO), produced mainly in the kidney by interstitial cells in peritubular capillaries of the renal cortex. (It is a 165-amino acid glycoprotein which technically is a haematopoietic cytokine.) Some extrarenal EPO production takes place in the liver (10%). EPO stimulates the production of erythroblasts, which are stem cells that are committed to becoming erythrocytes. It also stimulates angiogenesis and has an anti-apoptotic action. Recombinant EPO can be used to raise haematocrit; legitimately in patients and illegitimately in athletes seeking to enhance performance. As a separate effect it also increases the time to exhaustion. It has a relatively short elimination half-life of 4–13 hours after intravenous administration and can be detected in blood and urine. The rate at which the haematocrit will increase depends on the indication for the drug and the dose regimen employed.

- **Compensatory responses to anaemia:** the response to the anaemia of acute blood loss is detailed under 'Massive Haemorrhage: Compensatory Responses and Management'. In chronic anaemia, there is the same imperative to maintain oxygen delivery to the tissues but without the shifts of fluid between compartments and without activation of the rapid humoral responses. Cardiac output increases as do the production of erythropoietin (which can rise by several hundred times) and the stimulation of erythropoiesis. This may have little impact on the haematocrit, depending on the cause underlying the anaemia. Haemoglobin-oxygen affinity decreases so as to offload more oxygen, and tissue oxygen extraction also increases.

- **Red cell morphology:** It would be unreasonable to expect a detailed account of the numerous abnormal forms of erythrocytes, but the commoner ones are outlined here in the event that a simple description may be required from you as part of the overall discussion. The normal red blood cell is a biconcave, anuclear structure between 6 and 8 μm in diameter and with a volume of between 80 and 95 fl (this varies with different laboratory reference values). Of the many morphological abnormalities described, the commoner ones include **microcytosis** and hypochromia (typically due to iron deficiency anaemia); **macrocytosis** typically associated with megaloblastic anaemia due to vitamin B12 and folate deficiency, liver disease and some myelodysplastic syndromes; **target cells** with a dark centre with high haemoglobin content (liver disease, haemoglobinopathies); **spherocytes**, which are microcytic and circular (haemolysis, post-transfusion); **tear drop cells,** whose appearance is as described and which may be seen in severe anaemias; **sickle cells**, as in the anaemia of the same name; and **schistocytes**, which are fragmented cells seen after haemolytic processes and in severe coagulopathies.

- **Oral iron supplementation:** the largest reservoir of iron in the body is in blood, which contains around 500 mg in each 1,000 ml. Otherwise iron is stored in ferritin complexes which are most numerous in the liver, bone marrow and spleen. Total body iron is variously quoted as around 5 mg kg^{-1} in females and up to 10 mg kg^{-1} in males. Other sources quote a typical value in a healthy subject in the developed world of 4–6 g. Depleted iron stores can usually be corrected by oral iron, which is inexpensive, effective and safe. It is, however, associated with a number of low-level gastrointestinal side effects, including nausea, disturbed bowel function and epigastric discomfort. Absorption is increased if iron is in the ferrous form within an acidic medium and so may be reduced in patients whose gastric pH is reduced by proton pump inhibitors or histamine H_2 receptor antagonists. Iron metabolism is regulated by hepcidin, a polypeptide produced in the liver which controls absorption across the gut by inhibiting ferroportin (the iron export channel on gut enterocytes) and which also controls iron export from macrophages. If hepcidin concentrations are elevated, which happens in response to various inflammatory processes, then iron absorption from the gut will fall. Effective repletion of iron stores is also reduced by compounds present in some foods which bind iron and prevent absorption. These include phosphates and phytates (for example in whole grains, legumes and nuts) as well as all calcium-containing foods and liquids. The maximal rate of elemental iron absorption after oral administration is around 25 mg daily.
- **Intravenous iron supplementation:** in contrast to oral iron, intravenous iron can replenish body iron stores after a single infusion, depending on the deficit. Its use is indicated in those who either cannot tolerate or absorb oral iron. These would include some pregnant women, individuals with malabsorption syndromes and those who have undergone bariatric surgery such as gastric bypass procedures and sleeve gastrectomy. Its effectiveness is not in doubt, and meta-analysis of controlled trials of oral versus intravenous iron has shown a lower frequency of blood transfusion in the intravenous group.
- **Dose regimens:** although dose calculation tables are available which take into account factors such as body weight and haemoglobin concentration, it is more common to give a dose of 1,000 mg (higher doses confer no clinical benefit). This would be sufficient for the initial treatment of an iron deficit of 500–1,000 mg.
- **Side effects of intravenous iron:** anaphylactic reactions are very rare although possible, as are non-allergic and non-life-threatening reactions such as urticaria and lumbo-nuchal discomfort. The incidence of these is quoted as <1%. Patients with inflammatory arthropathies may experience exacerbations during treatment and may require pretreatment with increased doses of glucocorticoid. The mechanism underlying these exacerbations is not clear. Iron is a substrate for bacterial growth and so should theoretically be avoided in those with active infection. In practice the risks are generally considered to be low.

Postpartum and Massive Obstetric Haemorrhage

Commentary

Life-threatening obstetric haemorrhage is not uncommon; a typical district general hospital maternity unit with 3,000 annual deliveries could expect to see around 15 cases a year. The number of women who die in the UK is now very small, and maternal haemorrhage no longer features as a leading cause of mortality, which may reflect its better understanding and management. This is likely to be the focus of this oral. (In the developing world the situation is depressingly different. In sub-Saharan Africa, maternal mortality is estimated at 1%, with more than half that mortality attributable to haemorrhage.)

Core Information

Causes of Postpartum and Massive Obstetric Haemorrhage

- **Incidence:** this depends on the definition of postpartum and massive haemorrhage. By convention, postpartum haemorrhage (PPH) is defined as a blood loss of 500 ml within 24 hours of birth, but as 20% of women will lose that much blood routinely (and will regain it via the autotransfusion that occurs as the uterus contracts after delivery), this exaggerates the number who are at risk of significant haemodynamic disturbance. There is no single accepted definition of massive obstetric haemorrhage but suggestions include overall blood loss greater than 2,000 ml, blood loss at a rate of greater than 150 ml min^{-1}, a decrease in haemoglobin concentration of more than 40 g l^{-1}, 50% loss of maternal blood volume within 3 hours or the requirement for the acute transfusion of more than 4 units of packed red cells.
- **Uterine causes:** the most important immediate cause is uterine atony. The placenta receives almost 20% of the cardiac output at term (700–900 ml min^{-1}), which explains why acute haemorrhage may be catastrophic. In the UK, uterine atony accounts for around one-third of all deaths associated with maternal haemorrhage. Other causes include uterine disruption or inversion, complications of operative or instrumental delivery and retained products of conception. Retained placenta itself, although not invariably associated with bleeding, complicates some 2% of all deliveries. Abnormal placentation (placenta accreta, increta and percreta) occurs in 1 in 3,000 deliveries.
- **Non-uterine causes:** the main causes are genital tract trauma and disorders of coagulation.
- **Risk factors**
  - **Uterine atony:** there is a strong association with augmentation of labour. It may also follow uterine overdistension by multiple births, by polyhydramnios and by delivery of babies weighing greater than 4 kg. It is associated with protracted labour, with the use of tocolytic drugs and also with maternal hypotension. The relative ischaemia that may accompany uterine hypoperfusion or hypoxia will impair the ability of the uterus to contract effectively. There appears to be no link to multiparity.

— **Abnormal placentation:** a mother with an anterior placenta praevia overlying a previous Caesarean section scar has at least a one in four chance of placenta accreta.

— **Genital tract trauma:** this very vascular area may be damaged during delivery of a large baby, during delivery complicated by shoulder dystocia, or during a forceps delivery or vacuum extraction. Bleeding from the genital tract may be masked by normal post-delivery vaginal loss.

— **Coagulopathy:** this may be associated with abruption of the placenta (in 10% of cases), amniotic fluid embolism (up to 90% of cases), intrauterine death, pregnancy-induced hypertension (particularly HELLP syndrome) and gram-negative septicaemia.

Management of Major Obstetric Haemorrhage

The oral is likely to concentrate on the drugs that are used to treat uterine atony, as this is the most common cause (see under 'Uterotonics' in Chapter 4).

- **Arrest the bleeding.** This is the basic priority underlying the management of major haemorrhage from any cause. In obstetrics, however, in contrast to multiple trauma or a ruptured aortic aneurysm, the initial management of the commonest cause, uterine atony, is pharmacological. This is dealt with in more detail under 'Uterotonics' in Chapter 4, but the drugs that are used are oxytocin, ergometrine, misoprostol and prostaglandin 15-methyl $PGF_{2\alpha}$. Surgical control of bleeding will vary according to its source; genital tract trauma is obviously managed differently from abnormal placentation.

- **Volume resuscitation.** Obstetrics has followed the military model of trauma resuscitation by establishing formulaic regimens using 'major haemorrhage packs' (MHP). A typical regimen would be MHP 1 with red cells × 4 units; fresh frozen plasma (FFP) × 4 units; platelets 1 dose, to be followed as indicated by MHP 2 with red cells × 4 units; FFP × 4 units, platelets 1 dose; plus cryoprecipitate 2 packs if the fibrinogen concentration is less than 2.0 g l^{-1}. Tranexamic acid is also usually given. This empirical model is almost certainly inappropriate for the management of maternal haemorrhage. Pregnant women are hypercoagulable and can lose around 4,000 ml of blood before the prothrombin time (PT) and activated partial thromboplastin time (APTT) become deranged. In addition, the plasma fibrinogen concentration of at least 90% of women undergoing a PPH remains above 2 g l^{-1}, which is higher than that contained in FFP. In pregnancy normal fibrinogen levels are 4–6 g l^{-1}. This does call into question the wisdom of using trauma-type regimens with the risk of, amongst other complications, circulatory overload (TACO, see under 'Complications of Blood Transfusion'.).

- Point of care coagulation testing allows more targeted infusion of appropriate blood components (see under 'Point of Care Tests [and ROTEM] in Chapter 5).

- **Cell salvage in obstetrics:** this is now well established, with ample evidence from clinical studies to allay the fears that cell-salvaged blood could be contaminated with amniotic fluid. It is now routine in many centres to use a single sucker for the entire procedure rather than trying to use separate suction for liquor, and the advantages of the technique are well recognized. It may remove the need to transfuse allogeneic blood, with all its attendant complications, and it has economic benefits because in the context of maternity services, cell salvage is cost-effective. However, it is not entirely without its problems.

- **Problems with obstetric cell salvage. Rate of blood replacement**. The blood supply to the uterus at term is very high at up to 900 ml min^{-1}, and so in a situation of rapid uncontrolled bleeding a mother may lose half her blood volume within a matter of minutes. Cell salvage processing is just not quick enough to keep pace with such a rapid rate of blood loss. **Rhesus sensitization.** This may be a problem because reinfused blood may contain sufficient fetal red blood cells to stimulate an antibody response in mothers who are rhesus negative. If intra-operative cell salvage is used during caesarean section in rhesus D-negative women, and the baby is known to be rhesus D-positive, or more commonly has unknown rhesus status, then a minimum of 1,500 i.u. of anti-D should be given following the reinfusion of salvaged red cells. Blood should be taken for a Kleihauer test between 30–45 minutes after re-infusion. **Filters**. There are also potential complications associated with the use of the leucocyte-depleting filters (LDFs). The filters are fibreglass with a 40-micron pore size and are used to remove white blood cells and particulate components of amniotic fluid, particularly fetal squames and lamellar bodies. Whether this is necessary is open to doubt because these components have been identified in the maternal circulation of women who remain healthy and symptom-free. Nonetheless, their routine use is recommended by a variety of expert bodies including NICE, despite several case reports and an alert from the American Food and Drug Administration (FDA) regarding their propensity to cause profound hypotension. The filters work not only by passive sieving of matter and adherence to the material surface but also by the presence of an electric charge. This is usually negative. When platelets or Factor VIII adhere to the surface, their exposure to this negative charge is associated with significant bradykinin production. (Bradykinin is an inflammatory mediator, a vaso-active nonpeptide which binds rapidly to the vascular endothelium and mediates vasodilatation and hypotension via G-protein coupled receptors. It has a short half-life of around 15 seconds and is metabolized in passage through the lung.) In practice this should now be academic because, apart from the fact that the efficiency of LDFs is limited to a single unit of blood, the cell salvage process of modern machines is so effective that the presence of fetal material is negligible. Should hypotension occur it is safe to remove the filter and continue reinfusing the cell-salvaged blood.

Physiological Changes of Late Pregnancy Relevant to General Anaesthesia

Commentary

This is not designed to be a question about general anaesthesia for caesarean section, but as few other surgical procedures are performed at or around term, it will be a difficult subject to avoid. However, the examiners will initially try to do so, which will free you to take a standard systems approach to the subject. As all anaesthetists in training are exposed regularly to obstetric anaesthesia you will be expected to have a good understanding of its principles and practice. A discussion of the various systems is an appropriate way to start. Most of the information is little more than a list and you will be unlikely to cover any single aspect in great detail.

Core Information

- **Cardiovascular system:** during pregnancy there is a total weight gain that averages 12 kg. Half of this is accounted for by an increase in plasma volume and interstitial fluid. Plasma volume increases by up to 40% and total body water by around 7–8 litres. This volume loading is associated with mild cardiac dilatation, and so heart murmurs (for example, that of mitral regurgitation) are common. Cardiac output increases by 40–45% to near maximal at 32 weeks' gestation. The resting heart rate increases by 15%, and tachyarrhythmias are more common. The ECG shows left axis deviation caused by mechanical displacement by the gravid uterus, and minor T wave and ST segment changes may be seen. Blood pressure falls, with the diastolic drop of 10–15 mmHg making a bigger contribution than the systolic, and there is a decrease in systemic vascular resistance. There is reduced sensitivity to circulating vasopressors, although it appears that the uterine circulation may be more sensitive to these than the systemic.
  - **Aortocaval compression** (supine hypotension syndrome): this is of potential importance because it occurs to some degree in all women, although modern methods of assessment using, for example, femoral vein ultrasound, suggest that it is significant in around only 30%. The remainder are able to compensate by an increase in sympathetic tone and diversion of venous return through the effective collateral circulation of the azygos veins and the vertebral venous plexus. Supine hypotension in the patient anaesthetized either with neuraxial or general anaesthesia may not therefore be as great a problem as once was thought, but there will remain around 10% of women in whom it may occur but in whom it cannot be predicted. Compression by the gravid uterus of the great vessels affects mainly venous return, but it can also compromise aortic and uterine blood flow. Turning from the lateral to the supine position at term in some women may decrease cardiac output by up to 30%. Uterine blood flow may be compromised even in those who are asymptomatic and because the uteroplacental circulation does not autoregulate; that flow is crucially dependent on the pressure gradient. Most obstetric anaesthetists therefore continue to use a wedge or lateral tilt of up to 15°, although the Cochrane Collaboration (systematic reviews) has commented that there is little evidence to support this practice.
  - **Anaesthetic implications:** because it is not possible to predict those mothers in whom aortocaval compression will reduce cardiac output, there should still be appropriate positioning to avoid the possibility. Cardiac output and systemic blood pressure must be maintained to ensure continued perfusion of the uteroplacental unit, but equally the anaesthetist must be aware of the consequences of fluid-loading a mother who is in effect already waterlogged.
- **Respiratory system:** some of the data are contentious and much is based on older studies of small numbers of subjects, which show no signs of being repeated. There is an increase in minute volume by 40% at term, but this is initiated early in pregnancy

when progesterone-induced hyperventilation reduces $PaCO_2$ by around 1 kPa. This is associated with a mild respiratory alkalosis. This would shift the oxygen–haemoglobin dissociation curve downwards and to the left were it not for an increase in maternal 2,3-DPG, which offsets this effect. Increased metabolic demand for oxygen increases by around 50%, along with an increase in the work of breathing and a decrease in both chest wall and lung compliance. The increased demand for oxygen is more than compensated by the increase in cardiac output, and so there is a small rise in PaO_2 of about 1 kPa. There are anatomical changes which influence the upper airway; general fluid retention and oedema of pregnancy may complicate laryngoscopy and intubation. With regard to pulmonary volumes, the most important change is the 20% decrease in FRC, which, by the third trimester, may fall in the supine position to half its predicted value.

— **Anaesthetic implications:** the FRC must be filled with oxygen prior to induction to minimize risk of desaturation. This can be achieved either by preoxygenating the mother for 3 minutes with 100% O_2, or by asking her to take three vital capacity breaths. Slight head-up or ramped positioning will reduce encroachment of the closing volume on the FRC. The reduced FRC means that the onset of the effect of volatile anaesthetic agents will be more rapid, as will maternal desaturation.

— Relative hyperventilation and low-normal $PaCO_2$ should be maintained, although it is not until the $PaCO_2$ falls below about 2.7–3.3 kPa (20–25 mmHg) that uterine blood flow is compromised.

— The congested and more oedematous upper airway may be traumatized during instrumentation. A smaller tracheal tube (7.0) may be required.

- **Gastrointestinal system:** by the third trimester some 70% of mothers have symptoms of gastro-oesophageal reflux and heartburn. Oesophageal barrier pressure decreases with the loss of lower oesophageal sphincter tone, and there is also a fall in intestinal transit time and some duodenal gastric reflux. Gastric emptying itself, however, is not delayed in late pregnancy. Gastric residual volumes are increased, as is placental gastrin secretion. Whether this translates into maternal gastric hyperacidity remains disputed.

— **Anaesthetic implications:** the airway must be protected against the risk of pulmonary aspiration of gastric contents by antacid prophylaxis (H_2 antagonists, proton pump inhibitors and sodium citrate). Effective cricoid pressure applied during a rapid sequence induction is also considered essential.

- **CNS:** under the influence of progesterone and endogenous β-endorphins, the MAC of anaesthetic agents decreases by about one-third, and there is an increased sensitivity to all drugs which act centrally. (Requirements for local anaesthetics also decrease, which may be related to an increased availability of free drug and to hormonally enhanced neural sensitivity.)

— **Anaesthetic implications**: reduction in the doses of anaesthetic agents, sedatives and analgesics may be possible. Interpatient variability, however, is so great that it would be unwise to assume that anaesthetic awareness or severe postoperative pain are less likely.

- **Musculoskeletal system:** pregnancy increases ligamentous laxity owing to the rises in the hormones progesterone and relaxin. There is also an increased lumbar lordosis which helps to accommodate the enlarging uterus.

— **Anaesthetic implications:** scrupulous positioning of the patient with appropriate supports and protection may minimize the risk of postoperative backache or other joint problems.

- **Haematological:** pregnancy is a hypercoagulable state. There is an increase in all clotting factors, except for Factor XI, and fibrinolysis is impaired by a plasminogen inhibitor that is derived from the placenta.
  — **Anaesthetic implications:** the risk of venous thromboembolism is increased fivefold and routine preventative measures should be used (see under 'Drugs Affecting Coagulation' in Chapter 4). Should a mother have additional risk factors, then pharmacological intervention may be necessary, although in many units low molecular weight heparin is given routinely after caesarean section or other surgery.

- **Metabolic:** there is a 30% fall in the levels of plasma cholinesterase.
  — **Anaesthetic implications:** this fall has the greatest implications for those patients with atypical cholinesterases. It is often claimed that this decrease does not produce a clinically important increase in the duration of suxamethonium. Clinical experience would suggest, however, that the actions of suxamethonium are prolonged in many pregnant patients and that rapid offset with the resumption of spontaneous respiration is by no means guaranteed.

- **Drug handling:** increased renal blood flow and glomerular filtration enhances the clearance of drugs excreted renally. The reduction in maternal albumin may increase the amount of free drug present in plasma, which may enhance its effects.

- **Miscellaneous:** discussion of these various factors is likely to take up much of the time available. If you have covered many of the points discussed here, then the oral may move on to related topics, such as traditional rapid sequence induction and the role of cricoid pressure. A rocuronium/sugammadex technique has its advocates, but others cite the rapidity of suxamethonium's action (up to 35 s quicker) as the prime reason for its continued use in obstetrics. You would be brave to argue against the routine use of cricoid pressure in obstetric anaesthesia. It has often been argued that it is not used commonly in France, but this is something of an urban myth. By 1998, some 88% of French anaesthetists were employing the technique in obstetric general anaesthesia. Certainly, cricoid deformation can make intubation more difficult, but equally the backwards, upwards and rightwards pressure manoeuvre may well improve the view. Take a balanced approach in any discussion, enough to show that you are at least aware of the opposing arguments.

Non-Obstetric Surgery in Pregnancy

Commentary

It is not uncommon for pregnant women to require surgery for non-obstetric reasons such as acute appendicitis, torsion of ovarian cysts and trauma. There are implications both for mother and fetus of which anaesthetists should be aware, but the questions in the oral will be predictable. For a mother whose pregnancy is well advanced, the anaesthetic considerations are those which apply to caesarean section under general anaesthesia. For a mother in the first trimester, the main concerns relate to teratogenesis.

Core Information
- Non-obstetric surgery is required in 0.5–2.0% of women (the incidence varies with the survey). Acute appendicitis occurs in 1 in 2,000 confinements, and other surgical procedures include ovarian cystectomy and cervical cerclage. Maternal trauma may also necessitate surgery. The anaesthetic considerations vary according to gestational age.

General Principles
Maternal safety considerations are as for any general anaesthetic. In respect of the fetus, the timing of surgery should be such as to maximize fetal viability. The techniques used should minimize the risks of teratogenesis or the onset of premature labour, and prevent uterine hypoxia or hypoperfusion. The same principles apply to postoperative analgesia and to fluid and oxygen therapy.

First Trimester
- The major concerns are of teratogenesis and of spontaneous abortion. Up until 15 days of gestation the embryo is either lost or preserved intact, and so anaesthesia during this period cannot be teratogenic. The developing fetus thereafter is most vulnerable up to around 60 days (8–9 weeks) of gestational age. The largest single observational study looked at more than 5,000 Swedish women who had undergone non-obstetric surgery at different stages of pregnancy (41% in the first trimester). Neural tube defects were commoner (first trimester surgery), as was the incidence of low birth weights; otherwise there were no differences in the incidence of miscarriage or congenital abnormalities (*Am J Obstet Gynecol* 1989, 161: 1178–85). A more recent meta-analysis concluded that non-obstetric surgery and anaesthesia did not increase the risk of birth defects and spontaneous abortion (R. Cohen-Kerem *et al. Am J Surg* 2005, 190: 467–73). Although there is little evidence that any of the long-established anaesthetic agents are teratogenic in humans, mothers nevertheless should be offered regional anaesthesia where this is appropriate and/or elective surgery should be deferred. The teratogenic effects of nitrous oxide have been demonstrated only in rats, and risks to theatre personnel are negligible with modern gas scavenging systems.
- **Drug effects:** single doses of established agents as used during a general anaesthetic are unlikely to cause problems. Regular NSAIDs should be avoided because of the risk of premature closure of the ductus arteriosus. (Aspirin, however, appears to be safe.)

Later Pregnancy
- From about the third trimester of pregnancy, the anaesthetic considerations are little different from those which apply to caesarean section. As fetal delivery is not imminent, however, there is less concern about giving drugs such as opioids which might otherwise cause neonatal respiratory depression.

- **Physiological changes:** these are described under 'Physiological Changes of Late Pregnancy Relevant to General Anaesthesia'.
- **Summary of anaesthetic considerations:** avoidance of aortocaval compression (significant from around 20 weeks, depending on individual size); maintenance of uteroplacental perfusion; pre-oxygenation prior to induction; airway congestion, so consider smaller endotracheal tube; antacid prophylaxis and rapid sequence induction; quicker onset of volatile effect owing to reduced FRC; reduced MAC; ligamentous laxity, so care with moving and positioning; and hypercoagulability and increased risk of venous thromboembolism, so thromboprophylaxis is indicated. The physiological changes associated with laparoscopic surgery are more marked when superimposed on the maternal alterations imposed by pregnancy.

Factors Which Affect Placental Drug Transfer

- The placenta is in effect a lipid bilayer. Some nutrients cross this membrane by active transport processes, but drugs cross only by passive diffusion.
- Small hydrophilic molecules (up to a molecular weight of around 100) will diffuse across the placenta, but transfer of larger compounds that are poorly lipid-soluble depends largely on the concentration gradient (according to Fick's law of diffusion), on the permeability and on the area available for transfer. Permeability is inversely proportional to molecular weight.
- Transfer depends on the diffusion gradient, and this in turn is affected by the degree of protein binding and ionization on either side of the membrane. Local anaesthetics, for example, may concentrate on the fetal side of the circulation, due to ion trapping. The relative fetal acidaemia increases the proportion of drug in the ionized form, thereby reducing its transfer back across the placental membrane. The same is true of opioids such as pethidine and alfentanil.
- Lipophilic substances will cross the placenta according to flow-dependent transfer according to the rate at which they are delivered to the placental circulation.

Communicating Risks to the Mother

- **Teratogenesis:** major organogenesis is completed by the eighth week of pregnancy and, although the risk of other malformations persists briefly beyond that period, a mother who was 10 weeks into pregnancy can be reassured that the risks are negligible. Were she to require an anaesthetic in very early pregnancy, you could explain that you would use agents whose risks of causing fetal defects were extremely small. In practice, this would mean using the older agents which have been in long-established use. You would, however, recommend regional or neuraxial anaesthesia if feasible, as this effectively reduces any risk of congenital anomaly to zero.
- **Spontaneous abortion:** the increased risk of miscarriage is also very small, and probably bears no relation to anaesthesia. It is more likely that direct surgical stimulation might provoke premature uterine activity, but in practice this is unusual, even after pelvic surgery. The exception is following cervical cerclage, but in this case it should be the obstetric team rather than the anaesthetist who explains the risks and benefits.
- **General anaesthesia and developmental delay:** the concerns about neuronal damage associated with general anaesthesia in young children (see under 'Mechanisms of

Action of General Anaesthetics' in Chapter 4) have extended to the fetus. In the context of non-elective surgery for the mother, however, there is little that can be done to offset any potential risks, which do at the moment remain suggestive but unproven.

Pre-Eclampsia

Commentary

Pre-eclampsia complicates about 7% of all pregnancies in the UK, and is part of a spectrum of disease which includes HELLP syndrome, peripartum cardiomyopathy and possibly acute fatty liver of pregnancy. It is the second commonest cause of maternal death after thromboembolic disease. Patients with pre-eclampsia are more likely to require anaesthetic expertise than mothers with uncomplicated pregnancies, and so you need to be aware of its potential problems. You will have worked on a labour ward and seen this condition, and your experience is likely to be much more recent than many of the examiners, only a proportion of whom are obstetric anaesthetists. The oral will concentrate as much on the basic science as on the practicalities of managing these sick mothers.

Core Information

- **Definition:** pre-eclampsia is a systemic disorder of the vascular endothelium which has its origin in abnormal placental implantation.
- **Clinical features and diagnosis:** hypertension is the commonest presenting feature as defined by a systolic blood pressure of 140 mmHg or greater and a diastolic blood pressure of 90 mmHg or greater, measured on two separate occasions (at least 4 hours apart). Severe pre-eclampsia affects around 25% of total cases and is characterized by more extreme hypertension (systolic blood pressure >160 mmHg, diastolic DBP >110 mmHg and mean arterial pressure >125 mmHg), with proteinuria of >5 g in 24 hours. Patients may show renal impairment with oliguria (defined as output <500 ml in 24 hours), and they may complain of headache and visual disturbances. Distension of the liver capsule may cause epigastric and hypochondrial pain. Pulmonary oedema will impair gas exchange, and clotting may be deranged, particularly by thrombocytopenia. Hyperreflexia and clonus may presage the grand mal convulsions associated with eclampsia. Intrauterine growth retardation of the fetus is common.
- **Physiology of normal pregnancy:** in normal placental implantation, a subset of specialist cells known as invasive cytotrophoblasts migrate into the myometrium and replace the endothelium of maternal spiral arteries. This process is known as pseudovascularization. (Changes in the expression of a number of different signalling molecules are involved, but the details are likely to be beyond the scope of this oral.) As a consequence of this process, the maternal spiral arteries lose their typical vascular smooth muscle coat and are transformed into low-resistance capacitance vessels which enhance blood flow to the uteroplacental-fetal unit.

- **Pathophysiology in pre-eclampsia:** for reasons which are unclear, in pre-eclampsia this process is defective and there is incomplete trophoblastic migration into the spiral arteries with a reduction in placental perfusion. There is good correlation between the inadequacy of invasion and the degree of maternal hypertension, although the precise mechanism has not yet been elucidated. What is clear is that via this still opaque pathway there is a release of systemic vasoactive compounds which trigger the cascade of the inflammatory response, with endothelial damage, increased capillary permeability, vasoconstriction (partly mediated by an increase in thromboxane A_2 and a reduction in vasodilatory prostacyclin), platelet dysfunction and hypercoagulability. These systemic changes are global, and it is the multi-system nature of the condition that is responsible for the spectrum of clinical features that can be seen. The precipitants of this dysfunction remain speculative but include a maternal immune response to paternally derived fetal and placental antigens. It is believed that the characteristic endothelial cell abnormalities may be due to up-regulation of type 1 helper T cells in the maternal circulation with a resultant increase in cytokine production.

The typical hypertension which is the cardinal diagnostic feature of pre-eclampsia is a result of the production of endogenous vasoconstrictors as a means of ensuring that uteroplacental perfusion is sustained. It is mediated by circulating vasoactive humoral compounds (these have been identified in blood, placenta and amniotic fluid). The vascular damage may also be mediated via circulating immune complexes produced secondary to dysfunctional maternal immunomodulation. This occurs in response to the antigenic fetus, which in effect is a foreign allograft.

- This process can result in multi-organ failure, with fibrinoid ischaemic necrosis not only in the placenta but also in cerebral, renal and hepatic vessels. Microvascular thrombin is deposited throughout all vascular beds. This in turn can initiate primary disseminated intravascular coagulation.
- HELLP syndrome (described in 1982) is a variant of the parent disorder, which is characterized by **H**aemolysis, **E**levated **L**iver enzymes and **L**ow **P**latelets. There is hepatic ischaemia with periportal haemorrhage, which can proceed to frank necrosis. Microangiopathic haemolytic anaemia is accompanied by thrombocytopenia. Other parts of the coagulation process may be unaffected. Liver dysfunction is characterized by elevated transaminases (AST, ALT and γ GT), and renal impairment is manifest by elevated urea and creatinine, and, in severe cases, haemoglobinuria secondary to haemolysis. These complications may require critical care; although delivery initiates reversal of the disease, platelets may continue to fall for up to 72 hours.

Supplementary Information and Clinical Considerations

Anaesthesia for Caesarean Section in Pre-Eclampsia

- The choice of anaesthetic technique for caesarean section in mothers with pre-eclampsia has been controversial. The potential airway and haemodynamic problems associated with general anaesthesia are well recognized, but the choice between spinal and epidural anaesthesia is contentious. Traditional teaching has it that well-controlled incremental epidural anaesthesia should be used to avoid the precipitous falls in blood pressure which, it is claimed, will accompany spinal anaesthesia. There is no evidence to support this; indeed, there are at least four recent studies which dispute the presumption that severe hypotension accompanies spinal anaesthesia in mothers with pre-eclampsia. There is even a well-designed study now more than 50 years old and unethical by current standards, which examined the effect of high spinal block on pregnant, pregnant hypertensive, and non-pregnant controls. Profound hypotension affected only those mothers without hypertension. This is not surprising given that humoral rather than neurogenic factors mediate hypertension in pre-eclampsia.

- **Fluids and vasopressors:** these patients have the typical intravascular depletion of a vasoconstricted hypertensive circulation. An infusion of up to 10 ml kg^{-1} is accepted practice. Hypertensive mothers are said to be much more sensitive to the effects of catecholamines, and so although there are little data, it is prudent to 'decrease the dose' of prophylactic vasopressors (although no authority ever commits to advising by how much).

- **Other anaesthetic implications:** coagulopathy (which only complicates very severe cases) precludes neuraxial blockade. Treatment may include anti-hypertensive agents (such as labetalol) which can influence the response to epidural and subarachnoid block. Treatment may also include $MgSO_4$, which can potentiate neuromuscular blocking drugs. There may be renal dysfunction, and these mothers can easily be fluid-overloaded to the point at which they develop pulmonary oedema secondary to permeable pulmonary capillaries. Laryngoscopy, tracheal intubation and extubation can provoke an extreme pressor response, with surges in systolic blood pressure which may exceed 250 mmHg. Pre-eclampsia is associated with laryngeal and upper airway oedema.

Circulatory Changes at Birth (Congenital Heart Disease)

Commentary

This is not an area of clinical practice that involves anaesthetists very directly. Although congenital heart disease (CHD) is common, occurring in as many as 1 in 125 live births (the figure is from North American data), most abnormalities are identified early and the problems are referred on to specialist paediatric cardiac teams. Occasionally, patients do present later in life, but it is the applied pathophysiology itself which seems to be of particular interest to examiners, who will want to discover whether you understand the principles of rational management.

Core Information
Circulatory Changes at Birth (Figure 3.8)

- **Fetal circulation:** umbilical venous blood (SpO_2 80%) passes into the IVC (SpO_2 ~67%) via the ductus venosus (which traverses the liver). Most of this blood crosses into the left atrium via the foramen ovale. By the time this blood reaches the ascending aorta its saturation has fallen but some of this flow is destined for the

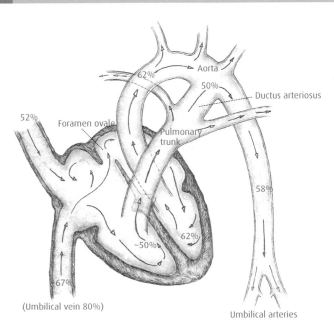

Fig. 3.8 The fetal circulation (showing oxygen saturations).

Aorta

62%

50%

Ductus arteriosus

52%

Foramen ovale

Pulmonary trunk

58%

62%

~50%

67%

(Umbilical vein 80%)

Umbilical arteries

cerebral circulation, and its saturation of around 62% is still higher than that in the ductus arteriosus (50%) and descending aorta (58%). These figures emphasize the fact that the fetus exists in a relatively hypoxic environment. Only about 10% of the cardiac output traverses the pulmonary vascular bed.

- In utero the right and left hearts pump in parallel. There are connections between the systemic and pulmonary circulations via the ductus arteriosus (which links the pulmonary artery to the aorta) and the foramen ovale (which is a communication between the left and right atria). The pulmonary circulation has high resistance, and the right and left ventricular pressures are equal, although the right ventricle ejects 66% of the combined ventricular output.
- With clamping of the umbilical cord there is a sudden rise in systemic vascular resistance (SVR) and aortic pressure.
- Respiration expands the lungs, and pulmonary vascular resistance (PVR) decreases in response to expansion, respiratory movements, increased pH and increased oxygenation. (PVR continues to decrease with recruitment of small arteries, and the reduction over weeks of pulmonary vascular smooth muscle.) Pulmonary blood flow increases. Enhanced pulmonary venous return into the left atrium raises the left atrial pressure above the right, and the foramen ovale closes by a flap valve effect. It is a functional closure which can be reversed if there is a sudden increase in right atrial pressure.
- The increase in left-sided pressure and the fall in right-sided pressures decrease, or even reverse, the shunting through the ductus arteriosus.
- The ductus closes in response to oxygen, to decreasing prostaglandin levels, to bradykinin and acetylcholine. The process takes up to 14 days to complete. It can be accelerated should the duct remain patent by giving a prostaglandin antagonist

such as indomethacin. In duct-dependent congenital cardiac disease it is important that the duct should be prevented from closing. Alprostadil (prostaglandin E_1) is the agent of choice. The dose in neonates, should the examiner pursue it this far, is 50–100 nanograms kg^{-1} min^{-1} titrated against effect.

Supplementary and Clinical Information

Congenital Heart Disease
- **Acyanotic:** the commonest conditions are atrial septal defect (ASD), accounting for 5–10% of all congenital lesions, and ventricular septal defect (VSD), occurring in up to 25%. Others include patent ductus arteriosus, coarctation of the aorta, aortic and pulmonary stenosis, and atrioventricular septal defect (AVSD).
- **Cyanotic:** The tetralogy (tetrad) of Fallot is the most frequently occurring cyanotic lesion (10%). Others are less common: transposition of the great vessels (5%), hypoplastic left heart syndrome (1–2%), total anomalous pulmonary venous drainage (1%), truncus arteriosus (<1%), tricuspid atresia, hypoplastic right ventricle and Ebstein's anomaly. The details of these complex lesions do not matter; what is of importance is the principle that deoxygenated blood bypasses the lungs and shunts directly into the systemic arterial circulation.
- Some of these terms have been superseded in the specialist literature by a nomenclature that is based on following the blood flow through the heart and on *concordant* (normal) or *discordant* (abnormal) anatomical relations. According to this system, transposition of the great vessels, for example, is described as 'ventriculo-great arterial discordance'. By all means describe CHD in this way if you have this expert knowledge, but be aware that most examiners will probably be more familiar with the traditional terminology.

Management of Patients with Congenital Heart Disease
The practical application of this information may lie in the rational management of children, and later adults, with uncorrected lesions. It is unusual to encounter adults with cyanotic CHD.

Acyanotic CHD
- The main problem in acyanotic heart disease is pulmonary hypertension, which develops as the circulation attempts to 'protect' itself from high pulmonary blood flows caused by intracardiac left-to-right shunting (e.g. through a septal defect) by developing hypertrophy of the media of vascular smooth muscle.
- With progressive disease the resistances in the left and right circulations become finely balanced so that an increase in PVR or a decrease in SVR may reverse the shunt (from left to right, to right to left). This is Eisenmenger's Syndrome.
- **Principles of anaesthesia:** rises in PVR or falls in SVR must be avoided.
  - **PVR:** the resistance in the hyperreactive pulmonary vascular tree is increased by hypoxia, hypercapnia, acidosis, nitrous oxide and catecholamine release.
  - **SVR:** this is decreased by various factors, among them sympathetic block, most forms of general anaesthesia, some anti-hypertensive drugs and vasodilators, high ambient temperatures and pyrexia.

- Left ventricular function is also impaired by chronic hypoxia and by increased pulmonary venous return. Mechanical efficiency may be impaired by the loss of some of the stroke volume through a VSD.
- There is substantial risk of paradoxical embolus, and so filters should be attached to intravenous lines to ensure that even the smallest amount of air does not gain access to the circulation. Patients are at greater risk of bacterial endocarditis, but routine prophylactic antibiotics are no longer recommended.

Cyanotic CHD

This will be identified more commonly in children, and exists when there is:

- Right-to-left shunt with pulmonary oligaemia, as in the tetrad of Fallot (VSD, overriding aorta, pulmonary stenosis and right ventricular hypertrophy).
- Parallel left and right circulations (transposition of the great arteries).
- Mixing of oxygenated and deoxygenated blood without decreased pulmonary blood flow (double outlet RV, single ventricle, total anomalous pulmonary venous drainage [TAPVD] and truncus arteriosus).

Problems

- The chronic hypoxia stimulates polycythaemia. This leads to suboptimal rheology which worsens with dehydration (sludging and thrombosis are possible), and a significant risk of cerebrovascular accident (CVA) at a haematocrit of greater than 65%.
- There is a risk of paradoxical emboli, as described earlier.
- There is a risk of bacterial endocarditis, as described earlier.
- If there is pulmonary oligaemia, inhalation induction will be slower.
- As a final pedantic observation: 'tetralogy' is any series of four related literary or dramatic compositions, just as a 'trilogy' is a set of three. A 'tetrad' is a group of four, just as a 'triad' is a group of three. So 'Tetralogy of Fallot' strictly speaking is a misnomer, but the terminology is unlikely ever to change.

Physiology and Clinical Anatomy of the Infant and Neonate

Commentary

The scope for asking basic science questions that are directly related to paediatric clinical practice is quite restricted, and so topics tend to be limited to aspects of infant anatomy and physiology. With the exception of questions about the paediatric airway, physiology is probably asked more commonly than anatomy because it is inherently more complex. The discussion may include overall physiological aspects but is more likely to concentrate only on one or two. Examiners will expect theoretical rather than practical knowledge because they will assume that you have not anaesthetized children as young as this.

Core Information

The general physiological characteristics of the infant (defined as a child aged between 1 month and 1 year) and neonate. The very youngest children exemplify the differences between paediatric and adult practice.

Surface Area to Mass Ratio

- The smaller the child, the larger is the ratio of surface area to mass, so that in the neonate it is 2.5 times that of the adult. The larger this ratio, the greater is the required increase in metabolic rate to maintain normal body temperature, and this is one of the core factors that explains many of the physiological characteristics.

Cardiovascular System

- **Anatomical features:** at birth there is right ventricular hypertrophy (owing to the fetal circulation). The limbs are smaller in relation to the body, so there is less reserve blood volume to mobilize from the periphery. The foramen ovale closes functionally at birth although it remains anatomically patent.
- This need to maintain body temperature via heat production results in a higher basal metabolic rate (BMR) and higher tissue oxygen consumption which, at 7 ml kg^{-1} min^{-1}, is twice that of an adult.
- Cardiac output, which at birth is 200 ml kg^{-1} min^{-1} (100 ml kg^{-1} min^{-1} in the adult), increases predominantly by an increase in heart rate rather than stroke volume.
- Blood volume is 80 ml kg^{-1} at term and 75 ml kg^{-1} at age 2 years. The haemoglobin concentration at birth is 160–180 g l^{-1} (80% HbF), dropping to 100 g l^{-1} at 3 months and rising again to 120–140 g l^{-1} at 1 year.
- Infants demonstrate increased sensitivity to vagal stimulation.

Respiratory System

- **Airway:** a number of characteristics have implications for airway management. The head is disproportionately large in comparison with adults; the angle of the jaw is 140° (120° in adults); and the dimensions of the upper airway are reduced by a larger tongue, by lymphoid tissue and by narrower nasal and pharyngeal passages. The epiglottis is U-shaped and, although it is stiffer than in the adult, lies more horizontally (at an angle of 45°). It is sometimes described as 'infantile'. The larynx is higher (the cricoid cartilage lies at the level of C_4) and not only lies more anteriorly but is also tilted anteriorly. The ring of the cricoid cartilage forms the narrowest part of the airway up to at least the age of 8 years. The trachea is short (around 4 cm in the infant) and narrow (about 5–6 mm in diameter). The angles of the left and right main bronchi are approximately equal, so that left endobronchial intubation is as likely as right.
- **Respiration:** the high BMR of infants is associated with a high respiratory rate. Respiratory compensation occurs via an increase in respiratory frequency more than increases in tidal volume. Infant ribs are more horizontal and so are mechanically less efficient. The compliant chest wall is unable effectively to oppose the action of the diaphragm to maintain the FRC, and the soft sternum retracts rather than providing support for respiration. Respiration is predominantly diaphragmatic, and

the intercostal and accessory muscles are relatively weak, being deficient in type 1 muscle fibres until around the age of 2 years. (Tidal ventilation is 7 ml kg^{-1}, the same as in older children and adults.) Infants respond to hypoxia with bradypnoea rather than tachypnoea.

- Alveoli at birth number 20–50 million, and they are structurally underdeveloped. By 18 months they total 300 million, and thereafter grow in size rather than number. The FRC is small and desaturation occurs quickly.
- Decreased compliance (because of poorly developed elastic tissue) means that ventilatory units have short time constants, so alveolar ventilation is maintained at the expense of a high respiratory rate, high work of breathing and high oxygen consumption (15% of the total).
- Closing capacity exceeds FRC (up to the age of 6 years), and infants generate physiological CPAP (of around 4 cm H$_2$O) by partial adduction of the cords during expiration. The 'grunting' of a premature neonate in respiratory difficulty is an exaggeration of this mechanism.
- Pre-term infants are at risk of sudden apnoeic episodes (defined as cessation of breathing for 15 seconds or more). This applies up to around 60 weeks of post-conceptual age, and is a manifestation of poor maturation of ventilatory control.
- More than 50% of total airways resistance in infants (and children up to the age of around 6 years) is provided by peripheral airways less than 2 mm in diameter. This is why conditions such as bronchiolitis are so problematic in this age group.

Temperature Control

- Thermoregulation is immature in the infant. A large surface area is associated with increased heat loss, and neonates are especially vulnerable to rapid hypothermia. Infants aged less than 3 months do not shiver, but generate heat via non-shivering thermogenesis from brown fat, which comprises up to 6% of the body weight of the term fetus. Heat is generated by the catecholamine-mediated metabolism of fatty acids.

Energy Metabolism

- Fetal, pre-term and neonatal glucose homeostasis is complex. It should be sufficient to know that the infant does not have the same capacity to mobilize glucose as the adult. Illness, trauma or the stress of pre-operative fasting can all combine with the high basal metabolic rate to deplete glycogen stores and produce hypoglycaemia (defined in this context as a blood glucose concentration below 2.2 mmol l^{-1}). Restricted fat reserves also reduce the mobilization of free fatty acids and the production of ketones (which are an important energy substrate).

Renal System

- Infant kidneys have a reduced glomerular filtration rate (which, at 65 ml min^{-1}, is half that of the adult), diminished tubular function and sodium excretion, and a decreased concentrating ability. Sodium loss is inevitable, and there is limited ability either to conserve or excrete water, so infants tolerate hypovolaemia or overtransfusion badly. The excretory load is mitigated partially by 50% of the nitrogen that is incorporated into growing tissue. Renal function is mature at about 2 years of age.

Central Nervous System

- Neurological development continues in the early years of life with the completion of myelination of the brain and spinal cord. The sympathetic nervous system is also incompletely developed, which explains the tolerance of children to the effects of central neuraxial blockade which in adults may cause significant hypotension. The blood–brain barrier is immature, which increases the neonate's, and to a lesser extent the infant's, sensitivity to opiates and other CNS depressants. By 6 months of age the response to morphine is probably the same as in adults. There is some concern, as yet unresolved, about possible deleterious effects of general anaesthesia on the nervous system of the young child (see under 'Mechanisms of Action of General Anaesthetics' in Chapter 4).

Gastrointestinal System

- The incidence of neonatal gastro-oesophageal reflux is high (coordination of swallowing with respiration does not mature until around 4–5 months), but this rarely proves to be a problem in clinical practice.

Drug Effects

- A combination of factors influences the response of the neonate and infant to drugs. CNS depressants may have enhanced effects, both because the blood–brain barrier is less effective and because cerebral blood flow accounts for a greater proportion of the cardiac output. Total body water is higher, and so water-soluble drugs have a larger volume of distribution and may require higher initial doses. (Suxamethonium is an example.) Fat-soluble drugs may have a longer clinical effect because lower stores of body fat decrease redistribution. Plasma proteins are lower, and so free diffusible drug levels may be higher. Enzymatic function, particularly that associated with hepatic phase II conjugation reactions, is also immature. This may delay metabolism and excretion of drugs.

Supplementary Information

Fluid Requirements in Children

- **Fluid balance – children:** maintenance fluid requirements in children can be calculated according to a simple formula: $4 \text{ ml kg}^{-1} \text{ h}^{-1}$ ($100 \text{ ml kg}^{-1} \text{ day}^{-1}$) for the first 10 kg body weight, $2 \text{ ml kg}^{-1} \text{ h}^{-1}$ ($50 \text{ ml kg}^{-1} \text{ day}^{-1}$) for the next 10 kg body weight and $1 \text{ ml kg}^{-1} \text{ h}^{-1}$ ($20 \text{ ml kg}^{-1} \text{ day}^{-1}$) for each additional kg body weight. This is only a guide; illness, pyrexia and prematurity are among many factors that influence fluid replacement (which should be oral wherever possible).
- **Fluid balance – neonates/infants:** the preceding calculation does not apply to neonates and young infants. By the fifth day of life, term neonates of weight >2.5 kg require $150 \text{ ml kg}^{-1} \text{ day}^{-1}$. Newborns, however, have a relative excess of total body water and extracellular fluid, and in the first few days their requirements are much less. A typical regimen would be $60 \text{ ml kg}^{-1} \text{ day}^{-1}$ on day 1, $75 \text{ ml kg}^{-1} \text{ day}^{-1}$ on day 2, $90 \text{ ml kg}^{-1} \text{ day}^{-1}$ on day 3, $120 \text{ ml kg}^{-1} \text{ day}^{-1}$ on day 4 and $150 \text{ ml kg}^{-1} \text{ day}^{-1}$ thereafter.

- **Fluid resuscitation:** the immediate management of a child with moderate or severe volume loss is a bolus of 20 ml kg^{-1} of colloid or NaCl 0.9% repeated as necessary. Infants not only have high total body water of 70–80% compared with around 60% in the adult, but they also have a higher proportion of extracellular fluid (>50% in the neonate compared to 33% in the adult). This increases their vulnerability to dehydration.

Laparoscopy

Commentary

From the early days in which it was essentially the preserve of the gynaecologists who used it mainly for diagnosis and for sterilization procedures, laparoscopy has expanded to encompass major, highly complex and sometimes very prolonged surgery. The physiological consequences and potential complications are of increasing importance, as anaesthetizing patients for laparoscopic surgery is now routine. The physiological changes are not however, unduly complicated, and it should not be too difficult to give a reasonable account during any discussion.

Core Information

- **Surgical indications.** The benefits of avoiding open surgery with substantial tissue trauma and significant postoperative pain are intuitively obvious. Increases in surgical experience and expertise now mean that the range of operations that can be performed either laparoscopically or with laparoscopic assistance encompasses major bowel resection, nephrectomy, Nissen's fundoplication, complex bariatric surgery and major gynaecological procedures. It is now routine to perform hernia repair, cholecystectomy and appendicectomy using the same technique.
- **Laparoscopy.** Central to laparoscopy is the creation of a pneumoperitoneum, most commonly with carbon dioxide, but rarely with other gases such as nitrous oxide, argon and helium. (Non-absorbable gases have a theoretically higher risk of causing problems such as pneumothorax and venous gas embolism.) The gas is insufflated into the peritoneal cavity at 4–6 litres min^{-1} to create an intra-abdominal pressure of between 10 and 20 mmHg (normal is 0–7 mmHg). Leakage through surgical ports means that a constant gas flow of 200–400 ml min^{-1} may be required to maintain to prevent deflation and loss of the surgical view.
- **CO$_2$ absorption.** There is speculation that some insufflated CO2 leads to the intraperitoneal formation of H_2CO_3 and increased pain due to the local acidity. Otherwise CO_2 is absorbed efficiently across the peritoneum and will increase PaCO$_2$. Modest hypercapnia has some physiological benefits in that the catecholamine release it provokes may support the circulation and promote bronchodilation. This will, however, increase myocardial oxygen demand. Significant hypercapnia will cause a respiratory acidosis and also directly depresses the myocardium.
- **Patient position.** This depends on the surgical procedure. In major gynaecology, for example, the patient will be in the head down (Trendelenberg) position in order to

move abdominal contents out of the pelvis, whereas the reverse head-up position is necessary for upper abdominal procedures. Positioning may have significantly different physiological effects, as outlined in the following.

- **Cardiovascular effects.** An initial autotransfusion of a few hundred ml of blood from the splanchnic circulation increases immediate circulating volume, but this is offset by the decreases in venous return secondary to raised intra-abdominal pressure compressing the inferior vena cava. Systemic vascular resistance increases as a direct result, and it also rises indirectly with catecholamine and vasopressin release and activation of the renin-angiotensin system. This may offset any decrease in cardiac output due to reduced venous return but at the expense of increasing myocardial work. The reverse Trendelenberg position risks marked venous pooling and effective hypovolaemia.
- **Respiratory effects.** Splinting of the diaphragm further reduces FRC, and the raised abdominal pressure can increase airway resistance and reduce pulmonary compliance. In rare instances this can lead to significant shunting and oxygen desaturation, but in most cases any falls in PaO_2 can be attenuated by judicious changes to the ventilation. The changes are less marked in the head-up position. Extreme and prolonged Trendelenberg positioning can be associated with facial and upper airway oedema.
- **Central nervous system effects.** The rise in intra-abdominal and venous pressure may cause a concomitant rise in intracranial pressure, but the consequences are likely to be modest. Prolonged head-down tilt, however, has been associated with the development of hydrostatic cerebral oedema, although there is nothing that can be done specifically to avoid this other than to hope for a swift and accomplished surgeon.
- **Gastrointestinal and renal effects.** Sustained intra-abdominal pressures greater than 20 mmHg create what in effect is an abdominal compartment syndrome with mesenteric and mucosal blood flow that reduces by almost half (40%). These pressures may already be high in the morbidly obese patient in whom they can be in the region of 14 mmHg. Regurgitation of gastric contents is a possible complication, although it is very unusual to actually find gastric contents in the pharynx at the end of a procedure. The possibility does mean that tracheal intubation is favoured by most anaesthetists, although simpler and shorter procedures can be done using a laryngeal mask airway. (You will have to justify this decision if it comes to a discussion of the options.) Renal vascular resistance is increased by high intra-abdominal pressures, and so glomerular filtration rate and urine output may decline.
- **Compartment syndromes.** A patient in prolonged lithotomy in the Trendelenberg position is at risk of lower limb compartment syndrome secondary to immobility, compression (including by graduated compression stockings) and venous congestion due to reduced femoral venous return caused by the position and by the increase in intra-abdominal pressure.
- **Complications.** These may be surgical and due to damage caused by the trocars, particularly at the beginning of the procedure when the gas insufflation needle is inserted blind. Otherwise the complications are related primarily to the creation of the penumoperitoneum. The peritoneum is insensitive to direct injury but highly sensitive to stretch, which can cause profound vagal stimulation leading in the

extreme case to asystole. Rapid abdominal decompression is the vital first step in retrieving this situation should it occur. Venous gas embolism has been described; immediate discontinuation of insufflation should precede generic resuscitation. CO_2 embolism is less dangerous than air and other gases because of its high solubility and rapid absorption. High gas pressures have also been known to cause pneumomediastinum and pneumothorax. These complications, or gas injection into the wrong planes may also be associated with subcutaneous emphysema.

The Prone Position in Anaesthesia

Commentary
A surgical request for prone patient positioning is usually met with an inward groan by the anaesthetist who then has to contend with a number of potential problems which go beyond the difficulties of inverting an anaesthetized patient and losing ready access to the airway. These are mechanical and physiological and the oral is likely to explore your understanding of both.

Core Information
The indications for managing critical care patients in the prone position are discussed in more detail under 'The Failing Lung'. The surgical indications are for those operations that can be done in no other way, such as lumbar microdiscectomy and more complex spinal surgery. Operations such as tendo Achilles repair and haemorrhoidectomy can be performed successfully in other positions, but some surgeons prefer to operate with the patient prone.

The issue is complicated slightly by the fact that there is no standard prone position, and variations such as the 'knee-chest' tucked position or the jackknife position are associated with different physiological effects. Some of what follows therefore is necessarily a generalization which applies primarily to a prone position in which the patient is straight and more or less flat, with the pelvis and shoulders supported to leave the abdomen free, and the head centralized and neutral.

Manual Handling Issues
- Turning the patient is often problematic, particularly in those with raised BMI. Several handlers will be needed to ensure that the patient is logrolled into position without any twisting of the lumbar and cervical spines. The head must move as one with the shoulders with obvious care not to dislodge whichever airway device is in place.

Airway Access
- It is accepted wisdom that restricted access to the airway once the patient is inverted mandates endotracheal intubation, probably with an armoured tube, and this would be the 'safe' exam answer. In clinical practice, however, by no means all anaesthetists

are quite as dogmatic. The prone position confers some respiratory advantages in a patient who is breathing spontaneously and a standard laryngeal mask airway is relatively easy to resite should it move, unlike a tracheal tube (or a reinforced laryngeal mask airway). It would probably be wise not to volunteer this option as it remains contentious, but be prepared to discuss it should an examiner raise the issue.

Mechanical Pressure Effects

- **Ophthalmic problems**. These range from relatively benign complications such as chemosis and subconjunctival haemorrhage through retinal detachment to complete visual loss (which is quoted as occurring in 0.02–0.2% following spinal surgery). Decreased ophthalmic perfusion pressure secondary to hypotension, hypovolaemia and an increase in direct orbital pressure can contribute to ischaemic optic neuropathy or central retinal artery occlusion, both of which may result in blindness. The central retinal artery can also thrombose secondary to a reduction in flow, but in some cases this may be unilateral. Intraocular pressure can rise in patients with narrow-angle glaucoma who are positioned prone.

- **Peripheral nerve injuries.** Nerves of the brachial plexus are at particular risk of traction injury because they are effectively fixed at the cervical vertebrae, and they may also be compressed at the level of the first rib, clavicle and head of the humerus as they pass down into the upper limb across these potentially mobile structures. The ulnar nerve is vulnerable both to ischaemia and to direct compression, as is the lateral cutaneous nerve of the thigh, which may be in prolonged contact with pelvic supports.

- **Pressure sores and compartment syndromes.** The prone position is no more likely to cause pressure sores than the supine, except that there are probably more bony prominences to put the overlying tissues at risk. These include the anterior ankle joints, knees, anterior superior iliac spines, thorax, chin and forehead. Ischaemia develops after around 2 hours of unrelieved pressure and tissue necrosis after around 6 hours. Duration of surgery is therefore the major risk factor along with increased skin fragility associated with advanced age or corticosteroid therapy. Obesity is also a contributing factor. Compartment syndromes have been described, but this has usually been in association with variations on the knee-chest position in which there is flexion of the knees and hips.

- **Surgical bleeding.** The venous drainage from the spine is via the vertebral valveless venous plexus of Batson. The absence of valves means that any increase in intra-abdominal pressure secondary to external compression is likely to cause a significant increase in operative bleeding and potential compromise of any planned spinal surgery.

Physiological Effects

- **Cardiovascular system.** A consistent finding across various studies has been a decrease in cardiac index. This fall in cardiac output is attributed primarily to a reduction in stroke volume secondary to reduced venous return, which is due largely to venous pooling but to which inferior caval obstruction can make a contribution if positioning is poor and the abdomen is compressed. Intermittent positive pressure ventilation (IPPV) also abolishes the contribution that negative intrathoracic pressure usually makes to venous return. The compensatory sympathetic response to this effective hypovolaemia is reflected by a tachycardia and a rise in systemic vascular resistance. Patients who are anaesthetized may also tolerate poorly rapid changes in position.

- **Respiratory system.** In contrast, most of the effects of the prone position on the respiratory system tend to be beneficial. Functional residual capacity decreases by around 45% from the conscious, upright position to the anaesthetized supine position, but only by 12% from upright to prone. The change from supine to prone therefore, with all other factors unchanged, is associated with an improvement in PaO_2 which is due to better matching of ventilation-perfusion. The reasons for this improvement, in contrast to the cardiovascular changes which are relatively simply explained, are rather more complex. The renowned respiratory physiologist John West formulated the familiar concept of the three pulmonary zones to explain how hydrostatic pressure differences influenced the distribution of blood flow, and accepted teaching ever since has attributed the ventilatory changes in the prone position to be primarily a gravitational effect. However, more sophisticated investigation has demonstrated that blood flow is much less altered with changes of position (and in weightlessness) than previously believed, and a different model based on the structural features of the airway and associated vasculature has been proposed. There is substantial heterogeneity of ventilation and of perfusion at isogravitational levels which is related to the fractal characteristics of the pulmonary architecture, but at any particular level there is appropriate V/Q matching. In nature, a fractal is a repeating pattern that is reproduced at every scale of increase or decrease in size. The branching of the airways (an average of 23 generations) and blood vessels (28 generations as the arterial supply advances further into the alveoli) reduce their size asymmetrically but consistently by a constant factor that can be described mathematically. It is therefore the shape and structure of the bronchioles and blood vessels that are the prime dependents of ventilation and perfusion. It should be fairly clear that this is already too complex a topic to be discussed in detail in the oral, and it is not intuitively obvious quite why this pattern of lung architecture itself should improve ventilation-perfusion matching. A factor that is simpler to understand is the fact that the dorsal lung areas receive preferential perfusion independently of position, and this may be related to an intrinsically lower pulmonary vascular resistance in those regions. In the injured lung, the proximal architecture of the bronchioles and vessels may be distorted by oedema and inflammation, and this mismatch can be amplified by the distal branching with substantial V/Q mismatch in the alveoli.

Intracranial Pressure

Commentary

There are several variations on this question about intracranial pressure (ICP). The oral may concentrate on ICP itself or divert to include the concept of cerebral perfusion pressure (CPP), or the protection of the brain against hypoxic or ischaemic brain injury. The diagnosis and rational management of raised ICP are important, and so knowledge of the basic underlying mechanisms will be expected.

Core Information

Factors That Influence ICP

- The skull of an adult is in effect a rigid box which contains brain tissue, blood and CSF. The brain itself has minimal compressibility and so there is very limited scope for compensation. An increase in the volume of one component invariably results in an increase in ICP unless the volume of another component decreases (This is the Monroe–Kellie hypothesis.) These intracranial contents consist of brain tissue (1,400–1,500 g), blood (100–150 ml), CSF (110–120 ml) and extracellular fluid (<100 ml). The intracranial compliance curve is shown in Figure 3.9.
- Normal ICP is 10–12 mmHg. Any increase may be significant because of the potential impact on cerebral perfusion. The CPP is determined by mean arterial pressure (MAP) minus the sum of the central venous pressure (CVP) and the ICP. CPP = MAP − (CVP + ICP).
- **Mass lesions:** ICP is raised by mass lesions which increase the volume of brain, bone or meninges. These include tumours of all three structures, as well as infection (with abscess formation).
- **Volume increases:** ICP is raised by conditions which increase non-CSF fluid volume. Intracranial aneurysm, arteriovenous malformation and trauma are all relatively common causes of subarachnoid or subdural haemorrhage. ICP is raised by cerebral oedema, which itself has many causes, including trauma, infection, metabolic dysfunction (such as hepatic encephalopathy or Reye's syndrome), hypoxia, venous obstruction and increased hydrostatic pressure (such as is caused by a steep or prolonged Trendelenberg position on the operating table). It may form part of the symptomatology of altitude sickness (high-altitude cerebral oedema, HACE). It may also be idiopathic, as in benign intracranial hypertension. (This is a clinical entity

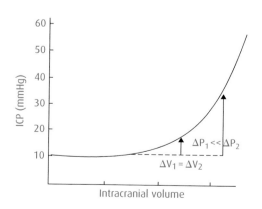

Fig. 3.9 Intracranial pressure–volume curve.

defined by an ICP greater than 15 mmHg (but which can reach three times that figure) in the presence of normal CSF composition, normal conscious level and with no evident pathological process). Increased ICP may be caused by a rise in intracranial venous pressure which is offset by intracranial and CSF pressure increases that restore the required gradient for CSF absorption into the venous system. Some cases can be managed with corticosteroids, diuretics and acetazolamide, but severe cases may require the insertion of a lumbothecal–peritoneal shunt.

- **Impaired drainage:** ICP is also raised by conditions which impede drainage of CSF (which is produced at 0.4 ml min^{-1}) and thus increase its intracranial volume. These include congenital and acquired hydrocephalus, which may also be associated with trauma, tumour or infection. A blocked ventricular shunt is another important cause.
- **Pathophysiology:** in the presence of raised ICP, CPP is given by MAP – ICP. Perfusion will be maintained until CPP starts to fall below 50 mmHg, with the onset of critical ischaemia at 30–40 mmHg. There may also be focal ischaemia in the region of a mass lesion. Raised ICP attenuates cerebral autoregulation to the point at which it is lost completely, after which cerebral blood flow follows MAP passively.

Measurement of Intracranial Pressure

- ICP can be measured by subdural or extradural transducers or via an intraventricular catheter. All these methods are invasive, requiring a burr hole, but they allow important quantification of cerebral perfusion pressure.
- **Subdural pressure transducers.** As the name describes, these devices are placed in the subdural space and fill with cerebrospinal fluid. After equalization, the pressures within the closed system can be transduced. They are less invasive than other methods, but are less accurate and do not allow sampling or drainage of CSF.
- **Intraventricular catheters**. These catheters provide the most accurate means of measuring ICP. They are usually placed into the lateral ventricle via a burr hole (most commonly in the right frontal area) and through the parenchyma of the brain. In addition to providing pressure measurements, the catheters can also be used to drain cerebrospinal fluid or to administer drugs such as antibiotics. The external transducer reference point is the external auditory meatus which approximates to the intracerebral centre, which is where the foramina of Munro link the lateral ventricles with the third ventricle. Complications include infection and blockage.
- **Intraparenchymal monitors.** These are useful when extreme ventricular compression makes the insertion of an intraventricular catheter impossible. They do not use a column of fluid (i.e. a saline-filled catheter) via which to transduce pressures but instead use a variety of other technologies. One example is the use of fibreoptic cables tipped with miniature mirrors whose displacement by raised ICP reflects light of varying intensity, which is then transduced into pressure. Another is the use of microchip sensors whose resistance alters as ICP changes. These systems cannot be recalibrated once they are in position, they cannot sample or drain CSF, and because of their location they may measure only local pressure changes rather than global ICP.

Supplementary Information and Clinical Considerations

The Clinical Features of Raised Intracranial Pressure

- **Symptoms:** these depend on whether the ICP rise is acute or chronic. Typically, patients complain of headache, nausea and vomiting. These symptoms are worse in the morning both because of increased hydrostatic pressure effects and because the $PaCO_2$ may be raised secondary to relative overnight hypoventilation. Patients may have changes in level of consciousness and visual disturbances (see following).
- **Signs:** patients may exhibit neurological signs caused by brain distortion or by one of the brain herniation syndromes (see following), including pupillary changes and failure of upward gaze. There may be papilloedema, hypertension, bradycardia and abnormal respiration. These last three constitute Cushing's triad.
- **Cerebral herniation:** several syndromes have been described, including central, cingulate and uncal herniation.
  - **Central herniation:** in this situation (which is the most important), the raised ICP forces the brain downwards through the foramen magnum as the cerebellar tonsils herniate and compress the medulla. This is known colloquially as 'coning'.
  - **Cingulate herniation:** the cingulate gyrus and part of the hemisphere are displaced beneath the falx cerebri. This primarily affects the anterior cerebral vessels.
  - **Uncal herniation:** the uncus (which is part of the hippocampal gyrus) herniates through, and is then compressed against, the tentorium.

Specific Clinical Signs (ICP Can Rise without These)

- **Cushing's reflex:** the triad comprises hypertension, bradycardia and abnormal respiration. This is a late and ominous sign that coning is imminent, as the carotid body receptors attempt to mediate an increase in perfusion pressure that is doomed to fail.
- **Pupillary signs:** these may follow uncal compression or kinking of the oculomotor nerve by distorted vessels. There is ipsilateral pupillary dilatation followed by motor paralysis of the extraocular muscles (excluding the superior oblique and lateral rectus muscles which are supplied by the fourth and sixth cranial nerves, respectively).
- **Eye signs:** the lateral rectus is also affected because of the displacement of the sixth cranial nerve (abducens), which has a long intracranial course. As it leaves the posterior margin of the pons, it is crossed by the anterior inferior cerebellar artery. Displacement of the cerebellum may distort these vessels such that they compress the abducens nerve. The clinical effect of such compression is failure of lateral gaze.

The Management of Raised ICP

- Moderate head-up position will reduce venous pressure without unduly affecting the MAP (provided there is no physical constriction to drainage by artefacts such as tracheal tube tapes). Moderate hypocapnia will reduce ICP, but the benefit is short-lived, and there is a risk of rebound hyperaemia. Mannitol 20% in a dose of

0.5 g kg^{-1} has a marked but transient effect. It may shift the patient back down the intracranial compliance curve and gain sufficient time for definitive treatment before a catastrophic rise in ICP (Figure 3.9), but it too is associated with rebound hypertension. If the blood–brain barrier is affected, mannitol may also cross into brain parenchyma and exert a reverse osmotic effect. High-dose dexamethasone reduces oedema secondary to intracranial tumours but has no effect on raised ICP following trauma. Hypertonic saline has a well-established role in the management of raised ICP secondary to brain injury and neoplasm, although not in other conditions. It also has a role in limiting secondary brain injury due to neurochemical changes. Hyperthermia will increase the cerebral metabolic rate for oxygen (CMRO$_2$) and cerebral blood flow and must be avoided. Hypothermia has the opposite effect and may confer some benefit. Intermittent cerebrospinal fluid drainage via an intraventricular catheter can be very effective. (Continuous drainage risks emptying the ventricles completely, which will then make ICP monitoring impossible.)

Cerebrospinal Fluid (CSF)

- **Formation:** its total volume is around 150 ml, about 80% of which is intracranial. Most of the extracranial (spinal) CSF is found distal to the conus medullaris. The choroid arterial plexuses form CSF either by secretion or by the quantitatively much less significant process of ultrafiltration. It is produced in the lateral, third and fourth ventricles, at a rate of around 0.4 ml min^{-1} (575 ml 24 h^{-1}). The rate of production is constant and is not related to ICP unless it is sufficiently high to compromise CPP and reduce blood flow to the choroid plexus.
- **Circulation:** CSF passes through the cerebral aqueduct to the fourth ventricle and thence through the midline foramen of Magendie and the two lateral foramina of Luschka to communicate with the subarachnoid space of the brain and spinal cord. It is either absorbed directly into cerebral venules (10%) or absorbed by the arachnoid villi (90%).
- **Functions:** it has a cushioning effect which protects the brain from injury. Supported by CSF, the effective cerebral weight is only 50g. By translocation from the intracranial to the extracranial subarachnoid space, CSF can partly buffer increases in ICP.
- **Composition:** it has a higher PCO$_2$ than plasma and a lower pH (7.33). The mean specific gravity is 1.006, with a range of 1.003–1.009. Its protein content is low (0.2 gl^{-1}), so buffering capacity is negligible. Glucose concentration is lower than in plasma. Sodium and chloride are higher, whereas potassium is lower (40%). This is because the formation of CSF requires the active transport of Na$^+$, Cl$^-$ and K$^+$ into the ventricles. Further Na$^+$ is then added in exchange for K$^+$ (mediated by Na$^+$/K$^+$ ATPase). The influx is maintained by the further exchange of H$^+$ and HCO$_3^-$ for Na$^+$ and Cl$^-$. H$^+$ and HCO$_3^-$ are generated from H$_2$CO$_3$ in a reaction catalysed by carbonic anhydrase.
- **Factors affecting rate of production:** acetazolamide, which is a carbonic anhydrase inhibitor, may reduce CSF production by as much as 50%. High-dose diuretics also reduce it by affecting the sodium transport process. (Corticosteroids may increase production, but not consistently enough to make them a reliable treatment for postdural puncture headache.)

Cerebral Blood Flow

Commentary

This is a standard question which has obvious relevance for general anaesthesia, for head injury, for techniques such as induced hypotension and for anaesthesia in patients with hypertensive disorders, including pre-eclampsia.

Core Information

Factors Which Influence Cerebral Blood Flow

- The brain weighs 2% of the human organism yet receives 15% of the cardiac output. The intracranial contents consist of brain tissue (approximately 1,400–1,500 g), blood (100–150 ml), CSF (110–120 ml) and extracellular fluid (<100 ml).
- **Normal cerebral blood flow (CBF):** normal CBF is 50 ml 100 g^{-1} of brain tissue per minute, and is determined by the Cerebral perfusion pressure (CPP). The CPP = MAP – (CVP + ICP). The normal CPP is 70–80 mmHg. Blood flow to grey matter is more than twice that to white matter.
- **Autoregulation:** over a wide range of MAP, typically between 50 and 150 mmHg, autoregulation maintains normal flow. The process is not instantaneous, and may take some seconds to complete. The classic cerebral autoregulation curve is an oversimplification; there is not a neat linear relationship between MAP and CBF at each end of the curve, and changes in perfusion pressure may be regional. Chronic hypertension shifts the autoregulatory curve to the right; drug-induced hypotension shifts it to the left (Figure 3.10). The mechanisms which underlie autoregulation are primarily myogenic, modulated by stretch receptors in vascular smooth muscle, and metabolic, in which hydrogen ions and substances such as nitric oxide and adenosine accumulate in the tissues at low flow and mediate vasodilatation.
- **PaCO$_2$:** there is a linear relationship between PaCO$_2$ and CBF in the range of partial pressures from 3.5 to 10.0 kPa. Below 3.5 kPa, cerebral vasoconstriction leads to tissue hypoxia (with subsequent reflex vasodilatation); at around 10.0–12.0 kPa there

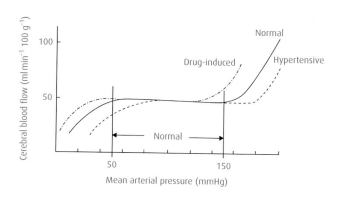

Fig. 3.10 Cerebral autoregulation.

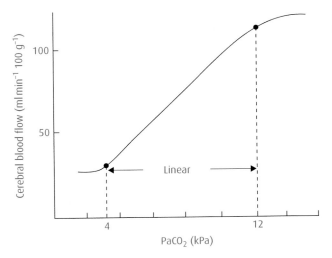

Fig. 3.11 Cerebral blood flow and $PaCO_2$.

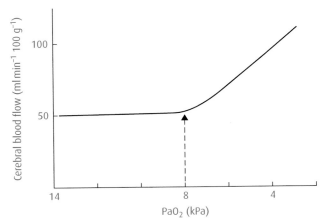

Fig. 3.12 Cerebral blood flow and PaO_2.

is a ceiling at which blood flow is maximal (at around 120 ml 100 g^{-1} min^{-1}) (Figure 3.11).

- **PaO_2:** decreases in the partial pressure of oxygen below 8 kPa are associated with sharp increases in CBF up to around 110 ml 100 g^{-1} min^{-1}. At 4.0 kPa, CBF is doubled. Hyperoxia is associated with decreases in CBF (Figure 3.12).
- **Temperature:** changes in temperature are associated with altered requirements for cerebral oxygen (the cerebral metabolic rate for oxygen, $CMRO_2$), although the relationship is linear rather than exponential. Thus, while at 37 °C, a 1 °C drop in temperature is accompanied by a fall in $CMRO_2$ of 6–7%; at a brain temperature of 15 °C (during deep hypothermic circulatory arrest, for example), a further 1 °C drop results in a decrease in $CMRO_2$ of only 1%.

- **$CMRO_2$:** CBF is linked to $CMRO_2$ by a mechanism that has not yet been fully elucidated. There is a short lag time of 1–2 minutes.
- **Rheology:** lower plasma viscosity is associated with enhanced capillary flow, although there is a balance between optimal rheology and oxygen delivery. A haematocrit above 50% risks intravascular sludging and a reduction in CBF, and a haematocrit below 30% is associated with decreased oxygen flux.
- **ICP:** The formula for CPP confirms that CBF is compromised by increases in ICP from its normal 10–12 mmHg.

Supplementary Information and Clinical Considerations

Measurement of Cerebral Blood Flow

- **Kety–Schmidt method:** this is an application of the Fick principle, which states that flow is equal to the amount of a substance taken up or excreted by an organ, divided by the arteriovenous (AV) concentration difference. (Hence CBF = Quantity of substance taken up by the brain/AV difference.) Nitrous oxide is used as the diffusible tracer. The subject breathes 10% N_2O for 10 minutes, during which time paired peripheral arterial and jugular venous bulb samples are taken. At the end of 10 minutes the concentrations are equal, at which point the venous concentration is the same as brain. The speed at which the arterial and venous curves equilibrate is a measure of N_2O delivery to the brain. The technique is invasive and gives only a global measure of flow. It is not a technique for clinical use.
- **Transcranial Doppler ultrasonography:** this gives a measure of the velocity of red cells flowing through large cerebral arteries, most commonly the middle cerebral, and can be used in clinical practice. The velocity can give an index of flow provided that the diameter of the artery is determined independently, and provided that this diameter changes little (as is the case with the major cerebral arteries).
- **Positron emission tomography (PET):** this (research) technique monitors the uptake by different areas of the brain of 2-deoxyglucose, which is labelled with a positron emitter.
- **Scintillography and SPECT scanning:** these techniques use radioactive xenon to trace regional blood flow, with or without enhancement by CT or MR imaging.

Anaesthesia and Cerebral Blood Flow

- **Intravenous induction agents:** all except for ketamine reduce $CMRO_2$, and as a result CBF falls in tandem. Autoregulation is not affected. Ketamine increases MAP, which leads to a rise in blood flow.
- **Volatile anaesthetic agents:** these uncouple CBF and $CMRO_2$. They reduce $CMRO_2$ but are associated with a rise in CBF secondary to their capacity to vasodilate the cerebral circulation and abolish autoregulation. The response to changes in $PaCO_2$ is unchanged. This action is dose-dependent but can partly be offset by the vasoconstrictor effect of hyperventilation. Autoregulation is abolished by 1.5 MAC of all the agents bar sevoflurane. This has only 30% of the vasodilatory potential of isoflurane and does not impair autoregulation. Nitrous oxide increases CBF by increasing the $CMRO_2$, while also affecting autoregulatory mechanisms.

- **Opioids:** opioids have little direct effect, but CBF will rise in response to CO_2 retention should respiratory drive be depressed.
- **Arterial pressure:** chronic hypertension shifts the autoregulatory curve to the right, while drug-induced hypotension shifts it to the left (Figure 3.10). If autoregulation is attenuated by the use of volatile anaesthetics, then CBF and ICP will rise in parallel with an increase in MAP.
- **Venous pressure:** Any of the many factors which increase venous pressure, such as position, coughing, straining against a ventilator, impeded drainage from the head and neck, volume overload or the use of IPPV and PEEP, will decrease CPP and reduce CBF.
- **Steal and inverse steal:** there will be focal areas of injured brain in which auto-regulation is lost, whereas elsewhere it is retained. Cerebral vasodilatation may further compromise these areas by diverting blood away ('cerebral steal'); conversely, the vasoconstriction associated with hyperventilation may divert blood from normal to damaged brain, where vasoconstrictor responses have been lost ('inverse steal').

Postoperative Cognitive Dysfunction and Delirium

Commentary

The three commonest disorders of mental function in the surgical and critical care patient are postoperative cognitive dysfunction (POCD), delirium and dementia. They are of course not exclusive, and the three may co-exist. Dementia is a state of chronic and progressive brain failure which is a significant risk factor for delirium and may well be exacerbated by the factors responsible for the other two conditions, but otherwise it is unlikely to feature in the oral. The risk factors for both the others are relatively straightforward, the underlying causes of POCD remain speculative, and the numerous confounding variables mean overall that the data are not robust. The oral may therefore feel rather superficial, but the information in the following account should be sufficient.

Core Information

- **Delirium:** this can most simply be defined as any acute disturbance of cognitive function. The most familiar postoperative presentation is the typical hyperactive psychomotor state with restlessness, irritability, inability to respond to requests or commands, and disconnection from the environment. Delirium, however, can also be hypoactive and may present in a patient who superficially is calm but who also has inattention and disconnection. This subdued affect can be misdiagnosed as post-operative fatigue or depression. Delirium can be precipitated by numerous causes, including metabolic derangements, acute febrile and critical illness, hypothermia, prescribed and illicit drugs, and by other factors such as sleep deprivation. It is associated with a threefold increase in postoperative mortality, increased infection rates and lengthened hospital stay.

- **Delirium in critical care:** this is believed to affect up to 60–80% of ventilated patients in intensive care. Hypoactive delirium is much more common than hyperactive, and is probably undiagnosed. (There are detailed diagnostic and assessment criteria that have been described, such as CAM-ICU, but any proper consideration of these would take up too much time in the oral.) Many of the risk factors are the same as those which predispose patients to POCD and include increasing age, pre-morbid abuse of alcohol or other substances, a history of depression or cognitive impairment, smoking (which may relate to nicotine withdrawal) and hearing or visual deficits which increase the probability of disorientation. In addition, there are the effects of the critical illness itself, such as sepsis, multi-organ dysfunction and metabolic derangement, on top of which are superimposed immobilization, prolonged sedation and sleep deprivation. It is estimated that patients in critical care 'sleep' for only 2 hours in 24, with about 5% rather than the usual 25% being rapid eye movement (REM) sleep. Critical care delirium can be reduced by substituting sedation with benzodiazepines such as dexmedetomidine, by instituting sedation breaks, by reinforcing orientation and by endeavouring to reinstitute a more normal sleep-wake cycle. None of this is easy.

- **Postoperative cognitive dysfunction (POCD):** this can also be defined as a disturbance of cognition, but it is one that is temporally related to surgery and anaesthesia. Moreover, a proper diagnosis of POCD can be made only if there has been a baseline pre-operative neuropsychiatric evaluation with which postoperative cognition can be compared. Technically this is important because POCD can be very subtle and it may affect only one or two domains of cognition, which include memory, perception, attention span, information processing, language understanding and abstract thinking.

- **Incidence:** the difficulty in accurate diagnosis means that the true incidence of POCD is hard to determine. Although postoperative mental deterioration has been recognized anecdotally for decades, it was not until the late 1990s that the phenomenon was investigated in detail. This came in the form of the International Study of Post-Operative Cognitive Dysfunction (ISPOCD-1) that was published in 1998 and which evaluated more than 1,200 patients aged over 60 years undergoing major non-cardiac surgery and, crucially, who had completed baseline pre-operative psychometric tests (*Lancet* 1998, 351: 857–61). Cognitive dysfunction was present in 25% of the patients at discharge and in 10% at 3 months. A later study using a similar trial design found an incidence of 30–40% (in 1,064 adults of all ages), which reduced to 13% at 3 months in the over-60 age group (*Anesthesiology* 2008, 108: 18–30)

- **Study problems:** even where studies have tried to match patients by age, co-morbidity and surgical complexity, there are numerous other factors which make valid conclusions difficult, if not impossible. One is the necessity of having a baseline evaluation and a standard definition of the condition; another is the requirement for uniformity of surgical and anaesthetic technique. A patient undergoing major orthopaedic surgery, for example, may be classified as having had a 'regional anaesthetic' technique, but might have been given intrathecal opioids or α-2 agonists plus intravenous benzodiazepine and target-controlled sedation with propofol.

- **Risk factors for POCD:** The pre-operative independent risk factors that studies have identified contain few surprises, other than perhaps the association of lower educational attainment with POCD. Others include increasing age (studies tend to concentrate on patients >60 years), major and prolonged surgery, high alcohol intake and/or other substance abuse and pre-existing degrees of mild cognitive impairment and co-morbidity (higher ASA grades).
- **Aetiology of POCD:** by definition POCD is due to neuronal pathology of some kind, and intuitively it would seem logical that hypotension and/or hypoxaemia could compromise cerebral perfusion and oxygen delivery. It would also seem possible that inhaled anaesthetics could contribute. There is continued interest and concern about the effects of general anaesthetics on both the developing and the ageing brain, and in vitro work has indicated, for example, that isoflurane activates enzymes (caspases) that may be instrumental in the formation of the neurofibrillary disarray that is characteristic of Alzheimer's disease. In cardiac surgery it has been suggested that the high incidence of POCD (which is quoted in some studies as being as high as 30–80% immediately post-surgery and 10–60% at 3 months) may be due to microemboli generated during cardiopulmonary bypass.

It is probable, however, that none of these factors is materially important. Somewhat surprisingly, the ISPOCD-1 study amongst others concluded that there was no correlation between episodes of perioperative hypotension or hypoxia and POCD. Long-term cognitive outcomes also appear to be unaffected whether or not patients have had general or regional anaesthesia, and so the impact of any volatile anaesthetic toxicity has to be minimal. In addition, there are several studies in cardiac anaesthesia which report that the incidence of POCD does not differ in patients who have been on cardiopulmonary bypass and those who have had off-pump surgery. With the causes described here having therefore largely been refuted, attention has now turned to the possibility that an inflammatory response may underlie the development of POCD.

- **Immunity and the role of inflammatory mediators:** animal models have demonstrated that surgical stress initiates a cascade of inflammatory mediators, starting with the release of tumour necrosis factor (TNF-α) and the production of cytokines, particularly interleukin-1β (IL-1β), which breach the blood–brain barrier and allow leucocyte migration into the hippocampus (with subsequent impairment of memory). Extrapolating these findings to humans, however, is more problematic. Biomarkers of neuronal injury such as S-100β protein (S-100β), neuron specific enolase (NSE) and interleukin-6 (IL-6) can be elevated, but although these do correlate with impaired cognitive function in some individuals, there appears to be no consistent relationship with the development of POCD. The interpretation of these findings is made yet more complicated by the fact that some inflammatory molecules are also neuroprotective (this applies, for example, to TNF-α and IL-6), and it may be other factors that could be more significant in distorting this balance. One such influence may be chronic low-grade neuroinflammation from any cause, which in effect primes the patient's system for an exaggerated inflammatory response. This would explain the greater propensity for the development of POCD in some of the identified higher risk groups. Overall, there seems to be tentative consensus that an inflammatory response probably does underlie some of these postoperative neurological manifestations.

- **Cerebral oxygen desaturation:** near infrared spectroscopy has demonstrated that 'silent' episodes of cortical oxygen desaturation can occur even while haemodynamic indices show little alteration and peripheral oxygen saturation remains unchanged. Should cerebral oxygen monitoring become routine then any causal link between silent hypoxia and POCD may become much clearer, but in the meantime it must remain speculative.

- **Management of POCD:** it may be that in due course pro-inflammatory modulators could have a role in attenuating POCD, assuming that the condition is dynamic and not due to a single temporal event. Until the aetiology of the condition has been better elaborated, its management is supportive, with the treatment of any obvious acute medical precipitants, including uncontrolled pain, and the avoidance of any interventions which might make it worse. This would usually include sedative or neuroleptic drugs. If a patient is acutely agitated (which makes delirium a more likely diagnosis), then haloperidol is the most commonly used agent. (It is a dopamine D_2-receptor antagonist with a prolonged half-life of 20–36 hours. The intravenous dose is 0.5–1.0 mg repeated every 15 minutes and titrated against response).

Intraocular Pressure

Commentary

Successful intraocular surgery requires a still, soft and quiet eye. Attention to the following principles should allow you to satisfy the examiners that you can provide this safely. However, remember that theory is not always mirrored by practice. Cataract surgeons will operate uncomplainingly on a patient breathing spontaneously through a laryngeal mask airway whose high end–tidal CO_2 should in theory raise intraocular pressure (IOP) to the point at which surgery is impossible. Your clinical answers can reflect this reality.

Core Information

Definition and Prime Determinants of Intraocular Pressure

- **Definition:** IOP is the pressure exerted by the contents of the globe on the scleral envelope that encloses them. Normal pressure is quoted as 16 ± 5 mmHg.
- **Choroidal blood volume:** the choroid is a thin, but dense, capillary plexus which covers most of the posterior chamber of the globe. It also contains small arteries and veins. It has a high baseline blood flow which is maintained over a wide range of pressures. Whether the choroidal vessels autoregulate has been disputed, but evidence suggests that there is some degree of myogenic and vasomotor autoregulation of the choroidal circulation. Choroidal blood volume does rise in response to elevations of venous pressure and is also sensitive to increases in $PaCO_2$ and to

hypoxia. A P_aCO_2 of 1.0 kPa is associated with a rise in choroidal blood flow of approximately 10%. Hypocarbia reduces CBV and also inhibits carbonic anhydrase.

- **Aqueous humour:** the production and drainage of aqueous humour are in dynamic equilibrium. Aqueous is produced under the influence of carbonic anhydrase, and is secreted via the ciliary processes in the posterior chamber, supplying oxygen and glucose to the cornea and lens, which are avascular. A smaller proportion (around 20%) is formed via plasma ultrafiltration. It circulates freely through into the anterior chamber before draining through spaces in the trabecular meshwork (the spaces of Fontana) to the canal of Schlemm. This drainage can be affected by increases in venous pressure or by any decrease in the area of the trabecular spaces. This is one of the mechanisms underlying chronic open-angle glaucoma. Relaxation of the iris can narrow the iridocorneal angle and impair drainage. In subjects in whom this angle is already narrow, the use of mydriatics can precipitate acute ('narrow-angle') glaucoma (see Figure 2.12). Drainage can be restored by constricting the pupil with miotic drugs such as pilocarpine and carbachol.

- **Central venous pressure:** this rises acutely (to as much as 40 mmHg) with coughing, straining, retching and the Valsalva manoeuvre. Other precipitants include head-down posture, obstruction to venous drainage from the head and neck, hypervolaemia, breathing against a ventilator and the use of IPPV and PEEP. This increase in pressure is paralleled by a similar rise in IOP with a reduction in aqueous drainage and an increase in choroidal blood volume.

- **Extrinsic compression:** IOP rises as a result of direct extrinsic pressure on the globe, caused, for example, by retrobulbar haemorrhage or by undue pressure on the eye when a patient is anaesthetized in the prone position.

- **Extraocular muscle tone:** any increase (such as is caused by a depolarizing muscle relaxant) is reflected in a rise in IOP; otherwise this is not a significant component.

- **Measurement of IOP:** the most complex (and accurate) method is Goldmann applanation tonometry, which measures the force that is required to deform (i.e. flatten) the cornea, but which requires topical anaesthesia, fluorescein dye and the use of a slit lamp. There is a simpler contact device (the Perkins applanation tonometer which is in effect a portable version of the Goldmann instrument). Probably more widely used (certainly by optometrists) are non-contact tonometers which direct a pulse of air against the cornea. Successful deformation is signaled by a reflected light beam and the instrument computes the IOP from the delivered force and the surface area.

Supplementary Information and Clinical Considerations

Anaesthetic Effects on Intraocular Pressure

- **Laryngoscopy and tracheal intubation:** if measures are not taken to obtund the sympathetic responses to laryngoscopy, the IOP can rise by 20 mmHg or more.

- **Drugs used in anaesthesia:** all intravenous anaesthetic agents except ketamine will reduce IOP, as will inhalational agents, assuming that the $PaCO_2$ is not allowed to rise. This effect is thought to be related to a direct central action rather than one secondary to hypotension. Etomidate can cause myoclonus and so should probably be avoided. Involuntary extraocular muscle contraction associated with suxamethonium transiently increases IOP by around 10 mmHg. In addition, the fine muscle intraocular muscle fibres demonstrate tonic contraction which lasts as long as the neuromuscular block. (The rise in IOP is not purely mechanical; an increase is seen even if the four recti muscles have been sectioned.)

- **Nitrous oxide:** N_2O will diffuse into gas-filled spaces, and this will include the eye if the vitreous has been replaced by gases such as sulphur hexafluoride (SF_6) or (di) carbon octafluoride (C_2F_8), which may take up to 70 days to resorb. N_2O is more than 100 times more diffusible than SF_6 and enters the vitreal cavity, thus increasing gas volume and IOP.

- **The open eye:** when the eye is open (either surgically or due to trauma) the IOP is lower than normal, and so the transluminal pressure on the choroidal vessels is greater. This means that any sudden increase in pressure in the choroidal circulation may be associated by prolapse of intraocular structures such as the iris and the lens, or by expulsive haemorrhage with almost certain loss of vision. Anaesthetic techniques should be such as to minimize this risk.

- **Drugs used to lower IOP:** these work mainly by reducing aqueous humour formation and include topical β-adrenoceptor blockers such as timolol, which inhibits adenylate cyclate-mediated production of aqueous, and systemic carbonic anhydrase inhibitors such as acetazolamide. Dorzolamide and brinzolamide are also sulphonamide derivative carbonic anhydrase inhibitors, but both can be used topically. Mannitol will reduce IOP by osmotic dehydration of the vitreous in the posterior chamber.

- **Pre-existing glaucoma:** patients with chronically raised intraocular pressures, such as those with narrow angle glaucoma, are less able to attenuate the effects of acute rises in IOP by increasing the rate of aqueous humour drainage, and in these subjects the acute IOP rise can be even more significant.

The Penetrating Eye Injury

- Anaesthesia for a patient with a penetrating eye injury involves balancing the risks of pulmonary aspiration of gastric contents against the risks of causing a rise in IOP that may further threaten sight. (The possibility of failed intubation is another consideration.) Assuming that the procedure is a surgical emergency and that the patient is not fasted, there are two main problems: the first is the use of suxamethonium and the second is the rise in IOP that may accompany laryngoscopy and tracheal intubation.

  — **Suxamethonium:** this causes a transient increase in IOP and in theory therefore should be avoided. In practice, there are no published reports of further eye damage associated with its use under these circumstances. However, most anaesthetists would prefer an alternative for rapid sequence induction, and high-dose rocuronium (0.9–1.0 mg kg^{-1}) will provide satisfactory conditions for intubation within 60 seconds.

  — **Laryngoscopy:** the sympathetic response to laryngoscopy also increases IOP (as noted earlier). Many different methods have been described for attenuating this pressor response, and if you try to embark on a detailed account of these then the examiner will almost certainly move you on. You may be asked, however, to give one or two examples. The long list of possible techniques includes pre-treatment with a β-adrenoceptor blocker, high-dose intravenous induction agent, nebulized lidocaine or intravenous lidocaine (2 mg kg^{-1}), topical local anaesthetic to the hypopharynx, intravenous opioid (such as alfentanil 20–40 μg kg^{-1} or remifentanil 1 μg kg^{-1}) and clonidine (5 μg kg^{-1}).

The Neuromuscular Junction

Commentary

If you are asked about the neuromuscular junction, it is almost inevitable that the oral will include questions about neuromuscular blockers and the assessment of neuromuscular blockade. If, however, you are asked about either of the two latter topics you may not be required to discuss the neuromuscular junction in any detail. It is for this reason that the following account is somewhat simplified. The subject may be introduced by a discussion about disorders affecting neuromuscular transmission.

Core Information

Anatomy of the Neuromuscular Junction

- ACh is formed in the motor nerve terminal (by the acetylation of choline, catalyzed by choline-O-acetyltransferase). Much of the synthesized ACh is stored in vesicles containing around 10,000 molecules and which lie just within the axonal prejunctional membrane.
- ACh release is triggered by the motor nerve action potential. In response to depolarization, voltage-gated channels permit an inward flux of calcium which stimulates release into the junctional gap. (This itself is complex, involving the activation of a number of improbably named proteins which facilitate the process: synaptotagmin, syntaxins, synaptophysin and synaptobrevin. Synaptobrevin is of passing interest because it is inhibited by botulinum toxin, which thereby prevents ACh release and muscle contraction.)
- Prejunctional nicotinic cholinergic receptors modulate further ACh mobilization and release via a positive feedback mechanism.
- ACh acts at the postjunctional nicotinic receptor, whose structure has been fully identified. It consists of five glycoprotein subunits characterized as α (2), β, δ and ε which form a central ionophore (ion channel). Binding of one molecule of ACh to one of the two α units facilitates the binding of a second, during which the receptor undergoes an evanescent conformational change and the ionophore opens. A net influx of sodium ions then depolarizes the muscle cell membrane.
- The ACh in the cleft will interact with an α unit only once before being broken down within 100 μsec by the acetylcholinesterase in the junctional folds of the muscle membrane.

Supplementary Information

Neuromuscular blocking agents (for greater detail, see under 'Neuromuscular Blocking Drugs (and Sugammadex) in Chapter 4).

- **Structures:** all are quaternary amines, whose potency is increased if the molecule contains two quaternary ammonium radicals. (Pancuronium is bisquaternary, whereas vecuronium is monoquaternary.)
- **Depolarizing block:** suxamethonium is the only therapeutic depolarizing neuromuscular blocker, but agonists at nicotinic cholinergic receptors can have a similar effect. Anticholinesterases given in the absence of non-depolarizing block, for example, may themselves cause blockade. Following depolarization of the muscle membrane, suxamethonium remains bound to the receptor for some minutes, during which time muscle action potentials are prevented.
- **Phase II block:** this is a postjunctional non-depolarizing ion channel block, which accompanies the prolonged action or accumulation of suxamethonium. The block is also characterized by impairment of prejunctional ACh release. This probably explains why anticholinesterases may reverse the block, although the advice to do so is not universal.
- **Non-depolarizing block:** non-depolarizing blockers are competitive inhibitors of ACh at the postjunctional nicotinic receptors. They bind to one or both of the α units to prevent ACh access, but they induce no conformational change in the receptor. Receptor occupancy needs to be at least 80%, depending on the surgery that is planned, and it is important to recognize that the sensitivity of muscle groups is very different. The pattern appears to be the same across all mammalian species such that the muscles of facial expression, including the ocular muscles, and the muscles of the distal limb (including the tail) are much more sensitive than the diaphragm. Thus, only 20% receptor blockade is sufficient to paralyze the tibialis anterior muscle, whereas the diaphragm requires 90%.

Clinical Considerations

Disorders of Neuromuscular Function

This may include myasthenia gravis and related diseases. These are more common in medical exams than in clinical practice.

- **Myasthenia gravis:** this is an autoimmune disease in which antibodies are formed to the postjunctional acetylcholine (ACh) receptor. (This is a simplification but will suffice for this exam.) The resulting decrease in the population of effective receptors means that muscles fatigue rapidly on repetitive exertion. Clinically, this can be demonstrated by asking a patient to chew gum; the muscles of mastication do not fatigue in normal individuals. Electromyographic stimulation of myasthenic patients will reveal fade. The diagnosis can be supported by testing with edrophonium, and first-line treatment is with another anticholinesterase, pyridostigmine (see under 'Anticholinesterases' in Chapter 4).
- **Anaesthetic considerations:** patients clinically may be weak, and postoperative ventilatory support may be required in as many as 30% of subjects. Myasthenic

patients demonstrate some resistance to depolarizing neuromuscular blockers, but a dose of suxamethonium 2 mg kg^{-1} will allow good conditions for intubation. Acute sensitivity to the effects of non-depolarizing blockers means that initial doses should be around one-tenth of normal. In practice, combinations of drugs such as propofol and remifentanil mean that muscle relaxants can usually be avoided.

- **Crises:** a **myasthenic** crisis, which can be precipitated by various physical and emotional stresses or which can be spontaneous, is manifest by an exacerbation of symptoms severe enough to cause respiratory failure. A **cholinergic** crisis is precipitated by an overdose of anticholinesterase. In addition to stimulating muscarinic receptors, the excess ACh acts as a neuromuscular blocker at the diminished number of receptors, thereby leading to muscle weakness and respiratory compromise. Edrophonium, which is a short-acting anticholinesterase with effects which last for about 5 minutes, will transiently improve a myasthenic, and transiently worsen a cholinergic crisis.

- **Eaton–Lambert syndrome:** in around two-thirds of cases this condition is associated with malignancy, classically with bronchogenic carcinoma. It appears to reduce the number of pre-synaptic quanta of ACh that are released (possibly by antibodies to voltage-gated calcium channels and to the associated protein synaptotagmin), but the post-synaptic membrane sensitivity is normal. Unlike myasthenia gravis, the muscle weakness improves with activity; however, these patients are acutely sensitive to the effects both of depolarizing and non-depolarizing muscle relaxants.

Postoperative Nausea and Vomiting

Commentary

Postoperative nausea and vomiting (PONV) is a common problem, and this is a standard question which can follow a predictable course. It combines physiology and pharmacology, and you will be expected to demonstrate that you understand the underlying physiological principles and that you can recognize patients who are at risk. You may also be asked about treatment, although this in itself is a large subject (see under 'Drugs Used in the Treatment of Nausea and Vomiting' in Chapter 4). If the examiner wants to cover all three areas, then time constraints mean that the questioning will be relatively superficial, but you may be examined in more depth on one or other aspects of the topic.

Core Information

Neural Pathways Which Mediate Nausea and Vomiting

- Nausea and vomiting are reflexes, with afferent and efferent pathways which are mediated by a number of anatomically ill-defined structures in the medulla oblongata of the brain stem. These are the vomiting centre, the chemoreceptor trigger zone and the nucleus tractus solitarius. The vomiting centre acts as a central integrator.

- **Vomiting centre (VC):** this receives afferents from a large number of sources, including the cerebral cortex, the viscera and the chemoreceptor trigger zone (CTZ). Its receptors are primarily cholinergic (muscarinic M_3), but it also contains some histaminic (H_1) receptors.
  - **Cortical afferents:** nausea and vomiting may be provoked by pain, fear and anxiety, as well as by association and by other psychological factors. It may also be precipitated by visual and olfactory stimuli. Cortical stimulation of the vomiting centre may also result from organic disturbance such as raised or lowered ICP, hypoxia (of which nausea is a sensitive early sign) and the vascular derangement that accompanies migraine.
  - **Visceral afferents:** the vomiting centre responds to stimuli such as peritoneal irritation, as well as a variety of visceral disorders, including inflammation, distension and ischaemia. Obvious causes include intestinal obstruction or perforation, gastric stasis and gastric irritation. Cardiac pain is also a potent stimulus to vomiting.
  - **CTZ afferents:** see following.
- **Chemoreceptor trigger zone (CTZ):** this is also located in the medulla, in the area postrema on the floor of the fourth ventricle. It lies outside the blood–brain barrier and responds both to afferents from various sources as well as to emetogenic substances in blood and cerebrospinal fluid. Its receptors are primarily dopaminergic (D_2) and serotoninergic (5-HT_3).
  - **Gastrointestinal and vagal afferents:** enterochromaffin cells in the gut produce 5-HT and vagal input is mediated by 5-HT_3 receptors.
  - **Vestibular afferents:** inputs are received from the vestibular apparatus via the cerebellum. Its receptors are cholinergic (muscarinic M_3) and histaminic (H_1).
  - **Drug effects:** numerous drugs exert a direct action on the CTZ. These include opioids (which also sensitize the vestibular apparatus to motion), cytotoxic drugs, cardiac glycosides, volatile anaesthetic agents and drugs with sympathomimetic effects.
- **Nucleus tractus solitarius (NTS):** this is also found in the area postrema in the lower pons and receives afferents from the CTZ (dopamine D_2 receptors), from the vagus, from the vestibular apparatus and from the limbic system. It precipitates vomiting by stimulation of several nuclei: the dorsal motor nucleus of the vagus, the nucleus ambiguous, the ventral respiratory nuclei and the rostral nucleus.

Supplementary Information and Clinical Considerations

There are groups of patients who are at particular risk of postoperative nausea and vomiting (PONV). (This information is duplicated under ['Drugs Used in the Treatment of Nausea and Vomiting' in Chapter 4] but is reproduced here for convenience).

- **Factors related to patients:** in terms of odds ratio, female gender is the most reliable predictive factor (OR 3). Although there are some studies that have suggested that PONV is decreased in the luteal phase of menstruation (during the second half of the cycle), the data are inconsistent and current consensus is that the phase of the menstrual cycle has no influence. A positive history of PONV is another predictive factor, which doubles its likelihood (OR 2), as does a history of motion sickness, and if ambulation after surgery is premature. Smoking appears to exert a protective effect with an odds ratio of 2 (in theory acting as a potent inducer of the cytochrome P450 system); so, to a lesser extent, does regular alcohol consumption. PONV is increased by preoperative anxiety. Body habitus has no impact on the incidence of PONV, and there is no association with obesity, as formerly was believed. There is an inverse relationship with increasing age in adults.

- **Factors related to surgery:** intra-abdominal, intracranial, middle ear and squint surgery have all been associated with a higher incidence of PONV, as have laparoscopic and gynaecological procedures. Multivariate analysis in large trials, however, suggests that there is no direct causation and that these operations (with the exception of squint surgery in children) do not represent independent risk factors for PONV. Empirical experience across this range of surgical procedures nonetheless suggests that the need for rescue antiemetic therapy does appear to be greater than for some others. Moderate to severe postoperative pain can also be a potent precipitant.
- **Factors related to anaesthesia:** volatile anaesthetics at least double the incidence of PONV, and as would be expected the risk is dose- and duration-dependent. It is believed that the emetic potential of volatiles (which is similar for all the halogenated hydrocarbons) is related to a decrease in serum concentrations of anandamide. (The word 'ananda' means 'bliss' in Sanskrit, and anandamide has been described somewhat ludicrously as 'the molecule of extreme pleasure'.) More prosaically it is a neurotransmitter with a wide spectrum of activity, including the suppression of emesis, and whose effects are mediated via CB_1 and CB_2 cannabinoid receptors. The increased risk of PONV of which nitrous oxide is frequently accused is actually modest (OR 1.4) and the ENIGMA II trial (Myles *et al.* Lancet 2014, 384: 1446–54) showed that this risk is nullified with concomitant anti-emetic therapy. Opioids increase the risk in a dose-dependent fashion. Drugs with sympathomimetic actions are also associated with increased risk. Hypoxaemia is a stimulus to vomiting.
- **Factors related to disease:** the list of potential causes is long and includes intestinal obstruction, hypoglycaemia, hypoxia, uraemia and hypotension.
- **Scoring systems:** these include the Apfel score, which estimates the likelihood of PONV according to the number of predisposing factors (see under 'Scoring Systems' in Chapter 5).

Management of PONV

- **Overall:** this includes prevention by avoidance of emetic drugs (this need not include nitrous oxide, as long as an anti-emetic is given), by the use of total intravenous anaesthesia (TIVA), by vigorous hydration and (contentiously) by high-inspired oxygen concentrations. There are also complementary techniques such as acupressure on the P_6 acupuncture point at the wrist.
- **Drug treatment:** the pharmacology is considered in detail under 'Drugs Used in the Treatment of Nausea and Vomiting' in Chapter 4. A multimodal approach uses combinations of H_1-antagonists (phenothiazines such as prochlorperazine), anticholinergic M_3-antagonists (atropine, glycopyrrolate), anti-dopaminergic D_2-antagonists (domperidone, metoclopramide, haloperidol, droperidol), 5-HT_3 antagonists (ondansetron, granisetron) and NK_1-antagonists (aprepitant,

fosaprepitant). This is necessary because the efficacy of single agents is disappointing, and the numbers needed to treat (NNT) are relatively high. The NNT for ondansetron, for example, is quoted as between 5 and 6. Other drugs with anti-emetic effects include corticosteroids, cannabinoids and propofol.

Obesity

Commentary

This topic is a perennial favourite, possibly because the nation is getter fatter, with at least 20% of adults now being classified as obese. There is potentially much to cover in the time available, but, equally, this is a subject on which it is quite difficult to fail. There is a lot of information to convey, but most of the data are relatively soft, and in reality there is little in the subject for the examiner to use as a discriminator. You will nonetheless be expected to address those areas where safety is crucial: the risk of regurgitation and aspiration, perioperative respiratory problems and prophylaxis against venous thromboembolism.

Core Information

- **Classification:** the most widely used method of classifying obesity is the body mass index (BMI), which is determined by the weight (kg) divided by the square of the height (m^2). A BMI of 18–25 kg m^{-2} is normal, 26–30 is overweight, 31–35 is obese, and more than 35 is morbidly obese. (Some authorities use a figure of 40 to define morbid obesity.) There are further categories of 'super obesity' (patients with a BMI of 50–60) and 'super-super obesity'. At this point the terminology risks becoming faintly ridiculous, but this latter category defines any patient with a BMI of more than 60. These divisions are necessarily arbitrary and need more nuanced interpretation, not only in heavily muscled individuals in whom the measurement is obviously misleading, but also in some ethnic groups. NICE, in their 2015 guidelines recommend the use of lower thresholds (BMI 23 low risk; BMI 27.5 high risk) to trigger intervention in black African, African-Caribbean, South Asian and Chinese. These ethnicities have a higher tendency to central abdominal obesity and type 2 diabetes.
- **Ideal weight:** there are simple empirical formulae to approximate a patient's 'ideal' weight. One such estimates the optimum weight by subtracting from the height in centimetres 105 (for women) and 100 (for men).
- **Neurohumoral mechanisms underlying obesity:** In addition to the array of social, psychological and cultural factors that are associated with food and eating, there are highly complex regulatory neurohumoral mechanisms that are processed in the hypothalamus. These control appetite and satiety, and substances so far identified include, leptin, ghrelin, adiponectin, peptide YY$_{3-36}$ and insulin. Leptin is produced by adipocytes and signals satiety. Obese subjects predictably have high plasma leptin concentrations secondary to their increased adipocyte mass, but they can have reduced leptin sensitivity. Ghrelin is an orexigenic peptide that is released in the stomach and inhibited by gastric distension. YY$_{3-36}$ has the same effect on stimulating appetite but is

released in the small bowel. As a simplification, there are anorectic and orexigenic neurohumoral factors which regulate energy balance. In obese individuals, the balance between the two systems is disrupted. It is probable that there is a genetic component.

- **Abdominal obesity:** there has been more interest recently in abdominal obesity as a predictor of cardiovascular disease, hypertension and diabetes. Visceral fat appears to provoke chronic low-grade inflammation that may trigger both insulin resistance and the hypertension, atherosclerosis and diabetes mellitus that characterize the metabolic syndrome. So-called perivascular adipose tissue is not inert: it produces factors that influence vascular tone and may contribute to cardiovascular morbidity. In patients with a BMI of 25 or less the waist circumference should not exceed 102 cm (40 in) in men and 88 cm (34.5 in) in women. Waist to hip ratios are also used and ideally should not exceed 0.9 in men and 0.85 in women.
- **Mortality:** the morbidly obese individual has only a 1 in 7 chance of reaching a normal life expectancy, and their mortality for all forms of surgery averages twice that of the non-obese population. Problems affect most systems.
- **Cardiovascular changes:** hypertension is found in 50–60% of subjects, and is severe in 5–10%. There is increased blood volume, with increased cardiac work. Although adipose tissue is relatively avascular, it has been calculated that each additional 1 kg of fat contains 0.6 km of blood vessels. There is an increased incidence of coronary artery disease and cardiomyopathy. The risk of deep venous thrombosis and pulmonary embolus doubles. Obese patients have less water per unit of body weight, they tolerate hypovolaemia badly and they may also compensate poorly for changes of position during anaesthesia.
- **Respiratory problems:** the increased adipose tissue of the neck and upper chest may make bag-valve-mask ventilation difficult. It does not of itself increase problems with tracheal intubation. There are a number of studies of patient undergoing bariatric surgery that demonstrate there is no greater incidence of Cormack and Lehane grade 3 and 4 views in the morbidly obese than in controls of normal body habitus. The work of breathing is increased because of the mass effect of chest weight, which reduces chest wall compliance. Spontaneous respiration is restricted, and the large abdominal mass can cause diaphragmatic splinting. There is a reduction in the FRC together with an increase in closing volume. Other lung volumes decrease (total lung capacity, inspiratory capacity and expiratory reserve volume), and there is also an increase in pulmonary 'shunting' with mild hypercapnia and perioperative hypoxia. Equilibration with inhaled volatile anaesthetic agents may be slow. Some 5% of obese subjects have obstructive sleep apnoea (see under 'Control of Breathing'). Seriously obese patients may hypoventilate and manifest the 'Pickwickian syndrome', which consists of obesity, somnolence, polycythaemia, pulmonary hypertension and right heart failure. (This is not named after Mr Pickwick in *The Pickwick Papers* by Dickens, but after the fat boy, Joe.) All these factors put the morbidly obese at risk of postoperative respiratory failure, particularly with a combination of obstructive sleep apnoea and opioid analgesia.
- **Gastrointestinal system changes:** obesity predisposes to hiatus hernia, gastro-oesophageal reflux with potential pulmonary aspiration of gastric contents, and cholelithiasis. Fatty change in the liver is also common, progressing in extreme cases to cirrhosis.

- **Endocrine problems:** there is a fivefold increase in the likelihood of developing diabetes mellitus. There is an increase in plasma insulin levels which is linked to high calorie intake, but binding to cell receptors decreases (this is insulin resistance).

Clinical Considerations

- **Bariatric surgery:** ('baro-' comes from the Greek for 'weight'). The financial costs of obesity are such that bariatric surgery is becoming more common in the NHS. There is good evidence that it can reverse some of the complications such as hypertension and diabetes mellitus. Following roux-en-Y gastric bypass surgery, for example, 60% of patients with type 2 diabetes will revert to normal glycaemic status. Procedures are usually laparoscopic and include gastric banding, in which an adjustable band encircles the upper part of the stomach to create a small pouch; surgical gastroplasty, which reduces the effective size of the stomach; sleeve gastrectomy which leaves a small residual stomach; gastric bypass surgery, which causes weight loss by malabsorption; duodenal switch surgery; and intragastric balloon insertion. NICE has drawn up a list of criteria for eligibility for weight reduction surgery. Specifically their recommendations state that surgery is an option if all of the following criteria are fulfilled: BMI >40 or >35 with co-morbidity that may improve with weight loss (such as hypertension and diabetes), all appropriate non-surgical methods have been tried without success, the individual is receiving intensive management in a Tier 3 (weight assessment and management) service, they are fit for anaesthesia and surgery and they commit to long-term follow-up. In patients with BMI greater than 50 kg m^{-2}, bariatric surgery 'is the option of choice, instead of lifestyle interventions or drug treatment . . . when other interventions have not been effective'.
- **Miscellaneous physical and technical problems:** these patients are difficult to move, lift and nurse. Venepuncture is challenging, and all practical procedures, including local and regional anaesthetic blocks, can be technically demanding. The accurate estimation of drug dosage can be problematic, although as a general guide lean body mass does not exceed 70 kg in women and 90 kg in men. Non-invasive arterial pressure monitoring may be inaccurate. Surgeons as well as anaesthetists face technical problems, and the duration of surgery is frequently prolonged.
- **Summary of anaesthetic problems:** potentially difficult airway management, higher risk of regurgitation of gastric contents, problematic determination of drug dosage (should titrate against lean body mass rather than total body weight), difficulty in maintaining perioperative oxygenation, increase in difficulty of all practical procedures; problems with manual handling, wide range of potential co-morbidities, risk of postoperative respiratory failure and high risk of venous thromboembolism.

The Physiology of Ageing

Commentary

This subject, like obesity, is another question which is quite difficult to fail. In this topic also there is a lot of information that can be conveyed, but much of it is predictable and again there may be little in the subject for the examiner to use as a discriminator. It will help if you can quote some numerical data; it may appear otherwise that you are simply recounting the obvious fact that every physiological variable deteriorates. An alternative strategy is to make clear that you are focusing your answer on the areas of higher anaesthetic priority.

Core Information

Physiological Changes with Increasing Age

- **General points:** progressive and global decline in physiological function is measurable after about the fourth decade of life, and more rapid deterioration occurs when patients reach their seventies.
- **CNS:** there is progressive structural change with cerebral atrophy (the weight of the brain decreases by more than 10%), a decrease in neurotransmitter concentrations, diminished cerebral blood flow and a fall in oxygen consumption. MAC decreases with age both for general and for local anaesthesia. It declines by about 5% per decade after the age of 40 years, and if this curve is extrapolated, it reaches zero at the age of 137. Basal metabolic rate is said to decline by 1% per year after the age of 30 years. There may be some increase in receptor sensitivity, for example to benzodiazepines, while the effect of opioids may be enhanced because of decreased protein binding.
- **Autonomic nervous system:** there is a gradual functional decline as evinced by orthostatic hypotension owing to impairment of baroreceptor function. This occurs in 25% of subjects older than 65 years. Temperature control is impaired, and heat generation is reduced by the decline in BMR. The frail and elderly may also have less subcutaneous fat for insulation. The autonomic changes have been described as 'physiological beta blockade'.
- **Cardiovascular system:** there is gradual functional decline; cardiac output decreases (by 20% at age 60), with decreases in heart rate, stroke volume and myocardial contractility. A decline in receptor numbers means that there is decreased sensitivity to inotropes. The risk of pulmonary thromboembolism is increased, both because of age itself, and because of the nature of the surgery for which elderly patients may present, particularly orthopaedic fractures and intra-abdominal procedures. Anaemia is common and a preoperative haematocrit of less than 24% is associated with worse outcomes.
- **Respiratory system:** there is a progressive decline with age. The closing volume matches functional residual capacity (FRC) in the upright position at around the age of 65 years but encroaches on FRC by age 44 if supine. Increased V/Q mismatch leads to a widening of the alveolar–arterial oxygen gradient (A–aDO$_2$), there is decreased sensitivity to hypoxia and hypercapnia, and there is a decrease in lung compliance.
- **The airway:** elderly patients are more likely to be edentulous, with mandibles that are osteoporotic. Oropharyngeal muscle tone is lax, and cervical spondylosis and osteoarthritis are common problems.
- **Gastrointestinal system:** elderly subjects have slower gastric emptying, parietal cell function is impaired and hiatus hernia and gastro-oesophageal reflux are more common.

- **Renal system:** renal blood flow diminishes and glomerular filtration rate is decreased by 30–45% in the elderly. Renal concentrating function is diminished, fluid handling is impaired and preoperative dehydration is more likely.
- **Drugs:** hepatic and renal function decline with a decrease in the clearance of drugs, protein binding is reduced and receptor sensitivity alters. It is increased for CNS depressants, but decreased for inotropes and for β-adrenoceptor blockers. The response to α-agonists is similar to that seen in younger patients.

Clinical Considerations

Factors of Particular Relevance to Anaesthesia

- **Coexisting disease is common:** the list is potentially very long and includes ischaemic heart disease, hypertension, chronic airways disease, cerebrovascular disease, osteoarthritis, diabetes mellitus, dementia (which has an incidence of 20% in those aged over 80 years), Parkinson's Disease, physical frailty, malnutrition, polypharmacy and sensory impairment.
- **Surgical mortality is high:** about 15% of the population of the UK is aged over 65, and the population is continuing to age. This is a group in whom surgery is more common, and in whom mortality rates are higher. In the 1999 National Confidential Enquiry into Perioperative Deaths (NCEPOD) report, which looked at the extremes of age, 75% of reported deaths were more than 70 years, and the overall mortality rate was 10%.
- **Regional anaesthesia:** given the neurological and physiological impairments seen with increasing age, regional and neuraxial techniques are an appropriate alternative, assuming that the advantages are not negated by excessive sedation. Hypotension is a potential problem with neuraxial blocks and is associated with a poorer outcome in surgery such as fixation of femoral neck fracture. Anaesthetists' thresholds for management of low pressure do vary, but it is prudent not to let the intraoperative mean arterial pressure fall by more than 20% of baseline. Fluid administration as a means of countering hypotension is rarely effective without concurrent administration of a vasopressor and risks circulatory overload. Apart from replacement for surgical losses, it is recommended that fluid infusion should not usually exceed 8–10 ml kg^{-1}.
- **Summary of anaesthetic considerations:** there is a high probability of coexisting disease, an increased regurgitation risk (but not enough to mandate rapid sequence induction), an increased sensitivity to effects of hypnotic and opiate drugs, greater difficulty in maintaining perioperative oxygenation, skin fragility and high susceptibility to pressure effects of prolonged immobility, reduced temperature control, an increased likelihood of POCD (see following) and thromboembolic events.
- **Postoperative cognitive dysfunction (POCD):** this describes a spectrum of deficits which include short-term memory lapses, acute disorientation and confusion, longer-term personality changes and difficulties with tasks requiring organization of thought. Some form of POCD occurs in about 25% of the elderly surgical population. Intuitively, it would be easy to attribute this to alterations in cerebral perfusion and oxygenation associated with anaesthesia and surgery, but there is no

evidence to support this contention. POCD is almost certainly multifactorial. For more details see under 'Postoperative Cognitive Dysfunction and Delirium'.

The 'Stress Response' to Surgery

Commentary

The stress response to injury is a subject of continued, although perhaps diminishing, interest to anaesthetists, if not to examiners. There is no consensus about the desirability of abolishing it, but considerable research effort has been expended into studying the attenuating effects of general and regional anaesthesia. Much remains speculative and so the subject eludes focus. You will be able to give the impression of knowing sufficient information about the topic if you have grasped the overall picture and can reproduce some of the key concepts, and it should not be difficult to provide a broad overview.

Core Information

- The 'stress response' is the term used to describe the widespread metabolic and hormonal changes which occur in response to trauma, including surgical trauma. It is a complex neuroendocrine response whose net effect is to increase catabolism and release endogenous fuel stores while conserving body fluids. In evolutionary terms, it is a natural mechanism which increases an injured animal's chances of survival. In the context of modern surgery, however, it is viewed as detrimental.
- The degree of catabolism is related to the severity of the surgical insult or traumatic tissue injury. In practice, the plasma concentrations of most substances increase, and it is unlikely that the examiner will ask you specifically about a single hormone. If this does happen, and you do not immediately know the answer, then try to answer it from first principles. Do not be concerned if your reply does not seem that logical; it is not clear, for example, why prolactin concentrations should increase while thyroid hormone should rise little, if at all.

Endocrine Response

- **Autonomic nervous system – sympathoadrenal response:** this is mediated via the hypothalamus with the stimulation of adrenal medullary catecholamines. There is also increased presynaptic noradrenaline release. This leads to cardiovascular stimulation with tachycardia and peripheral vasoconstriction. The renin–angiotensin system stimulates aldosterone release, leading to sodium and water retention.
- **Hypothalamic–pituitary–adrenal (HPA) axis:** hypothalamic releasing factors respond to major surgical trauma by stimulating the anterior pituitary. This in turn leads to increases in adrenocorticotrophic hormone (ACTH) which stimulates adrenal glucocorticoid release as well as somatotrophin (growth hormone). This enhances protein synthesis and inhibits breakdown, stimulates lipolysis and antagonizes insulin. Prolactin release is also evident, although its purpose is not obvious. The other anterior pituitary hormones, including thyroid hormone, change little.

The posterior pituitary produces increased amounts of arginine vasopressin (antidiuretic hormone, ADH) which acts on V_2 receptors in the kidney to increase water reabsorption.

- **Cortisol:** release from the adrenal cortex after stimulation by ACTH may increase fourfold, and this leads to intense catabolism in which there is protein breakdown, increased gluconeogenesis and lipolysis, with inhibition of glucose utilization. Cortisol is anti-inflammatory; it inhibits leucocyte migration into damaged areas and inhibits synthesis of various inflammatory mediators, including prostaglandins. It is also gluconeogenic, and abnormally high blood glucose levels impair wound healing and increase the risk of infection. In health, there is negative feedback control of ACTH release which ceases to function after major trauma.
- **Insulin:** this is the major anabolic hormone of which there is a relative perioperative deficiency. Its effects are unable to match the catabolic response. There is also evidence of increased insulin resistance. Hyperglycaemia occurs secondary to high cortisol levels, to lipolysis and to the anti-insulin action of growth hormone.
- **Inflammatory response:** after major tissue trauma, a number of cytokines are released (including IL-1, IL-6, TNF-α and interferons). IL-6 is the cytokine mainly responsible for the development of the systemic 'acute phase response'.

Modification of the Response by Anaesthesia

- Catabolism provides endogenous fuel from carbohydrate, fatty acids and amino acids, with the loss of body nitrogen. The process is accompanied by sodium and water retention. In the elderly surgical population with patients with significant co-morbidity, the stress response may have obvious adverse effects. Whether or not anaesthetists robustly should be trying to ablate the response, however, remains contentious.
- **Opioids:** these suppress hypothalamic and pituitary secretion, and high-dose opioids (for example, morphine in a dose of 4 mg kg^{-1} or fentanyl in a dose of 100 μg kg^{-1}) may attenuate the response substantially, but this is at the cost of profound sedation and respiratory depression. The effect does not endure.
- **Etomidate:** this drug is an effective inhibitor of cortisol and aldosterone synthesis via its inhibition of the 11-β and 17-α hydroxylase steps of steroid synthesis. This inhibition persists for 6–12 hours after a single dose. It might be logical to use etomidate deliberately to attenuate the response, although this has never been done, presumably because of anxieties about an agent whose use as an infusion in intensive care patients is associated with increased mortality.
- **Benzodiazepines:** these also inhibit cortisol production, probably via a central effect.
- **α-2 agonists:** these attenuate the sympathoadrenal responses, and lead indirectly to a decrease in cortisol production.
- **Regional anaesthesia:** this is of continued interest because it has been demonstrated that extensive extradural block ablates the adrenocortical and glycaemic responses to surgery. It may be more difficult to achieve in upper gastrointestinal tract and thoracic surgery, but there is increasing acceptance of the claim that targeted and sustained regional anaesthesia has beneficial effect on surgical outcome. This, however, may be related as much to earlier ambulation and improvements in respiratory function as to the abolition of the stress response itself.

The Glucocorticoid Response to Surgery

Commentary

The stress response to injury may be important in patients who are receiving corticosteroids. The traditional concern relates to the danger of precipitating an Addisonian crisis in patients whose hypothalamic–pituitary–adrenal (HPA) axis is suppressed. Many clinicians believe that these anxieties are overstated. Certainly there is now little justification for the use of potentially dangerous supraphysiological replacement regimens.

Core Information

Steroid Response to Surgery

- **Sympathoadrenal response:** this is an autonomic response which is mediated via the hypothalamus, and which results in an increase in medullary catecholamines. There is also an increase in the presynaptic release of noradrenaline. Aldosterone release is stimulated by the renin–angiotensin system, leading to sodium and water retention.
- **HPA axis response:** hypothalamic releasing factors stimulate the anterior pituitary, with resultant increases in ACTH via corticotrophin-releasing hormone (CRH).
- **Cortisol production:** ACTH stimulates adrenal glucocorticoid release. This is mediated by a specific cell-surface receptor, with G protein activation, adenyl cyclase stimulation and increased intracellular cAMP. The effects of cortisol are catabolic, with protein breakdown, gluconeogenesis, inhibition of glucose utilization and lipolysis. The hormone is also anti-inflammatory; it inhibits leucocyte migration into damaged areas and decreases the synthesis of inflammatory mediators such as prostaglandins.
- **Cortisol output:** This varies according to the degree of surgical stress. There is normally a maximal rise at 4–6 hours, with peak cortisol usually subsiding within 24 hours. After major surgery it may be sustained for up to 72 hours. Normal blood levels are around 200 nmol l^{-1}, but the increase following surgery may range from 800 to more than 1,500 nmol l^{-1}. Normal 24-hour cortisol output is around 150 mg; minor surgery such as hernia repair will stimulate extra production of less than 50 mg in 24 hours, whereas following thoracotomy or laparotomy, between 75 and 100 mg will be released.

Supplementary and Clinical Information

Perioperative Steroid Replacement

- Patients who are receiving corticosteroids are often assumed to have suppression of the HPA axis. This occurs via a feedback inhibition of hypothalamic and pituitary function.
- This adrenal suppression means that patients cannot mount a normal steroid response to surgery and may develop an Addisonian crisis in the postoperative period. This is characterized by cardiovascular instability and electrolyte

derangement. Patients have hypotension, which may be refractory to routine treatment, and can be hypokalaemic, hyponatraemic and hypoglycaemic. Review of trials to date, however, suggest that steroid replacement regimens are unnecessary except in those patients who are being treated with glucocorticoids for primary disease of the HPA axis (e.g. primary adrenal failure, adrenal insufficiency secondary to hypopituitarism, congenital adrenal hyperplasia).

- Ideally any replacement regimen should be based on laboratory evaluation of the HPA axis (by conducting short synacthen or insulin tolerance tests if possible) and an assessment of the likely degree of surgical stress. Corticosteroid supplementation minimizes the risk of perioperative cardiovascular instability.
- Patients who are taking less than prednisolone 10 mg daily (or the equivalent) have a normal response to HPA testing and require no supplementation. Patients who have previously been taking an HPA suppressant dose, but have discontinued this within 3 months from surgery, should be assumed to have residual suppression. They should be tested wherever possible because exogenous steroid supplementation is not innocuous. Patients on high immunosuppressant doses must continue these perioperatively.
- Steroid equivalence: prednisolone 10 mg equates to methylprednisolone 8 mg; hydrocortisone 40 mg and dexamethasone 1.6 mg.
- In the light of the reviews outlined here, it is rarely necessary to do other than ensure that the patient continues taking their normal dose. Corticosteroid supplementation is, however, well embedded in clinical practice, and the following are typical replacement regimens.
- If taking more than 10 mg prednisolone daily and undergoing minor to moderate surgery:
  — Continue the usual dose preoperatively.
  — Give hydrocortisone 25 mg intravenously at induction.
  — Prescribe hydrocortisone 100 mg in the first 24 hours (by continuous infusion).
- If taking more than 10 mg daily and undergoing major surgery:
  — Continue the usual dose preoperatively.
  — Give hydrocortisone 25 mg intravenously at induction.
  — Prescribe hydrocortisone 100 mg per day for 48–72 hours (by continuous infusion).

The dangers of supraphysiological doses of exogenous corticosteroids. Complications of steroid therapy make for a long list. Although this question pertains to problems related to acute administration, the problems of long-term therapeutic use are also summarized.

- **Complications of acute (supraphysiological) therapy:** increased catabolism, hyperglycaemia, immuno-suppression, peptic ulceration, delayed wound healing, myopathy (which can occur acutely), steroid psychosis (which is related to sudden large increases in blood levels), fluid retention and electrolyte disturbance, including hypokalaemia.
- **Complications of chronic glucocorticoid therapy:** these include immunosuppression, hypertension, increased skin fragility, posterior subcapsular cataract formation, osteoporosis, hypocalcaemia caused by reduced gastrointestinal absorption, negative nitrogen balance and Cushing's Syndrome.

Adrenaline (Epinephrine)

Commentary

Adrenaline is a key drug in anaesthesia, intensive care and resuscitation. The questioning will include some clinical aspects of its use, but these are rooted firmly in the basic physiology of the compound, and so it is this with which you must be familiar.

Core Information

Basic Pharmacology

- Adrenaline is one of the body's principal catecholamines (a catechol is a benzene ring with two adjacent hydroxyl groups) and is produced via a short biosynthetic pathway in the adrenal medulla, from where it is secreted. Phenylalanine undergoes two hydroxylation steps to form first tyrosine, and then dihydroxyphenylalanine (dopa). Dopa is decarboxylated to form dopamine, which is hydroxylated to produce noradrenaline. Methylation of noradrenaline produces adrenaline (full chemical name: dihydroxyphenylmethyl aminoethanol). In summary:

$$\text{Phenylalanine} \rightarrow \text{Tyrosine} \rightarrow \text{Dopa} \rightarrow \text{Dopamine} \rightarrow \text{Noradrenaline} \rightarrow \text{Adrenaline}$$

- Adrenaline is inactivated by oxidative deamination (monoamine oxidase) and methylation (catechol-O-methyltransferase, COMT). COMT is much the more significant pathway. Metabolism is very rapid and adrenaline's elimination half-life is <60 s.
- Unlike noradrenaline, which is responsible for maintaining normal sympathetic tone, it is not a 'routine' neurotransmitter but is released instead in response to physiological crisis.
- Adrenaline has effects at both α- and β-adrenoceptors, of which there are several subclasses: α_1, α_2 (each with a further three subtypes) and β_1, β_2 and β_3.
- These adrenoceptors are G protein-coupled, and are associated with different second messenger systems. The α_1 actions are mediated via phospholipase C, and α_2 effects via a decrease in cyclic AMP. β effects are all mediated via an increase in cAMP.
- **Cardiovascular effects:** in lower doses, the β_1 effects predominate, but there is still a rise in systolic blood pressure caused by the increase in cardiac output. Even at low blood concentrations (the normal level is around 25 picogram ml^{-1}), there is still a β-receptor-mediated fall in diastolic pressure, and so the pulse pressure widens with only a small rise in mean arterial pressure. α_2 vasodilatation in skeletal muscle and in the liver also counteracts any rise in peripheral vascular resistance. There is an α_1-mediated increase in the force and rate of myocardial contraction, coupled with an increase in stroke volume secondary to enhanced venous return. Cardiac output increases. Direct myocardial stimulation is partially opposed by inhibitory baroreceptor reflexes which act to modify the rises in blood pressure. The transplanted heart, which is denervated, shows a more exaggerated response to circulating

adrenaline than would otherwise be the case. The same is true if the actions of the vagus nerve have been blocked by high doses of atropine, or if ganglion-blocking drugs have been given. (In both normal and denervated hearts, adrenaline enhances the excitability of myocardial cell membranes.) As the dose of adrenaline increases, so both α and β effects are seen, whereas at high doses α_1 vasoconstriction predominates. It may also cause α_1-mediated vasoconstriction in the main coronary arteries, which is offset by β_2-mediated vasodilatation in the smaller vessels. From an evolutionary point of view it would seem curious were the net effects of adrenaline to compromise the coronary circulation, although the evidence for that proposition remains elusive.

- **Respiratory effects:** adrenaline is a potent bronchodilator, acting via β_2 receptors to inhibit smooth muscle contraction in the airways.
- **Metabolic effects:** adrenaline increases oxygen consumption by up to 30%. Blood glucose rises both because of increased glycogenolysis in muscle and liver and decreased insulin secretion. This is an α_2 effect.
- **CNS effects:** in higher doses adrenaline is a cerebral stimulant which causes arousal. If administered intrathecally, adrenaline acts on α_2 receptors to produce analgesia.
- **Gastrointestinal effects:** smooth muscle of the gastrointestinal tract relaxes, although the sphincters contract (α_1 effect).

Supplementary and Clinical Information
Potential problems associated with adrenaline.

- **Ischaemic necrosis:** injection of adrenaline-containing solutions into digits or appendages may jeopardize the blood supply.
- **Cardiac arrhythmias:** adrenaline appears to increase the automaticity of the ventricular conducting system. The ECG may show runs of ventricular premature beats, leading in the worst case to ventricular fibrillation. This effect is enhanced by hypercapnia, by hypoxia and by acidosis. In conjunction with the use of some volatile agents, particularly halothane, this could be a fatal combination, although newer agents are much safer.
- **Cardiac disease:** adrenaline should be infiltrated with caution in those patients who have pre-existing hypertension or ischaemic heart disease. The combination of adrenaline and monoamine oxidase inhibitors (MAOIs) may also be hazardous.
- **Alternative vasopressors:** these include agents such as felypressin (Octapressin), which is a vasopressin (ADH) analogue. This is a potent local vasoconstrictor which is less likely to provoke cardiac arrhythmia.

Indications for Its Use
- **Cardiac resuscitation:** adrenaline is the main drug in the cardiac arrest algorithms. Its main action is to constrict the peripheral circulation into which the much-reduced cardiac output produced by external cardiac compression is being delivered. (CPR delivers at best around 10–15% of normal output.) This central redistribution of the available cardiac output increases coronary perfusion pressure and coronary arterial flow. The standard dose in adults is 1 mg (1 ml of 1 in 1,000 or 10 ml of 1 in 10,000).

- **Circulatory support:** its use to support the failing circulation is popular in some intensive therapy units. Some cardiologists also favour it as the drug of choice for cardiogenic shock. It is given by continuous infusion via a central vein at a rate of $0.05–2.0\ \mu g\ kg^{-1}\ min^{-1}$.

- **Bronchodilation:** adrenaline can be used in acute severe and refractory asthma in a dose range similar to that used for circulatory support.

- **Anaphylaxis:** adrenaline is the drug of first choice. It is given either by deep intramuscular injection in a dose of 500 μg (0.5 ml of 1 in 1,000) or by intravenous injection at a rate of $100\ \mu g\ min^{-1}$ until the patient responds.

- **Upper airway obstruction:** nebulized adrenaline can reduce upper airways oedema, due, for example, to croup in children or allergic reactions in adults. A dose of 1–2 mg diluted with saline can be used in adults, while children may receive $400\ \mu g\ kg^{-1}$ up to a maximum dose of 5 mg.

- **Vasoconstriction:** adrenaline can be added to solutions of local anaesthetic to reduce local bleeding, to prolong the duration of action and to reduce the rapidity with which the drug is absorbed. Surgeons may use pre-prepared solutions containing adrenaline 1 in 80,000 up to 1 in 200,000, but they may also prepare their own mixtures for use, for example, in plastic surgical procedures in which large areas of subcutaneous tissue are infiltrated. It is important to be aware of how much adrenaline is being given in these circumstances. The total dose should not exceed 500 μg. (Solutions of 1 in 1,000 contain $1,000\ \mu g\ ml^{-1}$, 1 in 10,000 contain $100\ \mu g\ ml^{-1}$, 1 in 80,000 contain $12.5\ \mu g\ ml^{-1}$, 1 in 100,000 contain $10\ \mu g\ ml^{-1}$ and 1 in 200,000 contain $5\ g\ ml^{-1}$.) Some surgeons may also use vasoconstrictors such as cocaine (in nasal surgery) and phenylephrine. The pressor effect of these drug combinations can be very hazardous.

5-Hydroxytryptamine (Serotonin)

Commentary

This is a basic science topic that you might expect to encounter in the Primary FRCA rather than the Final. Although serotonin does mediate a large number of physiological functions via a family of receptors and subtypes, the direct anaesthetic applications nonetheless are quite modest. Much remains to be elucidated about the receptor types, which, as always, will relieve the pressure on you to deliver precise factual answers. You cannot, for example, be expected to know details of $5\text{-}HT_6$ and $5\text{-}HT_7$ receptors when their functions remain unclear.

Core Information

- 5-hydroxytrytamine (5-HT), or serotonin, is one of four aminergic neurotransmitters (the others being dopamine, noradrenaline and histamine), which has its highest CNS concentrations in the midbrain, but which is also present in the spinal cord, retina, cerebellum, hypothalamus and limbic system. At 1%, this is a tiny proportion of total body 5-HT, the remainder of which is found peripherally. It is most abundant in the enterochromaffin cells in the walls of the stomach and the small bowel, and it is also found in platelets. In the gastrointestinal myenteric plexus it functions as an excitatory neurotransmitter.

- 5-HT is synthesized by hydroxylation and decarboxylation of tryptophan (an essential amino acid, the dietary intake of which can influence 5-HT levels) and is metabolized by monoamine oxidase. Its main metabolite is 5-hydroxyindole acetic acid (5-HIAA). 5-HT is stored in cytoplasmic vesicles. Reuptake is the primary mechanism whereby the compound is recovered following release.

- There are numerous receptor subtypes, further examples of which continue to be characterized. Currently there are 5-HT$_1$ (with five subtypes 1_A, 1_B, 1_D, 1_E, 1_F), 5-HT$_2$ (with subtypes 2_A–2_C), 5-HT$_3$, 5-HT$_4$, 5-HT$_5$ (with subtypes 5_A–5_B), and 5-HT$_6$ and 5-HT$_7$ receptors, totalling 14. All of these, apart from 5-HT$_3$ receptors, are coupled to G proteins. The effects of the 5-HT$_3$ receptor are mediated via a rapid sodium/potassium ligand-gated ion channel. The receptors are variously presynaptic and postsynaptic depending on subtype. They appear to mediate a large number of different and sometimes contradictory effects.

- Many, but not all, 5-HT$_1$ receptors are inhibitory in effect. 5-HT$_{1A}$ receptors are the main target of drugs used to treat depression, thus drugs such as fluoxetine (Prozac) are selective serotonin re-uptake inhibitors (SSRIs) at these sites. Buspirone, which is a 5-HT$_{1A}$ agonist, is used as an anxiolytic. Sumatriptan and related drugs are 5-HT$_{1B/D}$ agonists which are very effective treatments for migraine. The primary site of action appears to be selective carotid artery vasoconstriction mediated by 5-HT$_{1B}$ receptors.

- 5-HT$_2$ receptors appear to exert excitatory postsynaptic effects and are abundant in the cortex and the limbic system (the hallucinogen LSD is a potent agonist). Platelet aggregation and smooth muscle contraction is mediated by 5-HT$_{2A}$ receptors, and CSF production by 5-HT$_{2C}$. Gastrointestinal secretion and peristalsis is enhanced by a 5-HT$_2$ stimulatory effect on smooth muscle. 5-HT$_{2A}$ receptors mediate vascular smooth muscle contraction and vasoconstriction. Methysergide, which is an ergot alkaloid used to treat refractory migraine as well as diarrhoea associated with carcinoid syndrome, is a 5-HT$_{2A}$ and $_{2C}$ antagonist. (The use of this drug is limited by its well-recognized potential to cause devastating endocardial, valvular and retroperitoneal fibrosis.)

- 5-HT$_3$ excitatory ionotropic receptors in the area postrema mediate nausea and vomiting. They are also excitatory to enteric neurons. Ondansetron, granisetron and tropisetron are effective 5-HT$_3$ antagonists.

- 5-HT$_4$ receptors are found in the gut, and centrally in the striatum of the brain. They may have a presynaptic facilitatory effect on acetylcholine release and so may be involved in cognitive function. They are also excitatory to enteric neurons. Metoclopramide is a 5-HT$_4$ agonist.

- The remaining receptor types have functions which remain incompletely understood. 5-HT$_5$ and 5-HT$_6$ receptors in the limbic system appear to be involved with the control of mood, and 5-HT$_6$ receptors in particular have a high affinity for antidepressants. 5-HT$_7$ receptors may have some role in sleep and arousal.

Systems Effects

- **CNS:** these include mood and affect, arousal, circadian rhythms and CSF. Serotoninergic pathways are similar to noradrenergic systems which inhibit some dorsal horn pain tracts. Discharge in the dorsal raphe nucleus precipitates migraine. 5-HT influences autonomic function, including temperature and blood pressure.
- **Cardiovascular system:** 5-HT causes platelet aggregation and can mediate both vasoconstriction and vasodilatation. Intravenous serotonin causes a fall in blood pressure owing to arteriolar vasodilatation, which is preceded by an initial rise. In blood vessels, $5\text{-}HT_{2A}$ receptors mediate vasoconstriction ($5\text{-}HT_1$ agonism leads to constriction of larger intracranial vessels). Other 5-HT receptors, however, cause vasodilatation which is mediated via the release of nitric oxide (NO) and by the inhibition of noradrenaline release from sympathetic nerve terminals.
- **Respiratory system:** 5-HT causes bronchial smooth muscle contraction.
- **Gastrointestinal system:** 5-HT increases gastrointestinal secretion and peristalsis. It is also involved with nausea and vomiting.
- **Genitourinary system:** 5-HT increases uterine muscle tone.

Supplementary and Clinical Information

- **Carcinoid syndrome:** this occurs as a result of enterochromaffin tumours which secrete not only 5-HT but other neuropeptides such as substance P, vasoactive intestinal polypeptide (VIP), prostaglandins, histamine and bradykinin. More than 80% of these tumours originate in the gut, and so symptoms do not appear until they metastasize to the liver. Prior to metastasis these substances are degraded to inactive metabolites. Once they gain direct access to the circulation, either from primary sites in the lung or from metastases, then the problems of flushing, hypotension, tachycardia, wheeze, abdominal cramps and diarrhoea may supervene. Endocardial and valvular fibrosis (which affects the right side of the heart more frequently than the left) may also complicate the condition, as may pellagra. This is due to nicotinamide (vitamin B2) deficiency, which is caused by the excessive consumption of dietary tryptophan by the tumour. The symptoms of carcinoid are due not solely to serotonin secretion, but those which are mediated via 5-HT can be treated with the $5\text{-}HT_2$ antagonist cyproheptadine. Octreotide, which is a long-acting somatostatin analogue that suppresses 5-HT and other hormone secretion, can also be used.
- **Serotonin syndrome:** this describes the effects of excessive stimulation of central $5\text{-}HT_{1A}$ and $5\text{-}HT_2$ receptors due either to overdose by serotoninergic drugs such as tramadol, selective serotonin reuptake inhibitors, monoamine oxidase inhibitors or to a combination. It can also be precipitated by the perioperative administration of methylene blue, which as a phenothiazine derivative can increase plasma 5-HT concentrations. Its manifestations are mental, with agitation and disordered cognition; autonomic, with tachycardia, hypertension, pyrexia and diaphoresis; and neurological, with exaggerated muscle rigidity, clonus and tremor. (There are formal criteria for its diagnosis, known as the Sternbach criteria, which require four major symptoms/signs or three major and two minor, but that is likely to be detail too far).
- **Management:** in general, the treatment of serotonin toxicity is supportive because its optimal management remains uncertain. The $5\text{-}HT_{2A}$ antagonist cyproheptadine has been used, as have drugs such as dantrolene, propranolol and diazepam.

Cytochrome(s) P450

Commentary

This kind of question does risk giving the College and the examination a bad name. It is not as though cytochrome P450 is a single well-defined entity; on the contrary, it comprises numerous key forms with yet further genetic variations. Nor is it a topic of searing anaesthetic relevance; certainly it is of academic interest, but ignorance of most of its functions is little impediment to the delivery of safe and sophisticated anaesthesia. As a subject that is perceived both as intellectual and topical, however, it is no surprise to find it appearing in the Final FRCA. If the question is asked of you, just reproduce some of what appears in the following (which itself is a substantial oversimplification of a complex and very detailed topic), and you will probably know more than your examiners. If, however, you should happen to be discussing this with an examiner whose special interest this happens to be, then do not worry. Their specialist knowledge will inhibit the line of questioning because they will be conscious of a potential loss of objectivity.

Core Information

- **Description:** cytochrome or, more accurately, cytochromes P450, comprise a superfamily of enzymes which are concerned with the metabolism of a wide range both of endogenous and exogenous compounds. They are involved in biosynthesis as well as breakdown and catalyze, for example, the formation of hormones such as testosterone and oestrogens. They contain a pigment (hence cyto-*chrome*) and are characterized by maximal absorption in the presence of carbon monoxide, at 450 nm. This cytochrome–carbon monoxide compound is pink, which explains the 'P' in the nomenclature.

- **Biochemistry:** they are haem-thiolate proteins, and they act as mixed function mono-oxygenases, now known as 'Phase I enzymes' because they mediate the Phase I metabolism (mainly oxidation and hydroxylation) of numerous compounds. Most drugs are metabolized by cytochrome proteins. These utilize the haem iron moiety to oxidize molecules and render them more hydrophilic so as to facilitate renal excretion. The typical reaction can be represented by:

$$R - H \text{ (substrate)} + O_2 + NADPH + H^+ \rightarrow R - OH + H_2O + NADP^+$$

Phase I reactions render a compound hydrophilic by the addition of hydroxyl group or similarly, hydrophilic sulphydryl or amine groups. Phase II reactions eliminate reactive metabolites produced by Phase I reactions, together with compounds that have not been cleared. Phase II also increase hydrophilicity, usually by adding polar groups such as glucuronides. The reactions are catalyzed predominantly by transferases.

- **Numbers:** in humans there are 18 families, 43 subfamilies and 57 enzymes, each encoded by a separate gene. This manifests as a wide variation in the susceptibility of different individuals to particular drugs and toxins. Despite these large numbers, it is estimated that six main CYP enzymes are responsible for more than 90% of all drug oxidation.

- **Sites:** these ubiquitous microsomal enzymes are sited on the smooth endoplasmic reticulum of cells and on the inner membrane of mitochondria, but they are found in highest concentrations in the liver and small bowel. Individual hepatocytes may contain several forms of the enzyme.
- **Nomenclature:** the enzymes are divided into main families according to similarities in their amino acid sequences (possessing 40% or more structural homology) and are named CYP1, CYP2 and so on. It is families CYP1, CYP2, CYP3 and CYP4 which appear to be responsible for most drug biotransformation. These groups are then further classified into subfamilies (possessing 55% or more homology), which are described using capital letters following the family designation. Individual enzymes of the subgroup are designated using arabic numerals, for example, CYP3A4: (CYP3 [family], A [subfamily], 4 [individual enzyme]).
- **Important subtypes:** the most abundant cytochrome enzymes are members of the CYP3A subfamily, which comprise 70% of the cytochrome enzymes in the gastro-intestinal system, and 30% of those in the liver. The enzyme that metabolizes the greatest proportion of drugs in the liver is cytochrome CYP3A4. This enzyme and CYP3A3 are the major isoforms of the small gut, while the variant that is found in the stomach is CYP3A5. (This is absent in 70% of Caucasians and 50% of individuals of Afro-Caribbean origin, but its functions are replicated in such cases by CYP3A4.) Another important subtype is CYP2D6, which is estimated to be responsible for the metabolism of up to a quarter of the available prescription drugs. Some 5–10% of the Caucasian population has CYP2D6 deficiency, and numerous mutations in the CYP2D6 gene have been identified (see under 'Pharmacogenomics' in Chapter 4).

Supplementary and Clinical Information

- **Induction of enzymes:** as plasma concentrations of drugs increase, so enzyme synthesis may increase to match it, and numerous substances induce cytochrome P450. These include barbiturates, anticonvulsants, alcohol, glucocorticoids and some antibiotics. (This is a generalization, because these agents induce different groups; alcohol, for example, induces CYP2E1. You will not be expected to recount this level of detail.) Tobacco, or at least its polycyclic aromatic hydrocarbons, is also a potent inducer of cytochrome P450 (CYP1A1 and CYP1A2), and this is of anaesthetic interest because smoking appears to confer a protective effect against PONV. This may be because of the more rapid metabolism and elimination of volatile agents which are associated with PONV, although the hypothesis remains speculative. (Smokers also show less sensitivity both to the effects of aminosteroid neuromuscular blockers as well as to morphine, although probably not by mechanisms associated with cytochrome P450.)
- **Inhibition of enzyme action:** competitive inhibition occurs when two (or more) drugs are metabolized by the same enzyme. The process can be complex, with reversible and irreversible binding to the haem binding site, either by drugs or by their metabolites. Such interactions may have serious consequences. An example is the cardiac arrhythmias associated with the antihistamine terfenadine. The drug can lead to a prolonged QT interval, with the development of torsade de pointes (a malignant form of ventricular tachycardia characterized by a changing QRS axis). Terfenadine itself is a cardiotoxic prodrug with an active metabolite which is not.

A number of diverse substances, such as the bioflavonoids in grapefruit juice and antibiotics such as erythromycin, inhibit the function of CYP3A4 and its metabolism of terfenadine with the risk of precipitating dangerous arrhythmias. Drugs such as metronidazole and amiodarone inhibit CYP2C9, which is the enzyme involved in the metabolism of warfarin. Both can produce significant prolongations of prothrombin time. The analogous effects of cimetidine, which is a non-specific inhibitor of cytochrome P450, are relatively weak in comparison.

Nitric Oxide

Commentary

There are at least 5,000 research publications on this ubiquitous molecule, whose importance has been recognized only since the 1980s. It is an enormous body of work, so the 8 minutes of the oral will only allow a broad overview. Although it appears to mediate a large number of functions, its direct implications for anaesthesia are disappointingly modest. You will, however, need to know some of the basic details of its synthesis and chemistry, as well as those areas of anaesthetic practice and pharmacology for which nitric oxide (NO) does have relevance.

Core Information

- **NO** is a free radical gas which is formed in a reaction between molecular oxygen and L-arginine. The reaction is catalyzed by nitric oxide synthetase (NOS) and leads to the formation of NO and citrulline.
- **NOS isoforms (iNOS, eNOS and nNOS):** there are three NOS isoforms. The single inducible form, iNOS, is expressed in response to pathological stimulation in a variety of cells, including macrophages, neutrophils and endothelial cells. It is induced by several chemical mediators, such as interleukins, β-interferon and tumour necrosis factor (TNF). The two constitutive forms are eNOS, which is present in endothelium (and some other cells such as cardiac myocytes and platelets), and nNOS, which is present in neurons. The activity of the constitutive isoforms of NOS is governed by intracellular calcium-calmodulin, whereas iNOS is calcium-independent. The quantity of NO generated by iNOS exceeds by about 1,000 times that which is formed by the constitutive enzymes.
- **Actions:** NO is a central signalling molecule which modulates many aspects of physiological function. As an endothelium-derived relaxing factor (EDRF), it regulates blood pressure and regional blood flow, as well as limiting platelet aggregation. As a neurotransmitter, NO may have a role centrally in memory, consciousness and CNS plasticity. Its peripheral roles include gastric emptying. An absence of nNOS is characteristic of infants with hypertrophic pulmonary stenosis. It has a non-specific role in the immune system, and by mechanisms such as the inactivation of haem-containing enzymes and nitrosylation of nucleic acids can destroy pathogens and tumour cells.

- **Cardiovascular effects:** it is a small lipophilic molecule which diffuses rapidly across cell membranes to combine with thiol groups to form nitrosothiol compounds. It binds to the iron moiety to activate soluble guanylyl cyclase. This enzyme catalyses the formation of cyclic guanosine monophosphate (cGMP) with the activation of protein kinases, protein phosphorylation and finally the relaxation of vascular smooth muscle.
- **Inactivation:** as a free radical gas, NO has a half-life measured in seconds (variously quoted as 0.50–1.0 s, up to 5 s). It is inactivated after forming complexes with haemoglobin, and with other haem-containing molecules. The affinity of haem for nitric oxide is more than 10,000 times greater than its affinity for O_2. It is also inactivated by a series of oxidation reactions that produce nitrate. This is then excreted renally.

Supplementary and Clinical Information

- **Vasodilators:** the nitrovasodilators such as glyceryl trinitrate (GTN) and sodium nitroprusside (SNP) act by producing exogenous NO in a reaction mediated by glutathione-S-transferase and cytochrome P450. Vascular smooth muscle is constantly in a state of NO-mediated vasodilatation, the compound being formed in response to shear stresses in the vessel wall. The venous circulation has a lower basal release. This is the reason why drugs such as GTN and SNP are more effective dilators of the venous rather than the arterial circulation. NO deficiency may contribute to hypertension or organ ischaemia.
- **Interactions with volatile anaesthetics:** volatile agents inhibit NOS and so reduce production from endothelial cells. The end effect of volatile administration is not vasoconstriction, however, because NO inhibition is offset by direct mechanisms which influence vascular smooth muscle tone. It has been argued, although not universally accepted, that NOS inhibition by volatiles may decrease MAC, that NO influences conscious level and that it may have a role as one of the mediators of general anaesthesia.
- **Inhaled NO:** its half-life is very short, and so when the gas is inhaled it acts to reduce pulmonary vascular resistance without exerting any systemic effects. This is because it binds so rapidly to haem and so in effect is scavenged by haemoglobin. It may therefore be of use in patients with intrapulmonary shunts typical of conditions such as ARDS. Systemic administration causes indiscriminate pulmonary vasodilatation, which can only worsen the ventilation–perfusion mismatch. Inhaled NO, in contrast, is delivered to better-recruited alveoli where it dilates the associated pulmonary vessels and reduces shunt fraction. It is also a bronchodilator. In theory, its use should benefit patients with impaired right heart function and those with pulmonary hypertension. Clinical experience is probably greatest in the treatment of neonates with respiratory distress syndrome. Although NO has also been used to treat ARDS, there is no evidence that it is superior to other strategies such as prone ventilation, and difficulties with safe delivery systems have also limited its use.
- **Delivery:** this can be problematic because, at concentrations greater than around 100 parts per million (ppm), the free radical gas is highly reactive and toxic. It is stored in nitrogen in a concentration of 1,000 ppm, and has been given in doses that range from 250 parts per billion up to 80 parts per million.

Plasma Proteins

Commentary

This is a rather non-specific topic which could branch off into unpredictable directions for which you may not be prepared. A reliable strategy may be to dwell on the core subject in as much descriptive detail as you can muster, but it may not be possible to avoid being asked, for example, about the functions of one of the many hormones that are transported by plasma proteins or more likely, about the immunology of γ-globulins. The oral may include a question about therapeutic implications and touch on intravenous immunoglobulin treatment and plasmapheresis.

Core Information

Proteins That Are Normally Present in Plasma

- Plasma is the non-cellular component of the intravascular space and comprises around 3,500 ml in a 70-kg adult man, accounting for about 5% of total body weight.
- Amongst the considerable quantity of ions, inorganic and organic molecules (including electrolytes, urea, creatinine, fats, amino acids, sugars, metals, vitamins and enzymes) are a large number of plasma proteins. These comprise albumin, the globulins and fibrinogen. All of these apart from the γ-globulins are synthesized in the liver.
- **Albumin:** albumin has a molecular weight of around 69,000 and is quantitatively the most important, with a plasma concentration of 5 g dl^{-1} (35 g l^{-1} in blood), around 55% of the total. Albumin makes the greatest contribution (20 mmHg) to the plasma oncotic pressure and is a versatile carrier protein for numerous substances, including bilirubin, calcium, metals, fatty acids, amino acids, enzymes, hormones and drugs. It is synthesized in the liver at a rate of 0.2 g kg^{-1} day^{-1}.
- **Globulins:** the globulin fraction is divided further into α_1, α_2, β_1, β_2 and γ subtypes. Their molecular weights average around 200,000, but they are quantitatively less significant with a plasma concentration of 1.5 g dl^{-1} (10 g l^{-1} in blood). They contribute about 5 mmHg to plasma oncotic pressure. The α and β fractions are synthesized in the liver and include coagulation factors, transport proteins such as α_1-acid glycoprotein (which binds bupivacaine, amongst others) and precursors such as angiotensinogen. They also include steroid and thyroid hormone binding globulin as well as acute phase proteins, such as C-reactive protein. Complement is a series of plasma proteins which are also produced in the liver.
- **γ-globulins:** the γ-globulins are antibodies which are synthesized in plasma cells. There are five different classes: immunoglobulin (I$_g$) G, which is the most abundant and which, together with IgM, is responsible for complement fixation; IgA, which is a secretory antibody; IgD, which mediates the recognition of antigens by lymphocytes; and IgE, which is found on the cell membranes of mast cells and which mediates the

classic anaphylactic type 1 hypersensitivity reaction (see under 'Immunology and Drug Reactions'). IgG, IgM and IgA are 'natural' antibodies because they are independent of antigen exposure and can be induced without sensitization.

- **Fibrinogen:** this is a large molecule of molecular weight variously quoted as between 340,000 and 500,000, which has a plasma concentration of 0.5 g dl^{-1} (3.5 g l^{-1} in blood), contributing about 1 mmHg to plasma oncotic pressure. As coagulation factor I, it is a crucial part of the final coagulation common pathway.
- **Other functions:** plasma proteins are weakly ionized because of their carboxyl ($-COOH$) and amino ($-NH$) groups, which dissociate to form anions at body pH. This gives them a buffering capacity which amounts to about 5% of the total. (Some texts quote 15%.)

Supplementary and Clinical Information

- These include **coagulation** (see under 'Drugs Affecting Coagulation'), **immunological function** (see under 'immunology and Drug Reactions'), **oncotic pressure** (see under 'Osmosis' in Chapter 5), **buffers** and **disease states** associated with abnormalities of plasma proteins (such as multiple myeloma, which is a malignancy affecting plasma cells which produce IgG, IgA and IgM paraproteins).
- **Intravenous immunoglobulin (IVIG).** This is produced from the pooled plasma of a thousand or more donors and contains predominantly IgG immunoglobulins. Initially IVIG was used to treat primary immunodeficiency but it is now also given to patients with haematological diseases such as autoimmune idiopathic thrombocytopaenic purpura (ITP), thrombocytic thrombocytopaenia (TTP), graft versus host disease and Guillain-Barré syndrome. It suppresses a number of inflammatory mediators including cytokines and modulates the activity of complement. An autoantibody-mediated cytopaenia such as ITP occurs because opsonized platelets bind to the Fc receptor sites on splenic phagocytes and are destroyed. IVIG appears to work by competitive inhibition at the Fc receptor. (Its further complex and detailed actions are beyond the likely scope of the oral.) Side effects are uncommon and are relatively non-specific, including headache, flushing, myalgia and nausea. Standard dose regimens are either 400 mg kg^{-1} for 5 days or 1,000 mg kg^{-1} for 2 days.
- **Plasmapheresis.** This describes a variety of techniques in which the extracorporeal separation of blood components yields a filtered plasma product. Centrifugation techniques utilize the different specific gravity of substances, whereas membrane plasma separation techniques filter plasma components according to their size. Filtered plasma is either treated or discarded, and red blood cells together with colloid for volume replacement are reinfused into the patient. Plasmapheresis and plasma exchange are used to remove damaging macromolecules. There are some conditions for which it is first-line therapy and include thrombotic thrombocytic purpura (which as soon as the diagnosis is confirmed requires immediate treatment), Guillain-Barré syndrome, myasthenia gravis and Goodpasture syndrome. Second-line indications include Lambert-Eaton myasthenia, multiple sclerosis, severe systemic lupus erythematosus (SLE) and autoimmune haemolytic anaemia.

Thyroid Function

Commentary

This oral may include a discussion of the anaesthetic implications of thyroid disease, but it will also cover the basic physiology of thyroid function. Even if details of the biochemistry elude you, at least ensure that you can outline the effects of thyroxine.

Core Information

- **The thyroid gland** produces thyroid hormone, which is an iodine-containing amino acid that is central to metabolism. In essence it maintains the metabolic rate that is optimal for normal cellular function.
- **Production:** the production of thyroxine first involves iodide trapping within the gland by a process of active transport. Iodide is rapidly oxidized to iodine prior to the iodination of tyrosine with the formation of diiodotyrosine (DIT). Two molecules of DIT condense to form T_4. Thyroxine is then stored in the colloid of the thyroid bound in a peptide linkage as part of the large thyroglobulin molecule. It then undergoes proteolysis and release into the circulation. Most of the hormone is released in the form of T_4 with only about 5% secreted as T_3. Once in the circulation about one-third of T_4 is converted to T_3.
- **Secretion:** secretion is controlled by the thyroid-stimulating hormone (TSH) of the anterior pituitary, which in turn is regulated by thyrotropin-releasing hormone (TRH) from the hypothalamus. The process is subject to negative feedback control by thyroid hormones which act both at the pituitary and hypothalamus. The proteolysis of stored thyroid hormone is inhibited by iodide.
- **Binding:** carriage in the circulation is via binding to albumin and thyroxine-binding globulin (TBG). TBG has very high affinity, and so most circulating T_4 is bound. T_3 is bound equally by TBG and by albumin. Free T_3 and T_4 concentrations in plasma are very low.
- **Functions:** in summary, thyroid hormones stimulate oxygen consumption, act as a regulator of carbohydrate and lipid metabolism, and have an important role in normal growth and maturation. The hormones enter cells and T_3 binds to thyroid receptors in the nuclei. T_3 acts more rapidly and is three to five times more potent than T_4. The hormone–receptor complex then binds to DNA and changes the expression of a variety of different genes that code for enzymes that regulate cell function. Thyroxine is calorigenic, increasing the oxygen consumption of almost all metabolically active tissues. (Exceptions include the brain, anterior pituitary, testes, uterus, lymph nodes and spleen.) T_4 actually depresses pituitary oxygen consumption, presumably via a negative feedback mechanism. It increases the force and rate of myocardial contraction, increases the number and affinity of β-adrenergic receptors and enhances its response to circulating catecholamines. As a catabolic hormone, it increase lipolysis and stimulates the formation of low-density lipoprotein receptors. It increases protein breakdown in muscle and enhances carbohydrate absorption from the gut.

Supplementary Information and Clinical Considerations

Anaesthetic implications of thyroid disease: (overt thyrotoxicosis and myxoedema are rare, but anaesthetic mismanagement of either condition may be disastrous).

- **Airway problems:** all forms of thyroid disease may be associated with large goitres, which may extend retrosternally and cause airway problems secondary to compression of the trachea, in some cases down to only a few millimetres in diameter.
- **Hyperthyroidism:** the well-known clinical features are predictable from knowledge of the actions of the hormone. Excess thyroid hormone hyperstimulates almost all metabolically active tissue. Severe cases may have cardiac arrhythmias and heart failure. The cardinal principle underlying the anaesthetic management of thyrotoxic patients is to render them euthyroid prior to surgery and to avoid the risk of 'thyroid storm' caused by an acute hypermetabolic state.
- **Hypothyroidism:** in contrast, hypothyroid patients need much smaller doses of anaesthetic drugs. The BMR is greatly reduced, and with it cardiac reserve. Uncorrected myxoedema may be associated with amyloidosis, with consequent cardiac and renal impairment.

Medical Management of Thyroid Disease

- **Hyperthyroidism:** these patients should be rendered euthyroid before surgery. One approach is to achieve this over 2–3 months using propylthiouracil, which decreases thyroid synthesis and inhibits the peripheral conversion of T_4 to T_3. Carbimazole can be used as an alternative. This also decreases synthesis of thyroid hormone, possibly by inhibiting iodination of tyrosine residues in thyroglobulin. For 10 days or so prior to surgery patients are also given potassium iodide to reduce the vascularity of the gland.

An alternative and less time-consuming option is to control the manifestations of thyroid overstimulation using β-adrenoceptor blockers for 2–3 weeks preoperatively, together with potassium iodide as described. Emergency surgery in hyperthyroid patients carries the risk of a thyrotoxic crisis, also known as 'thyroid storm', in which there is a sudden further extreme surge of metabolic stimulation, with hyperpyrexia, diaphoresis, tachycardia and arrhythmias. Intravenous β-blockade using propranolol (or esmolol if there is concern that the patient is in cardiac failure), together with intravenous potassium iodide, should allow adequate control. Larger doses of anaesthetic agents may be required to compensate for their more rapid distribution and metabolism.

- **Hypothyroidism:** the opposite of thyroid storm is myxoedema coma, which is characterized by obtunded cerebration, marked hypothermia, alveolar hypoventilation and bradycardia. Correction of hypothyroidism is usually undertaken slowly, giving oral thyroxine, although intravenous T_3 can be used in emergency situations. This risks provoking myocardial ischaemia and should be avoided if possible. T_4 can be given, but its conversion to T_3 under these circumstances is greatly depressed.
- Skin contains various proteins combined with polysaccharides, hyaluronic acid and chondroitin sulphuric acid. In hypothyroidism these complexes accumulate, and so promote water retention along with a characteristic coarsening of the skin, which

becomes puffy. When treated with thyroid hormone these complexes are metabolized with resolution of the 'myx' (mucus/mucin) -oedema.

- **Thyroid eye disease** Thyroid Exophthalmos is a characteristic of autoimmune Graves' disease and is caused by swelling of the muscles and connective tissues of the orbit, which leads to proptosis. This effect is due not to thyroid hormone but to autoimmune attack on the tissues by cytotoxic antibodies. These are formed in response to antigens that are common to the eye muscles and to the thyroid. The changes are not completely reversible with treatment.

Nutrition

Commentary

Nutrition has become a separate science, and in many hospitals there are specific teams which manage the needs both of the perioperative surgical patient as well as the critically ill. You will nevertheless need to know something about the subject because nutrition is a topic that reappears in the exam. You will not have to know specific details of trace element or vitamin concentrations, although you may be asked about the daily requirements of the major minerals. You can anticipate a broad discussion of the effects of starvation, of the indications for nutritional support, of the major components of feeds, and the place of enteral and parenteral routes of administration.

Core Information

Indications for nutritional support in the surgical and critically ill patient, and the physiological changes that are associated with starvation.

- **Indications for nutritional support:** cachectic patients with a preoperative weight loss of 15% or more, or who have effectively been starved for more than 10 days (for example, because of dysphagia), have improved outcomes if they receive nutritional support before surgery. There are numerous other indications, including malabsorption owing to small bowel resection, small bowel fistulas, radiation enteritis, intractable diarrhoea and vomiting, and hyperemesis gravidarum.
- **Starvation:** this can be defined as the result of a severe or total lack of nutrients needed for the maintenance of life. In the absence of adequate intake, hepatic glycogen stores are depleted within 24–48 hours, after which adipose tissue becomes the source of fatty acids for use as an energy substrate. A small number of cell types, amongst which are erythrocytes and cells in the renal medulla, can utilize only glucose, and this has to be provided via amino acids that are produced from protein breakdown. The CNS normally depends on glucose but can function using ketones as an energy substrate. During prolonged fasting, there is an obligatory protein loss of at least 20 g daily. (Catabolism is a form of accelerated starvation with glycogenolysis, lipolysis and proteolysis.)

- **Nutritional requirements – energy:** basal expenditure can be judged from the Harris–Benedict equation (which links weight, height and age) or from nomograms. Kilocalorie needs range from around 30 kcal kg^{-1} in the non-stressed ambulatory state to 60 kcal kg^{-1} in sepsis or following major trauma. After severe thermal injury, which exemplifies an accelerated catabolic state, patients may require 80 kcal kg^{-1}.
- **Nutritional requirements – protein:** this can be estimated empirically. Demands may range from 0.5–1.0 g kg^{-1} in the non-stressed state to 2.5 g kg^{-1} under conditions of extreme stress.
- **Assessment of nitrogen balance:** each gram of nitrogen is equivalent to 6.2 g of protein or 30 g of muscle. In catabolic states patients are in negative balance. Losses can be determined over each 24-hour period by measuring urinary urea and incorporating the value into a formula, a typical example of which is 24-hour nitrogen loss = (Urinary urea mmol $24hr^{-1} \times 0.028$) + 4. 0.028 is a factor that converts urea in mmoles to grams of nitrogen, and 4 grams is the approximate total lost daily in faeces, skin, hair and urine as non-urea nitrogen.
- **Nutritional requirements – fluids:** a simple formula for basal requirements in a temperate climate is 100 ml kg^{-1} for the first 10 kg body weight, 50 ml kg^{-1} for the next 10 kg and then 20 ml kg^{-1} thereafter. To this total must be added the various losses as appropriate. (This formula can also be used to approximate normal kilocalorie requirements.)
- **Calorie sources:** carbohydrate (glucose) and protein (amino acids) provide 4 kcal of energy per gram, fat provides 9 kcal g^{-1}. (Alcohol provides 7 kcal g^{-1}.) Glucose-rich solutions are associated with hyperglycaemia and fatty infiltration of the liver, with excess CO_2 production which increases the respiratory quotient (RQ) to unity, with hyperinsulinaemia and fluid retention, with hypophosphataemia causing reduced tissue oxygenation, and with decreased immune function. Lipid administration (10% or 20% emulsion) reduces reliance on glucose as a calorie source with its attendant problems and provides essential fatty acids. Hyperlipidaemia can complicate its administration. Protein is given in the form of crystalline amino acids.
- **Additives:** these include extra electrolytes, where appropriate, together with phosphate and magnesium; trace elements, including zinc, copper, manganese, chromium and selenium; and the full range of fat-soluble and water-soluble vitamins.
- **Daily requirements:** Sodium: 1.0 mmol kg^{-1}. Potassium: 1.0 mmol kg^{-1}. Calcium: 0.1 mmol kg^{-1}. Magnesium: 0.2 mmol kg^{-1}. Phosphate: 0.7 mmol kg^{-1}. (These are simplified for ease of memorization, as most authorities list a range).
- **Other supplements:** glutamine appears to improve energy utilization and protein synthesis in skeletal muscle as well as enhancing both gut immunity and lymphocyte function. Arginine also improves lymphocyte function, as well as influencing wound healing. Omega-3 fatty acids may modulate the inflammatory response to trauma and in sepsis.
- **Parenteral nutrition:** total parenteral nutrition (TPN) may be necessary in specific cases such as short bowel syndrome, but under most circumstances enteral feeding is preferred. Complications associated with the parenteral route include all those associated with central venous catheterization, as well as the problems of impaired gastrointestinal structure and function, a decrease in splanchnic blood flow, a loss of

normal bowel flora with increased bacterial translocation, hepatic steatosis and acalculous cholecystitis. Infection is a significant risk, and TPN has the added disadvantage of high cost.

- **Enteral nutrition:** in contrast, enteral feeding improves splanchnic blood flow, maintains better gastrointestinal tract integrity and is associated with greater nitrogen retention and enhanced weight gain. It also improves immune defences by increasing the secretion of IgA. The splanchnic hyperaemia associated with resumed nutrition can in theory precipitate ischaemia secondary to increased oxygen consumption, and may divert blood from core organs. This may be problematic should the patient be haemodynamically unstable. The benefits of enteral feeding outweigh these risks in the majority of patients.
- **Complications:** in summary, they include the complications of central venous access, hyperglycaemia, fatty infiltration of the liver, increased CO_2 production with implications for weaning from mechanical ventilation, hyperlipidaemia, bacterial translocation and cholecystitis.

The Refeeding Syndrome

- The refeeding syndrome describes the severe metabolic derangements that can occur when nutrition is reintroduced to individuals who have been starved or severely malnourished, and to patients with severe illness who are profoundly catabolic. It presents typically within 4 days of the start of replenishment and is characterized by metabolic derangement and acidosis, together with variable symptoms and signs. These include gastrointestinal symptoms, muscle weakness and myalgia, impaired cerebration, cardiac arrhythmias and myocardial dysfunction. It is because these are relatively non-specific that the condition may go unrecognized.
- Individuals at risk include patients with cachexia due to malignancy; those with malabsorption due, for example, to inflammatory bowel disease; and those with long-term nutritional deficiencies including chronic alcoholics and those with anorexia nervosa. Specific mineral depletion can occur such as the hypophosphataemia associated with chronic antacid use (aluminium and magnesium bind to phosphate and prevent its absorption), or the hypokalaemia in patients on long-term diuretic therapy.
- When a subject is starved, hepatic glycogen is fully depleted within 24–48 hours (depending on energy expenditure), after which the body becomes dependent on fatty acids and amino acids as the primary energy source. The brain is able to use ketones as an energy source and blood levels do rise as muscle preferentially switches to fatty acid utilization. As starvation continues, there is increased protein catabolism together with the intracellular depletion of various essential substances, including potassium, magnesium and phosphate, whose serum concentrations, however, may remain within the normal range. Insulin secretion is suppressed and glucagon release is increased. The basal metabolic rate decreases by up to 25% in order to conserve energy stores.
- As soon as nutrition is reintroduced (either enterally or parenterally) there is sharp rise in metabolic rate as the increase in blood glucose stimulates release of insulin, which as an anabolic hormone increases the synthesis of glycogen, fat and protein.

This anabolism requires various minerals, in particular phosphate and magnesium, together with co-factors of which thiamine (vitamin B_1) is probably the most important. Insulin drives potassium and glucose into the cells via the Na^+-K^+ ATP-ase symporter. Phosphate and magnesium also move into the intracellular compartment. These processes reduce the plasma concentrations of all these substances whose total body levels are likely to be substantially depleted. It is these fluid and electrolyte shifts superimposed on total body mineral depletion that are responsible for the clinical features of the syndrome.

- **Glucose:** the glycaemia that occurs with refeeding stimulates insulin release with the suppression of gluconeogenesis. Acute hyperglycaemia may follow with predictable sequelae of osmotic diuresis and metabolic (ketotic) acidosis.
- **Sodium and water:** the sudden return of carbohydrate metabolism is accompanied by sodium and water retention. If the relative oliguria is then treated with fluid restoration, there is the risk of circulatory overload with a myocardium that may already be impaired by depleted ATP.
- **Phosphate:** this mineral is essential for all intracellular process, for maintaining the structure of the cell membrane and for activating a large number of enzymes and second messenger systems. In its incorporation in 2,3-DPG it controls oxygen-haemoglobin affinity and is central to energy storage as part of ATP. It functions as a buffer in the renal regulation of acid-base balance. Hypophosphataemia is therefore associated with erythrocyte, leucocyte and platelet dysfunction; metabolic acidosis; and hypercalcaemia. Severe ATP depletion can affect myocardial contractility, and is also associated with rhabdomyolysis. Normal cerebration can be impaired. Severe hypophosphataemia is defined as a plasma concentration less than 0.3 mmol l^{-1}. Initial acute replacement can be initiated with 18 mmol intravenously over 12 hours.
- **Potassium:** this is the major intracellular cation, and the rapid uptake by cells and consequent fall in plasma concentration can provoke potentially fatal cardiac arrhythmias.
- **Magnesium:** this is another important intracellular cation which is a co-factor in numerous enzyme systems, including those involved in oxidative phosphorylation and ATP production. It is described in more detail under 'Magnesium Sulphate' in Chapter 4. Severe hypomagnesaemia is defined as a plasma concentration less than 0.5 mmol l^{-1}. Acute replacement can be achieved by giving 24 mmol intravenously over 24 hours.
- **Thiamine:** this is an essential co-factor in carbohydrate metabolism. Its deficiency can cause acute neurological disturbance, including Wernicke's encephalopathy with confusion and ataxia.
- **Re-establishment of nutrition.** Guidelines, including those from NICE, recommend slow repletion at a maximum initial rate of 10 kcal kg^{-1} 24 h^{-1} and increasing to full energy requirements over 4–7 days. This will depend on the degree of malnutrition or the period of starvation; if this is severe, the initial rate should be halved to 5 kcal kg^{-1} 24 h^{-1}. There is no need for correction of electrolyte and mineral concentrations before refeeding begins. Vitamin supplementation should also be started immediately.

Electroconvulsive Therapy

Commentary

There are few shorter anaesthetics than those given for electroconvulsive therapy (ECT). This benefit is usually offset by the fact that the procedure is often undertaken in isolated sites with patients who may have relevant co-morbidity. The physiological effects may be transient, but they can be extreme, and are effects of which you should be aware. (If you are struggling to retrieve this information, then just try to remember instead the presentation and sequelae of a grand mal convulsion.)

Core Information

- Electroconvulsive therapy (ECT), in which an electric shock is used to induce a grand mal convulsion, is an empirical and somewhat controversial treatment. Its use is now confined mainly to patients with refractory psychiatric disorders, particularly psychotic depression but also catatonia, mania and schizophrenia.
- **Technique:** a shock of about 850 mA is delivered across the cerebral hemispheres by a stimulator that delivers a pulsatile square wave discharge. Pulses of 1.25 ms at 26 Hz are delivered for up to 5 seconds. Unilateral ECT is sometimes performed on the non-dominant hemisphere with the aim of minimizing post-procedure cognitive dysfunction. Memory impairment is substantially reduced with this technique.
- **Grand mal convulsion:** a short latent phase is followed by a tonic phase of general contracture of skeletal muscle which lasts around 15 seconds. This is succeeded by a clonic phase which lasts 30–60 seconds. The central electrical seizure (as demonstrated by EEG) outlasts the peripheral myoclonus. The optimal duration of seizure activity has not been established, but the shock is usually repeated if the EEG changes are short.
- **Autonomic effects – parasympathetic:** the discharge is short-lived but is associated with typical parasympathetic effects. Their most extreme manifestations include bradycardia and vagal inhibition, leading to asystole.
- **Autonomic effects – sympathetic:** as the clonic phase of the seizure begins there is a mass sympathetic response which peaks at around 2 minutes. Plasma adrenaline and noradrenaline levels at 1 minute exceed baseline by 15 and 3 times, respectively. Predictable effects include tachyarrhythmias and hypertension, with increased myocardial and cerebral oxygen consumption.
- **Cerebral effects:** the cortical discharge is accompanied by a large increase in cerebral blood flow, which may increase more than fivefold, and cerebral oxygen consumption ($CMRO_2$), which may increase by four times. Intracranial pressure rises accordingly.
- **Musculoskeletal effects:** the grand mal convulsion is accompanied by violent contractions of all skeletal muscles, and has been associated with vertebral fractures and other skeletal damage. The Bolam principle, which has underpinned the law relating to medical negligence since 1957, followed from a case in which a patient suffered a dislocated hip as the result of an unmodified convulsion during a session of ECT.

Supplementary Information

- **Complications:** there are predictable problems associated with the convulsion, which include cardiac arrhythmias and hypertension. The risk of skeletal and tissue damage, for example to the tongue, is minimized by 'modifying' the convulsion with a small dose of suxamethonium. This attenuates the force of the muscle contraction on the skeletal system. Post-procedure disorientation, memory impairment and cognitive dysfunction occur in around 50% of patients and may persist for some weeks. Patients often undergo a 'course' of ECT, typically twice-weekly sessions for 3 to 4 weeks depending on response, and so the cerebral effects are likely to be cumulative.

- ECT should not be used in patients who have suffered a recent cerebrovascular or myocardial event (within 3 months), who have a CNS mass lesion or have raised intracranial pressure. It should probably be avoided in patients with osteoporotic bone disease because of the risk of fractures and should be used with caution in patients with glaucoma and severe ischemic heart disease. A symptomatic hiatus hernia does not contraindicate ECT but does mandate intubation following a rapid sequence induction.

- Anaesthetic implications relate to the physiological effects outlined previously, together with the problems of anaesthetizing often elderly patients in remote locations. The interactions of anaesthetic agents with concurrent mood modifying medication are rarely a problem due to the brevity of the procedure and the simple nature of the technique.

- **Anaesthetic technique:** intravenous anaesthetic induction is the norm, with propofol as the most commonly used and familiar agent. Although the EEG displays initial activation, it thereafter exhibits dose-related depression, and propofol may shorten seizure duration. Thiopental has less of an effect in this regard, while etomidate prolongs seizure duration and may reduce the excitatory threshold. Anaesthesia is usually maintained with intermittent bolus doses of induction agent as indicated. The grand mal convulsion is modified with a neuromuscular blocker, typically suxamethonium in a dose of 0.5 mg kg^{-1}. Should suxamethonium be contraindicated, then given the very transient nature of the procedure a rocuronium/sugammadex technique would be appropriate. Drugs to attenuate the parasympathetic and sympathetic stimulation do have theoretical advantages, for example in patients with ischaemic heart disease, but in practice these are rarely given. Airway management is usually simple with pre-oxygenation (if tolerated by the patient) followed by bag-valve-mask ventilation during the period of apnoea.

- **The Mental Capacity Act:** a patient is said to have capacity if (1) they are able to understand the information that is imparted to them, (2) are able to retain that information, (3) are able to weigh up the information before arriving at a decision, and (4) are able to communicate that decision (not necessarily verbally). Although patients who require ECT may have mental health issues which do not allow them to fulfill those criteria, that cannot be assumed to be the case, and so a proper assessment of capacity is mandatory. The involvement of an advocate is recommended but is not a legal requirement. Advanced directives made at a time when the patient did have capacity should not normally be overridden, although this is not absolute. Medical professionals may conclude, for example, that ECT could be life-saving in a severely depressed patient with suicidal ideation.

Pain Pathways

Commentary
The neuraxial processing of nociceptive afferent input is formidably complex, and many details both of anatomical pathways and of neurotransmitter systems have yet to be elucidated. You will not be able to take complete refuge behind that complexity, however, because it is obvious that pain management is a central part of anaesthetic practice. You will be expected to provide at least a simplified account of how a pain stimulus travels from the periphery to the centre, and how it may be modulated within the CNS. Because the information does remain incomplete, however, you may be able to satisfy the examiners with a relatively limited account. You would be able to suggest, for example, that a drug might exert its effects by activating descending inhibitory noradrenergic pathways. There is little danger of being asked to develop this much further, because you might find yourself otherwise discussing some of the 20 or more neurotransmitters that are believed to act at the dorsal horn.

Core Information
- The primary afferent nociceptors comprise free, unmyelinated nerve endings that are responsive to mechanical, thermal and chemical stimuli. These are relatively, but not completely, specific. Mechanoreceptors and temperature receptors, for example, are nociceptors only above a certain threshold. Following tissue trauma, the release of chemical mediators initiates nociception while activating an inflammatory response.
- Stimulation of these nociceptive afferents leads to propagation of impulses along the peripheral nerve fibres to the spinal cord by two parallel pathways. The first is via myelinated A-δ fibres, of diameter 2–5 μm, and rapidly conducting at between 12 and 30 m s^{-1}. This type of pain is fast, localized and sharp, and provokes reflex withdrawal responses. The second route to the spinal cord is via non-myelinated C fibres, of smaller diameter (0.4–1.2 μm) and which conduct impulses more slowly at between 0.5 and 2.0 m s^{-1}. C fibres mediate pain sensations that are diffuse and dull.
- The primary afferents terminate in the dorsal horn of the spinal cord. The cell bodies lie in the dorsal root ganglia. A-δ fibres synapse in the laminae of Rexed I and V, while the C fibres synapse in the substantia gelatinosa. (This comprises lamina II and a part of lamina III.) They relay with various classes of second-order neurons in the cord, some of which are 'nociceptive-specific', which respond selectively to noxious stimuli and are located in the superficial laminae, and others of which are 'wide dynamic range', are non-specific and are located in the deeper laminae.
- Most of the secondary afferents decussate to ascend in the lateral spinothalamic tract, although some pass up the posterolateral part of the cord. These fibres pass through

the medulla, midbrain and pons, giving off projection neurons as they do so, before terminating in the ventral posterior and medial nuclei of the thalamus.

- From the thalamus there is a specific sensory relay to areas of the contralateral cortex: to somatic sensory area I (SSI) in the post-central gyrus, to somatic sensory area II (SSII) in the wall of the sylvian fissure separating the frontal from the temporal lobes and to the cingulate gyrus, which is thought to mediate the affective component of pain. The separation between sensory–discriminative and affective areas of the cortex is likely to be an oversimplification.

- **Modulation:** one of the major complexities of pain pathways is the modulation of afferent impulses which occurs at numerous levels, including the dorsal horn where there is a complex interaction between afferent input fibres, local intrinsic spinal neurons and descending central efferents. Afferent impulses arriving at the dorsal horn themselves initiate inhibitory mechanisms which limit the effect of subsequent impulses. As pain fibres travel rostrally, they also send collateral projections to the higher centres such as the periaqueductal grey (PAG) matter and the locus ceruleus of the midbrain. Descending fibres from the PAG project to the nucleus raphe magnus in the medulla, and to the reticular formation to activate descending inhibitory neurons. These travel in the dorsolateral funiculus to terminate on interneurons in the dorsal horn. These fibres from the PAG are thought to be the main source of inhibitory control. Descending inhibitory projection also derives from the locus ceruleus. The inhibitory activity mediated from the PAG is also stimulated by endorphins released from the pituitary and which act directly at that site.

- **'Gate' control:** this represents one aspect of modulation. Synaptic transmission between primary and secondary nociceptive afferents can be 'gated' by interneurons. These neurons in the substantia gelatinosa can exert pre-synaptic inhibition on primary afferents and post-synaptic inhibition on secondary neurons, thereby decreasing the pain response to a nociceptive stimulus. The inhibitory internuncials can be activated by afferents which subserve different sensory modalities, such as pressure (A-β fibres). This phenomenon underlies the use of counter-irritation, dorsal column stimulation, TENS and mechanical stimulation ('rubbing it better'). Descending central efferents from the PAG and locus ceruleus can also activate these inhibitory interneurons.

- **Transmitters:** these are numerous. Excitatory amino acids such as glutamate and aspartate have a major role in nociceptive transmission at the dorsal horn, where there are NMDA, non-NMDA, kainite, glutamate, AMPA, neurokinin, adenosine, 5-HT, GABA, α-adrenergic receptors and μ, κ and δ opioid receptors. The primary afferents release various peptides, among them substance P, neurokinin A and calcitonin gene-related peptide (CGRP). There are different neurotransmitters in the various descending inhibitory pathways, which include neuropeptides (enkephalins and endorphins) in the PAG, metenkephalin and 5-HT in the nucleus raphe magnus pathway and noradrenaline in the locus ceruleus descending pathway.

Supplementary and Clinical Information

- The usual target for analgesics is via ligand–receptor blockade, and the large number of receptor types means that you will only be able to give one or two examples of where in the neuraxis analgesics exert their effects. Opioid receptors, for instance, are expressed in the cell body of the dorsal root ganglion and transported both centrally to the dorsal horn and peripherally. There are also receptors at higher centres such as the periaqueductal grey matter, and so opioids exert their actions at numerous sites in the CNS. Ketamine acts on the open calcium channel of the NMDA receptor, amitriptyline modifies descending noradrenergic pathways, clonidine and dexmedetomidine act at pre-synaptic and post-synaptic α_2-receptors, and NSAIDs predominantly have a peripheral action which attenuates the hyperalgesia associated with the inflammatory response. The future may lie in analgesics that will regulate gene expression and exert selective modification.

The Complex Regional Pain Syndrome (CRPS)

Commentary

Complex regional pain syndrome (CRPS) types I and II are important examples of neuropathic pain. The condition is seen almost exclusively in chronic pain management clinics, and you may well have little direct experience of its main features and management. Neuropathic pain, however, complicates many disease states, is severe and difficult to treat, and remains incompletely understood. For this reason it continues to appear as a popular examination topic.

Core Information

- **CRPS types I and II** are the names given to what were formerly known, respectively, as reflex sympathetic dystrophy and causalgia. In some, but not all cases, sympathetically maintained pain may be a prominent feature.
- **CRPS type I** (formerly known as reflex sympathetic dystrophy or Sudek's atrophy) is associated with injury to tissue – bones, joints and connective tissue – but not to major nerves. The trauma may be relatively trivial, and is most commonly precipitated by an orthopaedic injury to a distal extremity such as the lower leg or wrist.
- **CRPS type II** (formerly known as causalgia), by contrast, is characterized by significant nerve injury without transection. It is more commonly associated with proximal nerves in the upper leg and upper limb. Most frequently affected are the sciatic, tibial, median and ulnar nerves.
- **CRPS:** in type I there may be pain of a more diffuse nature, whereas in type II there may be more discrete localization to the distribution of a single nerve, but otherwise the differences between the two types are largely academic and most authorities no longer pursue the distinction. Overall the treatments are the same.
- **Sympathetic mediation:** the subdivision into sympathetically maintained pain (SMP) or sympathetically independent pain (SIP) applies to both types.
- **Pathophysiology:** this remains incompletely understood, but it has both peripheral and central components. A chronic peripheral inflammatory process is suggested by elevated local levels of inflammatory markers (interleukin-8 and tumour necrosis

factor-α) with suppression of some anti-inflammatory mediators (cytokines IL-4 and IL-10). The inflammatory actions of neuropeptides such as bradykinin and Substance P may also be enhanced. (This hypothesis arose from the observation that there may be a link between treatment with ACE inhibitors and CRPS. In addition to blocking angiotensin converting enzyme, this class of drug reduces the metabolism of other peptides, including bradykinins and Substance P.) There are, in addition, alterations of central afferent processing, such as 'wind-up', with the persistent perception of non-noxious afferent inputs as painful. The pain may also be maintained by efferent noradrenergic sympathetic activity as well as by circulating catecholamines, although the lack of any significant response to sympathetic blockade suggests that this is of lesser importance. The upregulation of α_2-adrenoceptors in local axons may be responsible for sudomotor dysfunction. There is usually no communication between sympathetic efferent and afferent fibres, but following injury it is apparent that modulation of nociceptive impulses can occur not only at the site of injury but also in distal undamaged fibres and the ipsilateral dorsal root ganglion itself, around which sympathetic axons may proliferate. It is speculated that reperfusion injury may also be a precipitant of a vicious cycle in which cytokines and free radical species damage endothelium with the further release of cytokines and persistent nociception.

Supplementary and Clinical Information

Typical Clinical Features

- Symptoms include burning and constant pain, allodynia (which is pain provoked by an innocuous stimulus and which occurs in about one-third of cases), hyperpathia (which is an abnormally intense painful response to repetitive stimuli) and hyperalgesia (which is an exaggerated pain response to a noxious stimulus).
- The pain is accompanied by signs of failure of autonomic regulation in the region affected. These include swelling and local oedema, temperature changes due to vasomotor instability, associated skin colour changes and abnormal sudomotor activity.
- There may be associated weakness and trophic changes, with loss of the normal healthy appearance of skin, which thins and becomes translucent; of hair; and of nails. There is also focal atrophy of underlying tissue, including muscle, and this in turn may precipitate focal osteoporosis.

Current Treatments

- **Early treatment and prevention:** there is some evidence from controlled trials that early stellate ganglion block following upper limb trauma prevents onset in some patients, as does treatment with vitamin C (ascorbic acid, 500 mg for 50 days), which antagonizes oxygen free radicals.
- **Sympathetic block (diagnostic):** if this is effective it will both diagnose the presence of sympathetically maintained pain and initiate its treatment, although the evidence for benefit is disputed. Procedures include stellate ganglion block as previously described, lumbar sympathectomy and plexus blocks.

- **Sympathetic block (therapeutic):** a series of blocks may confer benefit which increases in duration after each one, or which may confer only temporary relief which finally disappears. Several agents have been used in intravenous regional anaesthesia (IVRA). These include guanethidine, clonidine and bretylium. Randomized controlled trials have demonstrated IVRA with guanethidine to be worse than placebo (IVRA with NaCl 0.9%). Some patients may be considered for a permanent neurolytic procedure (best if performed within 12 months of injury), but symptoms can recur as early as 6 months.

- It has been recommended that all treatment be directed towards functional restoration, so any window during which analgesia is satisfactory should be used for rehabilitation and sensory desensitization. Physiotherapy is important to minimize functional disability.

- **Dorsal column stimulation:** spinal cord stimulation has been used both in CRPS types I and II. Low-frequency pulsed stimulation appears to be a successful method of attenuating the pain associated with CRPS type II. Results otherwise have been equivocal, partly because the frequency and duration of stimuli have varied significantly between studies.

- **Transcutaneous electrical nerve stimulation (TENS):** this may benefit some patients (unlike acupuncture, for which there is little evidence of efficacy).

- **Free radical scavengers:** some evidence from RCTs does support the use of the oxygen free radical scavengers dimethyl-sulphoxide and N-acetylcysteine, which dampen the inflammatory response.

- **Membrane stabilizers:** A controlled trial of gabapentin 1,800 mg day^{-1} showed no benefit, and there is no other convincing supporting evidence of the efficacy of this or related compounds. Evidence for the benefit of tricyclic antidepressants such as amitriptyline or membrane stabilizers such as phenytoin remains anecdotal, but their use is based nonetheless on a substantial body of clinical experience.

- **Calcium modulating drugs:** calcitonin and biphosphonates (both of which inhibit bone resorption) may ameliorate symptoms in early CRPS. Radiographic osteoporotic changes can be seen as soon as 2 weeks after the onset.

- **Simple analgesics:** codeine, co-drugs and non-steroidal anti-inflammatory drugs may give some patients relief. There are no robust data to support their prescription.

- **Opioids:** these are said to be effective in the early stages of the condition.

- **Glucocorticoids:** these may help the acute inflammatory stages of the disease process but are typically given in very high doses (e.g. methylprednisolone starting at 100 mg day^{-1} and reducing in pulses by 25 mg every 4 days).

- **NMDA antagonists:** there are reports that ketamine given by low-dose subcutaneous injection or infusion can be beneficial. Side effects associated with racemic ketamine have limited its use, but development of the S enantiomer may allow it to be evaluated more widely.

- **Intravenous immunoglobulin:** single low-dose infusion (0.5 g kg^{-1}) may improve pain transiently in patients with long-term symptoms.

- **Capsaicin:** topical capsaicin depletes peptide neurotransmitters from primary afferents and may be of benefit.

- **Psychotherapy and pain management programmes:** as with most chronic pain states, this is probably the most important part of the multidisciplinary approach.

(If you mention it too early, however, you do run the risk of appearing to give a generic and therefore potentially less convincing answer.)

Diabetic Ketoacidosis (DKA and HONK)

Commentary

This will be as much a question about the pathophysiology of these medical emergencies as their management. To discuss the formation of ketones in diabetic ketoacidosis (DKA) you will need to know some of the pathways of intermediary metabolism. Make sure at least that you can explain the final steps which lead to the characteristic metabolic acidosis. In practice, anaesthetists become involved only infrequently with cases of DKA because although they require intensive management, they rarely require intensive care. The other hyperglycaemic emergency, hyperosmolar non-ketotic acidosis (HONK), variously called hyperosmolar non-ketotic coma or hyperosmolar hyperglycaemic state (HHS), is less common than DKA but may also be part of the discussion.

Core Information

- **Definition:** DKA is a serious complication of diabetes mellitus. It can occur both in type 1 insulin-dependent, and type 2 non-insulin-dependent disease, although it is more common in the former. It is characterized by the biochemical triad of hyper-glycaemia, metabolic acidosis and ketonaemia and is a manifestation of an extreme disorder of carbohydrate metabolism.
- **Pathogenesis:** DKA follows a decrease in the effective levels of circulating insulin, sometimes secondary to acute illness which is accompanied by an increase in the plasma concentrations of glucose and also of counter-regulatory stress hormones, the most important of which are glucagon, catecholamines, cortisol and growth hormone.
- **Gluconeogenesis:** in the presence of insulinopaenia, hyperglycaemia occurs as a result of gluconeogenesis, accelerated glycogenolysis and impaired glucose utilization by peripheral tissues. Gluconeogenesis is enhanced by a large number of gluconeo-genetic precursors, which include amino acids from proteolysis. Increased glycogen-olysis in muscle also produces lactate (CH_3–$CHOH$–$COOH$), which is converted in the presence of lactate dehydrogenase to pyruvate (CH_3–C=O–$COOH$), whose concentration rises as a consequence of all these effects. Glycerol from increased lipolysis, mainly in adipose tissue, makes a small contribution, but there is otherwise no pathway of conversion of lipid to glucose. There is also an increase in the activity of a range of gluconeogenetic enzymes. (These are numerous, but as an example, catecholamines increase the activity of glycogen phosphorylase.) Of these various mechanisms which lead to hyperglycaemia, it is hepatic and renal gluconeogenesis which quantitatively are the most important.
- **Lipid and ketone metabolism:** pyruvate is at the gateway of the citric acid cycle (Krebs cycle, tricarboxylic acid cycle) of aerobic metabolism. Two molecules of pyru-vate become incorporated into each molecule of acetyl-coenzyme A (acetyl-CoA),

and so the concentration of acetyl-CoA increases. At the same time, insulin inhibits hormone-sensitive lipase, while counter-regulatory hormones, particularly adrenaline, activate it. There follows at least a doubling of the plasma concentrations of free fatty acids (FFAs), whose metabolic utilization also takes place via acetyl-CoA. When the pathways are saturated, excess acetyl-CoA condenses to form acetoacetyl-CoA. This is then converted in the liver (via a deacylase) to free acetoacetate, which in turn is a precursor of β-hydroxybutyrate, acetoacetate and acetone. These three compounds are known as ketone bodies. β-hydroxybutyrate and acetoacetate are the anions of the strong acids acetoacetic acid and β-hydroxybutyric acid. (β-hydroxybutyrate is the more important of the two, being three times as abundant.) The acids fully dissociate at body pH and are buffered. When the buffering capacity is exceeded, metabolic acidosis supervenes. (In health, ketones are a useful energy substrate, being utilized by brain, heart and muscle.)

Hyperosmolar Non-Ketotic Acidosis (HONK)

- **Hyperosmolar hyperglycaemic acidosis:** this is more accurately called hyperosmolar hyperglycaemic non-ketotic state, because one of the diagnostic features is a pH that is close to normal (>7.30). The condition is less common than DKA and typically presents in patients with type 2 diabetes and in an older age group, usually in their sixties (reported average age is 57–69 years) rather than in their thirties as is the case with DKA. It is usually precipitated by a dehydrating illness, most commonly by infection, but a large number of physiological and pharmacological stressors can provoke the same effect. In up to 40% of cases HONK is the first presentation of diabetes. Patients may present with altered cerebration (although coma is a feature of fewer than 20% of cases), clinical signs of severe dehydration and with deranged biochemistry: glucose >33 mmol l^{-1}, serum osmolality 320 mOsm kg^{-1} or greater, pH >7.30, HCO_3 >15 mmol l^{-1}, but with no ketonaemia. Quoted mortality is high at 10–20%.
- **Pathophysiology:** type 2 diabetics have either reduced levels of insulin, insulin resistance at the cellular level or both. An acute illness with the attendant physiological stress further reduces circulating insulin while stimulating a rise in counter-regulatory hormones. The resulting hyperglycaemic hyperosmolality leads to osmotic diuresis vigorous enough to cause sodium and potassium loss as well as intracellular dehydration. Although this cycle is similar to that which takes place in the genesis of DKA, these patients do not become ketonaemic or profoundly acidotic. The reasons are not fully understood, although it may be that there is sufficient residual insulin to prevent ketogenesis. Counter-regulatory hormone levels are lower in HONK than in DKA, and in addition hyperosmolar states inhibit lipolysis and thereby reduce the amount of substrate for the ketogenic reactions outlined earlier.

Supplementary and Clinical Information

- **Presentation:** a typical patient with DKA will present with the symptoms and signs of diabetes mellitus, namely polyuria, polydipsia, pronounced dehydration and weight loss. In addition, their mental state may be obtunded, and they may hyperventilate owing to the metabolic acidosis (Kussmaul breathing). Their breath is characteristically ketotic, owing to the exhalation of volatile acetone. Abdominal pain, diarrhoea, and nausea and vomiting may also be evident, most commonly in children. Dehydration of muscle, gastric stasis and paralytic ileus have all been advanced as possible causes for this, although the case is unconvincing. Patients with HONK are severely dehydrated but without the clinical symptoms and signs of ketosis and acidosis.

Management

- **Precipitants:** there is always a precipitating cause of DKA and HONK. Disparate factors can be involved, some of which are amenable to treatment. Onset can be provoked by infection, inadequate insulin treatment, alcohol abuse, trauma, myocardial infarction and the use of certain drugs, amongst them β-adrenoceptor blockers, corticosteroids and thiazide diuretics.
- **Assessment:** initial assessment can broadly follow the Airway, Breathing, Circulation algorithm, with particular emphasis on the patient's mental state and their volaemic status. Dehydration is usually severe, particularly in HONK. There are various methods of determining the fluid deficit. An orthostatic rise in heart rate without a change in blood pressure indicates an approximate 10% decrease in extracellular volume or a deficit of about 2 litres. An orthostatic fall in mean blood pressure of 10–12 mmHg indicates a 15–20% deficit (3–4 litres), while supine hypotension suggests dehydration greater than 20% (4 litres or more). Known acute weight loss is a more accurate guide.
- **Investigations:** those specific to DKA and HONK should encompass arterial blood gases, plasma glucose, electrolytes, ketones and serum osmolality. Other investigations may include urinalysis, a full blood count and differential, blood and urine cultures, chest X-ray and ECG. The blood lactate is usually normal.
- **Treatment aims:** the goals are to restore normovolaemia and adequate tissue perfusion, to reduce plasma glucose and osmolality towards normal, to clear ketones at a steady rate (in DKA) and to correct the deranged acid–base and electrolyte status.
- **DKA management – fluids and insulin:** management of DKA need not be complex and it need not be hurried; it may take 12–16 hours to get the condition well under control, and the metabolic acidosis may persist for some days. Initial resuscitation should be with NaCl 0.9% (unless the corrected Na^+ is greater than 150 mmol l^{-1}), given at a rate of 1.0–1.5 litres in the first hour. This can be reduced to 300–500 ml h^{-1} thereafter, titrated against response. Some authorities advocate giving bolus intravenous insulin (0.15 units kg^{-1}) followed by an infusion at a rate of 0.1 units kg^{-1} h^{-1}, while others recommend omitting the bolus dose. A rate of 0.1 units kg^{-1} h^{-1} is adequate to obtain high physiological levels of insulin, and there is no evidence that an initial bolus dose has any influence on outcome.
- **HONK management:** correction of dehydration is the first priority, initially with NaCl 0.9% 1.0–2.0 litres over 1–2 hours. Insulin should not be given until the volaemic status has improved, otherwise the cellular uptake of K^+, glucose and water will further deplete the intravascular compartment. Thereafter, glucose 5% should be given to further replete intracellular dehydration, at which point insulin (with K^+) can be given at a starting rate of 0.1 units kg^{-1} h^{-1} and aiming initially for a blood glucose concentration of around 15 mmol l^{-1}, and keeping it at between 10–15 mmol

l^{-1} for 24 hours. Too rapid a correction can be associated with the development of cerebral oedema, particularly in the rare cases of HONK in children.

- **Phosphate:** phosphate, like potassium, shifts from the intracellular to the extracellular compartment, while the osmotic diuresis contributes to urinary losses. During treatment of DKA the phosphate re-enters cells to unmask the total body depletion. There are theoretical problems associated with hypophosphataemia which include muscle weakness, haemolytic anaemia, cardiac depression and depleted 2,3-DPG, but there is no evidence that supplemental phosphate improves outcome in these cases. The mean phosphate deficit is around 1 mmol kg^{-1}.

- **Bicarbonate:** the administration of HCO_3^- remains contentious. Bicarbonate does not cross the blood–brain barrier, and so, if given, it will worsen intracellular cerebral acidosis. It can also reduce extracellular potassium and may provoke cardiac arrhythmias. If the patient's pH is >6.8, there is no evidence of any outcome benefit.

- **Complications:** cerebral oedema can supervene if glucose concentration drops too fast. It may also follow excessive fluid therapy as well as the administration of bicarbonate.

- **'Euglycaemic ketoacidosis':** This is a described entity whose name is misleading. By 'euglycaemic' is meant a blood glucose concentration of less than 16.7 mmol l^{-1}, and so in some patients the sugar will still be relatively high. The key factor in its pathogenesis appears to be the patient's recent oral intake. If the patient is well fed, then liver glycogen stores are high and ketogenesis is suppressed. If the patient has been unable to eat, for example because of intractable vomiting, then glycogen stores are depleted and the liver is primed for ketogenesis.

Spinal Cord Injury

Commentary

This question occurs more commonly in the exam than in most anaesthetists' clinical practice. The incidence of traumatic spinal cord injuries in the UK is quoted as around 13 cases per million head of population per year, and so two to three individuals are paralysed each day. Anaesthetists may be involved in their immediate care, but the more difficult and, from the examiners' point of view, more interesting aspects of spinal cord injury, tend to occur once they have been transferred to specialist centres. Your own knowledge, as well perhaps as that of your examiner, is likely to be largely theoretical, and the emphasis of the oral will be on the applied anatomy and pathophysiology of the condition, with some emphasis on the effects of lesions at different spinal levels.

Core Information

Acute Spinal Cord Injury

- The clinical signs depend on the level of injury. More than 50% of spinal injuries occur in the cervical region because in comparison with the thoracic and lumbar spines, it is mobile and unprotected. In adults, the fulcrum of the cervical spine is at $C_{5/6}$, which is the commonest site of cord damage. (In children the fulcrum is higher.) The remaining injuries are divided equally between the thoracic, thoraco-lumbar and lumbosacral regions. Primary damage is due to several mechanisms: traction forces occurring particularly at junctions where the spinal conformation changes, haemorrhage and direct cord compression, most commonly by subluxed vertebrae. Injuries involving the cervical cord are associated with tetraplegia; those at T_1 and below result in paraplegia.

- **Patterns of spinal cord injury:** Data from the USA, where the incidence of acute spinal cord injury appears to be almost three times greater than in the UK, indicate that there is complete tetraplegia in 19% of injuries, complete paraplegia in 28%, incomplete tetraplegia in 30% and incomplete paraplegia in 21%. In tetraplegia, it is C_5 which is the commonest level of neurological injury. In paraplegia, it is at T_{12} and L_1.

- **Neurogenic shock:** Immediately following acute cord injury there is a massive catecholamine surge with associated hypertension and tachycardia. (This is more marked with cord damage at higher levels). This rapidly gives way to the phase of 'neurogenic shock', which denotes the marked peripheral vasodilatation, hypotension and bradycardia consequent on the loss of sympathetic efferent pathways. Unopposed vagal tone is high, and should there be further vagal stimulation the risk of asystolic cardiac arrest is high unless vagolytics such as atropine or glycopyrronium are given. Hypotension can be fluid resistant, and in common with intracranial catastrophes, acute spinal cord injury may also precipitate neurogenic pulmonary oedema (up to 40% in some series). Management therefore needs to be cautious, with vasopressors rather than excessive fluid used to increase systemic blood pressure. This period of neurogenic shock is variable and may be short-lived; equally it may persist for some weeks.

- **Spinal shock:** A subsequent phenomenon is that of 'spinal shock', which is the period during which all spinal cord reflexes are profoundly depressed or abolished. There is complete flaccid paralysis below the level of the lesion, including loss of bowel and bladder function. Usually within days, however, the reflex spinal arcs begin to regain function, and this in due course develops into the phases of early and late hyperreflexia.

Immediate Management of Spinal Cord Injury

- The early management of cord injury includes immobilization and a standard approach to Airway, Breathing and Circulation. (There may also be associated trauma to other structures.) As with acute head injury management, the emphasis is on minimizing secondary damage by avoiding hypoxia, hypertension, hypercapnia and acidosis. Tracheal intubation may be necessary if there is any suggestion of respiratory compromise, and patients with lesions at C_3, C_4 or C_5 are likely to have lost some or all diaphragmatic function. Vital capacity at best will be 5–10% of normal with absent cough. A lower cervical injury spares the diaphragm, but breathing is still affected with vital capacity around 20% of normal. The expansion of the ribcage via the intercostals and accessory muscles of respiration is responsible for up to 60% of normal tidal volume. High thoracic lesions (T_2, T_3, T_4) reduce vital capacity to 30–50% of normal, but injury at lower levels of the cord will spare the intercostal muscles and so respiratory compromise is much less of a problem. If ventilation is impaired, sputum retention and chest infection may follow, and this is the commonest cause of death in the first 3 months after injury. In the spontaneously breathing tetraplegic patient, it is the supine position that is associated with the greater diaphragmatic excursion (the abdominal contents help move the diaphragm rostrally during expiration), and so these patients initially should be nursed flat.

- **Level of injury.** Summarized (and outlined previously): **High cervical** (C_3, C_4 or C_5) injuries compromise some or all diaphragmatic function. Vital capacity at best will be 5–10% of normal with absent cough. **Low cervical** (C_6, C_7) injuries spare the diaphragm but reduce vital capacity to 20% of normal. **High thoracic** injuries (T_2, T_3, T_4) reduce vital capacity to 30–50% of normal. **Low thoracic** injuries spare the intercostals and interfere least with respiratory function. Autonomic and spinal hyperreflexia are more pronounced the higher the level of cord injury.

- Spinal cord injury is a dynamic process in which secondary injury begins immediately with haemorrhage, vasogenic oedema and the release of inflammatory mediators and the formation of damaging free radical oxygen species. This risks enlarging the area of damage, and it is common for the injury level to rise by one or two segments in the first few days. This may be crucial; a C_5 lesion that rises to C_3 may mean the difference between spontaneous respiration and a lifetime of ventilator dependency. Apart from avoiding the physiological insults described earlier, however, there are no specific measures available to treat this cascade of problems.

- **Corticosteroids:** evidence from the North American Spinal Cord Injury study (NASCIS II), supported by a Cochrane review, suggested that high-dose methylprednisolone 30 mg kg^{-1} showed some benefit in reducing the extent of injury. This was offset by an increase in sepsis and possibly by a higher mortality rate, and as a result this intervention is not recommended by UK specialists in the field, and high-dose steroids are not given routinely.

Supplementary Information and Clinical Considerations

Anaesthesia in the Patient with Spinal injury

In the **acute phase**, anaesthesia can proceed as for any other emergency while giving consideration to the autonomic dysfunction described previously.

- **Suxamethonium:** this can be used to facilitate emergency tracheal intubation, but only in the acute phase, because within about 48–72 hours after the acute injury, there is proliferation of acetylcholine receptors in extrajunctional areas of the denervated muscle. Administration of suxamethonium results in a large efflux of potassium into the circulation. This dangerous hyperkalaemic response is proportional to the amount of muscle that is involved and may persist for as long as 9 months.

In the **chronic phase** of spinal injury, anaesthesia can be problematic.

- When spinal reflexes start to return, they are hyperreflexic. The normal supraspinal descending inhibition of the thoracolumbar autonomic outflow is lost, and so there occurs a mass reflex sympathetic discharge in response to stimulation below the level of the spinal lesion. There are changes in denervated muscle as well as the development of collateral neurons in the various reflex pathways. With time, the threshold appears to drop, together with the spread of stimulation across reflex centres. This explains why the mass response may be provoked by relatively minor stimuli.

- Both cutaneous and visceral stimuli (particularly associated with bladder distension, other genitourinary stimulus and bowel disturbance) can provoke this reflex response. It is confined to the area below the level of transection, where the autonomic nervous system is not subject to any inhibitory influences; proximally there is compensatory parasympathetic overactivity. It is rare in lesions below T_{10}.
- The clinical features of this response include muscle contraction and increased spasticity below the lesion. There may be vasoconstriction and severe hypertension that can be accompanied by tachycardia or compensatory bradycardia. Other cardiac arrhythmias may occur. Above the level of the lesion there may be diaphoresis and flushing. The more distant the dermatome that is stimulated from the lesion, the more emphatic is the sympathetic response. Autonomic hyperreflexia is more pronounced the higher the lesion in the cord, and the more limited the capacity for parasympathetic compensation.
- Patients may require surgery following cord injury, and autonomic hyperreflexia will complicate anaesthetic management. Reflex discharges can be prevented reliably by neuraxial block, although if an epidural is used it is important to ensure that the sacral segments are anaesthetized. Dense subarachnoid anaesthesia will prevent hyperreflexia completely. Deep anaesthesia or the use of vasoactive drugs to treat developing hypertension are less successful.

Immunology (and Drug Reactions)

Commentary
This is potentially a large topic but does include an aspect of particular interest to anaesthetists, namely severe adverse drug reactions. (The results of NAP 6, the Sixth National Audit Project, will in due course give more epidemiological information about perioperative anaphylaxis in the UK.). Allergic reactions is the area where the oral may end up, but not before you have been asked to give an overview of the immune system. Detailed discussion of T lymphocyte function or of cytokines would itself take up most of the time, and so questioning on these subjects is likely to be superficial. The basic science emphasis does mean, however, that you will have to demonstrate familiarity with the major components of immunity. What follows is necessarily a simplification of what is an entire medical sub-specialty.

Core Information
Basic components of the immune system.

Innate or Non-Specific Immunity
- The body has a number of non-specific defences against infection. These include the skin; the antimicrobial secretions of sweat, sebaceous and lacrimal glands; and the

mucus of the gastrointestinal tract and the upper airway to which organisms may adhere. The acidic environment of the stomach is hostile, and the lower gut is populated with commensals which prevent the overgrowth of less benign species.

- **Non-specific immune defences** do not recognize the substance that is being attacked and are activated immediately in response to potential threats, for example, from infectious agents. These defences include the activation of the alternative complement pathway (see following), phagocytosis by neutrophils, macrophages and mast cells, and the inflammatory response itself.
- **Inflammatory response:** this allows cells and proteins to reach extravascular sites by increasing the blood supply by vasodilatation, by increasing vascular permeability, by encouraging the movement of various inflammatory cells to the site of injury and by activating the immune system.
- **Leucocytes:** these comprise neutrophils (60–70% of the total), which are responsible for phagocytosis and inflammatory mediator release; basophils (1%), which are the circulatory equivalent of tissue mast cells; monocytes (2–6%), which function in the blood like macrophages; eosinophils (1–4%), which destroy helminths and other parasites, and which may mediate hypersensitivity reactions; and lymphocytes (20–30%). Most lymphocytes mediate specific immune defences, but NK (natural killer) lymphocytes bind non-specifically to tumour cells and to virus-infected cells.
- **Macrophages:** these are ubiquitous cells that are derived from monocytes. They destroy foreign particles by phagocytosis, mediate extracellular destruction via the secretion of toxic chemicals and also secrete cytokines. These are a complex set of soluble protein messengers that regulate immune responses and include the interleukins, tumour necrosis factor, colony-stimulating factors and interferons.

Acquired or Specific Immunity

- **Lymphocytes:** specific immunity involves recognition of cells or substances to be attacked, and lymphocytes are the mainstay of the specific immune system. B lymphocytes differentiate into plasma cells which synthesize and secrete antibody. T lymphocytes comprise helper cells (T-helper, *Th*) and killer cells (cytotoxic, *Tc*). NK cells are non-specific. *Th* cells produce a large number of cytokines in a process that links the innate and specific components of the immune system.
- **Antibodies:** these immunoglobulins are proteins which bind specifically with antigens, which contain two identical light and two identical heavy chains, and which are characterized as IgA, IgD, IgE, IgG and IgM. IgG is the most abundant and is the only immunoglobulin which crosses the placenta.

Supplementary and Clinical Information

You may be asked about adverse reactions to drugs. Not all of the described hypersensitivity reactions are necessarily involved in drug reactions, but a summary is included for completeness. This is because whenever Type I reactions are mentioned, the examiners will want to see if you are familiar with the rest of the classification.

- **Hapten formation:** most drugs are of low molecular weight and are not inherently immunogenic; they can, however, act as haptens by interacting with proteins to form stable antigenic conjugates.

The traditional classification of hypersensitivity into four types was originally described by Gell and Coombs, and is outlined here.

- **Hypersensitivity reactions:** these are abnormal reactions involving different immune mechanisms, often with the formation of antibodies. They occur on second or subsequent exposure to the antigen concerned. Four types have been described.
  - **Type I (immediate):** this is the classic anaphylactic, immediate hypersensitivity reaction, which is mediated by IgE. IgE is synthesized by B cells on first exposure to the antigen and binds to mast cells. On repeated introduction, the antigenic drug–protein complex degranulates mast cells with the release of a number of preformed vasoactive substances. These include histamine, heparin, serotonin, leukotrienes and platelet-activating factor. (Mast cells are numerous in skin, the bronchial mucosa, in the gut and in capillaries.) The term 'immediate' may mask the fact that Type I reactions can be biphasic, with a secondary response occurring up to 72 hours after the initial event but without re-exposure to the antigen.
  - **Type II (cytotoxic):** in this reaction, circulating IgE and IgM antibodies react in the presence of complement to mediate reactions which cause cell lysis. Such reactions can lead to haemolysis (caused, for example, by sulphonamides), thrombocytopenia (heparin, thiazide diuretics) and agranulocytosis (carbimazole, NSAIDs, chloramphenicol).
  - **Type III (immune complex):** the reaction of antibody and antigen produces a circulating immune complex (precipitin), which deposits in small vessels, in the glomeruli and in the connective tissue of joints. These precipitins also activate complement via the classical pathway. Type III reactions underlie many autoimmune diseases, including rheumatoid arthritis and systemic lupus erythematosus (SLE).
  - **Type IV (delayed):** this is the delayed hypersensitivity reaction, which is cell-mediated without complement activation and without the formation of antibodies. The reaction results from the combination of antigen with T (killer) lymphocytes and macrophages attacking the foreign material. This mechanism underlies the development of contact dermatitis. Granuloma formation in diseases such as tuberculosis and sarcoidosis is a result of a large antigen burden or the failure of macrophages to destroy the antigen. This 'granulomatous hypersensitivity' is also a Type IV response.

An alternative classification has since been proposed (by Sell and co-workers) which expands the reactions into seven categories: antibody reactions due to activation or inactivation (Gell and Coombs Type I), antibody reactions leading to cell lysis (Type II), immune complex reactions (Type III), T-cell cytotoxic reactions (Type IV), delayed hypersensitivity reactions (Type IV), granulomatous reactions (Type IV) and other 'allergic reactions'. This classification accommodates some of the overlap between components of the immune system but has not yet displaced the original.

- **Complement:** complement is an enzyme system consisting of 20 or more serum glycoproteins which, in combination with antibody, are activated in a cascade that results in cell body lysis. In summary, the complement system coats (opsonizes) bacteria and immune complexes, activates phagocytes and destroys target cells.

The final pathway is the amalgamation of complement proteins C5–C9 into a complex that disrupts the phospholipids of cell membranes to allow osmotic cytolysis. The classical complement pathway is a specific immune response that is initiated by the reaction of antibody with complement protein C1 and its subcomponents. The alternative pathway is a non-specific response that can be activated in the absence of antibody, but in the presence, for example, of anaesthetic agents, drugs or bacterial toxins.

- **Anaphylactoid reactions:** clinically, these may resemble anaphylactic reactions, but they involve the direct release of vasoactive substances (histamine, serotonin) from mast cells or from circulating basophils rather than release mediated via an antigen–antibody response.

Investigation of a Suspected Drug Reaction

- **Investigation of a reaction:** non-specific markers include urinary methyl histamine, which increases in the first 2–3 hours following a reaction, and mast cell tryptase. This enzyme is responsible for activating part of the complement cascade (it cleaves C3 to form C3a and C3b), and serum concentrations are elevated for about 3 hours after a reaction. A clotted blood sample should therefore be taken as soon as possible after emergency resuscitation and another 1 hour later. Patients can further be investigated by skin testing (at 6 weeks or longer after the event) and by assays of drug-specific antibodies using radioallergoabsorbent (RAST) tests. Negative skin tests do not exclude allergy, and patients should then be given an oral or intravenous challenge, with all resuscitation facilities immediately available.
- **Management of an anaphylactic (and anaphylactoid) reaction:** see under 'Latex Allergy' in the immediate next section.

Latex Allergy

Commentary

Latex allergy was first recognized in the late 1970s, since which time the use of latex in the surgical environment has become ubiquitous. More than a decade ago it was identified as a cause of anaphylaxis, and is the second commonest cause under anaesthesia (20% of cases). Secondary to prolonged exposure to latex-containing products, the prevalence of sensitivity amongst healthcare workers has been estimated at between 7 and 13%. It is an important cause of unexplained intraoperative collapse.

Core Information

- Latex is natural rubber produced from the milky sap of the rubber plant (*Hevea brasiliensis*). It consists not only of proteins but also contains lipid and carbohydrate molecules. It is the soluble proteins that cause severe allergic responses. The powder in some surgical gloves can bind to these latex proteins which are then released into the operating theatre atmosphere, where they can remain for several hours. It is for this reason that patients with severe latex allergy should be first on the operating list. Latex proteins can be inhaled, absorbed across mucous membranes or injected intravenously via equipment that inadvertently has been contaminated.

- The reactions to latex products include simple irritant contact dermatitis, and allergic contact dermatitis, which is a Type IV T cell–mediated hypersensitivity reaction to the chemicals used in manufacture. The potentially fatal response to latex exposure is a Type I IgE-mediated hypersensitivity reaction. Sensitized individuals produce IgE antibodies to latex proteins which, on re-exposure, may lead to an anaphylactic reaction with massive histamine release from mast cells and basophils (see under 'Immunology (and Drug Reactions)').

Identification of Patients at Risk, and Peri-Operative Management

- **Identification:** Type I hypersensitivity is best diagnosed by skin-prick testing. As long as the testing solutions contain a range of specific latex allergens, this has a sensitivity of 97% and specificity of 100%. Radioallergoabsorbent tests (RAST) may identify latex-specific IgE but have a 25% rate of false positive and false negative results. In the absence of such evidence the diagnosis is clinical. There may be a history of sensitivity to rubber products; also at risk are individuals who have been exposed repeatedly to latex products. Healthcare workers, patients undergoing repeated urinary catheterization such as those with spina bifida or others who need to self-catheterize, and patients who have undergone multiple surgical operations are included in this group. The patient may have a history of atopy and multiple allergies. There is cross-reactivity with a number of foods, among them kiwi fruit, avocado, papaya and chestnuts. Patients may also describe allergy to poinsettia plants.
- **Perioperative management:** all latex-containing products must be identified and avoided. Latex is ubiquitous and is found in trolley mattresses, pillows, TED stockings (those for the lower leg are latex-free), surgical gloves, elastic bandages, urinary catheters and surgical drains. Anaesthetic equipment which may contain latex includes the rubber bungs in some drug vials, which should therefore be removed before they are made into solution, some giving sets, blood pressure cuffs, face masks, nasopharyngeal airways, breathing systems and electrode pads. Recognition of this problem, however, has meant that latex-free equipment is now so widely available that many hospitals no longer need a separate trolley or box containing specific items for the latex-allergic patient. It is routine to insist that such patients should be placed first on a list to minimize the risk of exposure to airborne latex particles released during previous surgical procedures.

Supplementary and Clinical Information

- **Diagnosis:** the onset of a reaction to latex is typically much slower than those associated with intravenous drugs, and it may take 30–40 minutes to manifest.
- **Diagnosis:** in an established anaphylactic reaction the patient will be hypotensive, with angio-oedema or an urticarial rash, and have severe bronchoconstriction. Hypotension is commoner as a main feature than bronchoconstriction, but the latter may be much more refractory to treatment. Only one system may be involved,

and few patients will manifest the full range of clinical features. The onset of an anaphylactic reaction can sometimes be heralded by more subtle signs such as sneezing or coughing (precipitated by histamine release), and by the slower development of cutaneous signs.

- **Management:** after discontinuing contact with the trigger substance, management can follow the **A**irway, **B**reathing, **C**irculation algorithm. The patient should be given 100% oxygen and positioned supine with the legs and pelvis elevated to enhance venous return. The mainstay of treatment is adrenaline, which can be given initially in a dose of 0.5 mg (0.5 ml of 1:1,000) by intramuscular injection into the lateral thigh. Anaesthetists are likely to prefer intravenous administration; typically 50–100 μg over a minute and repeated according to response. Severe cases may need adrenaline by infusion at a rate of 100 μg min^{-1}. Secondary treatment can include corticosteroids, antihistamines and bronchodilators, although these are much less important than adrenaline, which is potentially life-saving.

- **Confirmation:** a blood sample should be taken for mast cell as soon as possible after the reaction begins followed by another between 1 and 2 hours but no later than 4 hours. A further sample can be taken 24 hours or longer after the event to measure levels during the 'convalescent' phase. (Tryptase is a protease that is found in all human mast cells and is a reliable marker of mast cell activation.)

Jaundice

Commentary

In routine practice it is rare to encounter deeply jaundiced patients. The outline science of the topic will occupy part of the oral, and its relevance to clinical medicine is obvious. Hepatic disease is a large subject, but you will be expected to recall the important implications for anaesthesia, among which are the hepatorenal syndrome and coagulopathy.

Core Information

- Jaundice (icterus) is the yellowing of skin, sclera and mucous membranes which occurs as a result of the accumulation of bilirubin (either free or conjugated) in the blood. The normal bilirubin concentration is less than 17 μmol l^{-1}, and jaundice is not usually detectable clinically until it reaches around 35 μmol l^{-1}. (Some authorities quote a higher figure of 50 μmol l^{-1}.)

- Bilirubin is formed from the breakdown of haemoglobin in the reticuloendothelial system. The polypeptides of the haemoglobin molecule (the 'globin') are separated from the haem moiety, which in turn is catabolized to biliverdin. Haem is an iron-containing porphyrin derivative. Biliverdin is converted to bilirubin prior to excretion in bile.

- Fat-soluble unconjugated bilirubin binds to albumin in the circulation and is transported to the liver, where it dissociates prior to conjugation with glucuronic acid.

As the water-soluble bilirubin diglucuronide, it is excreted via the bile canaliculi. A small amount gains access to the circulation to be excreted in urine.

Causes of Jaundice

There are four potential causes of hyperbilirubinaemia. It may be caused by excess production, by defective uptake into hepatocytes, by deficient intracellular binding or conjugation and by problems with secretion of bilirubin into the biliary system.

- **Increased bilirubin production:** the major cause is haemolytic anaemia. Free bilirubin concentrations rise, but rarely exceed 50 μmol l^{-1} because the liver has substantial reserve capacity to handle the excess.
- **Decreased hepatic bilirubin uptake:** diminished intake of bilirubin into hepatocytes occurs in Gilbert's disease, which causes unconjugated non-haemolytic hyperbilirubinaemia. It can also occur during the resolving phase of viral hepatitis. Free bilirubin concentration is rarely >50 μmol l^{-1}.
- **Defective bilirubin binding or conjugation:** this is characteristic particularly of premature neonates whose enzyme systems may be immature. It also occurs in rare (and usually fatal) diseases such as Crigler–Najjar syndrome. Free bilirubin concentrations rise.
- **Diminished secretion into the biliary system:** there are both extrahepatic and intrahepatic causes of a rise in conjugated bilirubin concentrations. Biliary outflow may be obstructed by gallstones (common), and by biliary and pancreatic carcinoma (rare). Intrahepatic cholestasis is associated with numerous conditions. It occurs in infective and alcoholic hepatitis, in severe cirrhosis of the liver, and as a result of primary biliary cirrhosis and sclerosing cholangitis. Cholestasis can occur in pregnancy (it is usually mild and is of unknown cause) and can be drug-induced. Implicated agents include oral contraceptives, anabolic steroids, sulphonamides and some neuroleptic agents, including chlorpromazine and haloperidol.
- These causes may combine: hepatocellular damage, for example, increases serum bilirubin by all four mechanisms.

Supplementary and Clinical Information

The Peri-Operative Implications of Jaundice

- **Aetiology:** the cause may be important because of accompanying morbidity; cirrhosis, for example, may be associated with alcoholic cardiomyopathy.
- **Coagulopathy:** the liver synthesizes many of the protein clotting factors, including prothrombin (factor II) and the other vitamin K-dependent factors (VII, IX and X). Jaundice may be associated with derangements of coagulation.
- **Myocardium:** bile salts can depress the myocardial conduction system and cause significant bradycardia.
- **Renal system:** anaesthesia in the presence of liver dysfunction can be followed by the hepatorenal syndrome, in which acute renal failure may supervene in the immediate postoperative period. The cause remains unknown, although it is presumed to be due to a hepatic endotoxin that the damaged liver can no longer contain. Management recommendations include the use of generous fluid therapy with the use of mannitol

to enhance urine output. The risk is particularly great if bilirubin concentrations exceed 180 μmol l^{-1}.

- **Infective hepatitis (B and C):** anaesthesia in the acute phase is invariably deleterious to hepatic function. Theatre staff must also be protected against the risks of contamination.
- **Drug elimination:** the reserve even of the damaged liver is great, but the normal mechanisms by which drugs are excreted may be impaired. Cytochrome P450 enzymes are converted to the inactive cytochrome P420. Hypoproteinaemia may increase the proportion of free active drug.
- **SpO$_2$ monitoring:** the absorption coefficient of bilirubin is similar to that of deoxygenated haemoglobin, and so SpO$_2$ will read artificially low. (This applies both to peripheral and cerebral oxygenation monitoring.)
- **Postoperative jaundice:** causes *de novo* include haemolysis following blood transfusion and adverse drug reactions. All volatile anaesthetics are metabolized in the liver, and halothane hepatitis is a well-recognized entity. The use of halothane is now negligible in the UK, but hepatitis of unknown aetiology has been reported rarely following the use of enflurane, isoflurane and sevoflurane.

The Arterial Tourniquet

Commentary
The arterial tourniquet seems at first sight to be a mundane piece of equipment on which to be examined. Its use is so widespread that it is easy to become complacent. The tourniquet is, however, associated with a range of potential complications, not all of which are immediately obvious, and so you will need to show both that you are aware of these and that you are able to minimize the risks.

Core Information
The indications for, and contraindications to, the use of an arterial tourniquet.

- **Indications:** the arterial tourniquet is used primarily to produce a bloodless field for extremity surgery. It also allows intravenous regional anaesthesia (IVRA, 'Bier's block') and intravenous regional sympathectomy with drugs such as guanethidine. As part of the isolated forearm technique, it has been used as a tool for researching anaesthetic awareness (see under 'Depth of Anaesthesia Monitoring' in Chapter 5) and in specialist oncological centres for isolated limb perfusion with high-dose chemotherapy for patients with localized soft tissue cancers.
- **Contraindications:** these are mainly relative. Tourniquets should be avoided in patients with major trauma to the operated limb, in patients with localized infection or tumour (both of which in theory can be disseminated) and in those with peripheral vascular disease (particularly affecting the leg). They should be used with caution in those with poor cardiac reserve or a fixed output state. Sickle cell disease has

traditionally been viewed as an absolute contraindication, but a number of studies have reported uneventful use of tourniquets providing that the general principles of sickle cell management have been observed and the limb has been exsanguinated effectively. The ischaemic tissue nonetheless still provides the hypoxic, hypothermic and acidotic environment most likely to promote red cell sickling, and so the risk of using a tourniquet must be evaluated carefully. Pulmonary embolism may complicate their use in patients who are at high risk of venous thrombosis.

The Physiological Consequences and Complications of Its Use

- **Arterial tourniquet:** the system comprises a cuff, a gas source and a pressure gauge which keeps cuff pressure at a preset value. The limb can be exsanguinated using arterial pressure and elevation, a pneumatic air exsanguinator or an Esmarch bandage (which is the most effective method).
- **Mechanical pressure effects:** these affect skin, muscles, nerves and blood vessels. Skin is most likely to be damaged by the shearing stresses caused by a tightly wound Esmarch exsanguinator. These can generate pressures as high as 1,000 mmHg and are also more likely to cause nerve injury than pneumatic devices.
- **Neurological damage:** nerves under the cuff itself are vulnerable; intraneural microvascular injury and oedema can lead to axonal degeneration. Injury is secondary both to ischaemia and to pressure. Direct mechanical compression effects are most likely at the edges of the cuff where shearing forces are highest and where there is a high differential pressure between compressed and non-compressed nerves. The radial is the nerve most at risk in the upper limb; the sciatic nerve in the lower. Impaired nerve conduction may not recover completely for 6 months.
- **Muscular and vascular damage:** Muscles directly beneath the cuff are also subject to pressure effects but are more likely than nerves to be adversely affected by ischaemia. There is evidence of microvascular damage and muscle fibre necrosis after only 2 hours of tourniquet ischaemia. The overall spectrum of injury that has been reported includes persistent post-tourniquet weakness, swelling due to local oedema and generalized discomfort. This is the result of reactive hyperaemia which increases blood flow to the muscles on deflation of the cuff, but into a circulation with increased vascular permeability. This constitutes the 'tourniquet syndrome', which can last up to 6 weeks. Compartment syndrome and rhabdomyolysis have also been described, but both are very rare. Atheromatous vessels can be traumatized, particularly in the lower limb, and peripheral vascular disease increases the risk of thrombus formation.
- **Duration:** a safe limit has not been established, but a 2-hour tourniquet time is a commonly recommended maximum, both to limit direct pressure effects and the potential damage to distal tissues owing to prolonged ATP depletion and progressive tissue acidosis. Risks are higher in the elderly, in those with peripheral vascular disease and if the limb is injured. The cuff can be deflated periodically as long as a reperfusion time of at least 10 minutes is allowed. Pre-tourniquet cooling of the limb can double 'safe' tourniquet time, but in practice this is rarely done.
- **Systemic effects – inflation:** limb exsanguination is a form of rapid autotransfusion. A single thigh tourniquet, for example, may divert 400 ml of blood into the circulation. This sudden increase in blood volume is usually well tolerated, but it may

threaten haemodynamic stability in patients with precarious cardiac function or a fixed output state such as mitral stenosis.

- **Systemic effects – deflation**
  - **Cardiovascular:** upon deflation of the cuff there is a fall in systemic vascular resistance, with decreases in arterial and central venous pressures as blood moves back into the now hyperaemic circulation of the reperfusing limb. This may last for 10–15 minutes.
  - **Respiratory:** as residual hypercarbic blood in the ischaemic limb rejoins the systemic circulation, there is a brief increase in the expired CO_2 tension which peaks at around 1 minute. The $FeCO_2$ (fractional concentration of expired CO_2) can rise by as much as 2.5 kPa but falls to baseline levels within a few minutes. Predictably these changes are more marked with lower limb tourniquets.
  - **CNS:** this transient increase in $PaCO_2$ is associated with an increase in cerebral blood flow, blood volume and intracranial pressure. Although this is usually insignificant, it can be important in trauma patients with closed head injuries.
  - **Reperfusion syndrome:** see under 'The Blood Supply to the Lower Limb' in Chapter 2.
- **Metabolic changes:** accumulation of lactate and potassium proportional to the duration of ischaemia results in transient plasma rises during reperfusion and causes a mild metabolic acidosis that corrects within around 30 minutes. (The limb venous pH is typically 7.0 after 2 hours' inflation time.)
- **Coagulation:** increased platelet aggregation owing to tissue compression and catecholamine release is offset by enhanced systemic thrombolysis (caused by release of tissue plasminogen activator) after tourniquet deflation. Emboli formation during all lower limb surgery is common; however, there is a fivefold increase in the risk of large venous thrombosis in patients undergoing total knee replacement in whom a tourniquet is used.
- **Temperature changes:** heat transfer from the core to the exsanguinated area is negligible and so central temperature can rise. This process is reversed following cuff deflation. Redistributed blood loses heat to the cool limb, which quickly becomes hyperaemic. Transient temperature falls of up to 0.7 °C have been reported.
- **Tourniquet pain:** in the awake patient, this is a dull, poorly localized but intense discomfort that intensifies with time. In both awake and anaesthetized patients, it is associated with hypertension and tachycardia. Pain may persist even in the presence of dense neuraxial or deep general anaesthesia. Its likely mechanism is complex. High pressure appears to prevent nerve conduction in fast A-δ pain fibres, while having less effect on the smaller non-myelinated slow-conducting C fibres which continue to transmit cutaneous impulses.
- **Complications secondary to leakage:** faulty or incorrectly applied cuffs can allow unintended access of drugs to the systemic circulation during IVRA. This is particularly dangerous with large volumes of local anaesthetic or with high-dose cytotoxic chemotherapeutic agents. Rapid injection through small syringes (which generate higher pressures than larger ones) may allow venous pressure to exceed cuff pressure.
- **Incidence of complications:** despite this list of potential problems the incidence of significant complications is low. In one large Norwegian survey of more than 63,000 cases, the reported rate of persistent complications was only 0.04%.

- **Safe practice and minimizing risk:** much of this is common sense. Equipment must be well maintained. Occlusion pressures and tourniquet inflation time should be minimized. The gauge pressure can be misleading; what is important is the pressure per unit area. This will be higher in a narrow cuff, or in a large limb where the pressure will be greatest at its widest point. Ideally the cuff that is used should be conical, thus exerting pressure more evenly around the limb. At the least it must be the correct size. Inflation pressure need be little higher than that needed to occlude arterial flow. Some have recommended using Doppler probes to detect the loss of peripheral flow before inflation to 50 mmHg above that level. In routine practice the tourniquet is usually inflated to around 100–150 mmHg above the systolic pressure, with the higher pressures reserved for the lower limb. Finally, tourniquets must be protected from contamination.

Arterial Cross-Clamping

Commentary
Arterial cross-clamping may be used in various operations, including carotid end-arterectomy and lower limb revascularization procedures. The most significant physiological effects, however, are seen after clamping of the aorta, and it is these on which the oral is likely to focus.

Core Information
Pronounced physiological changes occur both on the application and the release of the cross clamp, but these vary substantially according to the level at which the aorta is clamped. They will also vary according to any associated myocardial pathology. This is highly likely in patients with abdominal aortic aneurysms and peripheral vascular disease, but much less so in patients who have, say, connective tissue abnormalities which weaken the media of the thoracic aorta.

Application of an Aortic Cross Clamp
- **Cardiovascular effects: increased afterload.** Clamp application leads to an immediate increase in afterload, with a sudden increase in proximal arterial blood pressure, a reflex increase in myocardial contractility (the Anrep effect) and a concomitant increase in myocardial oxygen demand. This may partially be offset by increased coronary blood flow (depending on the patency of the coronary circulation) and a decrease in heart rate mediated by baroreceptors. There is also an increase in preload, which is attributed both to the passive elastic recoil of arterial vessels distal to the clamp that effectively autotransfuses blood into the venous circulation and to sympathetic vasoconstriction in the splanchnic bed which occurs in response to the effective hypovolaemia and which can redistribute as much as 800 ml of blood centrally. This manifests as an increase in left ventricular end diastolic volume and

pressure. If renal afferent arteriolar perfusion pressure falls, there is activation of the renin-angiotensin system with increased renin production. This appears to occur even if the clamp is infrarenal.

- **Aortic clamp level. Infrarenal.** An infrarenal clamp is probably the commonest site in vascular surgical practice and is associated with the least haemodynamic instability. Afterload increases only by around 5–7%, and a heart with reasonable left ventricular function is relatively unaffected. (Any increase in preload is also modest.) If, however, the patient does have ischaemic heart disease, then they may develop significant ventricular wall motion abnormalities. If the ventricle dilates, an increase in wall tension may initiate a vicious cycle of increased myocardial oxygen demand and the potential for further ischaemia. **Suprarenal/infracoeliac.** If the clamp is applied more proximally at a suprarenal but infracoeliac level, the increase in afterload is more marked, with a rise in mean arterial pressure (MAP) of up to 10%. **Supracoeliac.** If the clamp is supracoeliac, however, MAP can increase by more than 50% with a 35–40% decrease in left ventricular ejection fraction. **Descending thoracic aorta.** At even higher levels of cross clamping, such as in the descending thoracic aorta, MAP can rise by 80% and central venous pressure by 35%. These changes may partly be attenuated in those patients who have occlusive aortic disease and who may have developed a collateral circulation.
- **Associated complications:** these include myocardial ischaemia as described previously, distal arterial occlusion secondary to embolic plaques of atheroma which can be dislodged as the clamp is applied and ischaemia of the spinal cord. Figures for cord damage vary but have been quoted as 0.2% for elective procedures involving an infrarenal clamp, from 5–8% for elective and as high as 40% after emergency thoracic aneurysm repair (see under 'The Blood Supply to the Spinal Cord in Chapter 2). Suprarenal clamps are associated with acute kidney injury. All of these problems increase with the duration of cross-clamp time.

Release of an Aortic Cross Clamp

The haemodynamic effects of releasing an aortic cross clamp are qualitatively the same as those that follow any situation in which a previously ischaemic area is reperfused. An obvious example is the deflation of an arterial tourniquet following lower limb surgery. The quantitative effects, however, vary substantially depending on the duration of ischaemia, which in a difficult aneurysm repair may be prolonged.

- **Reperfusion injury:** see under 'The Blood Supply to the Lower Limb' in Chapter 2.
- **Haemodynamic changes:** the anaerobic metabolism in the ischaemic areas generates significant vasoactive metabolites, including hydrogen ions, lactate and potassium. Once these enter the general circulation, they mediate a significant fall in peripheral vascular resistance. Typically this may fall by as much as 70–80% with a concomitant drop in blood pressure of 40–60%. This is due both to the effective hypovolaemia (distal blood flow can increase fourfold with the sequestration of blood in reperfused tissues) as well as to the direct myocardial depressant effects of cytokines and other molecules. Coronary blood flow and left ventricular end diastolic volume can drop by 50% unless measures are taken to preempt the problem. Arrhythmias may accompany the transient hyperkalaemia.

Supplementary Information and Clinical Considerations

Attenuation of Haemodynamic Insults

- **Application of clamp.** Attenuation of the increase in afterload can be achieved using a venodilator such as glyceryl trinitrate (GTN at a starting rate of 0.5 μg kg^{-1} min^{-1}), by increasing the inspired concentration of volatile anaesthetic or both. Some anaesthetists use opioids, but these are more difficult to titrate against response and depending on the agent used may still be exerting an effect when the clamp is released. The increased capacitance proximal to the clamp also allows a degree of fluid loading to prime the system.
- **Release of clamp.** Any vasodilator infusion should be stopped in advance. Depending on the height of the clamp and its duration, rapid fluid administration will usually be needed to mitigate the problem of functional hypovolaemia. Vaso-pressors can be effective, but only in the presence of adequate fluid resuscitation. In theory, an increase in alveolar ventilation may partially offset the induced metabolic acidosis, although this is not routine.

Pharmacology

Mechanisms of Action of General Anaesthetics

Commentary

This has long been the focus of fundamental research which this oral will not have time to explore in depth. The subject matter is complex, and although selective effects on CNS proteins appear to offer the most complete explanation, much remains unexplained.

Core Information

Theories about Mechanisms Underlying General Anaesthesia

- Compounds that cause reversible insensibility range from xenon, which is chemically unreactive and whose monoatomic structure could not be simpler, to barbiturates and phenols, whose structures are both more complex and completely dissimilar. This makes the search for a unifying theory of action with particular emphasis on a specific structure–activity relationship more difficult. The Unitary Hypothesis acknowledges this but simply asserts that whereas the molecular structures may be very diverse, all general anaesthetic agents must exert their effects via a similar, although as yet a not fully understood, mechanism.

- **Meyer–Overton hypothesis:** Meyer and Overton (separately) were the first to relate the potency of anaesthetic agents to their lipid solubility. They argued further that the onset of narcosis was evident as soon as the particular substance had attained a certain molar concentration in the lipids of the cell, and that the lipid layers of the cell membrane represented the main site of action. Much early research was based on the hypothesis that disruption of the lipid bilayer affected the function of membrane proteins and mediated an interruption of neuronal traffic. As a unifying theory, however, it was undermined by the observations that temperature rises disrupt lipid membranes without inducing a state of general anaesthesia, and that there are many compounds with high-lipid solubility which exert no anaesthetic effect. Nonetheless, there remains a clear relationship between anaesthetic potency and lipid solubility which any theory of action must accommodate.

- **Clathrate theory:** it was proposed that anaesthetic agents form hydrates (clathrates) and from these microcrystals which aggregate in cell membranes to affect their function. At body temperature, however, very high pressure is needed for clathrate formation, and this alone makes the hypothesis unsustainable.

- **Pressure reversal:** it was discovered that anaesthesia induced with halothane in tadpoles and in mice could be reversed by subjecting them to pressure, a process which was assumed to restore the normal configuration of the cell membrane. The pressures required to reanimate these creatures, however, were in excess of 50 atmospheres, and so the volume expansion theory is also untenable.

- **Voltage-gated ion channels:** general anaesthetic agents appear to exert minimal effect at voltage-gated ion channels.

- **Transmitter-gated ion channels (TGIC):** ligand-gated membrane ion channels have been the focus of most recent investigations. They include the gamma-aminobutyric acid ($GABA_A$) receptor, as well as $5-HT_3$, acetylcholine, glutamate and glycine receptors. As membrane-bound proteins, these receptors contain integral anion-conducting channels, whose function is altered by the allosteric effects of a number of disparate compounds.

- **$GABA_A$:** $GABA_A$ is the major inhibitory neurotransmitter receptor system (accounting for around 30% of all inhibitory synapses), which makes it a prime candidate for a major site of action of general anaesthetics. Experimental work confirms that various compounds, including volatile and intravenous induction agents, enhance the ability of GABA to open the $GABA_A$ receptor ion channel. Almost all general anaesthetic agents, with the exceptions of xenon and ketamine, appear to influence the $GABA_A$ receptor at therapeutically relevant concentrations. The receptor consists of a pentameric arrangement of different subunits around the central ion channel pore. There are 18 subunits (α_{1-6}, β_{1-3}, γ_{1-3}, δ, ε, π, ρ_{1-3}) and a total of around 30 receptor isoforms. Complex research techniques have shown that single amino acid substitutions within the receptor subunit have a marked influence on anaesthetic effect, which confirms the highly specific interaction of drug and receptor. In respect of benzodiazepines, for example, it appears as though the α_1 subunit mediates sedation and amnesia, whereas the α_2 subunit is responsible for anxiolysis.

- **Two-pore domain K^+ channels:** these channels are found both pre- and post-synaptically throughout the nervous system. They are voltage-independent and appear to become hyperpolarized by some anaesthetic agents, particularly the volatile halogenated hydrocarbons.

- **Glycine receptors:** the glycine receptor is the spinal cord and brain stem analogue of the $GABA_A$ receptor of the brain. This too contains an integral chloride channel and is affected by general anaesthetic agents.

- **$5-HT_3$ and neuronal nicotinic acetylcholine receptors:** general anaesthesia affects cationic currents through these receptors, but further than this the function of these central receptors is not fully understood.

- **Glutamate receptors:** these consist of the N-methyl-D-aspartate (NMDA) and non-NMDA receptor classes, which comprise the primary excitatory neurotransmitter system in the brain. Inhibition of their function is therefore consistent with a theory of general anaesthesia. Ketamine, xenon and nitrous oxide all inhibit the NMDA receptor. The non-NMDA glutamate receptors are divided into various subclasses (AMPA and kainate), which are both strongly affected by ethyl alcohol but not by volatile anaesthetics.

- **Neurotoxicity:** there has been emerging concern about the effects of anaesthetic drugs, including the volatile agents, on the developing and on the ageing brain. Almost all the data have been derived from animal studies, primarily in rodents, and so can be extrapolated to humans only with extreme caution. Nonetheless, some studies have shown substantial increases in neuroapoptosis (programmed cell death) in animals exposed to NMDA-type glutamate receptor antagonists and GABA$_A$ agonists, along with evidence of persistent neurocognitive defects. The effects appear to be dose-dependent and additive with the use of multiple agents. There is, in addition, at least one study in primates to suggest that a single prolonged exposure to general anaesthesia before neurodevelopmental maturity can be associated with long-term cognitive impairment. There are, however, minimal human data. There are a number of retrospective cohort studies in children which have suggested an association between anaesthesia before the age of 4 and developmental or behavioural abnormalities, but overall the findings do not demonstrate a consistent effect, and clearly there are several confounding variables, including the dose and duration and nature of the agent(s) used and in what combination, the nature of the surgical insult and patient co-morbidities. Isolating the effects of anaesthetics on the elderly brain is equally problematic, particularly as there is some evidence of a neuroprotective (ischaemic preconditioning) effect conferred at lower doses. The chronic neurodegeneration that results in dementia is characterized by, amongst other processes, the accumulation of fibrillary tangles that consist of hyperphosphorylated microtubule-associated tau protein. Many anaesthetic agents appear to accelerate this process, although in the elderly there are even more confounding variables than in the neonate or infant. Given that clinical evidence for these adverse effects is weak, it would be premature to modify general anaesthetic techniques, but at both extremes of age it might assist the arguments of those who favour regional or neuraxial techniques. Studies in the elderly look predominantly at outcomes, but there are currently a number of prospective trials under way. The GAS (General Anesthesia Spinal) study is a multicenter trial in infants undergoing herniorraphy who are randomized either to general or to spinal anaesthesia. The subjects will be subjected to developmental and cognitive tests at ages 2 and 5 years. The PANDA (Pediatric Anesthesia and Neurodevelopment Assessment) study aims to recruit 1,000 children, or 500 sibling pairs, who undergo single-exposure general anaesthesia for herniorrhaphy before the age of 36 months, with assessments at 8 and 15 years of age. (The MASK [Mayo Safety in Kids] study is another large retrospective comparison of children receiving general anaesthesia before the age of 3 with a set of controls.) The eventual importance of these studies is self-evident and may well have a significant impact on future paediatric anaesthetic practice.

- **Conclusion:** those who searched originally for a unifying theory of general anaesthetic action could not have envisaged the research techniques that have begun to identify the highly complex structures of CNS receptors. Although many details remain to be elucidated, it now seems clear that the spectrum of altered physiological states characterized by anaesthesia is mediated by highly specific interactions of anaesthetic compounds with receptor proteins.

Chirality

Commentary

The science of chirality is somewhat indigestible, and you might feel aggrieved were this to be the only pharmacology that you were given the opportunity to discuss in the exam. The widespread use of levobupivacaine, and to a lesser extent ropivacaine, however, has given this subject some relevance (as suggested by the trade name 'Chirocaine'), and so even if you cannot unravel the nomenclature convincingly, you will have to be prepared to talk about drugs which can be presented as pure enantiomers. (If you are struggling for facts it may help if you remember that in the case of the newer drugs, 'R' stands for 'riskier' and 'S' stands for 'safer'.)

Core Information

Chirality and Isomerism

- 'Chirality' is derived from the Greek, means 'having handedness', and defines a particular type of stereoisomerism. Right and left hands are mirror images of each other but cannot be superimposed when the palms are facing in the same direction. There are many drugs which exist as right- and left-handed forms that are mirror images but which cannot be superimposed. These particular isomers are known as 'enantiomers' ('substances of opposite shape'), and this form of stereoisomerism is dependent on the presence of one more chiral centre; typically a carbon atom with four groups attached. These enantiomers have the capacity to rotate polarized light and so are also known as optical isomers. Their physicochemical properties are otherwise identical. Confusion can arise because of the differing nomenclature that has been used to describe chiral substances.
- One convention describes optical activity: enantiomers that rotate plane polarized light to the right are described as (+). This is the same as (dextro) or (d). Enantiomers that rotate plane polarized light to the left are described as (−), which is the same as (laevo or levo) or (l).
- Another convention, which is largely historical but nonetheless confusing, is based on the configuration of a molecule in relation to (+) glutaraldehyde, which was arbitrarily assigned a 'D' (not 'd') configuration. Compounds were denoted 'D' or 'L' according to comparison with the model substance, and the optical direction added where appropriate. This method of description is limited to stereoisomers of amino acids and carbohydrates.
- The currently accepted convention assigns a sequence of priority to the four atoms or groups attached to the chiral centre. The molecule is described as though it were

being viewed from the front, with the smallest group extending away from the viewer. If the arrangement of the largest to the smallest groups is clockwise, then the enantiomer is designated 'R' for 'rectus'. If the arrangement is anticlockwise, it is designated 'S' for 'sinister'. The optical direction is then added to complete the description. This gives, for example, S (+) prilocaine, and R (+) tramadol. Drug manufacturers have contributed to residual confusion about nomenclature by calling S (−) bupivacaine 'levobupivacaine', whereas logic (but not commercial interest) dictates that it should have been called 'sinister bupivacaine'.

- A racemic mixture is one which contains equal numbers of isomers or enantiomers.

Supplementary and Clinical information

Drugs such as bupivacaine and prilocaine are racemic mixtures. The more favourable safety profile of single enantiomer preparations has given chirality more immediate anaesthetic relevance.

- Chiral drugs that are found in nature are usually single enantiomers because they are synthesized enzymatically in reactions that are stereospecific. Such drugs include adrenaline (epinephrine), atropine, cocaine, ephedrine, hyoscine, morphine and noradrenaline (norepinephrine). All are levorotatory and still have the designation (l).
- Most synthetic chiral drugs are racemic mixtures and are less potent than the pure enantiomers because the d-forms are much less active. This is not surprising, because drug receptor sites are likely to contain chiral amino acids which are stereoselective.
- The clinical behaviour of the enantiomers, and in particular their toxicity, is related to the chiral form, which is of particular relevance to a number of anaesthetic-related compounds.
- **Bupivacaine:** the S (−) enantiomer has less affinity for, and dissociates quicker from, myocardial sodium channels. The risk of cardiovascular and CNS toxicity is reduced. The S (−) enantiomer also exerts some vasoconstrictor activity.
- **Ropivacaine:** this is the pure S (−) enantiomer of propivacaine. It also has a safer cardiovascular profile in overdose.
- **Prilocaine:** the S (+) enantiomer is a stronger vasoconstrictor and is metabolized more slowly than the R (−) form, which therefore produces higher concentrations of o-toluidine and a greater risk of methaemoglobinaemia.
- **Lidocaine:** this is achiral.
- **Ketamine:** the S (+) enantiomer has a greater affinity for its main binding site (the NMDA receptor) and is up to four times as potent as the R (−) form. Its administration is also associated with fewer emergence and psychotomimetic phenomena.
- **Etomidate:** this presented as the pure R (+) enantiomer ('R' in this case standing for 'required effect' rather than 'risk').
- **Isoflurane, enflurane, desflurane, halothane:** these are all chiral compounds that show some stereoselectivity in action. This selectivity is too modest to warrant their production as pure enantiomers. **Sevoflurane** is achiral.
- **Tramadol:** tramadol is a racemic mixture of R (+) and S (−) enantiomers. The (+) enantiomer appears to have relatively low activity at μ receptors, but the higher

affinity of its main M1 metabolite results in a sixfold increase in analgesic potency. (The μ effects in humans are unimpressive.) The S (−) enantiomer inhibits the CNS re-uptake of noradrenaline and 5-HT.

Propofol

Commentary

Propofol is the most commonly used agent for induction of anaesthesia in the UK. It is also used in total intravenous anaesthesia (TIVA) and for sedation in intensive care. This makes it a core drug and so detailed knowledge will be expected. You may be asked to compare it either against the 'ideal' or against the other main intravenous hypnotics.

Core Information

- **Chemistry:** propofol is a substituted stable phenolic compound: 2,6-di-isopropyl-phenol. It is highly lipid-soluble and water-insoluble and is presented as either a 1% or 2% emulsion in soya bean oil. Other constituents include egg lecithin (which is a phospholipid) and glycerol. This would make it a potential culture medium, but whereas it is not an antimicrobially preserved product according to US Pharmacopeia reference standards (USP), the addition of the bacteriostatic disodium edetate (EDTA) reduces the risk of bacterial contamination. It is a weak organic acid with a pKa of 11. It is not contraindicated in patients who are allergic to eggs. Egg albumen is antigenic, whereas egg lecithin is not. (As suggested by the etymology, the word 'lecithin' is derived from the ancient Greek for 'egg yolk'.)
- **Mechanisms of action:** it enhances inhibitory synaptic transmission by activation of the Cl^- channel on the β_1 subunit of the $GABA_A$ receptor. This inhibits acetylcholine release in areas such as the prefrontal cortex and parts of the limbic system. It also inhibits the NMDA subtype of the glutamate receptor (see under 'Mechanisms of Action of General Anaesthetics'), and may have additional effects at cannabinoid receptors.
- **Clinical uses:** these include induction and maintenance of anaesthesia in adults and children, sedation in intensive care and sedation during procedures under local or regional anaesthesia. Its anti-emetic effects can benefit chemotherapy patients when given by low-dose infusion (although the evidence for this is disputed by some).
- **Dose and routes of administration:** the drug is used only intravenously. A dose of 1–2 mg kg^{-1} will usually induce anaesthesia in adults. Children may require twice this dose. TIVA infusion rates vary greatly, but would typically range between 4 and 12 mg kg^{-1} h^{-1} (or 4–8 μg ml^{-1} effective site concentrations). Propofol is an effective anti-emetic when given at a rate of 0.5–1.0 mg kg^{-1} hr^{-1}.
- **Onset and duration of action:** an induction dose of propofol will lead to rapid loss of consciousness (within a minute). Rapid redistribution to peripheral tissues (distribution half-life is 1–2 minutes) leads to rapid awakening.

- **Pharmacokinetics:** propofol is highly protein-bound (98%) and has a large volume of distribution (2–10 l kg^{-1}). As is frequently the case given the heterogeneity of human subjects, the reported pharmacokinetic data vary considerably with its distribution half-life quoted at between 1 and 8 minutes and the elimination half-life at 4–12 hours. It has a relatively short context-sensitive half-life which is quoted as being 40 minutes after infusions of duration up to 8 hours, which therefore makes it a suitable drug for total intravenous anaesthesia. Its metabolism is mainly, although not exclusively, hepatic, with the production of sulphate and glucuronide conjugates and other inactive metabolites which are excreted in urine.

Main Effects and Side Effects

- **CNS:** propofol causes CNS depression and hypnosis. CMRO$_2$ is decreased, as are cerebral blood flow and intracranial pressure. It may be associated with excitatory effects and dystonic movements, particularly in children. Hiccups are common after rapid injection. The electroencephalogram (EEG) displays initial activation followed by dose-related depression. In higher doses it is an effective anti-convulsant, so most anaesthetists ignore the data sheet assertion that it is contraindicated in patients with epilepsy.
- **Cardiovascular system:** systemic vascular resistance and preload fall, yet it is relatively unusual to see compensatory tachycardia. Relative bradycardia is more common. Propofol is a myocardial depressant, partly via the inhibition of calcium channels, so the reduction in contractility also reduces oxygen demand.
- **Respiratory system:** propofol is a respiratory depressant which also suppresses laryngeal reflexes. (Without this attribute it is unlikely that the use of the laryngeal mask airway would have become so well established. According to the inventor of the device, Dr Archie Brain, his early demonstrations using thiopental for induction did not go at all well.)
- **Gastrointestinal system:** when given by infusion (at a rate of 0.5–1.0 mg kg hr^{-1}) the drug attenuates chemotherapy-induced emesis.
- **Other side effects:** propofol causes pain on injection. Preparations which include medium-chain triglycerides in the formulation have reduced this problem. Long-term infusion, particularly in children but also in adult critical care patients, has been associated with 'propofol infusion syndrome'. In severe cases this is characterized by hyperlipidaemia, profound metabolic acidosis and rhabdomyolysis which can lead to renal and cardiac failure. The syndrome may be due to effects on mitochondria, either by direct inhibition of the respiratory chain of oxidative phosphorylation or by compromising mitochondrial metabolism of free fatty acids. This remains unproven. It is recommended that infusions should be limited to no more than a rate of 4 mg kg^{-1} h^{-1}, although this does not eliminate the risk of the syndrome. The data sheet for propofol states that it should not be used in pregnancy, but this increasingly is ignored, and many maternity units routinely use propofol for general anaesthesia for caesarean section.
- **Miscellaneous:** propofol is not a trigger for malignant hyperpyrexia, and it may also be used safely in patients with porphyria. It does not release histamine, and adverse reactions are very rare. It does not have any marked modulating effects on the immune system. (This is in contrast to volatile anaesthetics).

- **Propofol derivatives:** Fospropofol is a pro-drug that is converted to active propofol some minutes after intravenous injection, with the result that induction of anaesthesia or the onset of sedation is delayed. It has the benefit of not causing pain on injection, but like propofol, it can cause perineal pain or dysaesthesia (the mechanism of which remains unclear). It would appear therefore to have no material advantages over propofol and is unlikely ever to become a mainstream agent. More promising is the agent PFO713, which is a similar substituted phenol but with larger 2,6, side chains. It is not associated with pain on injection and causes less cardiovascular instability.

Supplementary Information
Target-controlled infusion (TCI) and total intravenous anaesthesia (TIVA)

- **Advantages:** many of these are based on opinion rather than evidence, but include good recovery characteristics, avoidance of inhalational agents and their pollution, less nausea and cardiostability.
- **Disadvantages:** perceived problems include the risk of awareness, linked to the wide variability between subjects, the complexity and cost of equipment and the importance of secure intravenous access.

Suitability of Propofol as an Agent for TCI
- It is a highly lipophilic hypnotic that distributes rapidly from blood to the effector site. It then undergoes further rapid redistribution to muscle and fat before being metabolized.
- The initial distribution half-life, α, of propofol is short (2–3 minutes), whereas intermediate distribution, β_1, takes 30–60 minutes. The terminal phase decline, β_2, is less steep and takes 3–8 hours. The immediate volume of distribution is 228 ml kg^{-1}, but the steady state volume of distribution in healthy young adults is around 800 litres.
- **Context-sensitive half-life (half-time):** this is the time taken for the plasma concentration to halve after an infusion designed to maintain constant blood levels is stopped. This is different not only for dissimilar drugs but also for the same drug depending on the duration of infusion. The context-sensitive half-life for propofol is 16 minutes after 2 hours of infusion, and 41 minutes after 8 hours. Although this compares less well with remifentanil (4.5 minutes and 9.0 minutes), it means, nonetheless, that accumulation is modest when the drug is infused for moderate periods.
- **Clearance:** the whole body clearance of propofol is 2,500 ml min^{-1}.

Ketamine

Commentary
Ketamine is unique amongst anaesthetic agents in that, by causing 'dissociative anaesthesia', a single dose can produce profound analgesia, amnesia and anaesthesia.

It finds its way into the exam more frequently than its clinical use might deserve, but investigation of the S (+) isomer as an agent with fewer side effects has renewed the drug's promise. Its dissimilarity from the other induction agents means that it may be the sole subject of the oral.

Core Information

- **Chemistry:** ketamine is a cyclohexanone derivative of phencyclidine (PCP), which is an anaesthetic agent used in veterinary practice and which is also a drug of abuse ('angel dust'). Ketamine is water-soluble and is presented in three different concentrations. The solution is acidic, at pH 3.5–5.5. Its pKa is 7.5. Most formulations now contain preservative, which precludes its use in central neural blockade, although preservative-free preparations can be obtained to allow its neuraxial injection. It is usually presented as a racemic mixture of two enantiomers, although the pure S (+) enantiomer is available in (and from) Europe. The S (+) enantiomer is three to four times as potent as the R (−) enantiomer, and is associated with shorter recovery times and with fewer psychotomimetic reactions. This is primarily because a lower dose of S (+) ketamine is required to induce anaesthesia. At equal plasma concentrations the recovery times and the incidence of psychological disturbance are the same.
- **Mechanisms of action:** ketamine is a non-competitive N-methyl-D-aspartate (NMDA) receptor antagonist at the Ca^{2+} channel pore. The NMDA receptor is an L-glutamate receptor in the CNS (glutamate being the major excitatory neurotransmitter in the brain) and incorporates a cation channel to which ketamine binds. In addition, it reduces pre-synaptic glutamate release. Ketamine also has effects on opioid receptors, acting as a partial μ (MOP) antagonist and as a partial agonist at κ (KOP) and δ (DOP) receptors. It may therefore exert its analgesic effects after intrathecal or extradural injection at spinal κ receptors. These opioid effects are not antagonized by naloxone. It also acts as an antagonist at serotoninergic, muscarinic, nicotinic and monoaminergic receptors. It may also inhibit sodium channels in neuronal tissue and so in high doses has local anaesthetic actions.
- **Onset and duration of action:** an induction dose of ketamine does not lead to hypnosis within one arm–brain circulation time. Consciousness will be lost after 1–2 minutes, but the patient may continue to move and to make incoherent noises. Intramuscular administration will take 10–15 minutes to take effect. The duration of action is between 10 and 40 minutes.
- **Doses:** The reported dose ranges are wide, but typically an intravenous dose of 1–2 mg kg^{-1} will induce anaesthesia. The intramuscular dose is 5–10 mg kg^{-1}. Sub-hypnotic doses for sedoanalgesia are usually up to 0.5 mg kg^{-1}. The addition of 0.5 mg kg^{-1} to a sacral extradural block in children with local anaesthetic will increase the duration of action fourfold, although concerns about neurodevelopmental toxicity preclude its use via this route in young children (aged 3 or less) (see under 'Mechanisms of Action of General Anaesthetics']). Nasal and oral doses are 6–10 mg kg^{-1}, and the rectal dose is 10 mg kg^{-1}. (Dose regimens for pain syndromes are varied and complex; patients with CRPS, for example, have been treated by infusions of 0.1–0.2 mg kg^{-1} h^{-1} over 5 days, but details will be well beyond the scope of this oral.)
- **Pharmacokinetics:** ketamine is highly lipid-soluble but weakly protein-bound (25%). It has high intramuscular bioavailability (93%), but oral bioavailability is only

20–25%. Via the nasal route bioavailability is reported as being around 50%. Metabolism is hepatic; demethylation and hydroxylation produce norketamine, which is an active metabolite of one-third the potency of ketamine, and dehydronorketamine, which is very weakly active at the NMDA receptor. Further metabolism produces conjugates which are excreted in urine.

- **Central nervous system effects:** ketamine is unique amongst anaesthetic agents in that it produces what is known as 'dissociative anaesthesia', which describes what in effect is a state of catalepsy. Corneal and pupillary reflexes, for example, are preserved, and the patient's eyes may remain open, but there is no purposeful response to stimuli. The 'dissociation' is essentially between the thalamus, which relays afferents from the reticular activating system, and the cerebral cortex and limbic systems. Its action both in the thalamus and in the limbic system is excitatory and not inhibitory. Afferent input is not affected, but essentially the central processing at thalamocortical and limbic levels is distorted. Ketamine is also a potent analgesic at doses much lower than those required to induce anaesthesia. It is amnesic. Anecdotally, it is reported that ketamine is less effective in brain-damaged patients. Unlike other induction agents, it increases $CMRO_2$, cerebral blood flow and intracranial pressure, but does not influence autoregulation.
- **Cardiovascular system:** ketamine is sympathomimetic and increases levels of circulating catecholamines. On isolated myocardium, however, it acts as a depressant. Indirect effects result in tachycardia, increases in cardiac output and blood pressure, and a rise in myocardial oxygen consumption.
- **Respiratory system:** it is a respiratory stimulant which is said to preserve laryngeal reflexes and tone in the upper airway (this is not always obvious at high doses). It is an effective bronchodilator.
- **Gastrointestinal system:** it causes salivation. As with most sympathomimetic anaesthetic agents, the incidence of nausea and vomiting is increased.
- **Other effects:** the use of ketamine has been limited by its CNS side effects. It is associated both with an emergence delirium and also with dysphoria and hallucinations. Emergence delirium is a state of disorientation in which patients may react violently to minor stimuli such as light and sound. The psychotomimetic effects are a separate phenomenon, which can become manifest many hours after apparent recovery from anaesthesia. Benzodiazepines may attenuate the problem.

Supplementary Information

- **Differences from other induction agents:** as detailed earlier, ketamine is both anaesthetic and analgesic, producing these effects by actions across a range of receptors. In contrast to propofol, thiopental and etomidate it is sympathomimetic, elevating levels of circulating catecholamines and increasing cardiac output and systemic vascular resistance. Ketamine is a respiratory stimulant which preserves laryngeal reflexes and tone in the upper airway. It antagonizes the effects of ACh and 5-HT on the bronchial tree and causes clinically useful bronchodilatation. It is used in the management of severe asthma that is refractory to other agents. The R (−) enantiomer appears to be a more effective antimuscarinic in this regard than the S (+) form. It is also different in that it is not limited to the intravenous and rectal routes but can also be given intramuscularly, orally, nasally, extradurally and intrathecally. Consensus has it that ketamine can probably (with caution) be used in patients with porphyria.

- **Clinical uses:** ketamine can be used for the induction of anaesthesia in adults and children, for so-called field anaesthesia as a single anaesthetic agent outside the hospital setting, for bronchodilatation and for sedoanalgesia during procedures performed under local or regional anaesthesia. Given extradurally or intrathecally it prolongs by three to four times the duration of analgesia provided by local anaesthetic alone. It is finding increasing use as a perioperative 'co-analgesic' when given in sub-hypnotic doses (for example, 25 mg intravenously) It can also be used in the treatment of chronic pain syndromes (see under 'The Complex Regional Pain Syndrome (CRPS)' in Chapter 3).
- **Ketamine as an antidepressant:** for decades, the monamine system has been the therapeutic target of drugs to treat depression (major depressive disorder, MDD) but around two-thirds of patients have little sustained benefit from treatment. Interest more recently has shifted to the glutamate system, as various studies have shown that a single sub-anaesthetic dose of ketamine can have an immediate and persistent antidepressive action. This shows therapeutic promise, but long-term therapy may be limited by side effects, particularly those affecting the urinary tract.
- **Ketamine bladder:** ketamine is also a drug of recreational abuse and it has become apparent that chronic misuse is associated in some users with severe bladder damage, in the worst cases necessitating total cystectomy. Chronic inflammation by urinary ketamine and its metabolites can result in ulcerative cystitis and irreversible fibrosis.

Thiopental and Etomidate

Commentary

It may seem perverse to link thiopental (thiopentone) and etomidate in the same question, but it may happen because thiopental is no longer the core agent that it once was. Its use, like that of etomidate, has shrunk to the point where in many units it is used mainly for emergency anaesthesia. Etomidate is the only other mainstream drug that is used solely as an induction agent (unlike propofol and ketamine), and so it is logical to explore their differences. (You may nonetheless be asked about one or the other.)

Core Information

- **Specific uses**: it can be argued that both thiopental and etomidate are now almost niche drugs that are used for very definite purposes. Both lead to rapid loss of consciousness in one arm–brain circulation time. Etomidate has the advantages of cardiostability, minimal histamine release and a low incidence of hypersensitivity reactions. It is used mainly in emergency cases in patients who may be hypovolaemic, in those in whom haemodynamic stability is of particular importance and in those with limited cardiac reserve. (Some anaesthetists take the view that the same outcome can be accomplished with appropriately low doses of thiopental.) Thiopental is still the default choice for rapid sequence induction of emergency anaesthesia. It is also a potent anticonvulsant and when given by continuous infusion is probably the most effective treatment for refractory status epilepticus.

- **Disadvantages:** etomidate is painful on injection, causes myoclonus and in many patients is emetic. Another major drawback is its potent inhibition of steroidogenesis. Thiopental is a myocardial and haemodynamic depressant, does not suppress airway reflexes and is antanalgesic. It is highly irritant, and inadvertent intra-arterial injection is more dangerous than with other induction agents. Hypersensitivity reactions are rare (1 in 15–20,000) but when they occur are severe. Neither thiopental nor etomidate is safe in patients with porphyria.

Comparative Pharmacology

- **Chemistry:** etomidate is a carboxylated imidazole. It is water-soluble but has been formulated in propylene glycol 35% to improve the stability of the solution. This is a high osmolarity organic solvent which may be responsible for some of the adverse effects. A newer preparation presents etomidate in a lipid formulation containing medium chain triglycerides. It is a pure R (+) enantiomer. Thiopental is the sulphur analogue of the barbiturate pentobarbitone and in solution has a pH of 10.4. The ampoules contain nitrogen to prevent any reaction with atmospheric CO_2.
- **Mechanism of action:** both drugs act by enhancing inhibitory synaptic transmission by activation of the Cl^- channel on the β_1 subunit of the $GABA_A$ receptor.
- **Clinical uses:** both are used for the induction of general anaesthesia in adults and children. Etomidate cannot be used for maintenance of anaesthesia, nor for sedation in intensive care because of its effects on steroid metabolism (see the following). Thiopental can be given by infusion (but usually only in the management of status epilepticus as described earlier).
- **Dose and routes of administration:** both can be given by the intravenous and rectal routes. The intravenous dose of etomidate is 0.2–0.3 mg kg^{-1} (6 mg kg^{-1} rectally); that of thiopental is 3–5 mg kg^{-1} (50 mg kg^{-1} rectally).

Main Effects and Side Effects

- **CNS:** both drugs are CNS depressants. Etomidate may be associated with marked myoclonus, although the EEG displays no epileptiform activity. Thiopental is a potent anticonvulsant which decreases cerebral blood flow, ICP and $CMRO_2$. Etomidate also reduces these indices but does not significantly affect cerebral perfusion pressure.
- **Cardiovascular system:** etomidate is associated with negligible changes in arterial blood pressure or heart rate. It is said to maintain cardiac output and to have minimal myocardial depressant effects. There are, however, some Doppler studies which have shown that cardiac index actually falls, but systemic vascular resistance rises (mediated by α_{2B}-adrenoceptors in vascular smooth muscle). Etomidate produces the least alteration in the balance of myocardial oxygen supply and demand.

It is these characteristics that make the drug popular for induction of anaesthesia in patients with limited circulatory or cardiac reserve. Thiopental causes dose-related myocardial depression and hypotension.

- **Respiratory system:** etomidate has some respiratory depressant effects, but these are transient and much less marked than is seen with barbiturates or propofol. Neither agent inhibits hypoxic pulmonary vasoconstriction.
- **Gastrointestinal system:** etomidate is emetic and is associated with a high incidence of nausea and vomiting. Thiopental is not.
- **Pharmacokinetics:**
- Etomidate: it is 75% protein-bound and has a volume of distribution (V_d) of 2.0–4.5 l kg^{-1}. The distribution half-life ($t_{\frac{1}{2}\alpha}$) is 2–4 minutes, and the elimination half-life ($t_{\frac{1}{2}\beta}$) is 1–4 hours. It is metabolized by ester hydrolysis and N-dealkylation in the liver to inactive compounds which are excreted renally.
- Thiopental: this is 85% protein-bound and has a similar V_d of 2.5 l kg^{-1}. The distribution half-life ($t_{\frac{1}{2}\alpha}$) is very short, at 1–2 minutes, and the elimination half-life ($t_{\frac{1}{2}\beta}$) is 10 hours. It undergoes hepatic oxidation to an inactive carboxylic acid derivative and to pentobarbital, an active oxybarbiturate which is metabolized slowly.
- **Miscellaneous:** etomidate does not release histamine and the incidence of hypersensitivity reactions is extremely low (fewer than 1 in 50,000). Thiopental is associated with histamine release, and Type 1 hypersensitivity reactions are more common (1 in 15–20,000). Neither drug triggers malignant hyperpyrexia. Etomidate increases levels of δ-ALA synthetase and is considered unsafe in porphyria. Thiopental, being a barbiturate, is contraindicated.
- **Adrenocortical suppression:** etomidate is an inhibitor of steroidogenesis in the adrenal cortex. Its imidazole structure (a ring comprising three carbon and two nitrogen atoms) allows it to combine with cytochrome P450 to prevent cortisol production. Specifically it blocks two enzymes, 17-α hydroxylase and 11-β hydroxylase, which catalyze at least six of the reactions in the biosynthetic pathways from cholesterol to hydrocortisone (cortisol). The mineralocorticoid and glucocorticoid pathways are linked, and etomidate inhibits both the formation of corticosterone, which is a precursor of aldosterone, as well as hydrocortisone. It is unlikely that you will be asked to describe these pathways in any detail, but the enzyme inhibition does explain why etomidate is one of the most potent inhibitors of steroid production that has so far been synthesized. The immunosuppressant effects of etomidate were unmasked by studies in which mortality rates in intensive care patients were shown to be demonstrably higher in those who had been sedated with a continuous infusion. The effect is not limited to etomidate given by infusion; it is now clear that impaired adrenocortical function will follow even a single induction dose, and that, although the enzyme inhibition is reversible, it may still persist for up to 8 hours. Thiopental has no such effects.
- **Derivatives:** thiopentone has no modified analogues. There are analogues of etomidate: methoxy-carbonyl etomidate (MOC-etomidate), which has high cardiovascular stability and which interferes only transiently with steroidogenesis, and carboetomidate, which has a modified imidazole ring that also substantially attenuates adrenocortical suppression.

Inhalational Agents: Sevoflurane

Commentary

Sevoflurane is one of the standard volatile agents in use in the UK, and its greater cost notwithstanding, it is replacing isoflurane on most anaesthetic machines. As it is a core anaesthetic drug, detailed information will be expected, but the amount of such information that can be conveyed will be constrained by the time restriction imposed by the structure of the oral. You may not be asked about a single agent but rather asked to compare one or more of them. The outline (as with the accounts which follow the other available agents) does not aim therefore to be wholly comprehensive, but it should be sufficient. It does nonetheless include a brief summary of the effects of volatile agents on the EEG. This aspect is unlikely to feature in the oral but may inform a discussion about methods of assessing the depth of anaesthesia. (See under 'Depth of Anaesthesia Monitoring' in Chapter 5.)

Core Information

The Pharmacology of Sevoflurane

- **Physicochemical characteristics:** sevoflurane is a highly fluorinated hydrocarbon with the simple formula $C_4H_3F_7O$. boiling point 59 °C; blood–gas partition coefficient 0.68; minimum alveolar concentration (MAC_{50}) 2.0%; metabolism 3–5%.
- **Central nervous system effects:** sevoflurane is a hypnotic agent that can be used for the induction and maintenance of general anaesthesia. Theories about its mechanism of action are detailed in the following.
- **Cerebral blood flow:** sevoflurane is a vasodilator which increases cerebral blood flow and may thereby affect intracranial pressure. As the effects on the EEG would suggest, it also decreases the cerebral metabolic rate and oxygen consumption ($CMRO_2$). In addition, it uncouples the relationship between cerebral blood flow and P_aCO_2. There is a dose-dependent reduction in cerebral perfusion pressure secondary to its cardiodepressant effects. It confers a degree of neuroprotection via a process analogous to ischaemic preconditioning.
- **Effects on the electroencephalogram (EEG):** the changes are dose-dependent. At low concentrations (at MAC less than 1.0), sevoflurane (and the other volatile agents) reduce power in the alpha range (waves of frequency 8–15) and increase it in the beta range (16–30 Hz). There is thus a shift overall to greater frequencies. As anaesthesia deepens, however, the activity in these frequencies decreases towards the theta (4–7 Hz) and delta (<3 Hz) ranges. At MAC greater than 2.0, all the volatile agents induce EEG burst suppression.
- **Respiratory effects:** sevoflurane reduces alveolar ventilation by reducing tidal volume. This is accompanied by an increase in respiratory frequency. The rise in respiratory rate and resultant increase in dead-space ventilation leads to an increase in P_aCO_2, to which, however, the respiratory centres become less sensitive. Sevoflurane reduces bronchial tone. It is not an airways irritant and is a forgiving agent

when used for inhalation induction because even high inspired concentrations rarely provoke coughing, laryngospasm or breath-holding.

- **Cardiovascular effects:** sevoflurane acts both as a vasodilator which decreases systemic vascular resistance and as a myocardial depressant which reduces cardiac output and mean arterial pressure. It is minimally arrythmogenic but may prolong the QT interval and so is best avoided in patients with congenital or acquired long QT syndrome. It has been suggested that volatile anaesthetics confer a degree of cardio-protection in a manner analogous to ischaemic preconditioning (in which a minor degree of cardiac injury attenuates greater damage secondary to a subsequent insult). This phenomenon is highly complex and is discussed at the end of this section.
- **Hepatic effects:** sevoflurane undergoes minimal metabolism (3–5%) and is not degraded to antigenic trifluroacetic acid-protein complexes (as happens with the metabolism of halothane). It leads to a dose-dependent reduction in hepatic blood flow secondary to its cardiovascular depressant actions.
- **Renal effects:** sevoflurane has negligible effects on renal physiology, but because it is a fluorinated hydrocarbon, it does produce inorganic fluoride ions sufficient to raise serum fluoride levels in some subjects to more than 50 μmol l^{-1}. Although this is a level at which fluoride has been shown to cause polyuric renal failure (following prolonged anaesthesia with methoxyflurane, for example), it does not appear to be clinically significant when associated with sevoflurane administration, and the agent is not considered to cause renal toxicity.
- **Effects on the uterus:** sevoflurane causes a dose-dependent reduction in uterine tone.
- **Malignant hyperpyrexia:** sevoflurane is a trigger agent.
- **Compounds A and B:** sevoflurane reacts with strong monovalent hydroxide bases, such as those which are used in soda lime and barium lime CO_2 absorbers, to produce a number of substances, including compounds A (trifluoromethyl vinyl ether), B, D, E and G. Only compound A has been shown to have any toxicity, as it is degraded into a nephrotoxic metabolite. (The reaction with barium lime is about five times more rapid than with soda lime.) The dose-dependent renal damage noted in rats has never been seen in humans despite many millions of administrations, probably because of marked quantitative differences in rodent enzyme systems.
- **Mechanisms of action:** the volatile agents act at the central neuraxial level (brain as well as spinal cord); at axons and synapses; and at the molecular level, on pre- and post-synaptic membranes. As a generalization about their overall mechanism of action, however, it appears that these agents acts as potent agonists at the $GABA_A$ and glycine receptors and thereby inhibit the function of their post-synaptic ligand-gated ion channels of the $GABA_A$ receptor. (The glycine receptor is another neurotransmitter-gated ion channel. Activation hyperpolarizes the membrane by increasing chloride conductance and so inhibits neuronal discharge.) The agents also act pre-synaptically as antagonists to inhibit ion channel activity mediated by serotoninergic, glutaminergic and particularly the nicotinic acetylcholine receptors. They act at spinal cord level by diminishing nociceptive afferents ascending to thalamo-cortical tracts. Hypnosis is mediated at supraspinal level, with the areas particularly influenced being the thalamus and the reticular formation in the midbrain.
- **Cardioprotection: ischaemic and anaesthetic preconditioning.** Ischaemic precon-ditioning describes the protective evolutionary process whereby tissues that are

exposed to recurrent ischaemic, hypoxic or metabolic insults that injure, but do not kill, the cells, are better able to tolerate a subsequent and much more severe event. (Thus a patient who has had repeated episodes of angina pectoris due to myocardial ischaemia may have less ventricular damage after acute myocardial infarction than a patient who prior to sudden coronary artery occlusion has been symptom-free.) The intracellular signalling pathways that underlie this process are dauntingly complex and remain at least partly hypothetical rather than proven. It appears, however, that changes in gene expression are a core part of the mechanism with up and down-regulation of those genes that are associated with cellular stress. Activation of what has been described as the intracellular signalling cascade involves second messenger reactions catalysed both by kinases and probably also by nitric oxide synthases. The cascade results in the modulation of myocardial mitochondrial activity via activation of the ATP-sensitive potassium channels, which are found on the nuclear, mitochondrial and sarcolemmal membranes of cardiac myocytes, and activation of the mitochondrial permeability transition pore. (These channels are also abundant in cerebral tissue.) This leads finally to a reduction in intracellular calcium and a fall in myocardial contractility. Overall, this incompletely understood process reduces the fragmentation of DNA and myocyte apoptosis that otherwise are the consequences of ischaemia and reperfusion.

The preceding is a considerable simplification of what is still imperfectly understood, but its relevance for anaesthesia is that a number of agents, particularly halogenated inhalation anaesthetics, but also opioids, appear to trigger an analogous process, now described as 'anaesthetic preconditioning'. The effect is initiated at MAC values as low as 0.25 but is maximal at MAC 1.0–1.5. Sophisticated studies have confirmed that volatile agents prime some of these signalling pathways and initiate a cascade of reactions with alterations in cardiac gene and protein expression. These are the same as those associated with ischaemic preconditioning, and there is no apparent difference according to the volatile agent. This suggests that a common mechanism is at work.

Inhalational Agents: Desflurane

Commentary

This is another standard agent that is available in the UK, although it occupies more of a niche role. Its differences lie mainly in its physicochemical characteristics, its capacity to provoke airways irritation and its considerable potency as a greenhouse gas. Otherwise many of its features overall are not dissimilar from those of the other volatile agents, but some of these are reproduced in the following account for convenience.

Core Information

The Pharmacology of Desflurane

- **Physicochemical characteristics:** desflurane is also a highly fluorinated hydrocarbon with the simple formula $C_3H_2F_6O$. It is structurally identical to isoflurane apart from the substitution of a fluorine atom for the chlorine atom on the α-ethyl carbon. Boiling point 23 °C; blood–gas partition coefficient 0.4; MAC_{50} 6.0%; metabolism 0.02%.

- **Vaporizer requirements:** although operating theatre temperatures in the UK should not reach the 23 °C at which desflurane boils, there remains that risk. Were desflurane to be used in a conventional vaporizer at higher ambient temperatures, there would be unpredictable variations in the concentrations of vapour delivered to the patient. As the agent boiled, this concentration would rise substantially, only to fall as the agent cooled due to loss of latent heat of vaporization. Manufacturers decided that it would technically be easier to heat the agent rather than to cool it, and so the Tec 6 (Ohmeda) and other vaporizers heat desflurane to 39 °C. This raises its saturated vapour pressure to almost 2 atmospheres (194 kPa), which means that the gaseous desflurane can be added directly to the fresh gas flow via a separate chamber.
- **Central nervous system effects:** desflurane is a hypnotic agent that can be used for the induction and maintenance of general anaesthesia. For theories about its mechanism of action see under 'Sevoflurane'.
- **Cerebral blood flow (CBF):** desflurane is a vasodilator which may increase CBF, but it does not increase intracranial pressure (ICP) at 1.0 MAC and with normocapnia. As the effects on the EEG would suggest, it also decreases the cerebral metabolic rate and oxygen consumption ($CMRO_2$). In addition, it uncouples the relationship between cerebral blood flow and P_aCO_2. There is a dose-dependent reduction in cerebral perfusion pressure secondary to its cardiodepressant effects. It confers a degree of neuroprotection via a process analogous to ischaemic preconditioning.
- **Effects on the electroencephalogram (EEG):** the changes are dose-dependent. (See under 'Sevoflurane' in the previous section.)
- **Respiratory effects:** desflurane reduces alveolar ventilation by reducing tidal volume. This is accompanied by an increase in respiratory frequency. The rise in respiratory rate and resultant increase in dead-space ventilation leads to an increase in P_aCO_2, to which, however, the respiratory centres become less sensitive. Desflurane has no effect on bronchial tone. It is an airways irritant, particularly at higher inspired concentrations, which means that it is rarely used for inhalation induction, and many anaesthetists do not use it in patients who are breathing spontaneously. This is despite the fact that up to end-tidal concentrations of around 6%, there is no greater incidence of coughing, laryngospasm or breath-holding than with other agents.
- **Cardiovascular effects:** desflurane acts both as a vasodilator which decreases systemic vascular resistance and as a myocardial depressant which reduces cardiac output and mean arterial pressure. It is minimally arrythmogenic. As with other volatile anaesthetics, it may have cardioprotective effects.
- **Hepatic effects:** desflurane undergoes minimal metabolism (0.02% predominantly to trifluoracetic acid) and is excreted more or less unchanged. It leads to a dose-dependent reduction in hepatic blood flow secondary to its cardiovascular depressant actions.
- **Renal effects:** desflurane has minimal effects on renal physiology, although its circulatory effects may reduce renal cortical blood flow. Despite being a fluorinated hydrocarbon, its negligible metabolism means that it does not does produce inorganic fluoride ions. It is not toxic to the kidney.
- **Effects on the uterus:** desflurane causes a dose-dependent reduction in uterine tone.

- **Malignant hyperpyrexia:** desflurane is a trigger agent.
- **Carbon monoxide (CO) production:** desflurane can react with the hydroxide bases, which are used in soda lime and barium lime CO_2 absorbers, to produce measurable amounts of carbon monoxide. This is greater with barium-containing absorbents and is a more pronounced phenomenon if the absorbent is dry. Clinically, this has not been identified as a significant problem.
- **Environmental considerations:** the fraction of volatile anaesthetic agents that is not metabolized is usually vented unchanged to atmosphere via theatre-scavenging systems, and there is increasing awareness of the fact that these are so-called greenhouse gases which contribute to climate change. Based on criteria that include production methods, utilization and its effects in the upper atmosphere, it has been calculated that desflurane has the largest life-cycle greenhouse emissions of any volatile agent, some 20 times greater than sevoflurane.
- **Mechanisms of action of volatile anaesthetic agents:** see under 'Sevoflurane'.

Inhalational Agents: Isoflurane

Commentary

Isoflurane has been superseded by sevoflurane as the default volatile anaesthetic agent, except in those departments where the drug budget commands a high priority. Isoflurane is substantially cheaper, and proponents for its continued use argue that the minor advantages of sevoflurane do not justify its (up to) tenfold higher cost. Factors such as the 'greater ease' of use of sevoflurane are soft criteria for which it is hard to produce robust data. And if, for example, anaesthetist A claims that isoflurane causes too many airway problems on induction, then anaesthetist B will simply counter that that is because they do not know how to use the drug properly. So you can make your own judgement.

Core Information

The pharmacology of isoflurane.

- **Physicochemical characteristics:** Isoflurane is a halogenated chlorofluorocarbon with the simple formula $C_3H_2F_5O$. Boiling point 48 °C; blood–gas partition coefficient 1.4; MAC_{50} 1.15%; metabolism 0.2%.
- **Central nervous system effects:** isoflurane is a hypnotic agent that can be used for the induction and maintenance of general anaesthesia. Theories about its mechanism of action are detailed earlier under 'Sevoflurane'.
- **Cerebral blood flow:** isoflurane is a vasodilator which increases cerebral blood flow and may thereby affect intracranial pressure. As the effects on the EEG would suggest, it also decreases the cerebral metabolic rate and oxygen consumption ($CMRO_2$). In addition, it uncouples the relationship between cerebral blood flow and P_aCO_2. There is a dose-dependent reduction in cerebral perfusion pressure secondary to its cardiodepressant effects. It confers a degree of neuroprotection via

a process analogous to ischaemic preconditioning. (Described previously under 'Sevoflurane'.)

- **Effects on the electroencephalogram (EEG):** the changes are dose-dependent, as for the other volatile agents.
- **Respiratory effects:** isoflurane reduces alveolar ventilation by reducing tidal volume. This is accompanied by an increase in respiratory frequency. The rise in respiratory rate and resultant increase in dead-space ventilation leads to an increase in P_aCO_2, to which, however, the respiratory centres become less sensitive. Isoflurane reduces bronchial tone. It is a greater airways irritant than sevoflurane; it increases secretions and is associated with a higher incidence of coughing, breath-holding and apnoea.
- **Cardiovascular effects:** isoflurane acts both as a vasodilator which decreases systemic vascular resistance and as a myocardial depressant which reduces cardiac output and mean arterial pressure. It is a coronary vasodilator, with arterioles being particularly sensitive to its effects. It was considered therefore to be more likely than other volatile agents to cause a 'coronary steal syndrome' by diverting blood away from stenotic areas of the myocardial circulation which are unable to dilate. This appears to be of more theoretical than practical concern, but the hypotension and reflex tachycardia that isoflurane can precipitate may cause local ischaemia in subjects with coronary artery disease. (Sevoflurane in contrast does not cause a tachycardia or any local abnormalities of myocardial perfusion.) Isoflurane is minimally arrythmogenic. In common with other volatiles, it triggers anaesthetic preconditioning.
- **Hepatic effects:** isoflurane undergoes minimal metabolism to trifluoroacetic acid and fluorine. The quoted rate of 0.2% may be low, but there is no evidence that either of these metabolites is associated with clinically deleterious effects. It leads to a dose-dependent reduction in hepatic blood flow secondary to its cardiovascular depressant actions.
- **Renal effects:** isoflurane has negligible effects on renal physiology. Its metabolism releases small amount of fluoride ions, but levels reach only 5–10 μmol l^{-1} even after several MAC hours of exposure.
- **Effects on the uterus:** as with the other halogenated agents, isoflurane causes a dose-dependent reduction in uterine tone.
- **Malignant hyperpyrexia:** isoflurane is a trigger agent.
- **Mechanisms of action:** see under 'Sevoflurane'.

Inhalational Agents: Xenon

Commentary

Xenon is the inhaled anaesthetic agent that most clearly approaches the ideal , but the high costs of production (around £10 litre^{-1}) means that it is unlikely ever to become a mainstream drug. Even when used in ultra-low flow systems (0.3 l min^{-1}), it costs in the order of £180–200 an hour. It also means that your knowledge (and that of the examiner) is likely to be entirely theoretical.

Core Information

- **Physicochemical characteristics:** Xenon (Xe) is a monoatomic inert gas. Boiling point −108 °C; blood–gas partition coefficient 0.12; MAC_{50} 71%; metabolism 0%.
- **Central nervous system effects:** xenon is one of the so-called noble gases that is present in the atmosphere. It can induce and maintain general anaesthesia. It has the lowest blood–gas partition coefficient of any inhalational agent (0.12), which results in a very rapid onset and offset of anaesthesia. It confers neuroprotection via its inhibition of glutaminergic NMDA receptors, activation of which appears to be a precursor of neuronal death following hypoxic, ischaemic or traumatic cerebral insults. Unlike other agents with purported neuroprotective characteristics, xenon does this at sub-anaesthetic concentrations.
- **Cerebral blood flow (CBF):** xenon increases cerebral blood flow and may thereby increase intracranial pressure. Unlike the other inhalation agents, however, it does not uncouple CBF from P_aCO_2.
- **Mechanism of action:** the predominant action of xenon is as a high-affinity glycine site NMDA receptor antagonist which inhibits post-synaptic excitatory transmission. This also means that it is a potent intra-operative analgesic. Its antinociceptive effect at spinal cord level is more potent than that of nitrous oxide, but it does not stimulate the release of endogenous opioid receptor ligands in the same way and so is likely to have a different mechanism of action. In common with nitrous oxide, however, it does activate the two-pore domain potassium channel (TREK-1). (This is one of a large group of potassium ion channels which in general exert influence over the resting membrane potential and cell excitability. Their regulators include O_2, GABA, 5-HT and noradrenaline.) It has no effect on $GABA_A$ receptors. Xenon acts as an agonist at nicotinic acetylcholine α_4 β_2 receptors, which amongst other functions mediate spinal antinociception, and it also appears to be a competitive antagonist at the $5-HT_3$ receptor (and so is anti-emetic).
- **Respiratory effects:** in contrast to the volatile hydrocarbons which depress tidal volume and increase respiratory rate, xenon does not depress respiration but instead maintains minute ventilation mediated via an increase in tidal volume and a decrease in respiratory frequency. At concentrations of 1.0 MAC (Xe 71%: O_2 29%), it is a relatively dense gas mixture that increases the work of breathing. It is not an airways irritant.
- **Cardiovascular effects:** xenon has minimal effects on the cardiovascular system and can accurately be described as cardiostable, even in patients with significant cardiac co-morbidity.
- **Haematopoiesis:** via activation of a transcription factor (HIF-1-alpha), xenon inhalation increases erythropoietin production. (In that regard it is a performance-enhancing drug which has been banned by the World Anti-Doping Agency, WADA. This is academic, however, as the nature of the compound means that there is no test for its detection.)
- **Hepatic effects:** as a monoatom, xenon undergoes no metabolism, and as a cardio-stable agent, it has no effect on hepatic blood flow.
- **Renal effects:** xenon has no influence on renal physiology.
- **Effect on uterine tone:** none.
- **Malignant hyperpyrexia:** xenon is a not trigger agent.

- **Environmental considerations:** xenon is exhaled unchanged and so returns to its source – the atmosphere. It therefore has no environmental impact in respect of greenhouse gas emission, although its production (by the liquefaction of air) is energy-intensive.

Inhalational Agents: Nitrous Oxide

Commentary

Not that long ago there were some candidates for the Final FRCA who were thoroughly discomfited by a written question on the 'pharmacology of nitrous oxide' (N_2O). This was hardly surprising, because few anaesthetists then had much interest in the drug, and it was ignored largely as being simply a carrier gas with modest analgesic properties. This perception did the complex pharmacology of the drug a disservice, and there followed an upsurge of interest, both in its potential toxicity as well as in its mechanisms of action. This interest appears now to be waning, but, given the continued and ubiquitous use of N_2O, it remains a core anaesthetic agent about which detailed knowledge will be expected. Some anaesthetists never use the drug, and it polarizes opinion. Your assessment should therefore be dispassionate.

Core Information

Anaesthesia

- **$GABA_A$ (mainly inhibitory) and NMDA (mainly excitatory) receptors in the CNS:** N_2O appears to have no effect on $GABA_A$ receptors but strongly inhibits NMDA-activated currents. There is concern that NMDA antagonists can be neurotoxic, which is a potential problem only if N_2O is used alone under hyperbaric conditions (which is a mainly theoretical scenario). If $GABA_A$ agonist agents or facilitators (such as benzodiazepines) are used in addition, they may exert a protective effect to offset this damage.
- **Dopamine receptors.** N_2O stimulates some dopaminergic neurons; this may mediate release of endogenous opioid peptides and explains why the effects of N_2O are partly antagonized by naloxone.

Analgesia

- **Opioid peptide release:** the release of endogenous ligands for opioid receptors occurs in the peri-aqueductal grey matter of the midbrain, and stimulates descending inhibitory noradrenergic pathways which modulate pain processing via noradrenaline release. Noradrenaline acts at α_2-receptors in the dorsal horn.
- **Other theories:** N_2O may also activate a supraspinal descending pain inhibition system with an increase in encephalinergic interneurons in the substantia gelatinosa of the cord. These endogenous encephalins inhibit transmission via substance P-dependent synapses.

- **Physical properties:** N_2O has a rapid onset and equilibration because of its very low blood–gas partition coefficient (0.47). Its boiling point is $-88.5\ °C$; critical temperature $36.5\ °C$; and MAC 105%. It is manufactured in a simple process of heating ammonium nitrate to a temperature of 240 °C (at higher temperatures the exothermic reaction risks detonation); $NH_4NO_3 \rightarrow 2H_2O + N_2O$.
- **Metabolism:** N_2O undergoes a negligible amount of metabolism by gut bacteria (0.004%) so in effect is excreted unchanged.

Supplementary Information and Clinical Applications

Advantages in Clinical Practice
- It is a useful carrier gas for more potent anaesthetic agents.
- It has a rapid onset and equilibration (blood–gas partition coefficient of 0.47).
- The induction of anaesthesia is accelerated via the second gas effect, in which the rapid uptake of N_2O from the alveoli increases the alveolar concentration of other agents.
- It is a potent analgesic whose effects are usually underestimated. The drug acts partly at opioid receptors and transiently has the potency of morphine. This is not surprising, given survey data showing that Entonox (N_2O/O_2) affords better pain relief during labour (effective analgesia in around 50% of mothers) than pethidine (effective analgesia in about 35%). It is associated with a significant reduction in chronic post-surgical pain.
- It is a weak anaesthetic (MAC_{50} is 105%), but, in combination with its analgesic actions, it decreases the MAC of other inhalational agents.
- It may offer some neuroprotection via the reduction of NMDA-induced glutamate excitatory toxicity.

Disadvantages in Clinical Practice
- **Effect on air-filled spaces:** the diffusing capacity of N_2O relative to nitrogen is high ($\times 25$).
  - In non-compliant air-filled spaces, pressure increases (in the middle ear, in nasal sinuses and in the eye if it has been filled with gas such as SF_6 after vitreoretinal surgery). The pressure change is related arithmetically to the alveolar partial pressure of N_2O, so that administration of 50% N_2O leads to a pressure increase of 0.5 atmospheres.
  - In compliant air-filled spaces, volume increases (significant for pneumothoraces, bullae, bowel, air embolus, cuffs of tracheal tubes). After 4 hours of 66% N_2O, the volume of the bowel increases by 200%. The volume change is related geometrically to alveolar partial pressure of N_2O; the percentage increase is given by the % N_2O divided by $(1.0 - FiN_2O)$. So, at 50%, the final percentage volume increase is $50/0.5 = 100\%$. At 75%, a pneumothorax will triple in size after 30 minutes of N_2O administration.
- **Emesis:** this is probably caused by a combination of its sympathomimetic and opioid effects, together with the effects of bowel distension.
- **Second gas effect:** this results in diffusion hypoxia (which is of modest clinical relevance; it lasts less than 10 minutes and can be readily overcome by giving supplemental oxygen).

- **Respiratory depression:** there is an increase in respiratory rate to offset decreased tidal volume; this is common to all volatile agents.
- **Cardiovascular system:** N_2O is a direct negative inotrope and chronotrope. Cardiac contractility is decreased if cardiac function is already impaired; its use exacerbating ischaemic change in any situation in which myocardial O_2 supply is exceeded by demand. It is an indirect stimulant (via its sympathomimetic action). It increases pulmonary vascular resistance in the presence of pre-existing pulmonary hypertension.
- **Greenhouse effect:** N_2O is a greenhouse gas which is some 300 times as potent as CO_2 in its potential to trap atmospheric heat; anaesthesia contributes about 1% of the global total. (Bacteria produce nitrous oxide naturally, and it is also generated by nitrate fertilizer use in agriculture.)
- **Bone marrow toxicity and neurotoxicity.**
  - A biochemical lesion in the liver (methionine synthetase inhibition) is demonstrable after only 40 minutes of N_2O administration.
  - N_2O oxidizes the cobalt atom in vitamin B12 (cyanocobalamin) from Co^{++} to Co^{3+} in a very simple reaction and thereby inactivates it. Vitamin B12 however, is a co-factor for the enzyme methionine synthetase.
  - Methionine synthetase catalyzes the transfer of a methyl group in a linked methyltransferase reaction. The methylation of homocysteine forms methionine, while the demethylation of CH_3-tetrahydrofolate leads to the formation of tetrahydrofolate (Figure 4.1).
  - Inhibition of methionine synthesis therefore prevents the production of methionine and tetrahydrofolate. Methionine is a precursor of S-adenosyl methionine (SAM). SAM is incorporated into myelin, and its absence leads to subacute combined systems degeneration of the cord. This is the classic lesion associated with chronic B12 deficiency. Acutely this inhibition can cause dorsal column function impairment (from experimental data after 48 hours of 20% N_2O administration). Tetrahydrofolate is an important substrate involved in nucleotide and DNA synthesis (hence the development of megaloblastic anaemia in folate and B12 deficiency).
  - The administration of methionine and folinic acid will provide substrates to allow biosynthesis to continue below the level of the enzyme block.

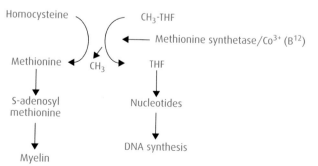

Fig. 4.1 Nitrous oxide toxicity; effect of methionine synthetase inhibition. THF, tetrahydrofolate.

- **Teratogenicity**
  — These mechanisms plus its other actions are believed to contribute to possible teratogenicity; α_1-adrenoceptor agonism is associated with disorders of left/right body axis development (such as situs inversus). The association is not strong; almost 25 million administrations of the drug take place in the USA annually without obvious sequelae.
- **Malignant hyperpyrexia**: there is one definite case report, so N_2O is considered to be a weak trigger.
- **Hyperbaric N_2O**: under these conditions the gas is excitatory, leading to a threefold increase in respiratory rate, diaphoresis and cardiovascular α-adrenergic stimulation. At increased pressure, N_2O becomes an anaesthetic (MAC is 105%), but it also causes CNS-mediated muscle rigidity and catatonic jerking.

Outcome after Major Surgery: ENIGMA and ENIGMA II

- The first ENIGMA trial recruited more than 2,000 patients who were undergoing major surgery expected to last more than 2 hours. (ENIGMA is a rather tortuous acronym: **E**valuation of **N**itrous oxide **I**n the **G**as **M**ixture for **A**naesthesia.) Its authors asserted that major complications were greater in the group that received N_2O than in the group that received 80% O_2 in air, and concluded that the routine use of the agent should be questioned. No patients received 30% O_2 in air, however, and so it was not possible to determine whether the purported beneficial effects were caused by a high FiO_2, the avoidance of N_2O, or both (P.S. Myles *et al. Anesthesiology* 2007, 107(2): 221–31). Subsequent to these methodological criticisms, the ENIGMA II trial recruited more than 7,000 patients of medium to high cardiovascular risk in a randomized single-blinded study. There were no differences in outcome between the two groups, although there was a 15% incidence of PONV in the nitrous oxide group. This difference too was eliminated by the administration of prophylactic antiemetics (P.S. Myles *et al. Lancet* 2014, 384: 1446–54).

Inhalational Agents: Comparison with the Ideal

Commentary
This is a standard introduction to a discussion of the agents that are available. After you have outlined the desirable characteristics of your ideal agent, you will be asked how one or more of the drugs in current use compare. The way this question is structured means that the subject tends to be discussed at a quite superficial level, although you will need to be prepared to explain some of the concepts in more detail. Much of the information is still relatively soft (in respect of airways irritation, for example), so include numerical data where you can. Be aware of the important purported differences in their effects on systems, but recognize also that comparisons have been established via studies of dissimilar methodology which have sometimes yielded conflicting results.

This means that you cannot be expected to discuss detailed comparative information. Nitrous oxide is not included because, although it is an inhalational agent, it differs from the halogenated hydrocarbons and xenon in that cannot be used as a sole anaesthetic agent.

Core Information

Characteristics of the ideal inhalational agent might include the following.

- **Safety:** the ideal agent would be safe by virtue of its specificity for the nervous system. It would, in other words, allow a controlled state of insensibility in which all other physiological indices such as cerebral and myocardial blood flow remained unchanged. It would also be advantageous were it to be analgesic. No such agent exists, and so patients receiving inhalational agents may be at potential risk from the secondary, undesirable effects of an agent, from direct toxic effects, or from toxic products of metabolism.
- **Respiratory effects:** the potential to cause airways irritation is discussed in more detail later in this section. All the drugs are respiratory depressants and cause a decrease in tidal volume with an increase in respiratory rate. They are effective bronchodilators. The ideal agent might be one that relaxes bronchial smooth muscle but which has no other effects on respiratory physiology.
- **Cardiovascular effects:** the ideal agent would exhibit complete cardiovascular stability; however, all the halogenated agents have cardiovascular effects, but none so marked as to preclude their clinical use. All the agents in current use are cardioprotective via a mechanism similar to that seen in ischaemic preconditioning. (See under 'Sevoflurane'.)
  - **Halothane** is the most arrhythmogenic. It causes a dose-related fall in mean arterial pressure (MAP) and may also cause bradycardia, junctional rhythms and ventricular premature beats. It sensitizes the myocardium to catecholamines, particularly in the presence of hypercapnia and acidosis, and under such circumstances may provoke much more malignant arrhythmias such as ventricular tachycardia. Experience with this agent in the UK has all but disappeared, but it is still used widely in the developing world.
  - **Enflurane** similarly causes dose-related cardiovascular depression, but is not arrhythmogenic. This agent similarly is almost obsolete in the UK.
  - **Isoflurane** leads to a dose-dependent reduction in systemic vascular resistance (SVR) and coronary vascular vasodilatation. Heart rate increases and cardiac output and contractility are maintained. Isoflurane was believed to cause a coronary steal syndrome in which coronary vasodilatation diverted blood away from stenotic vessels. Controlled trials have suggested that it is no worse than any other volatile in this regard.
  - **Desflurane** causes a similar fall in SVR and MAP, while heart rate rises and cardiac output is maintained.
  - **Sevoflurane** also leads to dose-dependent cardiovascular depression, with decreases in MAP, SVR and contractility. The heart rate does not increase and the agent causes less coronary vasodilatation than isoflurane.
  - **Xenon** is cardiostable.

- **CNS:** all the halogenated agents increase cerebral blood flow which can cause a rise in intracranial pressure that in some circumstances may be deleterious.
  - **Sevoflurane** preserves cerebral autoregulation better than the other agents.
  - **Desflurane**, in contrast, abolishes autoregulation at 1.5 MAC. Alone amongst the agents, it increases cerebrospinal fluid production.
  - At 1.0 MAC, **isoflurane** and **sevoflurane** are associated with minimal changes in CBF and ICP.
  - **Enflurane** is associated with abnormal epileptiform activity in the EEG, particularly if its administration is accompanied by hypocapnia.
  - **Xenon** increases cerebral blood flow and increases intracranial pressure.
- **Uterus:** all the agents, apart from nitrous oxide and xenon, cause dose-related uterine relaxation.
- **Malignant hyperpyrexia:** halothane is the most dangerous, although all the halogenated agents are reported triggers for this condition. Xenon is not.
- **Efficacy:** by definition, the agent has to be able to induce and maintain a state of anaesthesia, and all the halogenated agents produce dose-dependent narcosis. Some are more 'potent' than others in the sense that their effects are produced at lower concentrations, but clinically this is of little relevance. According to this criterion, for example, halothane is almost nine times as potent as desflurane. A much more significant property is the blood solubility, as quantified by the blood–gas partition coefficient. The less soluble the agent, the lower the amount required to produce a given partial pressure and the more rapid the onset of action. In ascending order, therefore, the agents can be ranked: xenon (whose blood–gas partition coefficient is only 0.12), desflurane (0.42), nitrous oxide (0.47), sevoflurane (0.68), isoflurane (1.4), enflurane (1.9) and halothane (2.3). 'Potency' in respect of inhalational agents is in effect defined by the MAC at which 50% of the population will not display reflex movement in response to a standard surgical stimulus. This is the MAC_{50}, but the MAC_{95} (the prevention of movement in 95% of subjects) is more useful. MAC_{50} values are halothane (0.75%), isoflurane (1.17%), enflurane (1.63%), sevoflurane (1.8%), desflurane (6.6%), xenon (71%) and nitrous oxide (105%).
- **Airways irritation:**
  - **Sevoflurane** is non-irritant to the upper airway and bronchi, and inhalational induction can be swift and effective in the most testing of circumstances.
  - **Halothane** shares the same characteristics, but is slightly more pungent.
  - **Enflurane** is not dissimilar, although inhalation induction is more prolonged.
  - **Isoflurane** is more irritant to airways and is associated with a higher incidence of coughing and breath-holding.
  - **Desflurane** is said to be the most inferior agent in this respect, its other benefits being offset by its effective capacity to provoke laryngospasm, excessive secretions and apnoea. This is not a problem at end-tidal concentrations up to 6%.
- **Toxicity**
  - **Nitrous oxide** depresses bone marrow function via its oxidation of the cobalt atom in the vitamin B12 complex as described previously.
  - **Sevoflurane** may produce the potentially, but not demonstrably, toxic compound A, as well as free fluoride ions.

- — **Enflurane** also produces fluoride ions, while halothane is implicated in post-exposure hepatic dysfunction.
- **Metabolism:** inhaled agents are eliminated through the lungs, but metabolism still occurs, principally by cytochrome P450 oxidation in the liver. None of the agents has active metabolites, but clearly the greater the proportion that undergoes hepatic metabolism the greater is the excretory load.
  - — **Xenon** is an inert gas which undergoes no biotransformation.
  - — **Nitrous oxide** undergoes minimal metabolism (0.004%), mainly by gut micro-organisms.
  - — **Desflurane** is resistant to metabolism (0.02%), and serum fluoride levels do not rise even after prolonged administration.
  - — **Isoflurane** metabolism is around 0.2%, which can lead to a small rise in fluoride concentrations.
  - — **Enflurane** metabolism is higher, at around 3%, and serum fluoride levels may reach 25 μmol l^{-1}, which may be of theoretical importance in patients with pre-existing renal impairment. (Fluoride is nephrotoxic at levels of 50 μmol l^{-1} and above.)
  - — **Sevoflurane** undergoes 3–5% metabolism and produces more fluoride ions than enflurane. Serum fluoride concentrations may reach 15–25 μmol l^{-1} after 1 MAC hour of administration. In theory, it should be used with caution in patients with renal dysfunction, but this is not regarded universally as a contraindication for its use. The chemical structure of sevoflurane is such that it cannot undergo bio-transformation to an acyl halide, and so, unlike halothane, enflurane, isoflurane and desflurane, its metabolism does not result in the formation of trifluoroacety-lated liver proteins and subsequent production of anti-trifluoroacetylated protein antibodies.
  - — **Halothane** is the most extensively metabolized of the inhalational agents, with 20–40% being degraded by both reductive and oxidative pathways. A trifluoroacetylated compound produced by oxidation can bind to liver proteins, triggering in susceptible patients an immune reaction which may precipitate hepatic necrosis. This is a separate problem from the transient postoperative rise in liver enzymes, which may be seen in up to 20% of patients.
- **Stability:** this refers to the molecular stability of the compound when exposed to the normal range of environmental conditions, and to the specific circumstances of its use in an anaesthetic breathing system. Ideally, it should be stable to light and to temperature, it should undergo no spontaneous degradation and require no preser-vatives, it should be non-flammable and non-corrosive and should be safe in the presence of soda lime and alkali. Most of the agents perform well against these criteria; some specific exceptions include the following.
  - — **Nitrous oxide** supports combustion.
  - — **Desflurane** has a low boiling point that is close to room temperature (23.5 °C).
  - — **Sevoflurane** reacts with strong monovalent hydroxide bases, such as those which are used in soda lime and barium lime CO_2 absorbers, to produce a number of substances, including compound A. (The reaction with barium lime is about five times more rapid than with soda lime.) Of the degradation products (compounds A, B, D, E and G), only A, which is a vinyl ether, has been shown to have any

toxicity, but the dose-dependent renal damage noted in rats has never been seen in humans despite many millions of administrations.

— **Halothane** may degrade when exposed to light and so is presented in amber bottles in thymol 0.01% as a preservative. Accumulated thymol can affect vaporizer function.

- **Xenon:** this gas most closely approaches the ideal agent. It provides effective hypnosis and analgesia together with some muscle relaxation. It is non-irritant and, although it can depress respiration to the point of apnoea, it is cardiostable. It undergoes no metabolism, is not toxic and does not cause allergic reactions. It is stable in storage, is non-flammable and is environmentally neutral. At present its cost is prohibitive, and so until an efficient xenon recycling system can be developed, this almost ideal inhalational agent will not find widespread use.
- **Methoxyflurane:** this is a fluorinated ether ($C_3H_4Cl_2F_2O$) whose use as a main-stream volatile anaesthetic agent was discontinued following recognition of its nephrotoxicity. This was associated with its metabolic degradation to inorganic fluoride and other compounds, particularly dichloroacetic acid. It is an agent with high-lipid solubility and a slow onset and offset of action. It is also, however, a potent analgesic, including at sub-hypnotic doses, and so it has been reintroduced particularly for the out-of-hospital management of acute pain secondary to trauma. (It is vaporized via a small handheld inhaler which contains only 3 ml of agent). When it was used as a general anaesthetic, methoxyflurane could be delivered at 1.0 MAC for up to 8 hours before nephrotoxicity would occur, and so it is likely that interest in potential of the agent as a useful rescue analgesic in a much wider context is likely to increase.

Neuromuscular Blocking Drugs (and Sugammadex)

Commentary

Questions on neuromuscular blocking drugs can be unpredictable. A single agent may form the basis of an oral, or you may be asked about one or more of the drugs during discussion of another subject such as the neuromuscular junction. What follows is not intended to provide a comprehensive monograph on each of the drugs. It aims simply to identify those particular aspects on which an examiner might concentrate, such as aspects of pharmacodynamics or pharmacokinetics that are of specific interest.

Core Information

- **The neuromuscular junction:** see under 'The Neuromuscular Junction' in Chapter 3.
- **Classification: Depolarizing muscle relaxants.** These drugs, of which **suxamethonium** is the only example in clinical use, act as agonists at the acetylcholine (ACh) receptor. Binding to the two α-subunits depolarizes the membrane, during which

process the voltage-sensitive sodium channels first open and then close. In this closed conformation they are inactivated. After a normal physiological depolarization, the membrane potential is restored within 1 ms by the action of acetylcholinesterase. As depolarizing relaxants are not metabolized in this way, the acetylcholine receptors remain activated and the sodium channels remain closed. The action of the drug is terminated as it diffuses away from the receptors down a concentration gradient to be hydrolyzed in plasma by plasma (butyryl) cholinesterase (pseudocholinesterase).

- **Classification: Non-depolarizing muscle relaxants.** These drugs in contrast are primarily competitive inhibitors of ACh at the post-junctional nicotinic receptors. They also antagonize prejunctional receptors and block the normal positive feedback cycle whereby acetylcholine stimulates its own release. The drugs are quaternary ammonium compounds with one or more quaternary nitrogen groups (the bisquaternary amines have greater potency than monoquaternary). The positively charged nitrogen-containing group, $N^+(CH_3)_3$, binds to one or both of the α-subunits to prevent ACh access, but induces no conformational change in the receptor. The α-subunits are separated by a distance of 1.4 nm, but it is not necessary for quaternary nitrogen radicals to have the same spatial separation for the drugs to exert their effect. The lipophilic bridge between the radicals varies with different non-depolarizing relaxants and is a prime determinant of their potency. The receptor binding is not static because the competitive antagonism is a continuous process of repeated association and dissociation. At the onset of block, there is a decremental reduction in the end-plate potential to the point at which it does not reach the threshold to generate an action potential for the initiation of muscle contraction.

- All of the non-depolarizing relaxants are quaternary amines, whose potency is increased if the molecule contains two quaternary ammonium radicals. There are two main groups: the benzylisoquinoliniums (drugs ending in '–urium'), and the aminosteroids (drugs ending in '–uronium'). The aminosteroids in general show greater cardiovascular stability and cause less histamine release.

- **Established agents:** (the duration of action that is quoted here is the time following an intubating dose at which there is 25% recovery and pharmacological reversal can be used.)

  — **Atracurium**: this is a bisquaternary amine, a benzylisoquinolinium mixture of 16 potential isomers. It has a medium duration of action which is reversible pharmacologically at 25 minutes. It may cause histamine release.

  — **Cisatracurium**: this is one of the isomers of atracurium, which has a slightly longer duration of action (45 minutes), and has greater cardiovascular stability because it is less likely to provoke histamine release. It is more potent than atracurium; a typical intubating dose is 0.1 mg kg^{-1}.

  — **Mivacurium**: this is a benzylisoquinolinium diester, with a short duration of action (15 minutes). Mivacurium undergoes ester hydrolysis and so, in theory, should not require reversing with anticholinesterases. In practice, residual curarization is still possible, and so conventional reversal agents can be used. Its capacity to cause histamine release is similar to that of atracurium. An intubating dose is 0.15 mg kg^{-1}.

  — **Pancuronium**: this is a bisquaternary aminosteroid whose vagolytic and sympathomimetic actions made its use traditionally popular in haemodynamically compromised patients. It is long acting (75 minutes) after an intubating dose of 0.1–0.15 mg kg^{-1}.

— **Vecuronium**: this is the monoquaternary homologue of pancuronium, which was developed in an attempt to create a 'clean' version of the older drug. Its structure includes a tertiary amine which becomes increasingly protonated in an acidotic circulation, thereby increasing both its potency and its duration of action. It has minimal cardiovascular effects and a short duration of action (30–35 minutes). Its effects are antagonized by sugammadex.

— **Rocuronium**: this is another monoquaternary aminosteroid which is very similar to vecuronium when used in equipotent doses. Its tertiary amine similarly becomes protonated in a patient who is acidotic. It provokes minimal histamine release and is cardiostable apart from modest vagolytic effects after large doses. When given in high doses (0.9 mg kg^{-1}) it provides good conditions for tracheal intubation within 60–75 seconds (hence its name: '**r**apid **o**nset *vecuronium*') and lasts for around 45 minutes. Lower doses of 0.6 mg kg^{-1} ($2 \times ED^{95}$, as is typical for muscle relaxants) last for around 35 minutes. It has a specific antagonist: **sugammadex**.

Sugammadex

— This is a γ-cyclodextrin (the 'su' prefix refers to 'sugar' and the '-gammadex' to the gammacyclodextrin moiety) modified by the addition of eight side chains to the cyclodextrin ring. The ring consists of cyclic dextrose units linked by 1–4 glycosyl bonds. This specific modification allows better accommodation of the aminosteroid molecule within what is described as a toroidal structure. (This is a mathematical term which describes a surface generated by a closed curve, rotating about, but not intersecting an axis in its own plane. More prosaically it is a structure shaped like a doughnut). The negatively charged hydroxyl groups on the outer surface are hydrophilic whereas the inner surface is lipophilic. Sugammadex chelates the lipophilic rocuronium molecule forming a stable structure which encapsulates the drug irreversibly. It does so in a ratio of 1:1. This specific action reverses the effect of rocuronium (and vecuronium) from any depth of neuromuscular block. This means that rocuronium can replace suxamethonium in a variety of clinical scenarios because it can be reversed within minutes of administration. A typical reversal dose, depending on the degree of residual neuromuscular blockade is 2–4 mg kg^{-1}. Reversal immediately after an intubating dose, however, requires 16 mg kg^{-1} which at current prices in the UK costs around £350 for a patient weighing 70 kg.

— **Metabolism and excretion:** The chelated complex is excreted unchanged by the kidneys. Its elimination half-life is reported as (an unusually precise) 2.2 hours.

— **Interactions:** the ability of cyclodextrins to encapsulate molecules is not confined to aminosteroids, and the compounds find non-medical uses (for example in air fresheners, specifically Febreze). Although sugammadex does not appear to effect endogenous hormones (which are usually strongly protein-bound), it may encapsulate exogenous progestogens such as those in oral contraceptive preparations. A small number of drugs have been identified as having the potential of displacing rocuronium from the sugammadex molecule; these are the antibiotics fusidic acid and flucloxacillin, and the anti-oestrogenic agent toremifine, which is used in the treatment of hormone-sensitive breast cancer.

- **Side effects:** there is little evidence of specific material complications with sugam-madex, although the data sheet lists cardiac arrhythmias as possible sequelae of its administration. Prolonged QT interval has also been cited as a potential problem, as have anaphylactic reactions. The use of sugammadex remains relatively low, and so the true incidence of these complications has yet to be established.
- **Other agents: Gantacurium** is also an isoquinolium (it is a tetrahydro-isoquinolium derivative of chlorofumarate) that has a rapid onset and offset of action (60–90 seconds and 10–14 minutes, respectively, following a dose of 0.2 mg kg^{-1}) and undergoes alkaline hydrolysis in the plasma by combination with L-cysteine. It does, however, release histamine, and so interest has shifted to a gantacurium derivative, currently referred to as CW002. Its defining characteristic is that is can be completely reversed by L-cysteine. Drugs such as rapacuronium, pipecuronium and doxacurium have either been withdrawn from use because of adverse effects or have faded from the market.
- **Metabolism and elimination:** most are eliminated by more than one mechanism.
  - **Suxamethonium:** this predominantly undergoes ester hydrolysis (by plasma cholinesterase); a small amount is hydrolyzed by non-specific plasma esterases, and 10% is excreted unchanged through the kidney.
  - **Mivacurium:** this is also metabolized by plasma cholinesterase at a slightly slower rate (88%) than suxamethonium. Abnormal cholinesterases will therefore increase its effective action more than suxamethonium. In E_uE_a heterozygotes (see under 'Suxamethonium' in the section that follows) it will last for 2 hours, and in E_aE_a homozygotes its action will be prolonged for 8 hours or more. The drug has no active metabolites.
  - **Atracurium:** about 10% is excreted renally, about 40–45% is hydrolyzed by hepatic esters and a further 45% undergoes Hofmann degradation at body temperature and pH (this reaction was first identified in industrial processes). The cleavage occurs at the linkage between the carbon chain and the quaternary nitrogen. Ester hydrolysis takes place at the site of the double carbon bond. Hofmann degradation produces laudanosine, a potentially epileptogenic metabol-ite which has not, however, been shown to cause problems in humans. Blood levels reach around 2 μg ml^{-1} after a standard bolus dose of 0.5 mg kg^{-1}. Its other product of metabolism is a monoquaternary acrylate compound.
  - **Cisatracurium:** qualitatively, the metabolism of cisatracurium is similar to atracurium, except a substantially greater proportion (up to 70%) undergoes Hofmann elimination, and ester hydrolysis is much less important. As the drug is five times as potent as atracurium, it is predictable that laudanosine levels similarly are lower at around 0.4 μg ml^{-1} after a bolus dose of 0.1 mg kg^{-1}.
  - **Pancuronium:** 60% is excreted renally, unchanged. The remainder is metabolized in the liver; the 3-hydroxy metabolite has 50% of the activity of the parent compound, and deacetylation also creates 3-desacetyl active metabolites which are rendered water-soluble by glucuronidation.
  - **Vecuronium:** about 30% is excreted renally, while the remainder undergoes hepatic deacetylation. Like pancuronium, it produces an active metabolite: 3-desacetylvecuronium.
  - **Rocuronium:** its elimination is mainly hepatic. It is metabolized to 17-desacetylrocuronium, which has around 5% of the activity of the parent compound.

Factors That May Potentiate the Action of Non-Depolarizing Muscle Relaxants

- A number of drugs can prolong the duration of action of NMBDs. Mechanisms include stabilization of the post-synaptic membrane, pre-synaptic inhibition of acetylcholine release or a combination of pre-and post-synaptic effects. Implicated agents include magnesium (pre- and post-synaptic inhibition) and those which have a direct effect on ion transport at the neuromuscular junction, such as calcium-channel blockers, β-adrenoceptor blockers and local anaesthetics. In higher doses, local anaesthetics can also exert a membrane stabilizing effect on the muscle membrane itself. Lithium potentiates neuromuscular blockade, as do some antibiotics – particularly the aminoglycosides – by pre-synaptic inhibition of acetylcholine. Given the ubiquity of gentamicin use for surgical prophylaxis, this is not simply a theoretical consideration.
- Other factors that potentiate NMBDs include hepatic and renal insufficiency, acidosis, hypokalaemia and hypothermia.

Suxamethonium

Commentary

Suxamethonium is arguably the only drug used in anaesthesia for which there is as yet no real alternative, although some might make the case for high-dose rocuronium as a substitute. It is a very familiar agent, and so in addition to an account of its actions you might, for example, be asked to justify its role in modern anaesthesia, which will inevitably involve a discussion of the significant potential problems associated with its use.

Core Information

- **Structure:** in common with all muscle relaxants, suxamethonium is a quaternary amine, which is the dicholine ester of succinic acid. This compound is almost identical to two molecules of acetylcholine (ACh). It is bisquaternary, and each of its ammonium radicals, $N^+(CH_3)_3$, bind to the α units of the ACh receptor.
- **Actions:** suxamethonium is the only currently available depolarizing muscle relaxant. It acts as an agonist at the ACh receptor, but, unlike acetylcholine, once having induced the conformational change that allows the ionophore to open (and then revert to a closed, inactivated conformation), it remains bound to the receptor for some minutes.
- **Indications:** it is an ultra-short-acting agent whose prime use is to allow rapid tracheal intubation in patients who are at risk of pulmonary aspiration of gastric contents. A typical intubating dose is 1.0–1.5 mg kg^{-1}. It can be used intermittently (with the purported problems of bradycardia with subsequent doses, although this is not always seen) and also by infusion. The maximum quoted total dose is 10 mg kg^{-1}, although it is likely that phase II block can be induced at lower doses.
- **Metabolism and elimination:** the primary metabolic route is ester hydrolysis in the presence of plasma cholinesterase. A small amount is hydrolyzed by non-specific plasma esterases, and 10% is excreted unchanged through the kidney.

Supplementary Information and Clinical Considerations

Does Suxamethonium Have a Future in Clinical Practice?

- The search for a 'clean' alternative to suxamethonium has lasted decades, so far without success. The drug provides the quickest means of achieving tracheal intubation. In severe laryngospasm in a patient without intravenous access, it can also be given intramuscularly or intra-lingually (in a dose of 4 mg kg^{-1}). At least one meta-analysis has asserted that, despite its many adverse effects, it is still the first-line agent in rapid sequence induction.
- Rocuronium has a much more benign side effect profile, and in a high dose of 0.9–1.0 mg kg^{-1} it can provide intubating conditions equivalent to those provided by suxamethonium, although up to 35 seconds slower. The problem of prolonged paralysis has been negated by the introduction of sugammadex, which can reverse the effect of rocuronium from any depth of neuromuscular block. (Albeit at a price: a 500 mg ampoule at current prices is around £150.)
- Suxamethonium – problems with its use:
  - **Bradyarrhythmias**: stimulation of muscarinic receptors in the sinoatrial node may lead to bradycardia, although the immediate administration of suxamethonium is frequently associated with transient tachycardia which often goes unnoticed or is attributed to the stress of laryngoscopy. Bradycardia is more common in children and other patients with a high resting vagal tone.
  - **Myalgia:** this should not be underestimated, as it can be very severe. Because it affects intercostal muscle and the diaphragm, it can have visceral characteristics which can even mimic symptoms of cardiac ischaemia. The mechanism is unclear; although suxamethonium causes fasciculations and an increase in muscle creatine phosphokinase (CPK), neither of these is directly related to post-administration pain. Myoglobin can also be detected in urine. Early ambulation, female gender, middle age and, it is said, lack of muscular fitness are all associated with a higher incidence, as are rapid injection and repeated smaller doses. Techniques used to attenuate the problem include pre-treatment with a non-depolarizing relaxant, dantrolene, lidocaine and phenytoin. None is universally effective.
  - **Muscle fasciculation and masseter spasm.** These are characteristics of the drug rather than specific problems, although both can be disconcerting. The phenomena are believed to be due to the prejunctional stimulation of acetylcholine receptors on the motor nerve, with transiently repetitive firing and ACh release.
  - **Hyperkalaemia:** serum potassium may rise about 0.5 mmol l^{-1} in the normal patient, but this increase can be dangerously high in patients in whom muscle cells are damaged or in whom muscles are denervated. Damaged muscle leaks potassium, while denervated muscle demonstrates an increase in extrajunctional ACh receptors. Conditions in which suxamethonium should be avoided, therefore, include renal failure, burns, spinal cord damage, polyneuropathies and crush injury. Dangerous rises can also occur in the critically ill, and the drug must be used with caution in intensive care patients.
  - **Prolonged action owing to decreased enzyme activity:** suxamethonium undergoes ester hydrolysis in a reaction that is catalysed by plasma cholinesterase.

Qualitative and quantitative changes in this enzyme have a substantial effect on the drug's duration of action. Enzyme activity is reduced by decreased enzyme synthesis due to liver disease, starvation, carcinomatosis, pregnancy, renal disease and myxoedema (hypothyroidism). Such reduction may increase by several times its normal duration of action of 3–5 minutes. Prolongation may also result from competition by other drugs metabolized by esterases, such as diamorphine, ester-linked local anaesthetics, esmolol and monoamine oxidase inhibitors. Anticholinesterases inhibit both plasma cholinesterase as well as acetylcholinesterase.

— **Prolonged action owing to abnormal enzymes**: qualitative differences result from inherited deficiencies of plasma cholinesterase. Its synthesis is controlled by autosomal recessive genes, of which 14 different mutations have so far been identified. The normal gene is characterized as E_u, and the commonest atypical gene as E_a (others include the fluoride gene, E_f, and the silent gene, E_s). The action of suxamethonium in a heterozygote, E_uE_a, will be prolonged by around 30 minutes, whereas in a homozygote, E_aE_a, this will extend to several hours and will be longer still in the case of E_aE_s and E_sE_s variations. Testing using inhibition by dibucaine and fluoride has been superseded by direct assay of cholinesterase activity. Suxamethonium apnoea is not life-threatening, assuming that it is recognized, but it is important to maintain anaesthesia in any patient who is receiving supportive ventilation.

— **Malignant hyperpyrexia and anaphylaxis**: it is a trigger for malignant hyperpyrexia, and, although allergic reactions are rare, anaphylaxis is more commonly seen with suxamethonium than with any other muscle relaxant, accounting for almost 50% of reactions. (For example, there were two fatal cases described in the 1991–1993 report of the *Confidential Enquiry into Maternal Deaths*.)

— **Phase II block**: repeated doses or prolonged infusions of suxamethonium (as was once a routine technique for caesarean sections under general anaesthesia) can result in the development of a Phase II block, which has all the characteristics of a non-depolarizing competitive block. A nerve stimulator will therefore show the typical fade of the train-of-four response, tetanic fade and post-tetanic potentiation. (Phase I describes the initial depolarizing block.) The mechanism has not been clearly elaborated, but theories include post-junctional receptor desensitization and pre-synaptic inhibition of acetylcholine synthesis and release. Phase II block is potentiated by inhalational anaesthetic agents. Although it can be reversed with standard anticholinesterases, the response is unpredictable.

Opiates/Opioids

Commentary

This may not appear as a question on its own, although it might be linked to the subject of patient-controlled analgesia (PCA), aspects of postoperative pain relief or even the properties of the 'ideal' opioid. Opiates are central to anaesthetic practice, and so you will be expected to have a comprehensive grasp of their pharmacology. There is some continued confusion over the terms 'opiate' and 'opioid'. The word 'opiate', strictly defined, is any drug that is derived from the opium poppy, *Papaver somniferum*. According to this definition, however, morphine and codeine phosphate are classed as opiates, whereas diamorphine (which is diacetylated morphine) is not. It is more logical therefore to use 'opiate' as the noun, and 'opioid' as the adjective, or alternatively, to use the term 'opioid' to mean any drug that acts at the opioid receptor. It would be more logical still to abandon the word 'opiate' altogether, but in the meantime the residual uncertainty means that you will not be disadvantaged if you tend to use the terms interchangeably. You will almost certainly be familiar with the drugs discussed, so have confidence in your clinical experience of their use.

Core Information

All the pure μ-agonists have similar pharmacodynamic effects; their differences are primarily pharmacokinetic.

- **Opioid receptors:** the nomenclature continues to evolve. The previously described three main opioid receptor subtypes were μ (mu), κ (kappa) and δ (delta), which were also referred to respectively as OP3, OP2 and OP1 receptors. In addition, there was the 'opioid receptor-like type 1' – ORL1 (OP4), which also inhibited calcium channels and increased cellular potassium efflux. These terms have been superseded by MOP (μ-opioid peptide receptor, with endomorphins as natural ligands), DOP (δ-delta opioid peptide receptor, with enkephalins as natural ligands), KOP (κ-opioid peptide receptor, with dynorphins as natural ligands) and NOP (nociceptin/orphanin FQ peptide receptor, with orphanin FQ as its natural ligand). Opioid receptors are distributed widely throughout the central nervous system. Opioids have a number of effects at the cellular level: they inhibit intracellular adenyl cyclase via G protein-coupling, they hyperpolarize cell membranes by facilitating the opening of post-synaptic potassium channels and they inhibit neurotransmitter release by decreasing the function of voltage-gated calcium channels. MOP (μ-) receptors are believed to mediate not only analgesic effects but also respiratory depression. KOP (κ-) receptors have more spinal and peripheral than central analgesic effects, as do the DOP (δ) receptors. The nociception NOP receptor is the most recently identified, and investigation has concentrated on its analgesic effects and its apparent neural processing of factors such as drug tolerance, reward and addiction. The σ (sigma)-receptor is not considered to be a true opioid receptor, but it does mediate psychotomimetic effects both of opiates and of other types of psychoactive agents.
- **Opioid actions:** these are almost too well known to repeat, but, to summarize, opioids have a mixture of inhibitory and excitatory effects. **Inhibitory actions: These** mediate sedation; anxiolysis, analgesia, respiratory depression (including inhibition of the respiratory response to hypoxia), inhibition of cough and loss of vascular smooth muscle tone. **Excitatory effects:** These explain miosis (stimulation of the Edinger–Westphal nucleus), nausea and vomiting via direct actions at the chemoreceptor trigger zone, ADH release from the posterior pituitary, urinary retention owing to enhanced detrusor muscle tone, bronchoconstriction caused by an increase in smooth muscle tone and constipation owing to increased activity in the circular

muscle of the bowel which prevents effective peristalsis. Other effects include histamine release, pruritus (which may not be mediated by μ-receptors, as it is not reliably reversed by naloxone) and chest-wall rigidity. This is associated with rapid injection of the more potent short-acting opioids but can occur with all of this class of drug. One possible explanation for the phenomenon is that it is due to the simultaneous inhibition of GABA release in the striatum of the basal ganglia together with a simultaneous but transient increase in dopamine production.

- **Morphine:** this can be given by various routes. There is a range of reported bioavailability: 100% (i.m.), 20–40% (oral), 35–70% (rectal). It is not always appreciated that it takes some time for a bolus intravenous dose to reach its maximal effect. Unlike all the other major opioids, at 20 minutes the drug has reached only 80% of its peak effect. Morphine is metabolized in the liver to morphine-6-glucuronide (5–15%), which is more potent than the parent compound (its precise relative potency has not been quantified because studies have looked at different aspects of opioid effect rather than at analgesia alone), and to morphine-3-glucuronide (50%), which has no analgesic effects.

- **Diamorphine:** this is a semisynthetic derivative of morphine, diacetylmorphine, which consists of two molecules of morphine. The compound has no activity at μ-receptors until it is metabolized to 6-monoacetylmorphine and thence to morphine (both are active). It is thus a prodrug with the same properties as morphine. Some clinicians are convinced nonetheless that anecdotally it is less emetic and more euphoriant than morphine. (When given intrathecally, its much higher lipid solubility does confer advantages.)

- **Pethidine:** the side effect profile is very similar to that of morphine, but pethidine is still regarded as an alternative opioid in patients who are intolerant of morphine. It has a rapid onset of action, but its effects are shorter. It differs in some other material respects. One of its metabolites is norpethidine, which is a convulsant. Prolonged or high-dose administration should therefore be avoided, and it should be used with care in patients with renal impairment. The drug is related structurally to atropine, which explains its anticholinergic actions. It relaxes bronchial and vascular smooth muscle and is antispasmodic. It is a membrane stabilizer and has a local anaesthetic effect. One useful property is its ability to attenuate or abolish anaesthesia-induced postoperative shivering (typically 25 mg by slow intravenous injection).

- **Fentanyl:** this is a phenylpiperidine (like pethidine), which itself is the parent compound of alfentanil and remifentanil. Onset of effect is at 1–2 minutes, with a peak action at 4–5 minutes and an effective duration of action after a single bolus of up to 30 minutes. It is highly lipid-soluble, and its metabolites are inactive. It is a drug that accumulates when given by infusion (or by repeated bolus injection); its context-sensitive half-time (CSHT) after 2 hours of constant infusion is 48 minutes, which, after 8 hours of infusion, extends to 282 minutes.

- **Alfentanil:** this is also a phenylpiperidine compound but with a shorter duration of action than fentanyl. After peaking at 1 minute after intravenous injection, its effects last for only 5–10 minutes. The drug accumulates when given by infusion, its CSHT being 50 minutes after 2 hours.

- **Remifentanil:** this is a phenylpiperidine ester whose action is terminated by nonspecific tissue esterases. Its main product of metabolism has minimal potency (<0.5%).

This gives it a short and predictable duration of action which is confirmed by its CSHT. It is effectively context-insensitive because the CSHT is 4.5 minutes after 2 hours of infusion, and only 9.0 minutes after 8 hours. Its very rapid offset of action makes it unsuitable for PCA for postoperative pain, but there are some obstetric anaesthetists who advocate its use for labour analgesia. (Bolus doses 20–40 μg with a 2-minute lockout. Associated problems include sedation and maternal desaturation.) One disadvantage of high-dose remifentanil infusion is its potential to cause postoperative hyperalgesia. This can be mitigated by low-dose ketamine, which suggests that the hyperalgesia is mediated via NMDA receptor activation.

- **Other pure μ-agonists:** these include **codeine phosphate** (which is metabolized to morphine), its semisynthetic derivative **dihydrocodeine**, **hydromorphone** (which is a potent morphine derivative used mainly in the treatment of severe cancer pain) and **oxycodone** (which has high oral bioavailability (up to 75%) and which is becoming more popular for the treatment of postoperative pain). Oxycodone has one weakly active metabolite, oxymorphone. (The usual oral dose of oxycodone is 5–10 mg given 3-4-hourly. There is also a sustained release preparation OxyContin; dose 10 mg 12-hourly).
- **Tramadol:** tramadol is a racemic mixture of R (+) and S (−) enantiomers, of which the R (+) enantiomer has low initial activity at μ-receptors; however, the higher affinity of its main metabolite (ortho-desmethyltramadol) results in a sixfold increase in analgesic potency. Nevertheless, the μ effects in humans are not impressive, although opioid side effects such as nausea, constipation and dysphoria are still apparent. The S (−) enantiomer inhibits the re-uptake of noradrenaline and 5-HT within the CNS. Tramadol has been used in PCA with 10–20 mg boluses and a 5-minute lockout. It causes less nausea than morphine but at the cost of inferior analgesia.

Supplementary Information

Patient-Controlled Analgesia (PCA)

- **Advantages:** PCA is popular with patients because of the autonomy and control that it gives them, which makes it particularly useful in those who might otherwise be reluctant to request analgesia and for those who dislike intramuscular injections. It is popular with nurses for the same reasons, and because it can save nursing time. It is popular with doctors because most PCA regimens by and large can cope with the very wide variability that characterizes patients' requirements for postoperative opioids. As a generalization, it is efficacious and safe.
- **Disadvantages:** it is important that a PCA does not lessen the direct personal contact between the patient and nursing staff. Electronic pumps can limit mobility, while disposable devices lack the facility to track demand and the total analgesic dose delivered. Security can also be a problem. PCA is still a system that delivers bolus doses, which results in peaks and troughs of effect. This can be overcome by adding a background infusion, but potentially this is at the expense of safety.
- **Drugs used in PCA regimens:** Morphine is commonly used in PCA regimens because it is seen to offer the best compromise between the combination of efficacy and duration of action. A typical regimen is 1.0 mg bolus with a 5-minute lockout time. Its pharmacokinetic profile, however, with the slow time to peak effect, suggests

that it is by no means the most suitable agent. Pethidine can be used; its peak effect is around 7–8 minutes after injection, and a typical regimen would be bolus doses of 10–20 mg with a 5-minute lockout. The peak effect of fentanyl occurs around 4–5 minutes, and its duration of action of about 30 minutes makes this a suitable, and underused agent (bolus doses of 10–20 µg; lockout time 5–10 minutes). The onset time of alfentanil and remifentanil is very short, at around 1–2 minutes, but rapid offset limits their suitability for PCA systems. Remifentanil PCA is nonetheless used in some maternity units for labour analgesia (20–40 µg bolus with a 2-minute lockout as described).

- **Opioid-induced hyperalgesia (OIH):** this describes the paradoxical increased sensitivity to pain in subjects given opioids – typically, although not exclusively, when taking high doses over a prolonged period. High doses of intraoperative opioids can also reduce nociceptive thresholds and cause secondary hyperalgesia. This appears to be a greater problem with remifentanil,. It is potentially problematic because hyperalgesia in the immediate post-operative period is associated with the development of chronic post-surgery pain syndromes. One theory had it that the metabolite morphine-3-glucuronide was antanalgesic, but that is an oversimplistic hypothesis that would limit the phenomenon to morphine-containing opioids alone, which is not the case. The precise mechanisms have not been elucidated, and as the postulated theories are complex they are unlikely to form the central focus of any discussion. As a brief and necessarily superficial explanation, however, it is possible first that there is an alteration of the opioid receptor itself such that the G-protein secondary messenger systems described undergo a switch from an inhibitory to an excitatory coupled mode. In addition, the prolonged use of opioids may cause down-regulation of glutamate transport at spinal cord level. The resultant increase in glutamate in glutamate activation of NMDA receptors may augment the sensitization of spinal neurons. Similarly, some descending inhibitory serotoninergic pathways may become pro-nociceptive. Other factors that have been implicated include changes in cytokine production, alterations in calcium channel functioning and the activation of Substance P. (This is a neuropeptide that at spinal cord level mediates nociception via binding to the neurokinin 1 receptor).

Local Anaesthetics: Actions

Commentary

Questions about local anaesthesia are popular because the subject can switch readily between basic science and its clinical implications. Mechanisms of action may not be a topic on their own but may instead form part of questions on the agents themselves and their toxicity, or as a supplement to a discussion of nerve blocks. There is considerable interest in the suggestion that effective neuraxial and regional anaesthesia may reduce tumour recurrence and prolong survival. This is outlined briefly at the end of this section, although the subject is more likely to arise as part of a discussion of thoracic epidural or paravertebral blocks. Intravenous lidocaine has also found a role as part of multimodal perioperative analgesia.

Core Information

- **Definition:** a local anaesthetic agent is defined as a compound which produces temporary blockade of neuronal transmission when applied to a nerve axon.
- **Drugs:** numerous drugs share this characteristic with conventional local anaesthetics. They include anticonvulsants, many antiarrhythmics, including bretylium and β-adrenoceptor blockers, some phenothiazines and some antihistamines, as well as drugs such as pethidine and ketamine. None is used as a local anaesthetic but all have a similar mechanism of action. The range of local anaesthetic agents used in the UK is small and is restricted largely to lidocaine, bupivacaine, prilocaine and, to a lesser extent, ropivacaine.
- **Basic structure:** all local anaesthetics are chemical descendants of cocaine and comprise a lipophilic aromatic portion, which is joined via an ester or amide linkage to a hydrophilic tertiary amine chain (Figure 4.2). Esters are hydrolyzed by non-specific plasma cholinesterase, and amides are metabolized in the liver.
- **Normal action potential:** local anaesthetic action is best described in the context of a normal nerve action potential. The axon maintains a voltage differential of 60–90 mV across the nerve membrane. At rest the membrane is relatively impermeable to the influx of sodium (Na^+) ions and is selectively permeable to potassium (K^+) ions. In the resting cell membrane, this selective permeability allows a small net efflux of K^+ ions, which leaves the axoplasm electrically negative (polarized). At rest, Na^+ ions tend to flow into the axon, both because the inside is electrically negative and because of the concentration gradient. This resting membrane potential is maintained by the Na^+/K^+ pump which continually extrudes Na^+ from within the cell in exchange for K^+, using ATP as an energy source. When specific sodium channels in the axonal membrane are opened, there is a selective permeability to Na^+ ions, and the membrane depolarizes. Repolarization takes place when voltage-dependent K^+ channels open to permit a large efflux of K^+. As the membrane becomes less negative, more Na^+ channels open, and open more rapidly; more Na^+ ions enter the cell, and depolarization is further accelerated.

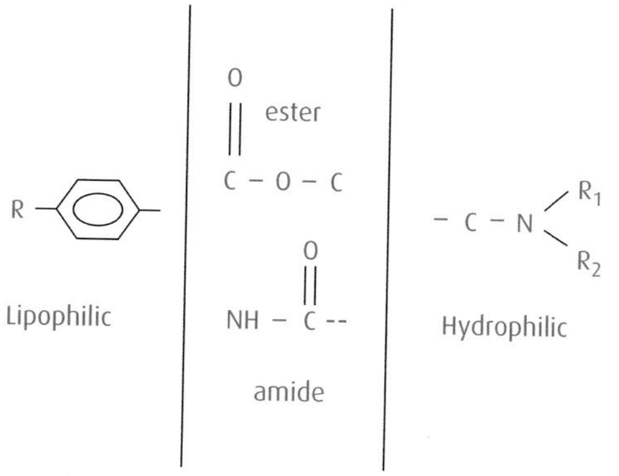

Fig. 4.2 Structure of local anaesthetics.

- **Impulse propagation:** the impulse is propagated by the spread of inward current through the conducting medium of the axoplasm to adjacent inactive regions. Inward currents from all the active nodes integrate as they spread, ensuring that impulse propagation will continue.

- **Local anaesthetic action:** these mainly block the function of the sodium channels, which exist in 'open', 'resting' and 'inactivated' conformational states. Local anaesthetic affinity is higher when the channel is in the open or inactivated state. The drugs exert no effect on cellular integrity or metabolism, but when a sufficient concentration is reached in the perfusing solution, depolarization does not occur in response to an electrical stimulus. Na^+ influx is blocked, although repolarization associated with K^+ efflux is unaffected. The agents in their cationic ionized form block the sodium channels on the inside of the axoplasm. External perfusion has no effect; the uncharged form must penetrate the cell wall before dissociating. The nerve blockade is concentration-dependent and ends when the local anaesthetic concentration falls below a critical minimum level. Local anaesthetics work by stabilizing the axonal membrane and will stabilize all excitable membranes, including those of skeletal, smooth and cardiac muscle. Local anaesthetics also block some potassium ion channels, broaden the action potential and enhance binding by maintaining the sodium channel in the open or inactivated state.

- **pKa:** local anaesthetics exist in equilibrium between ionized and non-ionized forms. The ratio of the two states is given by the Henderson–Hasselbalch equation (originally derived to describe the pH changes resulting from the addition of H^+ or OH^- ions to any buffer system). The Ka is the dissociation constant which governs the position of equilibrium between the charged and uncharged forms. By analogy to pH, the pKa is the negative logarithm of that constant. Rearranging the equation pH = pKa + log $[HCO_3^-]$ / $[H_2CO_3]$ gives: pKa = pH – log [base] / [conjugate acid]. This is the same as saying [base] / [conjugate acid] = 1.0, so the dissociation constant, or pKa, is the pH at which equal amounts of drug are present in the charged and uncharged state.

- **Clinical implications:** a pKa of 7.4 indicates that, at body pH, there are equal numbers of molecules in the charged and uncharged forms. Most local anaesthetics have pKa values higher than body pH, and the more distant the dissociation constant from body pH, the more molecules that exist in the ionized form. The pH scale is logarithmic; hence if a drug has a pKa of 8.4, it is 1 pH unit (i.e. a tenfold H^+ concentration) away from body pH. At 7.4 there is a 10:1 ratio, that is, the drug is 90% ionized and 10% non-ionized. At pKa 9.4 the difference is 100-fold, so at body pH of 7.4, 99% of the drug will be charged. Uncharged base is necessary for tissue penetration, and so drugs with lower pKa usually have a more rapid onset of action. Thus, lidocaine and prilocaine (pKa 7.7) have a shorter latency than bupivacaine (pKa 8.1). This dominance of the non-diffusible cation also explains the reason why local anaesthetics are much less effective in the presence of inflamed and acidotic tissue. Note, however, that pKa is not the only factor involved. Concentration and intrinsic potency are also important. Drugs also have to penetrate a perineural membrane of connective tissue, and this property has not been well quantified, thus

chloroprocaine (popular in the USA although not used in the UK) has one of the fastest onsets of action of all local anaesthetics, despite having a pKa of 9.1.
- **Barriers to drug passage:** peripheral nerves contain both afferent and efferent axons which are enclosed in a fine matrix of connective tissue which embeds the axons – the *endoneurium*. The fascicles of axons are enclosed within a squamous cellular layer, the *perineurium*, which is an effective semi-permeable barrier to local anaesthetics. The whole structure is surrounded by a sheath of collagen fibres, the *epineurium*, which permits easy diffusion of local anaesthetic. So, in the case of a myelinated sensory nerve, the local anaesthetic molecule may have to traverse four or five connective-tissue and lipid-membrane barriers. The most important of these is the perineurium, and this squamous cell layer, connected by tight junctions, is one of the main reasons why, under clinical conditions, only about 5% of the injected anaesthetic dose will actually penetrate the nerve.

Supplementary Information
Other factors that may influence local anaesthetic action.

- **Structure–activity relationships of local anaesthetics:** the site of local anaesthetic action is a protein structure in the Na^+ channel. The affinity of the drug to the channel, which determines its duration of action, is related to the length of the aliphatic (open carbon) chains on the compound. Small structural changes also influence factors such as lipid solubility and protein binding. These are summarized in Figure 4.3.

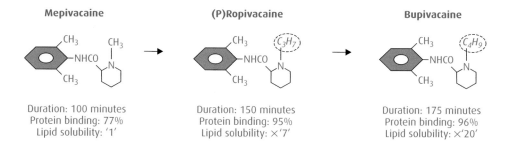

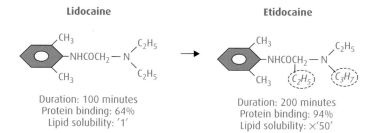

Fig. 4.3 Structure-activity relationship of local anaesthetics.

- **Lipid solubility:** this is a prime determinant of potency, which is increased by the substitution of longer side chains. The parent compound of ropivacaine and bupivacaine is mepivacaine, which has a single methyl group attached to the tertiary amine. Ropivacaine and bupivacaine are identical apart from propyl (C_3H_7) and butyl (C_4H_9) side chain substituents, respectively. (This makes for convenient recall, should you be asked: me-*methyl*-pivacaine; pro-*propyl*-pivacaine, ropivacaine being the pure enantiomer of propivacaine; and bu-*butyl*-pivacaine.) These small structural changes mean that bupivacaine has three times the lipid solubility of ropivacaine and twenty times that of mepivacaine. Etidocaine (a drug whose capacity to cause a preferential motor block has rather restricted its popularity) has a structure very similar to that of lidocaine; however, the addition of an ethyl (C_2H_5) group to the intermediate linking chain and substitution of a propyl group for the ethyl on the amide portion increases lipid solubility by 50 times. (This also doubles its duration of action; highly lipid-soluble agents are highly concentrated in tissue and dislodge slowly.) From least to most lipid-soluble, therefore, the local anaesthetics are ranked as follows: prilocaine, lidocaine, ropivacaine, bupivacaine and etidocaine. The relationship between lipid solubility and potency is not linear, and above a fourfold increase in partition coefficient there is a ceiling beyond which there is little observed increase in potency. (The esters procaine and chloroprocaine have low lipid solubility, and so are delivered in high 2–3% concentrations. Amethocaine and bupivacaine have high lipid solubility and produce effective anaesthesia at 0.25%.)
- **Protein binding:** this is also affected by structural differences in the molecule. Longer aliphatic substituents increase affinity for the sodium channel and prolong the duration of action. Bupivacaine and ropivacaine are both ~96% protein-bound. Lidocaine and prilocaine are much more weakly protein-bound (65% and 55%, respectively), with actions lasting for around 100 minutes. High protein binding decreases toxicity by reducing the proportion of free drug in the plasma.
- **MLAC:** the Minimum Local Analgesic Concentration model was developed by analogy to MAC (minimum alveolar concentration), which is routinely used to describe inhalational anaesthetic agents. It aims to allow a more sophisticated comparison of local anaesthetics in a particular context rather than simply looking at the drugs when given in what are potentially supramaximal doses. The model uses an 'up-and-down' sequential allocation of dose. The response of the subject is all or none; the concentration of local anaesthetic delivered being either effective or ineffective. If a specific concentration is effective, it is then reduced in a step-wise fashion to succeeding subjects until it is reported as ineffective. At that point the concentration is then increased in a step-wise manner by the same amount until the result identifies a threshold above which 50% of subjects will report that the drug is effective and below which 50% will say that it is not. This point represents the median effective concentration (EC_{50}) or dose (ED_{50}). The MLAC model has been used to examine the effect of adding adjuvants to neuraxial and plexus blocks and to identify, for example, the claims of sensory–motor dissociation that have been made for ropivacaine. **Resistance to local anaesthetics:** it appears probable that there is the rare possibility of both acquired and innate resistance to local anaesthetics. The antigen/antibody complex that is formed following envenomation (for example by scorpion stings) can interfere with the function of the sodium channel. In addition,

clinical experience reveals the very occasional patient in whom local anaesthesia is only partially effective or completely ineffective, which suggests the possibility of a mutation of the channel itself.

- **Frequency dependence:** you will be doing well if you get as far as discussing this phenomenon, which is discussed in more detail under 'Bupivacaine, Ropicaine, Lidocaine and Prilocaine' in a subsequent section.

Clinical Considerations

- **Intravenous lidocaine for perioperative analgesia.** A Cochrane review published in July 2015 concluded that there was 'low to moderate' evidence that intravenous lidocaine reduced early post-operative pain scores. The authors equivocated because of the small size of the studies that were reviewed, and they also commented on the lack of evidence about optimal dose regimens, timing and adverse effects. Nonetheless, the review did report that intravenous infusions of lidocaine reduced pain scores at up to 4 hours after laparoscopic and open abdominal surgery. There was no difference at 48 hours. It also appeared to have a beneficial effect on the recovery of bowel function. A lower incidence of post-operative nausea was attributed to its opioid-sparing actions. A typical dose regimen would be 2 mg kg^{-1} hr^{-1} (Cochrane Database of Systematic Reviews. Continuous intravenous perioperative lidocaine infusion for postoperative pain and recovery. July 2015).

Regional Anaesthesia and Tumour Recurrence

- **Influence of surgery and general anaesthesia on immune function:** The stress of surgery is immunomodulating. The details are complex, but in addition to factors such as the suppression of natural killer (NK) cell function and a global reduction in the reactivity of the immune system, surgery may enhance the release of substances such as the polypeptide transforming growth factor-β1 (TGF-β1), which is a cytokine important in establishing tumour blood supply and cell proliferation. Increased catecholamine levels themselves have also been shown to stimulate experimental tumour growth (a process that is inhibited by β-adrenoceptor blockers). Anaesthesia also modulates immune function, including that mediated by neutrophils, NK and T-cells. (Propofol, however, does not appear to have these effects.) Opioids depress humoral and cellular immune function, and in particular impair NK cell activity. NK cells are non-specific but bind to tumour cells and cells infected by viruses, and are probably the most important cell type involved in tumour surveillance. It is postulated that some of these effects, in particular the endocrine stress response and the adverse effects of opioids, may be attenuated by effective regional and neuraxial anaesthesia.

- **Regional anaesthesia and cancer surgery.** The evidence is drawn largely from retrospective reviews, in which inevitably there are numerous uncontrolled variables. Breast cancer, for example, is not a homogenous entity but includes several tumour types; equally heterogeneous are general anaesthetic techniques. These are invariably multimodal, and together with opioid analgesia, may well suppress immune surveillance of tumour cells. Other confounding factors include the concurrent use of chemotherapy and the need for allogeneic blood transfusions. Nonetheless, there are studies that suggest some regional anaesthetic techniques do increase recurrence-free survival in breast and prostate cancers. In one study looking at patients (n = 129) who had either paravertebral blocks or patient-controlled anaesthesia, there was a four times greater rate of recurrence-free survival in the block group (6% vs 24%). In another retrospective survey of 225 patients undergoing radical prostatectomy over a 10-year period, the use of epidural analgesia in combination with general anaesthesia was associated with a 57% reduction in biochemical cancer (using prostate-specific antigen as the marker). In other cancers, however, the results of studies are more equivocal. Analysis of the MASTER trial, for example, which prospectively studied a total of 503 patients with mainly cancers of the colon, revealed no difference in recurrence-free survival between the general anaesthesia/opioid and general anaesthesia/epidural groups. (P.S. Myles *et al. Lancet* 2002, 359: 1276–82). In contrast, a very large retrospective analysis of more than 42,000 patients with non-metastatic colorectal cancer found a significant association between overall survival and epidural anaesthesia but no difference in disease-free survival. (K.C. Cummings *et al. Anesthesiology* 2012, 116: 797–806. (This looked at data from the Surveillance, Epidemiology and End Results (SEER) programme which scrutinizes the incidence and survival rates of cancers in the USA). The evidence overall is conflicting, but there are some prospective randomized clinical trials that currently are in progress in breast, colon and lung cancers which should in due course inform the debate and indicate in the light of their findings whether anaesthetic techniques should be modified.

Local Anaesthetics: Toxicity

Commentary

The use of large drug doses for nerve and plexus blocks together with the potential for inadvertent intravenous injection means that local anaesthetic toxicity is not merely an academic possibility. In this oral you need to demonstrate that your practice is safe and that you have effective plan for management should the occasion arise.

Core Information

Factors that predispose a patient to local anaesthetic toxicity.

- **Site of injection:** the primary influences are the vascularity of the anatomical site of injection and the presence locally of tissue such as fat, which may bind local anaesthetics. There is a spectrum of absorption, which is greatest after intercostal and paracervical block, and thereafter, in descending order, sacral extradural (caudal) block, lumbar and thoracic extradural block, brachial plexus block, sciatic and femoral nerve block and subcutaneous infiltration. Absorption from this last site is so delayed that some authors have described using doses that far exceed recommended maxima. Lidocaine 35 mg kg^{-1}, for example, has been used during tumescent liposuction (but equally may be responsible for some of the disasters that have been reported in the USA following 'office' anaesthesia for cosmetic procedures).
- **Drug dosage and concentration:** it is not only the peak level but also the rate of rise that may contribute to local anaesthetic toxicity. The total mass of drug may also be

less important than its concentration; a dilute solution of the same dose is associated with lower peak levels. Because factors such as the rate of injection and the site of administration have such a substantial influence on blood levels, there is limited logic to the maximum doses of local anaesthetics that are usually cited. Be that as it may, the commonly quoted maximum doses are as follows: lidocaine 3.0 mg kg^{-1}, 7.0 mg kg^{-1} with adrenaline; bupivacaine 2.0 mg kg^{-1}; prilocaine 400 mg total dose (600 mg with adrenaline); and ropivacaine 150 mg total dose, with or without adrenaline. Plasma concentrations would be a more useful measure; convulsive activity supervenes when bupivacaine concentrations reach around 4 µg ml^{-1} and lidocaine levels reach 10–12 µg ml^{-1}. Early central nervous system symptoms and signs can manifest at much lower concentrations – at just over 2 µg ml^{-1} for levobupivacaine.

- **Vasoconstrictors:** the use of vasoconstrictors lowers the maximum blood concentrations but does not prolong the time to peak. There is also a complex interrelation with the inherent vasoactivity of local anaesthetics, all of which (apart from cocaine, which is a potent vasoconstrictor) demonstrate biphasic activity. At very low concentrations all enhance vascular smooth muscle activity and cause vasoconstriction. At clinical doses they demonstrate vasodilator activity that is dose-dependent and which varies for each drug. Racemic bupivacaine is a vasoconstrictor at low concentrations and is a less effective vasodilator than levobupivacaine 0.75%. Lidocaine also constricts at low concentrations but dilates at clinical levels. Increased blood flow increases vascular uptake and decreases duration of action.

- **Binding:** local anaesthetics bind mainly to α_1-acid glycoprotein, which is a high-affinity, low-capacity site and, to a lesser extent, to low-affinity, high-capacity sites on albumin. The binding decreases as pH decreases, and so toxicity is increased by hypoxia and acidosis. A decrease in intracellular pH will lead to increased ionization within the axoplasm and ion trapping. The convulsive threshold is inversely related to arterial PCO_2.

- **Mechanisms of toxicity:** the cardiovascular and CNS toxicities that may be seen are common to all local anaesthetic agents, and are predictable in light of the known mechanism of action of these drugs. Local anaesthetics work by stabilizing the axonal membrane, and will stabilize all excitable membranes, including those of skeletal, smooth and cardiac muscle. One of the main factors responsible for myocardial depression is the block of Ca^{2+} channels in the myocardium. Another is the lowering of Mg-adenosine triphosphate (Mg ATP) concentrations which in animal studies are associated with a reduction in myocardial contractility. Also important is the local anaesthetic inhibition of the carrier, carnitine acylcarnitine transferase which transports AcylCoA moieties (derived from FFAs, from ketones and indirectly from lactate) for utilization by myocyte mitochondria. This may explain why local anaesthetic–induced cardiac toxicity is so refractory.

Supplementary Information and Clinical Considerations

Symptoms, Signs and Immediate Management of Local Anaesthetic Toxicity

- **Clinical features:** the patient may complain of circumoral tingling and paraesthesia, light-headedness and dizziness. They may have visual and auditory disturbance manifested by difficulty in focusing and tinnitus. They may be disorientated. The objective signs are usually excitatory, with shivering, twitching, and tremors in the face and extremities preceding full grand mal convulsions. (This is due to preferential depression of inhibitory neural pathways.) Cardiac arrhythmias may be obvious on ECG monitoring, but these do not usually supervene until blood concentrations exceed by several times the convulsant levels.

- **Generic management:** the generic supportive ABC approach includes ventilation and inotropes as indicated.
- **Specific management**
  — **Cardiac arrhythmias**: if bupivacaine has been used, then resuscitation may be prolonged. Amiodarone (5 mg kg^{-1} in glucose 5% as the drug is incompatible with saline solutions) is the drug of choice for most induced arrhythmias, apart from ventricular fibrillation (VF). Historically, refractory VF was treated with bretylium (5 mg kg^{-1}), which is no longer available in the UK. Recent recommendations support the infusion of lipid emulsion. The effects of the intramyocardial inhibition of carnitine acylcarnitine transferase may be attenuated, if not reversed, by the increased concentration of free fatty acids which provide an enhanced energy substrate for myocardial mitochondria. There is also a 'lipid sink' hypothesis which suggests that the lipophilic drugs are bound preferentially by the locally high concentration of intravascular lipid rather than to tissues. This is rather less persuasive. If the lipid sink theory held true, then plasma local anaesthetic concentrations should rise. In preliminary studies it appears that in fact they fall. A typical lipid infusion regimen (as recommended by the Association of Anaesthetists of Great Britain and Ireland, the AAGBI) is to give intravenous Intralipid 20%, 1.5 ml kg^{-1} stat over 1 minute, followed by an infusion at a rate of 15 ml kg^{-1} h^{-1}. Two further 1.5 ml kg^{-1} bolus can be given 5 minutes apart and the rate of infusion doubled to 30 ml kg^{-1} h^{-1} if there has been no response or if there is deterioration after initial improvement. The total cumulative dose of Intralipid 20% should not exceed 12 ml kg^{-1} (so the anaesthetist would expect to give less than 1,000 ml in most situations).
  — **Grand mal convulsions**: phenytoin (usually given in a starting dose of 15 mg kg^{-1}) has a membrane-stabilizing local anaesthetic action. A better choice might be thiopental. It is a very effective anticonvulsant which, in small bolus doses of 50 mg, should suppress a fit that has been induced by local anaesthetic toxicity, but if necessary can be given as an infusion of 1–3 mg kg^{-1} h^{-1}. Diazemuls, midazolam or lorazepam can also be used to abort convulsive activity.
- **Pulmonary sequestration:** high blood levels may be attenuated by temporary sequestration of local anaesthetic within the lung. A high lung:blood partition coefficient encourages some uptake by the lung, and because the extravascular pH of lung is lower than that of plasma, this encourages ion trapping. Prilocaine is sequestered more effectively than bupivacaine, whose uptake in turn is greater than that of lidocaine.
- **Allergic reactions:** genuine allergy to amides is extremely rare, but is commoner with esters. Allergic reactions are due mainly to para-aminobenzoic acid (PABA), which is a product of the metabolism of ester local anaesthetics such as procaine, benzocaine, chloroprocaine and amethocaine.

- **Toxicity:** See earlier discussion. (The cardiovascular and CNS toxicities that may be seen are common to all local anaesthetic agents and are predictable in light of the known mechanism of action of these drugs. As already mentioned local anaesthetics work by stabilizing the axonal membrane and stabilize all excitable membranes, including those of skeletal, smooth and cardiac muscle.
- **CNS:** as the blood concentrations increase, an initial excitation gives way to generalized CNS depression with respiratory depression and arrest. The excitatory phase is caused by the selective blockade of inhibitory pathways in the cortex. Convulsive activity supervenes when bupivacaine concentrations reach 4 µg ml^{-1} and lidocaine levels reach 10–12 µg ml^{-1}.
- **Cardiovascular effects:** these are complex and vary between the agents. Lidocaine can be used as a primary treatment for ventricular arrhythmias. It decreases the maximum rate of depolarization but does not alter the resting membrane potential. In cardiac tissue, depolarization is related to sodium influx through fast channels and calcium influx through slow channels. The slow channels are responsible for the spontaneous depolarization of the sinoatrial node (SAN). Cardiac conduction slows with increasing blood levels, and this is manifest by an increased PR interval and duration of the QRS complex (ventricular depolarization). High doses depress SAN pacemaker activity, perhaps by inhibiting the slow calcium channels, and they also depress atrioventricular nodal conduction. In addition, local anaesthetics exert a dose-dependent negatively inotropic action on the myocardium. This effect relates directly to the potency of the agents. Bupivacaine is more dangerous than lidocaine in overdose by predisposing patients to arrhythmias and VF. The underlying mechanism for this effect is not known, but it appears to cause a unidirectional block with re-entrant tachyarrhythmias. Bupivacaine markedly reduces the rapid phase of depolarization, and recovery from this block is much slower than with lidocaine. The drug binds avidly to myocardial cells, and there is a decrease in the rate of depolarization and action potential duration, with subsequent conduction block and electrical inexcitability. Local anaesthetics inhibit carnitine acylcarnitine translocase as described previously.
- **Myotoxicity:** local anaesthetics will damage muscle into which they are injected directly. Skeletal muscle is a regenerating tissue, and so this is not usually a clinical problem, although persistent diplopia has been reported following the use of bupivacaine 0.75% concentrations for retrobulbar ophthalmic block.
- **Prilocaine toxicity:** prilocaine is considered to be one of the safest local anaesthetics. Its use in high doses may lead to methaemoglobinaemia.

Local Anaesthetics: Influences on Onset and Duration

Commentary

There are various ways of decreasing the onset time of local anaesthetic blocks and of increasing their duration of effective analgesia. This technique is of clinical interest because it shortens the onset time of effective anaesthesia and so is useful in patients having procedures under regional anaesthesia alone as well as in the context of extending an epidural block for urgent operative delivery. The subject allows exploration of the basic mechanisms of local anaesthetic action and to explain concepts such as pKa. Inevitably, there is some repetition of aspects discussed in related topics.

Core Information

Methods of decreasing the latency of local anaesthetic blocks.

- **Basic chemistry:** local anaesthetics are chemical descendants of cocaine and comprise a lipophilic aromatic portion, which is joined via an ester or amide linkage to a hydrophilic tertiary amine chain (see Figure 4.2). The presence of the amino group means that they are weak bases, existing in solution partly as the free base, and partly as the cation, as the conjugate acid. (They are usually presented as aqueous solutions of the hydrochloride salts of the tertiary amine. The tertiary amine is the base. They are therefore prepared as the water-soluble salt of an acid, usually the hydrochloride, which is stable in solution.) When the acid HA dissociates to H^+ and A^-, the anion A^- is a base because it serves as a proton receptor in the reverse reaction. The special relationship of base A^- to the acid HA is acknowledged by calling it the conjugate base of the acid.
- **Drug action:** the axoplasmic part of the sodium channel is blocked by the ionized part of the local anaesthetic molecule, but a charged moiety will not traverse the lipid and connective tissue membranes. It is only when existing in the uncharged form that the drug can gain access to the axoplasm.
- **Equilibrium and pKa:** drugs exist in rapid equilibrium between the non-ionized (N:) and the ionized species (NH^+). Both ionized and non-ionized drug forms can inhibit Na^+ channels, but access to the axoplasm is via the uncharged species. Once within the axoplasm, the local anaesthetic becomes protonated. Local anaesthetics have pKa values higher than body pH, and the further away the dissociation constant is from body pH the more molecules that exist in the ionized form.
- **Alkalinization:** the addition of bicarbonate will raise the pH of the weakly acidic solution nearer the pKa. (The pH of local anaesthetics is adjusted by the addition of sodium hydroxide (NaOH) and/or hydrochloric acid (HCl). Lidocaine, 6.5; Bupivacaine, 4.0–6.5; ropivacaine, 4.0–6.0; and prilocaine, 5.0–7.0. Methylparaben is added to lidocaine and bupivacaine as preservative; ropivacaine, or at least Naropin(the non-generic formulation) and prilocaine are preservative-free. The addition of 1.0 ml $NaHCO_3$ 8.4% to 10.0 ml of lidocaine 2% will raise its pH from 6.5 to 7.2. (With bupivacaine 0.5% the pH rise is only to 6.6.) More drug will exist in the non-ionized form, and so penetration will be more rapid. $NaHCO_3$ significantly reduces the latency of lidocaine, although its effect on bupivacaine is less impressive, with some studies reporting only a 2–3-minute improvement.
- **Carbonation:** this is a variation on alkalinization and is based on a similar principle but with a different site of action. Most local anaesthetics are marketed as hydrochloride salts; it is, however, possible to combine the base form with carbonic acid to form the carbonate salt rather than the hydrochloric acid. The H_2CO_3 is in equilibrium with dissolved CO_2. After infiltration of the drug, it is believed that the

increased amount of CO_2 moves into the axoplasm, where it increases the levels of the weak carbonic acid. This lowers the intracellular pH and thereby favours cation production. In clinical practice this theoretical promise has not been realized.

Methods of Extending the Duration of Local Anaesthetic Blocks

- **Adjuvants:** various agents can be added to local anaesthetics with the aim of prolonging their duration of action.
- **Dexamethasone:** the addition of this glucocorticoid to local anaesthetics for plexus and peripheral nerve anaesthesia is a popular current technique, and there are a number of systematic reviews to confirm that doses up to 8 mg can almost double the duration of some blocks. A dose-duration relationship has not been established. Similar prolongation times, however, have also been observed after intravenous administration, and so it is as likely that the effect seen may simply be the consequence of systemic absorption. Dexamethasone is also potentially neurotoxic (as are local anaesthetics), which suggests that intravenous administration might be the preferred option.
- **Clonidine:** this does appear to have a direct action on peripheral nerves, mediated via the hyperpolarization of cation channels, and is effective in increasing the duration of neuraxial blocks, at least partly by spinal α_2-agonism. High doses of adjuvant clonidine are associated with sedation and hypotension, which suggests that when added to peripheral nerve or plexus blocks there is also systemic absorption.
- **Buprenorphine:** this is a partial μ-agonist which may also block voltage-gated Na^+ channels and thereby exert a local anaesthetic effect. It also acts on κ- and δ-opioid receptors. It can in some reports almost double the duration of plexus blocks, and studies suggest that the effect is not due to systemic absorption. A typical quoted adjuvant dose would be 150 µg, but despite its reported efficacy this technique is not widespread in the UK.
- **Tramadol:** this also possesses cation channel (Na^+ and K^+) blocking properties and so reduces the transmission of nociceptive impulses. There are some studies to support its use as an adjuvant, but the greater part of the published literature reports minimal efficacy when tramadol is added to local anaesthetics for peripheral nerve and plexus blocks.
- **μ-opioid receptor agonists:** there are no consistent data to support any significant benefits of adding opioids such as morphine, fentanyl or alfentanil to peripheral nerve blocks.
- **Magnesium:** in addition to its multiple uses elsewhere (see under 'Magnesium Sulphate'), magnesium has been shown to be consistently effective in extending the duration of a variety of nerve and plexus blocks, both upper and lower limb. Typical reported doses are of the order of 150–200 mg. Magnesium is an NMDA receptor antagonist that alters the influx of calcium into neurons.
- **Adrenaline (epinephrine):** the addition of adrenaline is of very modest benefit, and when added to local anaesthetic for peripheral nerve block (typically 5–10 µg ml^{-1}) it extends sensory block by minutes rather than hours. When the mixture is given epidurally the local vasoconstrictor action does increase the effective concentration in the epidural space, and α_2-mediated analgesia may also result from intrathecal spread. Adrenaline reduces endoneural blood flow, however, and may thereby be neurotoxic. Its effect on onset time (or 'latency') is variable. Pre-mixed solutions have a lower pH

than plain solutions, and so the onset of block may actually be delayed. If the adrenaline is mixed with lidocaine immediately before epidural injection, then the latency is decreased, whereas if mixed with bupivacaine, it appears to make little difference.

- **Extending an obstetric epidural for operative delivery:** assuming that the starting point is a standard low-dose local anaesthetic/opioid epidural that has been established for labour, there are various options, depending on operative urgency. Typical regimens include levobupivacaine 0.5% × 20 ml, lidocaine 2% × 20 ml, and levobupivacaine 0.5% × 10 ml plus lidocaine 2% × 10 ml. It is common to add adrenaline 100 µg (5 µgml^{-1} is 1 in 200,000), and many anaesthetists add an opioid such as fentanyl or diamorphine. Some also alkalinize the solutions by adding sodium bicarbonate 8.4%, 1.0 ml per 10 ml, although with bupivacaine-containing solutions precipitation is a common problem.

Supplementary Information

- **Inflammatory modulation:** the inflammatory response is initiated partly by G-coupled receptor proteins. Local anaesthetics have been shown to interact with some of these proteins to modify the physiological response.
- **Protein binding and lipid solubility:** protein binding influences the duration of action of a compound, and lipid solubility is a prime determinant of intrinsic anaesthetic potency. Lidocaine has low lipid solubility, whereas that of bupivacaine is high.
- **Newer local anaesthetic formulations:** although plexus blocks frequently have a long duration of action (for example an interscalene or supraclavicular block may last for 16–24 hours), there is continued interest in sustained release local anaesthesia. Liposomes are one alternative formulation. A liposome is formed when amphipathic lipid molecules (i.e. ones which have both hydrophobic and hydrophilic properties) encounter an aqueous medium, and become so orientated as to form a phospholipid bilayer which is similar to a cell membrane. Within the sequestered aqueous phase, drugs of various kinds can be encapsulated. Their release varies according to the characteristics of the particular liposome. The duration of action of local anaesthetics may also be prolonged by the use of lipid emulsions (which increase the non-ionized proportion and release active drug more slowly) and by polymer microspheres. It has proved possible to modify local anaesthetic structures to form a permanently ionized molecule. The charged molecules do nonetheless penetrate the axonal membrane but at a very slow rate, after which they are then effectively sequestered within the neuron where they can exert a prolonged effect. None of these preparations is yet in widespread clinical use.

Bupivacaine, Ropivacaine, Lidocaine and Prilocaine

Commentary

It is hard to predict exactly how a question about local anaesthetics will be constructed, and it may be that the following information may arise as part of a discussion about local anaesthetic techniques or local anaesthetic toxicity. The examiner might take a conventional approach and ask you about the 'ideal local anaesthetic agent' and how the available drugs compare against this standard. Thereafter, the discussion will involve only agents that are in mainstream use in the UK, namely bupivacaine, ropivacaine, lidocaine (lignocaine) and prilocaine. (It is unlikely to include more niche drugs such as amethocaine and articaine.)

Core Information

Factors influencing the choice of local anaesthetic for peripheral nerve or plexus blocks.

- In general, the choice is influenced by considerations such as onset time, duration and toxicity. Potency is less of a practical issue; what is important is the behaviour of local anaesthetics at equipotent doses. Lidocaine and prilocaine have more rapid onset of action (shorter latencies) than bupivacaine and ropivacaine. Bupivacaine is more potent and has a longer duration of action than ropivacaine. The judgement that ropivacaine is associated with motor sparing is discussed later in this section. Levobupivacaine and ropivacaine have a similar toxicity profile; both are more hazardous in overdose than either lidocaine or prilocaine, which is the safest of all the amides, and which is the agent of choice for intravenous regional anaesthesia (IVRA).

You will then be asked about the physicochemical differences which are responsible for the variations in clinical behaviour. (In the interests of clarity these are separated out in the following account, although there is frequently some overlap. Duration of action, for example, is related both to lipid solubility and to protein binding.)

- **Definitions:** all four are local anaesthetics which produce a reversible block of neuronal transmission, and which are synthetic derivatives of cocaine. They each possess the same three essential functional units, namely a hydrophilic chain joined by an amide linkage to a lipophilic aromatic moiety (see Figure 4.2). Simple modifications to any of the three parts of this basic structure can have marked effect on the pharmacology of the drugs.
- **Structures:** The parent compound of ropivacaine and bupivacaine is **me**pivacaine, which has a single **me**thyl group attached to the tertiary amine. **Bu**pivacaine is identical apart from a **bu**tyl (C_4H_9) side chain. The structure of ropivacaine (which is effectively a derivative of bupivacaine and which is prepared as the pure S enantiomer of **pro**pivacaine) differs only in its shorter **pro**pyl (C_3H_7) substituent on the piperidine nitrogen atom. Prilocaine has a different structure in the lipophilic moiety with a single methyl group on the aromatic ring (unlike the 2,6-xylidine ring in the other amides). This makes this aromatic toluidine ring less stable and more rapidly metabolized (Figure 4.4). Lidocaine and prilocaine both have a tertiary amine rather than a piperidine ring at the hydrophilic end of the structure.
- **Onset time:** as discussed earlier the latency of local anaesthetics is related to their pKa and the ease with which drugs reach neural tissue. Drugs with a lower pKa usually have a more rapid onset of action, so lidocaine and prilocaine (pKa 7.7) work more quickly than bupivacaine and ropivacaine (pKa 8.1). (This may be only part of

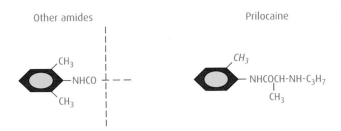

Other amides   Prilocaine   **Fig. 4.4** Toluidine ring: prilocaine and other amides.

the explanation; chloroprocaine has a swifter onset than any of these amides despite its pKa of 9.1.) (**Onset:** Chloroprocaine > Lidocaine/Prilocaine > Bupivacaine/Ropivacaine.)

- **Potency:** this is determined primarily by lipid solubility, which is increased by the substitution of longer side chains. Bupivacaine's longer butyl (C_4H_9) side chain increases at least threefold its lipid solubility in comparison with ropivicaine with its shorter propyl (C_3H_7) substituent.

- **Protein binding:** this is also affected by structural differences in the molecule. The affinity of local anaesthetics for the sodium channel is related to the length of the aliphatic chains. Affinity determines duration of action; hence ropivacaine, with its shorter propyl chain, has a duration of action of 150 minutes as compared with 175 minutes for bupivacaine. Both drugs are around 96% protein-bound. Lidocaine and prilocaine are much more weakly protein-bound (65% and 55%, respectively), with actions lasting for around 100 minutes. High protein binding decreases toxicity by reducing the proportion of free drug in the plasma. (**Duration:** bupivacaine 175' > ropivacaine 150' > lidocaine/prilocaine 100'.)

- **Toxicity:** ropivacaine was developed as a safer alternative to bupivacaine. Its myocardial and CNS toxicity has been quoted as being 25% less than racemic bupivacaine. The cardiovascular and CNS toxicity of bupivacaine, however, is a function of the R (+) enantiomer. The S (−) enantiomer has less affinity for, and dissociates faster from, myocardial sodium channels. Animal studies confirm a fourfold decrease in the incidence of ventricular arrhythmias and ventricular fibrillation. Symptoms of CNS toxicity in human volunteers such as tinnitus, circumoral numbness, apprehension and agitation are also less with infusions of the S (−) enantiomer. This is now available as levobupivacaine (Chirocaine), and would appear to be no more dangerous than ropivacaine. Both these drugs are, however, more toxic than lidocaine and prilocaine. Prilocaine is both less lipid-soluble and more weakly protein-bound than lidocaine, yet plasma concentrations are lower even when the same dose is given by the same route, and it is some 40% less toxic. The less stable toluidine ring is more rapidly metabolized to ortho (o)-toluidine. Some metabolism of prilocaine takes place in the lung. This would be a positive safety feature were it not for the fact that the ortho-toluidine metabolite causes methaemoglobinaemia by oxidizing the ferrous iron in haemoglobin to the ferric state. The loss of oxygen-carrying capacity shifts the oxygen–haemoglobin dissociation curve to the left. (SpO_2 readings are usually around 85%.) As methaemoglobin crosses the placenta, this further compromises oxygen delivery to the fetus, and so prilocaine is generally avoided in pregnancy. (The S [+] enantiomer of prilocaine is a stronger vasocon-strictor than the R [−] form, is metabolized more slowly and therefore produces lower concentrations of o-toluidine.) Normal methaemoglobin concentrations are <1%; toxicity is evident when this rises to >10%. It can be treated effectively with methylene blue, 1.0 mg kg^{-1}, which is a reducing agent. (**Toxicity:** bupivacaine > levobupivacaine > ropivacaine > lidocaine > prilocaine.)

- **Vasoactivity:** all local anaesthetics, apart from the potent vasoconstrictor cocaine, show biphasic activity, being vasodilators at high concentrations and vasoconstrict-ors at low. The vasoconstriction at low concentrations appears to be associated particularly with the S enantiomers. Ropivacaine probably exerts greater vasocon-strictor activity than bupivacaine, but it is no less toxic and has a shorter duration of action, so this vasoconstrictor activity probably confers little benefit. Prilocaine causes significantly less vasodilatation than lidocaine (so lasts longer despite being less lipid-soluble). At clinical doses the drugs have variable vasodilator activity. Bupivacaine dilates arterioles only at supraclinical levels, whereas lidocaine does so at clinical doses.

- **Sensory–motor dissociation:** this refers to the capacity of a local anaesthetic to block sensory nerves preferentially while sparing motor nerves. It is of particular advantage when the drugs are used in continuous epidurals for labour and for surgical anal-gesia. Selective block is a genuine phenomenon; etidocaine, for example, an agent which is no longer used in the UK, demonstrates more potent motor than sensory block. It is highly lipid-soluble and penetrates better than bupivacaine into the large myelinated A-α motor fibres. It also penetrates into the cord itself to provide long-tract anaesthesia. But what of the claim that ropivacaine exhibits greater sensory–motor dissociation than other local anaesthetics? This has been based largely on studies that have used doses that are supramaximal for sensory block, at which the greater motor blocking effect of bupivacaine is obvious. If the doses are reduced, then little motor block will be evident with either drug, but the differences in sensory block will be revealed. It is well known that this group of local anaesthetics demon-strates preferential sensory block; the purported superiority of ropivacaine is illusory and is based on the fact that it is simply a less potent drug.

- **Frequency dependence:** this is another factor which helps to explain true sensory–motor dissociation. Drug entry into the sodium channels occurs when the channel is open during the period of membrane depolarization. Nerves conduct at different frequencies; pain and sensory fibres conduct at high frequency, whereas motor impulses are at a lower frequency. This means that the sodium channels are open more times per second. Lidocaine, prilocaine, bupivacaine and ropivacaine all pro-duce a more rapid and denser block in these sensory nerves of higher frequency. This is not true of drugs such as etidocaine, which is associated with a much more profound motor block.

- **Metabolism:** amide local anaesthetics bind mainly to α$_1$-acid glycoprotein (high-affinity, low-capacity binding site), and to albumin (low-affinity, high-capacity). They undergo aromatic hydroxylation, amide hydrolysis and N-dealkylation (phase 1 reactions) in the liver. There is some suggestion of extrahepatic pulmonary metabol-ism (uptake and sequestration is greatest with prilocaine).

Spinal Adjuncts to Local Anaesthetics

Commentary

This is a question about the drugs that can be added to epidural or intrathecal solutions of local anaesthetics as a means of enhancing or prolonging their action. You may not have direct experience of non-opioid adjuncts apart from clonidine, and so this part of the discussion is likely to be purely theoretical. There can be some confusion about the term 'spinal' in the context of drug administration. Texts refer to 'spinal' opioids because that describes not their route of administration, but their site of action.

Core Information

Prolonging and augmenting the analgesic effect of a neuraxial block.

- **Spinal opioids:** the successful use of epidural morphine was first reported in 1979, and since that time several different opioids have been administered via the epidural and intrathecal routes. In the UK these include diamorphine, morphine, fentanyl, pethidine and methadone. Both onset and duration of action are related to the lipid solubility of the drug. Morphine has low lipid solubility, whereas that of fentanyl is high, and this is reflected in durations of action of 18 hours and 2–4 hours, respectively. The lipophilic drugs cross rapidly into the cord, while hydrophilic agents remain partly within the CSF, in which they may be carried rostrally to act on higher centres. This is the mechanism by which delayed respiratory depression may be caused. It is thus more common with morphine than with other drugs, and is better monitored by sedation scoring than respiratory rate. Pulse oximetry may be misleading because a high inspired oxygen concentration may mask ventilatory failure. Other complications of spinal opioids include nausea, vomiting, urinary retention and pruritus. Naloxone as a specific μ-antagonist will reverse some of these symptoms, but it may also reverse the analgesia. A logical alternative treatment, which can be useful for pruritus, is intravenous nalbuphine. This drug antagonizes μ-receptor-mediated effects while maintaining analgesia via κ-receptor agonism. (This is despite the fact that pruritus may not be mediated via μ-receptors, as it is not reliably reversed by naloxone.)
- **Opioid receptors:** opioid receptors were identified in the dorsal horn of the grey matter of the spinal cord in the mid-1970s, with early work confirming that epidural morphine was associated with prolonged analgesia. The site of action appears to be the specific receptors that are located in the dorsal horn of the spinal cord. They are most densely concentrated in the substantia gelatinosa, which comprises lamina II and part of lamina III of the laminae of Rexed. At least 75% of the receptors are pre-synaptic, and they mediate inhibition of the release of nociceptive transmitters such as substance P, following stimulation of the primary afferents.
- **Vasoconstrictors:** these have long been used to prolong the duration of anaesthesia provided by both intrathecal and epidural local anaesthetics, although the practice is much less common in the UK than in the USA. There is evidence from controlled trials which suggests that the practice is safe, in that it does not lead to spinal cord

ischaemia and neurological damage. There is also evidence that the addition of vasoconstrictors does not have a consistent action; the addition of adrenaline prolongs the action of intrathecal amethocaine, for example, but has little effect when added to bupivacaine or lignocaine. The reasons for this disparity are unknown. Vasoconstrictors that have been used include adrenaline, phenylephrine and octapressin.

- **α_2-agonists:** it was discovered more than 50 years ago that intrathecal adrenaline had a significant analgesic effect, which has since been shown to be due to its α_2-agonist actions at pre-synaptic and post-synaptic receptors in the spinal cord. Pre-synaptic activation inhibits noradrenaline release from the nerve terminal and thereby influences descending pathways, but this alone is insufficient to explain all the analgesic effects. Clonidine doubles the duration of action of intrathecal bupivacaine, prolonging both sensory and motor block. Its complications include hypotension, dry mouth and sedation. The dose–response curve for hypotension is complex because larger doses (as high as 450 µg) are associated with the smallest effects on blood pressure. This is attributed to a peripheral α_1 effect. Dexmedetomidine is both more potent and more α_2-selective.

- **NMDA receptor antagonists:** there are N-methyl-D-aspartate receptors in the dorsal horn of the spinal cord. **Ketamine** is effective by both extradural and intrathecal routes, and has been shown (in a preservative-free formulation) to quadruple the duration of effective analgesia in children when added in a dose of 0.5 mg kg^{-1} to sacral extradural (caudal) bupivacaine. (This is no longer accepted practice in young children because of concerns about potential adverse effects on neurodevelopment). **Magnesium sulphate** is also a physiological NMDA receptor antagonist which also inhibits voltage-gated calcium channels. When given intrathecally it increases the duration of effective block, but only in the presence of lipophilic opioids. A typical dose (the optimum has not been established) would be 50 mg. When magnesium is added to local anaesthetic alone its benefits are negligible.

Supplementary Information

There are some less commonly used adjuncts. The underlying receptor theory is both complex and incompletely understood, and a broad overview is likely to be sufficient.

- **Anticholinesterases:** part of the effect of α_2-agonists is mediated via the release of ACh from the dorsal horn, which indicates that cholinergic receptors are involved in endogenous modulation of pain sensations. The logic of this hypothesis means that the injection of an intrathecal anticholinesterase should have analgesic effects, and so it has proved with neostigmine. The technique has not passed into clinical practice because doses sufficient to permit the use of neostigmine as the sole anaesthetic agent are accompanied by severe nausea and vomiting. Sub-analgesic doses do exert an opioid-sparing effect with minimal nausea, and it may be that cholinomimetic drugs will be developed to exploit this mechanism further.

- **GABA agonists:** intrathecal midazolam produces analgesia which is antagonized by flumazenil, and it is assumed that it enhances the action of GABA on GABA$_A$ receptors. The effects of a single dose can be prolonged, which raises the suspicion that it may be neurotoxic. Intrathecal baclofen, which is another GABA agonist, is licensed in the USA for the treatment of spasticity, but it can also produce effective analgesia without any evidence of toxicity.

- **Non-steroidal anti-inflammatory drugs (NSAIDs):** spinal NSAIDs may inhibit presynaptic adenyl cyclase in the dorsal horn and decrease neurotransmitter release. (This is an oversimplification of a process that may also involve post-synaptic NMDA-stimulated gene expression.) Clinical experience is limited to sporadic case reports.
- **Monoamine uptake inhibitors:** Amitriptyline enhances noradrenergic and seroto-nergic inhibition at spinal level after intrathecal administration.

Induced Hypotension

Commentary
This is a question of continued interest and is a standard topic. You should be aware of the applied pharmacology, of the indications for the technique and of its potential complications.

Core Information
There is a difference between formal, induced hypotension, performed ideally with direct intra-arterial and cerebral function monitoring, and modest hypotensive anaes-thesia. The following account concentrates on the former, but the general principles do apply to both.

- **Indications:** an old adage avows that induced hypotension should be used only to make the impossible possible, and not the possible easy. There was a time when surgeons were largely oblivious to that injunction and requested hypotension for any procedure that involved blood loss. This included orthopaedic surgery, and particu-larly head and neck and some neurosurgical operations. Occasional surgeons will still insist that hypotension is essential – in cosmetic procedures such as rhinoplasty, for instance – but in reality, the genuine indications have now shrunk to the point at which the technique is confined to a very few, very specialized surgical procedures, one example of which is the removal of choroidal tumours of the eye. Moderate hypotension (as defined by a reduction in mean arterial pressure [MAP] by up to 30%) is used for various operations, including endoscopic sinus surgery, middle ear surgery and maxillary and mandibular osteotomies.

Intravenous Drugs That Can Be Used to Induce Hypotension
- The topic could be introduced by an invitation to describe the properties of an 'ideal agent' for inducing controlled hypotension. These would include pharmacological stability and ease of preparation and administration (unlike sodium nitroprusside, for example); very rapid onset and offset of action, with no rebound hypertension; rapid metabolism and excretion, with no direct or indirect organ toxicity; and a linear and predictable dose-response relationship.

- Otherwise the subject lends itself to a structured approach. You can, for example, talk either about their physiological sites of action or organize your answer according to the groups of drugs that are available. This is almost, but not quite, the same thing; labetalol, for instance, is a hypotensive drug with more than one site of action.
- The prime determinants of arterial blood pressure (BP) are cardiac output (CO), which is the product of heart rate (HR) and stroke volume (SV), and systemic vascular resistance (SVR). Drugs used to induce hypotension can affect one or more of these variables.

Drugs Which Affect Systemic Vascular Resistance (SVR)
α-Adrenoceptor Blockers

- **Phentolamine:** this is a non-selective α antagonist (the ratio of α1:α2 effects is 3:1), which also has weak β-sympathomimetic action. It decreases BP by reducing peripheral resistance owing to its peripheral α_1-vasoconstrictor blockade and mild β-sympathomimetic vasodilatation. The α_2-blockade increases noradrenaline release. The dose is 1–5 mg, titrated against response and repeated as necessary. The drug has a rapid onset of 1–2 minutes, with an effective duration of action of around 15–20 minutes.

Peripheral Vasodilators

- **Glyceryl trinitrate (GTN) nitroglycerine:** its hypotensive action is mediated via nitric oxide (NO). NO activates guanylate cyclase, which increases cyclic GMP (from guanosine triphosphate) within cells. This in turn decreases available intracellular Ca^{2+}. The drug causes more venous than arteriolar dilatation, and hence it decreases venous return and preload. Myocardial oxygen demand is reduced because of the decrease in ventricular wall tension. GTN has a rapid onset (1–2 minutes) and offset (3–5 minutes), which can allow precise control of BP. A typical infusion regimen would be to start at around 0.5 µg kg^{-1} min^{-1}, titrated against response. There is no rebound hypertension when the infusion is discontinued. The drug increases cerebral blood flow (CBF) and ICP. Tolerance to the effects of GTN may develop, which may partially be prevented by intermittent dosing.
- **Sodium nitroprusside (SNP):** SNP is another nitrovasodilator which mediates hypotension via NO. In contrast to GTN, it causes both arterial and venous dilatation, leading to hypotension and a compensatory reflex tachycardia. The drug has a complex metabolism that results in the production of free cyanide (CN$^-$), which, by binding irreversibly to cytochrome oxidase in mitochondria, is highly toxic, causing tissue hypoxia and acidosis. Toxicity is manifest when blood levels exceed 8 µg ml^{-1}. The maximum infusion rate is 1.5 µg kg^{-1} min^{-1}, and the total dose must not exceed 1.5 mg kg^{-1}. Treatment of toxicity is with sodium thiosulphate 50% (20–25 ml intravenously over 5 minutes) and/or cobalt edetate 1.5% (20 ml rapidly). SNP also increases cerebral blood flow and intracranial pressure. Coronary blood flow is increased. The rapid onset (1–2 minutes) and offset (3–5 minutes) of effect allows good control of BP, although patients may demonstrate rebound hypertension when the infusion is stopped. Tachyphylaxis may be seen in some patients; the mechanism is uncertain. The solution is unstable and so the giving set must be protected from light.

Ganglion Blockers

- **Trimetaphan (trimethaphan):** this agent is no longer available in the UK, but it was a popular hypotensive drug, particularly in neurosurgery. It will only come up as a topic in the oral as part of a discussion about sites at which drugs can act to produce hypotension. It is an antagonist at the nicotinic receptors of both sympathetic and parasympathetic autonomic ganglia, but it has no effect at the nicotinic receptors of the neuromuscular junction. It has some α-blocking actions and is a direct vasodilator of peripheral vessels. It is a potent releaser of histamine, which contributes to its hypotensive action. Reflex tachycardia is common, and this may present a problem during surgery which mandates a quiet circulation. Trimetaphan also antagonizes hypoxic pulmonary vasoconstriction. The drug is/was given by infusion at a rate of 20–50 µg kg^{-1} min^{-1}.

Direct Vasodilators

- **Hydralazine:** this produces hypotension by direct vasodilatation together with a weak α-antagonist action. This is mediated via an increase in cyclic GMP and decrease in available intracellular Ca^{2+}. The tone of arterioles is affected more than venules. Reflex tachycardia is common. It is less easy to titrate the dose against effect, and the drug finds its main use in the control of hypertension in pregnancy. The maximum infusion rate is 10 mg h^{-1}.

Drugs Which Affect Cardiac Output (CO)

- **β-adrenoceptor blockers:** there are many examples – all are competitive antagonists, but their selectivity for receptors is variable. Selective β_1-antagonism is clearly a useful characteristic. Their influence on BP is probably because of decreased CO via a decreased HR, together with some inhibition of the renin–angiotensin system. Unopposed α_1-vasoconstriction may compromise the peripheral circulation without causing hypertension.
- **Atenolol:** this is a selective β_1-antagonist except in high doses. It is long acting, with a $t_{1/2}$ of around 7 hours. Its use as a bolus (150 µg kg^{-1} over 20 minutes) is usually to treat cardiac arrhythmias rather than to induce hypotension.
- **Esmolol:** this is a relatively selective β_1-antagonist. It is ultra-short acting, with a $t_{1/2}$ of around 9 minutes. It is rapidly metabolized by non-specific ester hydrolysis. Its infusion dose is 50–200 µg kg^{-1} min^{-1}.
- **Labetalol:** this acts both as α- and β-antagonist (in a ratio that is quoted variously as 1:5 and 1:7), which mediates a decrease in SVR without reflex tachycardia. It is a popular drug in anaesthetic, obstetric anaesthetic and intensive therapy use. Its elimination $t_{1/2}$ is 4–6 hours. It can be given as a bolus of 50 mg intravenously, or at a rate of 1–2 mg kg^{-1} h^{-1}.
- **Propanolol:** this is a non-selective β-antagonist which is usually given as a bolus of 1.0 mg, repeated to a maximum of 5.0 mg (in a patient who is anaesthetized).

α_2-Adrenoceptor Agonists

- **Clonidine:** this is an α-agonist with affinity for α_2-receptors some 200 times greater than that for α_1. Its hypotensive effects are mediated via a reduction in central sympathetic outflow and by stimulation of presynaptic α_2-receptors which inhibit noradrenaline release into the synaptic cleft. It also possesses analgesic and sedative actions. Its elimination $t_{1/2}$ of around 14 hours is too long to allow its use for fine control of acutely raised BP, but it can be a useful adjunct in low doses.

Supplementary Information

Complications and Risks of Induced Hypotension

- **Dangers and complications:** these relate predictably to the consequences of hypoperfusion in key parts of the circulation. Precipitate falls in BP may lead to cerebrovascular hypoperfusion and stroke, and to myocardial ischaemia. Drug-induced hypotension usually shifts the autoregulatory curve to the left, and thereby confers a degree of protection. In patients who are previously hypertensive, however, the curve is shifted to the right, making them more vulnerable to catastrophic drops in perfusion of essential areas. (You may be asked to draw the curve of cerebral autoregulation to demonstrate these shifts (see Figure 3.10). The permissible reduction in blood pressure ideally should be matched to the patient. A young normotensive adult will tolerate a greater fall in mean arterial pressure than an elderly patient with hypertension. As a generalization, however, the accepted recommendation is to keep the MAP above 50 mmHg in the young and above 80 mm in elderly subjects.
- **Exacerbating influences:** the effects of induced hypotension will be enhanced by factors such as hypovolaemia, the use of other drugs with hypotensive actions such as volatile anaesthetic agents, the reduction in venous return associated with IPPV and drugs which release histamine. The head-up position may also further diminish effective cerebral perfusion.

Clonidine (and Dexmedetomidine)

Commentary

Clonidine is an old drug, which has been used in the treatment of hypertension and of migraine, in angina, as an anxiolytic, as a treatment for glaucoma and as a nasal decongestant. It has also been used in conditions as diverse as neuropathic pain, attention deficit hyperactivity disorder (ADHD), menopausal flushing ('menopausal vasomotor symptoms'), severe dysmenorrhea and postoperative shivering. Anaesthesia has found new uses for this agent, whose actions cannot totally be explained in terms of agonism at α_2-adrenoceptors. It is an interesting compound, but it is likely to be superseded by dexmedetomidine, which is now available in the UK.

Core Information

- Clonidine is an agonist at α_2-adrenoceptors (of which in humans there are three identified isoreceptors: α_{2A}, α_{2B} and α_{2C}). It has some minor activity at α_1-receptors (the ratio of α_1:α_2 is 1:200) and, because it is an imidazoline derivative, also acts at imidazole receptors. Two subtypes have so far been identified, the I_1 and I_2 receptors, which are located centrally and appear to mediate sedation and hypnosis. Clonidine is associated with a decrease in intracellular cyclic AMP via a Gi-protein receptor. Neuronal hyperpolarization appears to be the key mechanism by which α_2-adreno-ceptor agonists mediate their effects.

- It acts at presynaptic α_2-receptors, both centrally and peripherally, to inhibit the release of noradrenaline. In the hypothalamus, α_2-receptors are inhibitory to the vasomotor outflow. Clonidine also acts post-synaptically in the adrenal medulla.
- α_2-agonists activate receptors in the substantia gelatinosa in the dorsal horn of the spinal cord, which inhibits transmission down nociceptive neurons stimulated by $A\delta$ and C fibres. They also inhibit the release of the nociceptive neurotransmitter Substance P.
- At peripheral postjunctional α_2-receptors it mediates slow-onset vasoconstriction of long duration, to which its activity at α_1-receptors may contribute. This may explain why an intravenous dose may be associated with a transient rise in arterial BP.
- **Pharmacokinetics:** the oral bioavailability of clonidine is 70–80%, with peak levels attained at between 1 and 3 hours. Following intravenous administration, the distribution half-life is around 20 minutes and the elimination half-life quoted as between 12 and 16 hours. It undergoes hepatic metabolism, although 20–40% of an oral dose is excreted unchanged.

Supplementary and Clinical Information

The anaesthetic and medical uses of clonidine are numerous.

- **Stress and pressor responses:** clonidine can be used (in a dose of 5 µg kg^{-1}) to attenuate both the endocrine stress response to surgery and the pressor responses to laryngoscopy and tracheal intubation.
- **Adjunctive use in anaesthesia and analgesia:** a dose of 1–2 µg kg^{-1} intravenously reduces the MAC of inhaled volatile agents and decreases the requirement for systemic analgesics.
- **Hypotensive anaesthesia:** 1–2 µg kg^{-1} intravenously can produce modest and sustained hypotension which may improve operating conditions during which bleeding would otherwise mask the surgical field.
- **Antisialogogue effect:** a side effect of clonidine administration is reduced salivary secretion; this property can be useful in the perioperative period.
- **Alcohol withdrawal:** clonidine inhibits the exaggerated release of sympathomimetic neurotransmitters during acute alcohol withdrawal. It has also been used to attenuate the symptoms of opiate withdrawal.
- **Sedation and anxiolyis:** it has both sedative and anxiolytic actions. It finds use as pre-operative medication (up to 4 µg kg^{-1} in both adults and children), although the onset of action is relatively slow (30–45 minutes), and for sedation in critical care (typically 0.5–1.0 µg kg^{-1} h^{-1}).
- **Neuropathic pain:** clonidine can attenuate symptoms in some patients. It is particularly effective when given through an intrathecal drug delivery system.
- **Shivering:** a low dose (up to 0.5 µg kg^{-1}) may ameliorate postanaesthetic shivering.
- **Medical uses:** it has long been used as an anti-hypertensive agent whose usefulness is limited by the severe rebound hypertension that can follow discontinuation of

treatment. In a smaller dose it has a place in the prophylaxis of migraine. Some patients with attention deficit hyperactivity disorder (ADHD) respond well, and clonidine has also been used in the management of Tourette's syndrome.

- **Adjuvant use in regional anaesthesia:** there are α_2-receptors in the peripheral nervous system, but it is not clear whether they exist on the axons of peripheral nerves themselves. Nonetheless, the addition of clonidine to local anaesthetic does increase the duration of action of most blocks, partly due to the drug's ability to block voltage-gated calcium and other cation channels. It does produce a small decrement of nerve conduction at high concentrations, acting preferentially on C-fibres. Neuraxial clonidine does extend the duration of block; the addition of 2 μg kg^{-1} to local anaesthetic solutions for sacral extradural (caudal) block doubles the duration of effective analgesia. The same is true of clonidine given intrathecally. The side effects are those of sedation, dry mouth and, it is said, refractory hypotension, although this is not always an obvious problem in clinical practice. If intrathecal doses as high as 450 μg are given, then arterial blood pressure may even rise – secondary, it is said, to stimulation of peripheral α_1 receptors, although given the pharmacokinetics of intrathecal clonidine, that cannot be the only mechanism. Intrathecal α_2-agonists achieve analgesia partly through cholinergic activation, hence the brief interest in using spinal neostigmine as an adjunct.
- **Dexmedetomidine:** this is the R isomer of medetomidine, which has the advantage of being a more selective α_2-agonist than clonidine (with reported ratios of α_2:α_1 activity of 220:1 for clonidine and 1620:1 for dexmedetomidine); it also has more pronounced effects on central α-receptors. Their highest densities are found in the locus coeruleus which, amongst other functions, mediates alertness. It also contains a descending noradrenergic pathway which modulates nociceptive transmission. Dexmedetomidine has a much greater specificity for the α_{2A} receptor (8:1 ratio of activity) which may predominate in this region of the brain, making it a more effective anxiolytic, sedative and analgesic than clonidine. It otherwise has the same overall spectrum of activity, and the dose ranges are similar.
- **Pharmacokinetics:** following intravenous administration, dexmedetomidine has a rapid distribution half-life of 6 minutes and a terminal elimination half-life of around 2 hours. Its steady state volume of distribution is 118 L. It is highly protein-bound (94%), mainly to albumin, and undergoes hepatic metabolism via cytochrome P450 and by the formation of glucuronides. Elimination is predominantly renal (95%), with the remainder being excreted in faeces.

Antibiotics

Commentary

Antibiotics are not anaesthetic agents, but they are core medical drugs which anaesthetists administer to a large number of surgical cases, often for routine prophylaxis, as well as to the critically ill. Sepsis continues to kill, and bacterial resistance, which is a problem whose enormity has been recognized only tardily, threatens the effective treatment of infections as diverse as gonorrhea and tuberculosis. It is a topic of self-evident importance.

Core Information

There are more than 20 different classes of antibiotics, and so the oral is likely to focus on the mainstream agents that anaesthetists use and their broad mechanisms of action.

The Main Mechanisms of Antibiotic Action

- **Inhibition of bacterial cell wall synthesis.** Bacteria have an inner plasma membrane which is surrounded by a peptidoglycan wall. (Mammalian host cells do not have this structure and so are unaffected). Gram-negative species also have an outer lipid bilayer. Beta-lactams such as the **penicillins** and **cephalosporins** suppress peptidoglycan synthesis and so destroy the integrity of the whole cell wall. **Vancomycin** and bacitracin also interfere with peptidoglycan wall formation, as do the **carbapenems**, but the drugs act at different parts of the bacterial biosynthetic pathway. All these agents are bactericidal.
- **Inhibition of bacterial protein synthesis.** This is the most complex of the mechanisms due to the number of stages in the biosynthetic pathway. Prokaryotic ribosomes consist of a large number of proteins together with ribosomal RNA. Two subunits, 30S and 50S comprise the larger 70S ribosome. ('S' is not a unit of size but rather of sedimentation after centrifugation.) Eukaryotic cells have 80S ribosomes which are unaffected by these antibiotics. Antibiotics which interfere with protein synthesis work at different sites. **Aminoglycosides** block reactions at the 30S and 50S subunits. **Tobramycin** binds to the 30S ribosome but also suppresses initiation of the larger 70S complex. **Tetracyclines** also inhibit reactions at the 30S unit. The macrolide **erythromycin** affects the 50S subunit, as does **clarithromycin**. Protein synthesis is completed by a process of peptide elongation in a reaction catalyzed by peptidyl transferase. Drugs such as **clindamycin** and **lincomycin** are specific inhibitors of this enzyme.
- **Inhibition of bacterial DNA synthesis.** A class of enzymes known as the topoisomerases are required for bacterial DNA replication. Drugs such as the fluoroquinolones (**ciprofloxacin, levofloxacin**) inhibit the activity of topoisomerase II without affecting mammalian enzymes. **Metronidazole** interferes with DNA synthesis via the direct action of toxic metabolites.
- **Inhibition of bacterial RNA synthesis.** Suppression of RNA synthesis occurs via inhibition of RNA polymerases. **Rifampicin**, for example, blocks bacterial, but not mammalian enzymes. Some drugs which work in this way are not specific for bacteria and can be given as part of cytotoxic therapy for malignancy. Tumour cells have a much higher replication rate than normal cells and so a higher proportion will therefore be affected. Drugs of this class include **actinomycin D** and **doxorubicin**.
- **Inhibition of bacterial folate synthesis.** A small number of antibiotics work in this way. **Sulfonamides** compete with para-aminobenzoic acid (PABA) to inhibit folate synthesis, while **trimethoprim** blocks dihydrofolate reductase to achieve the

same effect. (These differences explain the rationale behind the use of co-trimoxazole [Septrin], which is a sulfamethoxazole/trimethoprim combination.)

Classes of Antibiotics

- **Beta-Lactams. Penicillins, Cephalosporins** (benzylpenicillin, amoxicillin, flucloxacillin, piperacillin, cefuroxime, cephalexin). As the name suggests, these antibiotics have a beta-lactam ring essential for their mode of action, which is to suppress the synthesis of peptidoglycan, a component of the bacterial cell wall. The drugs are bactericidal. Bacterial resistance is expressed mainly in the production of beta-lactamase enzymes which rupture the beta-lactam ring; hence the addition of a beta-lactamase inhibitor to co-amoxiclav (amoxicillin/clavulanic acid). They are effective against gram-positive organisms but not against gram-negative bacteria, most of which have an impermeable cell wall.
- **Sulfonamides** (sulfamethoxazole). A sulfonamide was the first commercially available antibiotic (1932). They act by inhibiting bacterial synthesis of folate and are broad-spectrum bacteriostatic agents.
- **Tetracyclines** (oxytetracycline, doxycycline). These inhibit bacterial protein synthesis and are bacteriostatic. They are broad-spectrum antibiotics which are active against both gram-positive and gram-negative species.
- **Glycopeptides** (vancomycin, teicoplanin). These act by inhibiting cell wall synthesis and are bactericidal at higher blood concentrations. Vancomycin is active against gram-positive organisms, but it is a large molecule that is unable to penetrate the outer lipid bilayer of gram-negatives. Teicoplanin is also mainly active against gram-positive species.
- **Carbapenems** (imipenem, meropenem). These are beta-lactams which inhibit bacterial cell wall synthesis but which have a wider spectrum of activity than the penicillins and cephalosporins, being active against gram-positive but particularly against gram-negative organisms. They are also effective against anaerobes.
- **(Fluoro)quinolones** (ciprofloxacin, levofloxacin). These act by disrupting bacterial DNA replication and transcription. They are broad-spectrum agents with particular activity against gram-negative organisms. They are generally less effective against gram-positive species. Fluoroquinolones are bactericidal, but the development of resistance is rapid.
- **Oxazolidinones** (linezolid). These inhibit bacterial protein synthesis and are effective against gram-positive organisms. They are bacteriostatic and are usually given as a third-line drug of last resort.
- **Macrolides** (erythromycin, clarithromycin) These inhibit protein synthesis and are bacteriostatic. They are commonly used in patients who are sensitive to penicillins and have a similar, although slightly broader spectrum of antibacterial activity.
- **Aminoglycosides** (gentamicin, tobramycin, neomycin). These inhibit protein synthesis and are used mainly against gram-negative bacteria. There is no absorption after oral administration so apart from neomycin are given parenterally. Oral neomycin is used for gut decontamination in hepatic encephalopathy. Whether they are bacteriostatic or bactericidal is dose-dependent. Their duration of action is prolonged beyond the time when blood levels have fallen. This is due to irreversible

binding to the intracellular bacterial ribosome. They are potentially nephrotoxic and ototoxic and potentiate the effects of neuromuscular blocking drugs.

- **Nitroimidazoles** (metronidazole, tinidazole). Metronidazole is the commonest drug of this class that is in clinical use in the UK. It undergoes reduction to produce toxic metabolites that suppress bacterial DNA synthesis. This reduction takes place only in anaerobic cells, and so the drug has no effect on aerobic organisms. Metronidazole is, however, also active against protozoa such as *Giardia lamblia* and *Entamoeba histolytica*.

Antibiotic Prophylaxis

Prophylactic antibiotics are now given routinely to reduce the risk of surgical site infection. This part of the oral may focus on patients at risk and the general principles underlying antibiotic administration.

- **Risk factors for surgical site infection.** Assuming appropriate asepsis and infection control measures these otherwise include insertion of any metalwork, implant or prosthesis; prolonged surgery; perioperative hypothermia; difficult haemostasis; and the insertion of surgical drains. Patients at greater risk include those at the extremes of age, those who are immunocompromised (for example receiving corticosteroids), those with diabetes mellitus, the obese (BMI >30 kg m^{-2}) and smokers.
- **General principles.** Narrow spectrum antibiotics should be selected, targeted to the most likely pathogens for the surgical procedure (and taking into account any local patterns of antibiotic resistance that have been identified). *Clostridium difficile* infection is a higher risk with cephalosporins, fluoroquinolones (ciprofloxacin), carbapenems (imipenem) and clindamycin. Alternative drugs should be considered. The antibiotic should have a half-life long enough to extend the duration of the operation after a single intravenous dose. This should be given as close to the time of surgical incision as possible and no more than 1 hour before. Following arthroplasty, antibiotics may be given for up to 24 hours. In long procedures such as revision arthroplasty, a second intraoperative dose may also be necessary. If operative blood loss is substantial (>1500 ml), additional doses should also be considered, on the assumption that the effective blood concentration will be lowered as a result. (This discussion is a summary of the Scottish Intercollegiate Network Guidelines [SIGN] recommendations that were published in 2015, but which are too lengthy to reproduce in full. The NICE guidelines of 2013 are less helpful, except that they do remove the requirement to give routine prophylaxis against infective endocarditis in patients with valvular and other cardiac structural abnormalities.)

Antibiotic Resistance

You will be unlucky if you find yourself discussing mechanisms of antibiotic resistance, but it is unlikely to be pursued in any detail. The basic processes are outlined here.

- **Mechanisms of resistance.** Acquired resistance to antibiotics is usually achieved by inhibition of the usual mode of action. The primary mechanisms include a simple decrease in the permeability of the bacterial cell wall, enzymatic degradation (of which beta-lactamase destruction of the active beta-lactam ring is the most obvious example) and changes in the proteins whose synthesis is the antibiotic target.

Anticholinesterases

Commentary

The use of drugs that inhibit the breakdown of acetylcholine is not confined to anaesthesia, and these agents find medical indications in conditions as diverse as dementia and myasthenia gravis. The oral is likely to focus both on the basic pharmacology of anticholinesterases (which is relatively straightforward) as well as their wider clinical applications.

Core Information

- **Cholinesterase enzymes:** There are two forms: acetylcholinesterase and butyrylcholinesterase (plasma cholinesterase). These enzymes were characterized as 'true' and 'pseudo' cholinesterase, but this terminology is no longer used. The physiological function of plasma cholinesterase is not fully elaborated, but its anaesthetic relevance lies in its metabolism of esters such as suxamethonium, mivacurium, diamorphine and aspirin. The actions of plasma cholinesterase are antagonized by anticholinesterases, and so the administration of neostigmine, for example, to a patient who is paralysed with suxamethonium would extend the duration of the block. This is not as improbable a clinical scenario as it seems; the short-acting anticholinesterase tacrine (tetrahydroaminacrine) used to be given specifically for that reason. The main relevance of anticholinesterases (sometimes referred to as choline esterase inhibitors) lies in their antagonism of acetyl cholinesterase.
- **Acetylcholine metabolism:** The breakdown and recycling of acetylcholine in the cholinergic junction is a highly dynamic process, with many thousands of molecules being hydrolyzed by acetylcholinesterase each second. Anticholinesterases prolong the survival of acetylcholine in the cleft of muscarinic and nicotinic junctions with effects that are predictable from the functions mediated by those receptors. The most extreme manifestations of acetylcholine excess are seen in cases of organophosphate poisoning.
- **Muscarinic effects:** These include bradycardia, bronchoconstriction and bronchorrhoea as well as increased gastrointestinal secretions and motility.
- **Nicotinic effects:** These are evident more in overdose or organophosphate poisoning than after administration of conventional doses. They include muscle fasciculations, weakness and cramping.
- **CNS effects:** These are also mainly apparent in overdose or poisoning. Features may include agitation, confusions, tremors, ataxia and, in extreme cases, convulsions and loss of consciousness.

Clinical Uses of Anticholinesterases

- **Reversal of neuromuscular blockade:** Competitive inhibition of the post-junctional receptor in the neuromuscular cleft by muscle relaxants is reversed by anticholinesterases which restore the levels of available acetylcholine. Neostigmine is the main agent that is used for this purpose.

- **Treatment of myasthenia gravis:** Myasthenia gravis is an autoimmune condition characterized by the formation of antibodies against post-synaptic acetylcholine receptors at the neuromuscular junction. As the number of effective receptors decrease there is a progressive reduction in muscle strength, particularly involving the bulbar muscles. Its estimated prevalence is 1 in 5,000 of the population, and it is twice as common in women than men. Edrophonium is used for diagnosis, while pyridostigmine is the primary cholinesterase inhibitor used for treatment.
- **Treatment of the central anticholinergic syndrome:** A relative or absolute reduction of cholinergic transmission in the central nervous system defines the central anticholinergic syndrome, which can occur following treatment or overdose with primary anticholinergic drugs such as atropine or hyoscine, or with drugs that have a secondary anticholinergic action such as the phenothiazines. Its clinical features are relatively non-specific and include agitation and disorientation with more predictable manifestations such as flushing, pyrexia, dry skin, mydriasis and sinus tachycardia. Physostigmine is given as first-line management.
- **Treatment of dementia:** Alzheimer's disease is characterized, amongst other things, by central depletion of acetylcholine in the cerebral cortex and the hippocampus. Anticholinesterases such as donezepil increase the concentration of acetylcholine and appear to slow the rate of deterioration. They do not cure or reverse the process of neurodegeneration.

Summary of Drugs in Clinical Use

- **Neostigmine:** This is the anticholinesterase with which anaesthetists are most familiar via its routine use for reversal of neuromuscular blockade. As a quaternary ammonium compound it does not cross the blood–brain barrier. After binding to the anionic site of acetylcholinesterase and then to an esteratic subsite, the drug is hydrolyzed, but in a process that takes some minutes, hence its sustained effect. Onset and time to peak effect are rapid (1 and 10 minutes, respectively), but the duration is relatively short-lived at around 20–30 minutes. It is usually given intravenously (the quoted dose is 50–70 micrograms kg^{-1}, but administration is better titrated to the degree of residual neuromuscular block). The oral form is poorly absorbed from the gastrointestinal tract, which makes it an unsuitable treatment for myasthenia gravis. Neostigmine has been used intrathecally as an adjunct to spinal anaesthesia. There are muscarinic receptors in Rexed laminae II and III of the spinal cord which mediate analgesia. The drug is an effective adjuvant but at the expense of dose-dependent nausea.
- **Pyridostigmine:** This is a neostigmine analogue which has 25% of its potency but which has a longer duration of action (4–6 hours). Its onset time is prolonged at up to 15 minutes, and so it is not a suitable agent for the reversal of neuromuscular block. It is, however, the preferred agent for the treatment of myasthenia gravis.
- **Physostigmine:** Unlike neostigmine and pyridostigmine, physostigmine lacks a quaternary ammonium group and so crosses the blood–brain barrier. It can therefore be used to treat the central anticholinergic syndrome (0.5–2.0 mg intravenously). It is a natural alkaloid metabolized by non-specific plasma esterases.
- **Edrophonium:** This is another quaternary ammonium compound, but one which has a very short duration of action of around 10 minutes. The effectiveness of

reversal of neuromuscular blockade is less predictable than with neostigmine, although in equipotent doses its muscarinic effects are less pronounced. Its predominant use is in the diagnosis of myasthenia gravis and as a means of predicting the patient's response to the longer-acting anticholinesterases.

- **Donepezil, rivastigmine and galantamine.** These three acetylcholinesterase inhibitors are approved by NICE for the treatment of mild and moderate dementia. Donepezil is a selective inhibitor of acetylcholinesterase and has no effect on plasma cholinesterase. It has a long half-life and can be given daily. Rivastigmine inhibits both forms of cholinesterase and with a shorter half-life is given twice daily. Galantamine is both a cholinesterase inhibitor and a presynaptic nicotinic modulator. Any clinical significance of this second action is unclear.

Supplementary Information

Organophosphate Poisoning

- Organophosphates are used particularly widely in agricultural settings where they are found in pesticides, insecticides and herbicides. They inactivate acetylcholinesterase by phosphorylation of the serine hydroxyl moiety that is located on each of the six active sites of the enzyme. The resultant accumulation of acetylcholine is accompanied by excessive cholinergic, nicotinic and central nervous system effects which, in cases of accidental poisoning, are frequently fatal.
- **Management:** In addition to supportive management, the treatment of organophosphate poisoning includes the use of anticholinergic drugs such as atropine or glycopyrronium, together with reactivation of the enzyme by pralidoxime. This binds directly to the organophosphate molecule and effectively reactivates the enzyme. It is ineffective once the organophosphate has bound irreversibly to acetylcholinesterase and so must be given at the latest within 48 hours of poisoning.

Anti-Arrhythmic Drugs

Commentary

There are still statements in textbooks to the effect that some form of arrhythmia (defined as the absence of normal sinus rhythm) complicates between 60 and 90% of all anaesthetics. The figures are based on studies which are now 3 decades old or more and which largely pre-date modern anaesthetic drugs and techniques. Yet, although the incidence seems high, it remains true that transient disturbances of cardiac rhythm are relatively common. Some of these are innocuous but others have the potential to evolve into more malignant rhythms that may threaten cardiovascular stability and which require urgent treatment. The rational management of arrhythmias is helped by some knowledge of cardiac electrophysiology, and it is this, more than the individual drugs themselves, which will probably be the scientific focus of the oral. The varying receptors, ion channels and ion pumps, many of which differ throughout parts of the conducting system and myocardium, contain vastly more detail than you will be expected to convey. A broad understanding of the principles of ion fluxes should be enough.

Core Information

The Cardiac Action Potential

- **Phase 4** – the 'pacemaker potential': in non-conducting tissue (atrial and ventricular myocytes, and Purkinje tissue), the negative resting membrane potential (RMP) of around −90 mV is maintained by high outward conductance of K^+ (gK^+) through open K^+ channels. During this time, fast Na^+ channels and slow (L-type) Ca^{2+} channels are closed. The membrane-bound ATP-dependent Na^+/K^+ exchange pump continues to extrude three Na^+ ions in exchange for two K^+ ions. In non-conducting tissue therefore the pacemaker potential is unimportant. In nodal and conducting tissue, however, there occurs a gradual depolarization owing to greater inward Na^+ (gNa^+) and Ca^{2+} (gCa^{2+}) conductance during late diastole. The negative membrane potential in early diastole also activates a cation channel that is permeable to both Na^+ and K^+ and which generates the inward I_f current (the i_f or 'funny' current is an inward pacemaker current which is activated by membrane hyperpolarization).
- **Phase 0** – rapid depolarization: at the threshold level of around −65 mV the fast sodium channels open with a large transient increase in gNa^+. (This is triggered in non-conducting tissue by an action potential [AP] in an adjacent cell.) The sudden influx in Na^+ generates a fast-response AP (meanwhile, the potassium channels close and K^+ efflux ceases).
- **Phase 1** – this is the period of rapid partial repolarization mediated by a short-lived hyperpolarizing efflux of K^+: the sodium channels close and inward gNa^+ drops.
- **Phase 2** – this is the plateau phase which lengthens the cardiac AP (in contrast to the much shorter APs generated in nerves and skeletal muscle) and which is produced mainly by the large influx of Ca^{2+} ions through slow (long-lasting L-type) calcium channels which open at a membrane potential of around −40mV. During phase 2, cardiac fibres are absolutely refractory to repeated depolarization. (This is the effective refractory period [ERP], which protects the heart from multiple compounded APs.)
- **Phase 3** – repolarization: this is caused by a large increase in gK^+ (efflux) and the inactivation of the Ca^{2+} channels (influx). The Na^+/K^+ pump re-establishes the resting membrane potential. Phase 3 is a relative refractory period during which a stimulus may generate an AP large enough to be propagated, but it will be conducted more slowly than usual.

In the light of the previous information, the questioning may move to classifications of anti-arrhythmic drugs.

- **Vaughan–Williams classification of anti-arrhythmic drugs:** the traditional Vaughan–Williams classification (1970) is convenient and still in use, but it is an oversimplification. It does not account for drugs that have more than one site of action (such as amiodarone), it fails to find a satisfactory classification for compounds such as adenosine and digoxin, and it is based on the assumption that all the agents are channel blockers, when in fact some drugs activate either receptors or ion channels.

— **Class I**: these drugs block sodium channels by binding to sites in the α-subunit, and reduce the maximum rate of depolarization during phase 0 of the cardiac AP. All share the same underlying mechanism of action but are further subdivided into classes Ia, Ib and Ic according to the specific characteristics of the Na^+ channel block that they produce. The electrophysiological differences are subtle and relate, amongst other complexities, to the different affinity of drugs to channels in the resting, open and refractory state. You are not likely to have to explain this in detail. Examples of the drugs include Ia, **disopyramide**; Ib, **lidocaine**; and Ic, **flecainide**.

— **Class II**: includes (some) β-adrenoceptor antagonists, including **propranolol**, **atenolol**, **metoprolol** and **esmolol**. These drugs increase the refractory period of the atrioventricular node and so may prevent recurrent supraventricular tachy-cardia, including paroxysmal atrial fibrillation (AF).

— **Class III**: this group includes drugs such as **amiodarone** and **sotalol**, which are now known to have more than one action. (The original definition encompassed drugs that prolonged the cardiac AP.) Their main mechanism of action is outward K^+ channel blockade which prolongs repolarization. This extends the Q–T inter-val, and, rarely, these drugs can precipitate torsade de pointes. Amiodarone (5 mg kg^{-1} iv) is useful both for supraventricular and ventricular arrhythmias. Sotalol is racemic, the S-enantiomer is a β-blocker, and both R and S forms prolong the AP. Other class III agents include **ibutilide** and **dofetilide** (used to convert atrial fibrillation).

— **Class IV**: these drugs block voltage-sensitive Ca^{2+} channels, thereby slowing conduction through the SA and AV nodes. Examples include **verapamil**, which is preferentially selective for cardiac tissues, and **diltiazem**. The drugs are ineffective in treating ventricular tachycardias, and verapamil given intraven-ously for this purpose has been fatal. **Magnesium sulphate** ($MgSO_4$) is a natural Ca^{2+} antagonist (an increase in intracellular Mg^{2+} inhibits Ca^{2+} influx through Ca^{2+} channels). It is effective at abolishing ventricular tachyarrhythmias, particularly torsade de pointes, and those induced by adrenaline, digitalis and bupivacaine.

— **Class V**: this added category includes those drugs that do not fit readily into the other four classes.

• **Adenosine** acts at the A^1 receptor (which is linked to the muscarinic K^+ channel). By enhancing K^+ efflux, adenosine hyperpolarizes cells and slows AV conduction. It has a very short duration of action (20–30 seconds) and, in a dose of 3–6 mg intraven-ously (repeated as needed), provides effective chemical cardioversion of supraven-tricular tachycardia (SVT).

• **Digoxin** and other cardiac glycosides increase contractile force and decrease AV node conduction, mainly via their inhibitory effect on the membrane Na^+/K^+-ATPase, and an increase in intracellular Ca^{2+}. Digoxin's long-term effect may be caused mainly by the increase in vagal tone.

Other Classifications

• **The 'Sicilian gambit' classification:** this represented an attempt in 1990 by a European Society of Cardiology working group to rationalize the actions of drugs according to the ion channels and the receptors on which they act. (It was described as a 'gambit', somewhat pretentiously, because it was viewed as an opening move rather than as a complete explanation.) The classification so far extends to blockers of Na^+ channels, Ca^{2+} channels, K^+ channels, the I_f current, α-adrenoceptors, β-adrenoceptors and muscarinic receptors, activators of the adenosine receptor, and suppressors of the Na^+/K^+ pump.

Supplementary and Clinical Information

The electrophysiological basis of common arrhythmias.

- **Sinus bradycardia:** the commonest acute cause is an increase in vagal tone, either unmasked by anaesthetic agents with no intrinsic vagolytic activity, or provoked by surgical stimuli such as traction on the peritoneum or the extraocular muscles. Vagal activation at the SA node increases gK^+ (outwards) and reduces slow channel gNa^+ and gCa^{2+} (inwards), decreases the slope of the pacemaker potential and suppresses the I_f current. Hyperkalaemia may stop pacemaker activity by increasing gK^+ (outward).
- **Sinus tachycardia:** this is not an arrhythmia, but is included for completeness. Sympathetic stimulation increases heart rate by decreasing gK^+. It also increases slow inward gCa^{2+} and gNa^+ and enhances the I_f current.
- **Drug effects:** calcium-channel blockers, as their name suggests, inhibit slow inward Ca^{2+} currents during phases 4 and 0, and some, such as diltiazem, can slow the heart rate. Digoxin enhances parasympathetic activity (and slows conduction through the AV node). β-adrenoceptor antagonists prevent the normal inhibition of vagal tone mediated by sympathetic activity (which normally increases heart rate by decreasing gK^+ outwards and increasing slow gCa^{2+} and gNa^+ inwards, thereby increasing the slope of the pacemaker potential during phase 4).
- **Hyperkalaemia:** this hyperpolarizes the cell, induces bradycardia and can even stop SA nodal firing completely.
- **Hypokalaemia:** this increases the rate of phase 4 depolarization by decreasing gK^+ and thereby increases the rate.
- **Hypoxia:** this is the most ominous cause of bradycardia. The lack of cellular oxygen can lead to complete cessation of pacemaker activity.
- **Ectopic pacemaker activity (ventricular premature beats):** non-conducting cells do not usually depolarize until activated by the pacemaker impulses. Under some circumstances, however, they do have a rising phase 4 which means that they can generate an AP spontaneously and themselves act as pacemakers. This occurs because of an increased inward movement of Ca^{2+} which reduces the membrane potential to threshold (−65 mV). Increased intracellular Ca^{2+} results particularly from myocardial ischaemia but is also associated with adrenergic stress and high-dose cardiac glycosides. Ischaemia also closes fast Na^+ channels and inhibits the Na^+/K^+ pump (which requires ATP [and oxygen] to maintain a low intracellular Na^+ against its concentration gradient).
- **Re-entry (pre-excitation) tachycardia:** these pre-excitation rhythms arise when a wave of depolarization that can travel down different conducting pathways

encounters a block. The impulse continues down the normal path, but should the paths then rejoin, the depolarization can travel retrogradely up the blocked segment only to depolarize the normal conducting pathway prematurely. The cycle repeats itself and thus gives rise to a tachyarrhythmia (typically supraventricular). Re-entrant circuits can be congenital (as in the accessory pathways of the Wolff–Parkinson–White syndrome) or acquired, following myocardial damage.

- **Atrial fibrillation (AF):** this is the most frequently encountered arrhythmia in clinical, although perhaps not in anaesthetic, practice. The commonest cause is myocardial ischaemia, but there are numerous others including sepsis, autonomic stimulation, hypomagnesaemia, hypokalaemia, hyperthyroidism, alcohol excess and mitral valve disease. Atrial fibrillation appears mainly to be a re-entry abnormality in which multiple propagating waves of depolarization are initiated by ectopic foci (most of which almost certainly originate from the pulmonary veins).

Management of Intraoperative Atrial Fibrillation

A patient's cardiac rhythm may flip into atrial fibrillation during the perioperative period. Given that they may then lose the atrial component of ventricular filling, which may be as high as 30–40%, there will be a reduction in cardiac output with potential haemodynamic instability. If this is severe then the immediate treatment is DC cardioversion. Otherwise the pharmacological options are as follows.

- **β-adrenoceptor blockers:** these will slow ventricular rate pending more considered treatment. The drug and dose will depend on what is immediately available, but as an example intravenous atenolol (starting with a small 1 mg dose and titrating against response) would be appropriate. But other drugs such as esmolol or metoprolol are equally effective in establishing rate control. All β-blockers should be avoided if the patient is on concomitant calcium channel blockers, and used with caution in patients with heart failure.
- **Amiodarone:** this is a valuable treatment for a range of acute arrhythmias including AF. The initial dose is 5 mg kg^{-1} (given by infusion in glucose 5%), followed by a stabilizing infusion of 900 mg over 24 hours.
- **Flecainide:** a dose of 2 mg kg^{-1} (to a maximum of 150 mg) may be enough to chemically cardiovert new onset AF, and will also help stabilize sinus rhythm that has been restored by DC cardioversion.
- **Digoxin:** this is used for medium- and long-term rate control rather than as an acute therapy. A loading dose (in the presence of normal serum K$^+$) of 500 μg given by infusion over 20–30 minutes can be repeated at 6–8 hours before maintenance treatment is initiated. Digoxin has a narrow therapeutic index and measurement of blood levels may be necessary.
- **(Ibutilide:** this is a class III anti-arrythmic which is not available in the UK but which has been used in the immediate management of AF [a typical loading dose would be 0.015 mg kg^{-1}]. In up to 8% of patients it may induce transient torsade de pointes which can last up to 1–2 hours.)

β-Adrenoceptor Blockers

Commentary

β-adrenoceptor blockers may form the subject matter for a whole oral, or they may be part of a more general discussion of anti-hypertensive drugs and anaesthesia. There are a large number of β-blockers, and you will not be expected to know about subtle pharmacological differences between them, although characteristics such as intrinsic sympathetic activity may form part of the questioning. You will need to know enough about the receptors on which they act to be able to address the question from first principles, but, as this is straightforward, much of the questioning will be clinically orientated.

Core Information

Clinical uses of β-blockers and mechanisms of action.

- **β-adrenoceptors:** the actions of β-blockers are predictable from what is known about β-adrenoceptors. The important effects (from an anaesthetic perspective) are that they mediate include increases in heart rate (β_1), myocardial contractility (β_1), conduction velocity ($\beta_2 > \beta_1$) and cardiac glycogenolysis ($\beta_1 > \beta_2$). β_2-receptors are responsible for relaxation of bronchial and vascular smooth muscle. β_3-receptors mediate lipolysis in adipose tissue.

Cardiovascular Uses

- **Angina pectoris:** the drugs are myocardial depressants which reduce cardiac work by blocking the effects of sympathetic stimulation. They decrease left ventricular wall tension, heart rate and resting contractility, thereby reducing myocardial oxygen consumption. β-blockers do not lead to coronary vasodilatation. Patients with myocardial ischaemia may benefit from long-term therapy, and survival following myocardial infarction (MI) is increased.
- **Arrhythmias:** β-blockers lead to a decrease in automaticity, an increase in the duration of the cardiac action potential and an increase in the effective refractory period at the AV node. They are useful in treating cardiac arrhythmias that are dependent on sympathetic activity, particularly SVTs. It is not advisable to use them to manage abnormalities of rhythm that have been induced by acute coronary ischaemia. β-blockers may worsen these arrhythmias and precipitate heart failure. (They are Vaughan–Williams class II anti-arrhythmics).
- **Hypertension:** the anti-hypertensive actions of β-blockers are not fully explained; peripheral resistance may remain unchanged, although cardiac output usually drops. There is no consistent relationship between treatments or with alterations in renin levels. The drugs may also inhibit 5-HT both centrally and peripherally.
- **Perioperative ischaemia:** a study by Mangano that was published in the *New England Journal of Medicine* in 1996 concluded that the administration of atenolol to patients undergoing non-cardiac surgery, and who were known to be at risk of ischaemic cardiac events, halved the incidence of silent postoperative myocardial

ischaemia, halved mortality and cardiac complication rates for up to 2 years, and reduced the incidence of perioperative infarction. The evidence was based on only 200 patients but, in conjunction with some other published work, was enough to convince a number of anaesthetists (and some surgeons) to adopt the practice (D.T. Mangano *et al.* 1996. *New England Journal of Medicine*, **335**: 1713–20). Others were more sceptical, commenting that it is rare for cardiovascular therapies to demonstrate relative risk reductions of greater than about 35%, because they target only some of the many pathogenic mechanisms that underlie cardiovascular disease. Mangano's study pre-dated the widespread (if transient) use of perioperative epidural analgesia, and it has also been pointed out that initial small trials that claim improbably large benefits are frequently superseded by much larger trials which typically show more modest or even no treatment effects. A decade or so later, the POISE trial (**Peri**O**perative IS**chaemic Evaluation trial) recruited more than 8,000 patients and investigated the effects of perioperative extended release metoprolol. To the surprise of many, this suggested that although it reduced the risk of myocardial infarction, it increased the risks both of serious stroke and overall death. (POISE trial. *Lancet* 2008, 371: 1839–47). For every 1,000 patients treated, metoprolol would prevent 15 MIs but at the cost of an excess of 5 disabling CVAs and 8 deaths.

- **Hypertrophic cardiomyopathy:** propranolol reduces the encroachment of the hypertrophic septum into the left ventricular outflow tract under the influence of sympathetic activity.
- **Pressor responses:** β-adrenoceptor blockers, particularly the ultra-short-acting esmolol, can be used to attenuate the pressor response to laryngoscopy.
- **Thyroid disease:** β-blockers are used to reduce the manifestations of a raised metabolic rate in thyrotoxic patients requiring curative thyroid surgery.

Supplementary and Further Clinical Information

Adverse Effects

- **Propranolol** was the first of many β-blockers to be synthesized. The clinical differences between them are probably less significant than is claimed. Some of the drugs are relatively cardioselective, but none is cardiospecific. This means that they will antagonize β_1-receptors at non-cardiac sites and in higher doses will also affect β_2-receptors. All have the potential to provoke bronchoconstriction in asthmatics, and they may worsen pulmonary function in patients with other forms of obstructive airway disease. These patients will then not respond to β_2-sympathomimetic treatment. Selective β_1-antagonists include **atenolol, acebutolol, esmolol** and **metoprolol**.
- Most of the other adverse effects are also related to their primary pharmacological actions. They may precipitate peripheral vascular ischaemia owing to unopposed α_1-vasoconstriction, and may mask the symptoms of hypoglycaemia. They may, in addition, contribute to hypoglycaemia by interfering with β_2-mediated glycogenolysis, carbohydrate and fat metabolism. Reduced exercise tolerance, dyspnoea and fatigue are other generic side effects. Drugs with membrane-stabilizing actions **(MSA)** such as **propranolol** and **metoprolol** are more likely to induce significant bradycardia or worsen pre-existing conduction abnormalities. **Sotalol**, which is a class III anti-arrhythmic drug, unlike other β-blockers, delays the slow outward potassium flux and extends the effective refractory period of the cardiac AP. This

prolongation of the QT interval is associated (rarely) with torsade de pointes. In patients in whom cardiac decompensation is being prevented by sympathetic drive, β-blockers may precipitate cardiac failure, unless a drug is used which possesses intrinsic sympathomimetic activity (**ISA**). Drugs with **ISA** are **oxprenolol, acebuto-lol, pindolol** and **celiprolol**. Fat-soluble drugs, particularly propranolol, are much more likely to penetrate the CNS and cause symptoms such as nightmares and sleep disturbance. This is less of a problem with the water-soluble compounds (such as atenolol, nadolol, sotalol and celiprolol).

Implications for Anaesthesia and Specific Anaesthetic Uses for β-Blockers

- The main clinical problem is that a β-blocked patient is one in whom sympathetic reflexes are blunted. This means that compensatory responses to actual or effective hypovolaemia (such as may accompany central neuraxial blockade) can be inadequate.
- Anaesthetists use the drugs for the urgent control of hypertension, including the pressor response to laryngoscopy. **Esmolol** is a cardioselective drug whose very short duration of action (the elimination half-life is 10 minutes or less) is terminated by non-specific plasma esterases. **Labetalol** can be used to provide control over a longer period. It has combined α- and β-adrenoceptor blocking actions (in a ratio that is quoted variously as 1:5 and 1:7), but of differing durations of effect. The α block lasts for 30 minutes, whereas the β block persists for 90 minutes.
- β-blockers can be used to provide moderate intraoperative hypotension, for the immediate treatment of tachyarrythmias (particularly supraventricular arrhythmias) and to reduce myocardial oxygen demand in the presence of cardiac ischaemia (although nitrates would be the first-line choice of many for this indication).

Anti-Hypertensive Drugs and Anaesthesia

Commentary

Hypertension is common and is treated by a wide range of drugs, often in combination. Most anti-hypertensive therapy has implications for anaesthesia, and current guidance is to withhold some agents, such as ACE inhibitors and angiotensin II antagonists, prior to surgery. Be prepared to demonstrate that you can make your own judgements based on an understanding of how the various drugs work.

Core Information

The implications for anaesthetic management of a patient who is receiving treatment for hypertension.

- **β-adrenoceptor blockers:** patients should continue taking these drugs and in some cases may be prescribed them *de novo*.
- **Diuretics:** the commonest diuretics are the thiazides, such as **bendrofluazide, chlorthalidone** and **indapamide**, which act on the distal tubule; and loop diuretics,

typically **furosemide**, which act on the loop of Henle. These drugs decrease the active reabsorption of sodium and chloride by binding to the chloride site of the electro-neutral Na^+/Cl^- co-transport system to inhibit its action.

— **Anaesthetic implications**: potassium loss can be significant, particularly in the elderly. Electrolytes should be checked prior to anaesthesia, and consideration should be given to withholding the drugs on the day of surgery.

- **Calcium channel antagonists:** therapeutically important calcium antagonists act on L-type calcium channels and are of three main classes: phenylalkylamines (**verapa-mil**), dihydropyridines (**nifedipine, amlodipine**) and benzothiazepines (**diltiazem**). All three groups bind to the α_1-subunit of the calcium channel and inhibit the slow inward calcium current in cardiac and smooth muscle cells. Verapamil has primarily cardiac effects and acts as a negative inotrope and chronotrope. Nifedipine and related drugs are more selective for vascular smooth muscle and so are usually used to treat hypertension. They are primarily arterial and arteriolar dilators and have minimal influence on the venous system. The effects of diltiazem are intermediate, but it, along with verapamil, is a class IV anti-arrhythmic. Both slow conduction through the SA and AV nodes where propagation of the AP is dependent on slow inward calcium flux. Verapamil terminates SVTs by causing partial AV block. Nifedipine may cause reflex tachycardia. Ca^{2+} channel blockers are all negative inotropes, but because they offload the myocardium by vasodilatation, cardiac output is usually maintained.

— **Anaesthetic implications**: there may be some synergistic action with volatile anaesthetic agents, which also affect slow Ca^{2+} channels in the myocardium and elsewhere. Nifedipine and verapamil may also potentiate the actions of non-depolarizing muscle relaxants.

- **Angiotensin-converting enzyme (ACE) inhibitors:** these drugs affect the renin–angiotensin system. Renin is a proteolytic enzyme secreted by the juxtaglomerular apparatus, which acts on angiotensinogen (a plasma globulin synthesized in the liver) to form angiotensin I. This inactive substance is converted to the potent vasocon-strictor angiotensin II by ACE. (Angiotensin II is then broken down further to angiotensin III and IV.) ACE is a membrane-bound enzyme on the surface of endothelial cells and is particularly abundant in lung with its huge area of vascular endothelium. The local formation of angiotensin II can occur in numerous different vascular beds. ACE inactivates bradykinin and several other peptides. Bradykinin is an inflammatory mediator and vasoactive peptide which causes vasodilatation and increased vascular permeability. It may also cause bronchial and other smooth muscle constriction. Angiotensin acts on receptors to mediate vasoconstriction (its pressor activity is 40 times as powerful as that of noradrenaline), and it also stimulates noradrenaline release from sympathetic nerve terminals, sodium reabsorption from proximal tubules and aldosterone secretion from the adrenal cortex. ACE inhibitors include **ramipril, captopril, enalapril, lisinopril** and **peri-ndopril**. These drugs mediate a significant fall in BP in hypertensive subjects and reduce cardiac load by affecting both capacitance and resistance vessels. They have no influence on cardiac contractility, although they do act preferentially on angiotensin-sensitive vascular beds in the myocardium, brain and kidney. Cough is a common side effect of their use, due to bradykinin accumulation.

— **Anaesthetic implications**: there are a number of studies that suggest that significant intraoperative hypotension may follow the concomitant administration of a general or regional anaesthetic in patients who are continuing to take an ACE inhibitor. The numbers in these studies are small, but it has become standard advice to discontinue ACE inhibitors 24–48 hours prior to anaesthesia. Discontinuation for 48 hours is probably too long a period; it is not uncommon to see rebound pre-operative hypertension in such patients. If the ACE inhibitor has not been omitted, then volume loading and vasopressors may be needed to maintain normal arterial blood pressure, but it has also been noted that patients may be resistant to the effects of vasopressors such as ephedrine and phenylephrine.

- **Angiotensin antagonists**: pure antagonists of the angiotensin II receptor (examples include **losartan, valsartan, irbesartan, candesartan**) should in theory have a similar spectrum of benefit as ACE inhibitors. They have a better side effect profile and do not cause persistent cough, although they are less effective in the treatment of heart failure.
  — **Anaesthetic implications**: these are broadly similar to those that apply to ACE inhibitors, although, if not discontinued prior to surgery, they are even more likely to cause profound and refractory intraoperative hypotension.

Hypotension and Its Management

Commentary
This may end up largely as an oral about drugs to treat hypotension, but it may be introduced from first principles. Vasopressors are the logical treatment for falls in BP that have been induced pharmacologically, but they also find deployment in a variety of clinical scenarios in which patients are hypotensive.

Core Information
Prime determinants of arterial blood pressure (BP).

- Arterial BP is determined by cardiac output (CO), which is the product of heart rate (HR) and stroke volume (SV), multiplied by systemic vascular resistance (SVR) (i.e. BP = [HR x SV] × SVR).
- CO is a function of HR and SV.
- Hypotension may result from an inadequately compensated decrease in any one or more of these variables.

Reduction in HR (BP = [HR × SV] × SVR)
- **Causes**
  — **Hypoxia**: pre-terminal hypoxia leads to bradycardia.
  — **Vagal stimulation**: profound bradycardia may follow traction on extraocular muscles, anal or cervical dilatation, visceral traction and, sometimes, instrumentation of the airway.

— **Drugs**: medication with drugs such as β-adrenoceptor blockers and digoxin may be responsible. Anaesthetic drugs may also contribute. Volatile agents in high concentrations (halothane in normal concentrations), suxamethonium, opioids and anticholinesterases can all be associated with bradycardia. Low doses of atropine may provoke a paradoxical bradycardia (the Bezold–Jarisch reflex).

— **Cardiac disease**: the commonest cause is ischaemic change affecting the conducting system.

— **Metabolic**: acute hyperkalaemia may hyperpolarize the myocardial cell membrane with a resulting fall in HR.

— **Spinal anaesthesia**: in theory, the block of the cardiac accelerator fibres from T_1 to T_4 should be associated with bradycardia. In practice, this is not often seen.

• **Management**

— Diagnose the cause, and if it is amenable to treatment then act accordingly. Is it hypoxia? Treat immediately. Is it surgical stimulus? Stop traction on the extraocular muscles or the mesentery. If drug treatment is required, the most effective immediate first-line drug is an anticholinergic agent, usually atropine or glycopyrrolate. Neither is a treatment for hypoxia.

Reduction in SV (BP = [HR × SV] × SVR)

• **Causes**

— The commonest cause is reduced venous return (VR). Determinants of VR include volaemic status, venous tone and the lower limb muscle pump, posture (VR is increased in the Trendelenberg head-down position), the respiratory cycle and the elastic recoil of the right ventricle. Volaemic status is the most important of these and may be reduced by an actual reduction in circulating volume secondary to blood loss or dehydration or to an effective reduction in circulating volume caused by sympathetic block or peripheral vasodilatation from some other cause (such as sepsis).

— Reduced contractility: SV may also be diminished because of a failing left ventricle.

• **Management**

— Diagnose the cause. Is it hypovolaemia? Resuscitate with the appropriate fluid. Is position contributing? Revert to recumbency or the head-down position; ensure lateral uterine displacement in the later stages of pregnancy. Beware aortocaval compression by the intra-abdominal mass that is not a gravid uterus. Is it a failing ventricle? Consider using inotropes to support ventricular function.

Reduction in SVR (BP = [HR × SV] × SVR)

• **Causes**

— The commonest cause of inadvertent profound hypotension is probably that which is induced by the sympathetic block associated with a spinal or epidural. It may also occur during anaesthesia in a patient in whom ACE inhibitors or angiotensin II antagonists have not been discontinued prior to surgery. In the context of critical care, the commonest cause is sepsis.

• **Management**

— The rational management of hypotension that has been induced pharmacologically is to treat it pharmacologically. The reduced SVR associated with sepsis is different, but it is still usually managed with a combination of vasopressor, fluids and inotropes.

Supplementary Information
Drugs available to treat hypotension.

Ephedrine
- **Pharmacology:** Ephedrine is a naturally occurring compound (from the Chinese plant *Ma Huang*), which is now synthesized for medical use. It is sympathomimetic and acts directly and indirectly, possessing both α- and β-effects. It also inhibits the breakdown of noradrenaline (norepinephrine) by monoamine oxidase. This mixture of effects means that its main influence on BP is via an increase in CO. Its α_1-effects mediate peripheral vasoconstriction, the β_1-effects are positive inotropy and chronotropy, and the β_2-effects are bronchodilatation (and vasodilatation). The bolus dose is 3–5 mg titrated against response and repeated as necessary. The drug has a rapid onset of action that is said to last for around 60 minutes, but which in practice appears to be less. The depletion of noradrenaline secondary to ephedrine's indirect action leads to tachyphylaxis.
- **Clinical usage:** traditionally, it has been favoured in obstetric anaesthesia because it does not cause α_1-mediated vasoconstriction in the uteroplacental circulation. It has now been superseded by α_1-agonists because it is associated with a greater fetal acidosis (probably by increasing fetal metabolic demand). Ephedrine increases myocardial oxygen demand and so should be used in caution in patients with a pre-existing tachycardia or with cardiac disease. It is also arrhythmogenic. It is an effective bronchodilator.

Phenylephrine
- **Pharmacology:** phenylephrine is an α_1-agonist with mainly direct actions but with some weak β-activity. Its primary influence on BP is via α_1-vasoconstriction and an increase in peripheral resistance. The dose is 50–100 µg titrated against response and repeated as necessary. Onset is rapid, but its duration of action is frequently less than the 60 minutes that is claimed.
- **Clinical usage:** it is an effective vasopressor which is especially popular in some cardiac units. It is also used more widely in obstetric anaesthesia despite traditional avoidance of all pressor drugs apart from ephedrine. Given by infusion after subarachnoid block, it maintains arterial blood pressure effectively. A typical starting rate before titrating against response would be 50 µg min^{-1} (60 ml hr^{-1} of a 50 µg ml^{-1} solution). Phenylephrine maintains maternal BP and neonatal cord pH better than ephedrine. It is not arrhythmogenic, but it can cause a reflex bradycardia which may require treatment with atropine or glycopyrrolate. It is useful in patients in whom a tachycardia should be avoided.

Metaraminol
- **Pharmacology:** metaraminol is a sympathomimetic with both direct and indirect actions and α- and β-effects (α-effects predominate). Its influence on BP is via

α_1-vasoconstriction and increase in CO with increased coronary blood flow. The dose is 1–5 mg titrated against response and repeated as necessary. The onset of action is rapid (1–3 minutes), and the duration of action is around 20–25 minutes.

- **Clinical usage:** it is a potent and effective vasopressor, which is particularly useful for the treatment of hypotension due to sympathetic blockade.

Noradrenaline (Norepinephrine)

- **Pharmacology:** noradrenaline is an exogenous and endogenous catecholamine. It is a powerful α_1-agonist with weaker β-effects. Its vasopressor effect is mediated via α_1-vasoconstriction and the increase in peripheral resistance. It is administered by intravenous infusion (0.05–0.2 $\mu g\,kg^{-1}\,min^{-1}$) and titrated against the desired level of arterial pressure. Its onset and offset of action are rapid.
- **Clinical usage:** noradrenaline is used more commonly in intensive care medicine than in anaesthesia, particularly to treat the low systemic vascular resistance associated with sepsis. Sudden discontinuation of an infusion may be accompanied by severe rebound hypotension. This explains the occasional requirement for the drug following removal of a noradrenaline-secreting phaeochromocytoma. Reflex bradycardia is common.

Adrenaline (Epinephrine)

- **Pharmacology:** adrenaline is also an exogenous and endogenous catecholamine, which acts both as an α_1-and β-agonist. In low doses, β-mediated vasodilatation predominates, but the BP rises because of the increase in CO. In high doses, adrenaline causes α_1-vasoconstriction. It is given either as a bolus (1.0 mg intravenously in the case of circulatory arrest) or as an intravenous infusion in the same dose range as noradrenaline (0.05–0.2 $\mu g\,kg^{-1}\,min^{-1}$).
- **Clinical usage:** the use of adrenaline as a vasopressor is effectively limited to catastrophic circulatory collapse and cardiac arrest.

Vasopressin

- **Pharmacology:** vasopressin acts on the V1 receptors of vascular smooth muscle in the systemic, splanchnic, coronary and renal circulations, where it is a potent vasoconstrictor. (In the pulmonary circulation there is nitric oxide–mediated vasodilatation). It is used to treat the hypotension associated with sepsis and in asystolic cardiac arrest. The infusion rate in sepsis would start at 0.01 I.U. hr^{-1} titrated according to response.

Inotropes

Commentary

Anaesthetists need to know how to support a failing myocardium. The use of inotropes in critical care is routine, and examiners will expect your knowledge of the applied clinical pharmacology to be sound. They will be aware that intensive care units have different preferred inotropes, and so you may well be given the opportunity to discuss the one with which you have had the most experience. You may also be asked to talk about a second-line inotrope. You will add credibility to your account if you can make it evident that these are drugs with whose clinical use you are very familiar.

Core Information

- **An inotrope.** The accurate definition of an inotrope is a substance that affects the force of muscular contraction, either positively or negatively. By common usage, however, the term 'inotrope' describes one of a range of drugs which increase myocardial contractility.
- Most inotropes act via a final common pathway to increase the availability of calcium within the myocyte. The activation of adenylyl cyclase leads to an increase in the production of cAMP from ATP, which in turn activates protein kinase A. This enzyme phosphorylates sites on the α_1-subunits of calcium channels, leading to an increase in open state probability, a rise in calcium flux and an increase in myocardial contractile force.
- The steps which lead to the activation of adenylyl cyclase are considerably more complex than this final pathway, there being at least 13 G protein-linked myocardial cell membrane receptors. β-adrenoceptors, 5-HT receptors, and histamine, prostaglandin and vasoactive intestinal peptide receptors interact with $G_{s(stimulatory)}$ proteins to activate ACh. Adenosine, ACh and somatostatin interact with $G_{i(inhibitory)}$ proteins to inhibit adenylyl cyclase activation, and α_1-adrenoceptors and endothelin receptors interact with G_q proteins to activate phospholipase C and thence protein kinases. (Unlike the 's' and 'i', the 'q' designation does not stand for anything specific but, essentially, was chosen arbitrarily from the later letters of the alphabet, the earlier ones having been reserved for classes of subunits that had already been identified.)
- Calcium leads to the final increase in contractility, and almost all the inotropes in common use have actions that are cAMP dependent. These include dobutamine, adrenaline, dopexamine, noradrenaline, dopamine, isoprenaline, enoximone, milrinone, ephedrine and glucagon. A much smaller group exerts its effects independently of cAMP. The most important are the cardiac glycosides digoxin and ouabain (no longer available in the UK).
- **Inflammatory response**: inotropes also appear to modulate the cytokine response. They inhibit secretion of TNF and alter the balance between pro-inflammatory cytokines, particularly IL-6, and anti-inflammatory molecules such as IL-10.

Inotropes

- **Dobutamine** is a synthetic catecholamine derivative of isoprenaline which is predominantly a β_1-adrenoceptor agonist. It also has dose-dependent effects at β_2- and α_1-receptors. It increases contractility, has minimal effects on heart rate and has little direct effect on vascular tone. It does not act at renal dopamine receptors, but may increase urine output by improving circulatory performance. The quoted dose range is 2.5–10.0 μg kg^{-1} min^{-1}, titrated against response, but much higher rates may be needed in the critically ill.
- **Adrenaline** is an exogenous and endogenous catecholamine, which is both an α_1-and β-agonist. It causes an α_1-mediated increase in the force and rate of myocardial contraction, coupled with an increase in stroke volume secondary to enhanced

venous return. In low doses, β_1-mediated vasodilatation is prominent, but the BP rises because of the increase in cardiac output. As the dose increases so both α- and β-effects are seen, whereas at high doses α_1-vasoconstriction predominates. In the context of critical care, adrenaline is given by intravenous infusion at a rate of 0.05–0.20 $\mu g\ kg^{-1}\ min^{-1}$.

- **Noradrenaline** is another exogenous and endogenous catecholamine. It is a powerful α_1-agonist with weaker β-effects which are most pronounced at low doses (<0.05 $\mu g\ kg^{-1}\ min^{-1}$). Technically, it is more a vasopressor than a direct inotrope, but it has become the first-line agent in many critical care units. (Rises in SVR are associated with increases in cardiac contractility. This is the Anrep effect.)
- **Dopexamine** is a dopamine analogue which also acts both at dopaminergic and β_2-adrenergic receptors. It has no effect at α-receptors. It is an inodilator which increases myocardial contractility while decreasing SVR. It also dilates the splanchnic circulation, acting on dopamine DA_1 and β_2 receptors, which is the main property that finds favour amongst intensivists. The dose range is 0.5–6.0 $\mu g\ kg^{-1}\ min^{-1}$.
- **Dopamine** is an endogenous precursor of noradrenaline, which acts on dopaminergic DA_1 and DA_2 receptors as well as at adrenoceptors. Its effects are dose-dependent: at low doses (up to 5.0 $\mu g\ kg^{-1}\ min^{-1}$) it stimulates mainly dopamine receptors, and it was believed that, because this caused renal vasodilatation, it conferred a renal protective effect. (There is no evidence for this purported benefit.) At infusion rates of between 5 and 10 $\mu g\ kg^{-1}\ min^{-1}$ it causes β_1-mediated increases in myocardial contractility and cardiac output. As the dose rises further, α_1-vasoconstriction becomes more predominant, although it may still provoke tachycardia. Few now believe that dopamine has any uniquely useful renal (or splanchnic) dopaminergic effects, and it is not a first-line inotrope.
- **Isoprenaline** is a synthetic catecholamine with very potent β-adrenergic effects (both β_1 and β_2), but with no α-adrenergic activity. Given in a dose of 0.02–0.2 $\mu g\ kg^{-1}\ min^{-1}$, it leads both to an increase in myocardial contractility and heart rate. It is the drug of choice for pharmacological treatment of complete heart block and for overcoming overdose with β-blockers.

Supplementary Information
Second-line drugs with different mechanisms of action.

- **Levosimendan** increases myocardial contractility by enhancing the sensitivity of cardiac myocytes to calcium (it binds to cardiac troponin C) and reduces systemic vascular and coronary vascular resistance (mediated via the opening of ATP-sensitive K+ channels in vascular smooth muscle, both venous and arterial). The drug does not increase intracellular free calcium and improves cardiac output without increasing oxygen demand. Its elimination half-life is around 60 minutes. (Levosimendan is diluted with glucose 5%, and a typical regimen is a loading dose of 24 $\mu g\ kg^{-1}$ followed by infusion at a rate of 0.1–0.2 $\mu g\ kg\ min^{-1}$).
- **Enoximone and milrinone** act via an increase in cAMP, which is mediated by inhibiting the action of phosphodiesterase-III (PDE-III). This enzyme is responsible for the intracellular degradation of cAMP. Both drugs increase contractility while causing peripheral vasodilatation. The dose of enoximone is 5–20 $\mu g\ kg^{-1}\ min^{-1}$ after a loading dose of 90 $\mu g\ kg^{-1}$; that of milrinone is 0.375–0.750 $\mu g\ kg^{-1}\ min^{-1}$ after a loading dose of 50 $\mu g\ kg^{-1}$. Because the effects of PDE-III inhibitors are not mediated

via adrenoceptors, these drugs can be useful if myocardial β-adrenoceptor down-regulation has occurred and the receptors have become desensitized. This process may be associated with long-standing heart failure and prolonged exposure to circulating catecholamines, but it can also occur acutely (within minutes).

- **Digoxin** is one of the cardiac glycosides (another being ouabain, worth citing if only for the name of the African tree, *Ouabaio akokanthera*, from which it derives), which also acts ultimately via an increase in calcium in the sarcoplasmic reticulum. Unlike other inotropes, however, it inhibits Na^+/K^+ ATPase. It does so by binding to an extracellular α subunit. The resulting increase in sodium concentration reduces the inwardly directed gradient across the cell membrane. One of the mechanisms by which free intracellular calcium levels are kept low is the Na^+/Ca^{2+} exchange transporter. One calcium ion is extruded from the cell in exchange for three sodium ions. More calcium is therefore available for release from the sarcoplasmic reticulum with each action potential.

- **Glucagon** exerts its positive inotropic effect via an increase in the synthesis of cAMP. It is rarely used for this specific purpose, but more commonly in the emergency treatment of hypoglycaemia. (It mobilizes hepatic glycogen.)

- **Ephedrine** is a sympathomimetic which has both direct and indirect α- and β-effects, but which is used primarily as a vasopressor. It inhibits the breakdown of noradrenaline by monoamine oxidase, and this mixture of actions means that its main influence on BP is via an increase in cardiac output. Its $α_1$-effects mediate peripheral vasoconstriction, while the $β_1$-effects increase the force and rate of myocardial contraction. Tachyphylaxis limits its effectiveness.

- **Vasopressin** is not a direct inotrope but has an accepted (and increasing) use as an adjunct vasopressor, particularly in the management of sepsis. It also finds use in asystolic cardiac arrest in which it may be a better agent than adrenaline, although inevitably the supportive data are not robust. In these contexts, the relevant action of this endogenous hormone is on the G protein–coupled V1 receptors of vascular smooth muscle in the systemic, splanchnic, coronary and renal circulations, where it is a potent vasoconstrictor. This property provides the rationale for its use in the management of oesophageal variceal haemorrhage. (In the pulmonary circulation there is nitric oxide mediated vasodilatation.) As a bolus in cardiac arrest a typical dose is 40 I.U., and by infusion in sepsis the starting rate would be 0.01 I.U. hr^{-1} titrated upwards according to response.

Drugs Used in the Treatment of Nausea and Vomiting

Commentary

The problem of postoperative nausea and vomiting is a core topic. The effective prescription of anti-emetics requires some knowledge about their diverse sites of action. This oral may be combined with general questions about the physiology of vomiting .

Core Information

Patients at particular risk of postoperative nausea and vomiting (PONV). (This information is largely duplicated elsewhere but is reproduced in this section for convenience).

- **Factors related to patients**: in terms of odds ratio, female gender is the most reliable predictive factor (OR 3). Although there are some studies that have suggested that PONV is decreased in the luteal phase of menstruation (during the second half of the cycle), the data are inconsistent, and current consensus is that the phase of the menstrual cycle has no influence. A positive history of PONV is another predictive factor, which doubles its likelihood (OR 2), as does a history of motion sickness, and if ambulation after surgery is premature. Smoking appears to exert a protective effect with an odds ratio of 2 (in theory acting as a potent inducer of the cytochrome P450 system); so, to a lesser extent, does regular alcohol consumption. PONV is increased by preoperative anxiety. Body habitus has no impact on the incidence of PONV, and there is no association with obesity, as formerly was believed. There is an inverse relationship with increasing age in adults.
- **Factors related to surgery**: intra-abdominal, intracranial, middle ear and squint surgery have all been associated with a higher incidence of PONV, as have laparoscopic and gynaecological procedures. Multivariate analysis in large trials, however, suggests that there is no direct causation, and that these operations (with the exception of squint surgery in children) do not represent independent risk factors for PONV. Empirical experience nonetheless across this range of surgical procedures suggests that the need for rescue antiemetic therapy does appear to be greater. Moderate to severe postoperative pain can also be a potent precipitant.
- **Factors related to anaesthesia**: volatile anaesthetics at least double the incidence of PONV, and as would be expected the risk is dose- and duration-dependent. It is believed that the emetic potential of volatiles (which is similar for all the halogenated hydrocarbons) is related to a decrease in serum concentrations of anandamide. This is a neurotransmitter with a wide spectrum of activity, including the suppression of emesis, and whose effects are mediated via CB1 and CB2 cannabinoid receptors. The increased risk of PONV of which nitrous oxide is frequently accused is actually modest (OR 1.4), and the ENIGMA II trial showed that this risk is nullified with concomitant anti-emetic therapy. Opioids increase the risk in a dose-dependent fashion. Drugs with sympathomimetic actions are also associated with increased risk. Hypoxaemia is a stimulus to vomiting.
- **Factors related to disease:** the list of potential causes is long and includes intestinal obstruction, hypoglycaemia, hypoxia, uraemia and hypotension.
- **Scoring systems:** there are various scoring systems, such as the Apfel score, which estimate the likelihood of PONV according to the number of predisposing factors. (Apfel uses previous history, non-smoking, female gender and administration of opioids). The incidence of PONV in relation to the number of factors is quoted as 0–10%, 1–20%, 2–40%, 3–60% and 4–80%. This suggests that a non-smoking female undergoing, say, routine day-case orthopaedic surgery, would have a 40% likelihood of PONV. Clinical experience suggests that this would seem unduly, if not improbably high, but validations of the various models suggest that they can be useful.

Applied Pharmacology of Anti-Emetic Drugs

- Nausea and vomiting are mediated by a number of sites with different receptors. This means that these symptoms can be treated by 'balanced anti-emesis' using drugs of differing actions. Although some drugs act at more than one receptor, their anti-emetic actions usually predominate at one.
- **Vestibular nuclei and the labyrinth:** these contain histamine (H_1) and muscarinic ACh (M_3) receptors. Drugs acting at this site include **cyclizine**, **promethazine** (H_1-antagonists), and **hyoscine**, **atropine** and **glycopyrrolate** (anticholinergic M_3-antagonists).
- **Visceral afferents:** these are mediated by serotonin (5-HT_3) receptors in the gut wall and myenteric plexus. Drugs acting at this site include ondansetron, granisetron, dolasetron (not available in the UK) and palonosetron (these are selective 5-HT_3 antagonists). Palonosetron has a more favourable side effect profile and also has a prolonged duration of action (it is reported to be effective for up to 72 hours).
- **Vomiting centre (VC):** this contains primarily muscarinic ACh (M_3) and some histamine (H_1) receptors. It may also contain μ-opioid receptors. Drugs acting at this site are the same as those which affect the vestibular apparatus.
- **Chemoreceptor trigger zone (CTZ):** impulses from the CTZ to the VC appear to be mediated mainly via dopamine (D_2) and serotonin (5-HT_3) receptors. It may also contain δ-opioid receptors. In addition, substance P, which is a slow excitatory neurotransmitter, may have a role by acting at neurokinin-1 (NK_1) receptors. NK_1-receptors are abundant in the brain stem where emetic afferents converge. Drugs acting at the CTZ include metoclopramide, domperidone, prochlorperazine, trifluoperazine, haloperidol and droperidol, which has recently again become available in the UK (D_2-antagonists). The newest agents are NK_1-antagonists of which aprepitant is the example now available in the UK. Its cost, if nothing else (each dose is approximately £15) makes it a second-line treatment.
- **Drugs of uncertain sites of action**
  - *Cannabinoids:* synthetic derivatives such as **nabilone** appear to antagonize the emetic effects of drugs which stimulate the CTZ. Because the cannabinoid effects can themselves be antagonized by naloxone, it is postulated that opioid receptors are involved in their actions. There are at least two endogenous cannabinoid receptors, CB_1 and CB_2, which modulate neurotransmitter release.
  - *Corticosteroids:* high-dose steroids such as **dexamethasone** or **methyl prednisolone** act as anti-emetics by mechanisms that are unclear.
  - *Propofol:* its antiemetic property is disputed, but its effective use in patients with chemotherapy-induced emesis suggests otherwise. It would appear therefore to act at the CTZ.

Supplementary Information

Significant side effects of anti-emetics.

- **Antimuscarinic drugs** (atropine, hyoscine, glycopyrrolate): all are potent antisialogogues, and so a dry mouth is almost invariable. Hyoscine is sedative. All three agents can cause the central anticholinergic syndrome, although it is very much less common with glycopyrrolate (as a quaternary ammonium compound, its ability to cross the blood–brain barrier is very limited).

- **Antidopaminergic drugs** (metoclopramide, prochlorperazine, haloperidol, droperidol): these may cause acute extrapyramidal and dystonic effects which are caused by a preponderance of the antidopaminergic stimulatory actions over anticholinergic inhibitory actions in other parts of the CNS. This imbalance can be restored almost instantly with an intravenous anticholinergic agent such as procyclidine 5–10 mg. The phenothiazines may also cause sedation. Droperidol is associated with prolongation of the QT interval (with the potential development of torsade de pointes) and so should be avoided in any patient with a prolonged QTc (corrected QT interval) or in patients taking one of the many other drugs that have the same effect. (These include Class Ia and Class III antiarrhythmic drugs, antihistamines such as terfenadine, some 5-HT$_3$ antagonists which might be prescribed as part of multimodal antiemetic therapy, and some antibiotics, quinolones and macrolides, including erythromycin). QT prolongation is, however, dose-dependent, and in the lower doses given for anti-emesis it does not present significant risk. Droperidol is also an α_1 antagonist and so may cause hypotension. It is a neuroleptic which has been used as pre-operative medication and can be dysphoric; patients appear outwardly calm but with intense internal agitation and anxiety which they are unable to communicate.
- **Antiserotoninergic drugs** (ondansetron, granisetron, palonosetron): ondansetron and granisetron are associated with QT interval prolongation, whereas palonosetron is not; otherwise their side effect profile is favourable, with headache being reported as the main side effect, complicating treatment in 3–5% of patients.
- **Cannabinoids** (nabilone, dronabinol): sedation is common, and the drugs may sometimes exert psychotomimetic effects similar to those induced by the parent compounds. Dry mouth and postural hypotension may also occur.
- **Corticosteroids** (methyl prednisolone, dexamethasone): the list of acute side effects includes steroid psychosis, which is related to a sudden increase in plasma levels of corticoids, and metabolic disturbance, including hyperglycaemia, fluid retention and hypokalaemia. Short courses of high-dose steroids may cause peptic ulceration.

Drug Overdose: Prescribed and Therapeutic Drugs

Commentary

Patients take overdoses of numerous different drugs. The clinical features of drug poisoning may result from exaggeration of their normal effects or from the direct toxicity of the parent compound and its metabolites. Effective management of drug overdose in many cases of poisoning depends on some understanding of the mechanism of action of the substances that have been ingested.

Core Information

Drugs commonly taken in overdose. (This may include a brief outline of emergency management. A generic Airway, Breathing, Circulation approach will not be adequate because specific details will be required where appropriate).

Antidepressants

The main classes of drugs are the tricyclic antidepressants (TCAs) such as **amitriptyline** and **imipramine,** and the selective serotonin re-uptake inhibitors (SSRIs) such as **fluoxetine** (Prozac), **paroxetine** (Seroxat), **sertraline** (Lustral), **citalopram** (Cipramil) and **escitalopram** (Cipralex).

- **Mechanisms:** TCAs are tertiary amines and are related chemically to phenothiazines. They act by blocking the re-uptake of amines, primarily noradrenaline and 5-HT, by competitive inhibition of a transport protein binding site. They have minimal influence on dopaminergic synapses but do affect muscarinic ACh and histamine receptors.

SSRIs are relatively selective for 5-HT uptake, have fewer anticholinergic side effects than TCAs and are safer in overdose. They can cause a 'serotonin syndrome' if used in combination with drugs such as monoamine oxidase inhibitors. Its features include hyperthermia, muscular rigidity and cardiovascular collapse.

- **Features of overdose:** the major problems are cardiovascular and neurological. Ventricular arrhythmias are common and are associated particularly with QT interval prolongation. In high doses they appear to block a specific cardiac potassium channel (the HERG channel). Ventricular fibrillation may supervene. Other potential arrhythmias include heart block and ventricular tachycardia. CNS effects include agitation and excitability, grand mal convulsions and coma. The muscarinic effects resemble those of atropine poisoning, with flushing, dry mouth, mydriasis and gastrointestinal stasis. Features of poisoning with SSRIs are analogous, but are generally less severe.
- **Management:** this is largely supportive. Benzodiazepines may abort convulsions. Cardiac arrhythmias should be treated only with extreme caution, if at all, because the combination of effects can be fatal. Magnesium is probably the least dangerous treatment, although intravenous lidocaine and amiodarone have been used. ECG monitoring is mandatory for at least 24 hours after ingestion. Induced alkalosis (plasma pH > 7.5) by the use of hyperventilation and intravenous $NaHCO_3$ may reduce the amount of free drug that is present.

Paracetamol

This is a simple analgesic in ubiquitous use.

- **Mechanisms:** paracetamol probably acts as an inhibitor of central prostaglandin synthesis, although its exact subcellular mechanism of action remains unclear. Evidence about any peripheral anti-inflammatory action is conflicting. It is rapidly absorbed from the small intestine. Its therapeutic index is narrow because the liver enzymes which catalyze the normal conjugation pathways rapidly become saturated.

A dose of 8–10 g in adults is toxic. The alternative metabolic pathway via mixed function oxidases produces a metabolite (N-acetyl-*p*-benzoquinine imine) which is toxic to cells both of the liver and of the renal tubules. This metabolite is normally conjugated with glutathione, but will accumulate when glutathione stores are depleted to cause centrilobular hepatic necrosis and renal tubular damage.

- **Features of overdose:** nausea and vomiting occur early; symptoms and signs of hepatic failure appear later.
- **Management:** definitive early treatment is with agents that will replenish glutathione stores and prevent hepatic damage. Methionine, which is a glutathione precursor, can be given orally, although the more common treatment is intravenous N-acetylcysteine. Fulminant hepatic failure can be treated only by hepatic transplantation.

Benzodiazepines

These anxiolytics and hypnotics, of which there are more than 20 available for clinical use, are common prescription drugs. Typical examples are temazepam, diazepam and clonazepam. (Midazolam is a drug whose use is restricted largely to hospital.)

- **Mechanism of action:** benzodiazepines facilitate the opening of GABA-activated chloride channels and thereby enhance fast inhibitory synaptic transmission within the CNS. They bind to a separate receptor, which effects an allosteric change that increases the affinity of GABA for the $GABA_A$ receptor.
- **Features of overdose:** these drugs are relatively safe in overdose because, taken alone, they cause profound sedation but without respiratory depression, haemodynamic instability or secondary toxicity. In combination with other CNS depressants, however, they may be associated with marked respiratory depression.
- **Management: flumazenil** (Anexate) is a specific benzodiazepine antagonist which displaces benzodiazepines from the binding sites and reverses their effects. The effective duration of action of flumazenil is shorter than that of many of the drugs which it antagonizes, and so the dose (typically up to 500 µg intravenously) may need to be repeated. The incautious use of flumazenil may also unmask convulsions caused, for example, by TCAs, otherwise suppressed by the benzodiazepine overdose.

Tramadol

This is a synthetic piperidine analogue of codeine. It is an oral analgesic which is used for moderate pain, but which is not associated with drug dependence or abuse. It is not, therefore, a controlled substance.

- **Mechanisms:** for details see under 'Opiates/Opioids' earlier in this chapter. Tramadol has relatively low activity at µ-receptors, but it also acts by inhibiting the re-uptake of noradrenaline and 5-HT within the CNS.
- **Features of overdose:** although activity at µ-opioid receptors is weak, after overdose patients may demonstrate typical features of sedation and respiratory depression. Of greater interest are the signs of a 'serotonin syndrome', which include agitation, tachycardia and hypertension, diaphoresis and muscular rigidity.

- **Management:** in general, the treatment of a tramadol overdose is supportive. Naloxone can be used to treat the opioid side effects, but the optimal management of a serotonin syndrome remains uncertain. The 5-HT$_{2A}$ antagonist cyproheptadine has been used, as have drugs such as dantrolene, propranolol and diazepam.

Alcohol

This is included because alcohol ingestion frequently complicates overdose with other drugs. TCAs, for example, can dangerously enhance the depressant effects of acute alcohol intake.

- **Mechanism of action:** ethanol facilitates the opening of GABA-activated chloride channels to increase fast inhibitory synaptic transmission within the CNS. It also acts to inhibit the NMDA receptor.
- **Features of overdose:** disinhibition is followed by CNS depression. The features of acute intoxication are too well known to warrant detailing. An important complication that must not be missed, however, is the effect of acute alcohol on glucose metabolism. Individuals who have recently ingested large volumes of alcohol are at risk of profound hypoglycaemia. The metabolism of alcohol to acetaldehyde is catalysed by alcohol dehydrogenase in a reaction which produces NADH from NAD$^+$. This effectively depletes NAD$^+$, which is an important co-factor (a hydrogen acceptor) in the gluconeogenetic conversion of lactate to pyruvate ($C_3H_6O_3 \rightarrow C_3H_4O_3$; NAD$^+ \rightarrow$ NADH + H$^+$).
- **Management:** at lower blood concentrations (up to 10 mg dl^{-1}) the metabolism of alcohol follows first order kinetics, but at higher levels it demonstrates zero order kinetics. Management is of alcohol overdose is supportive as there is no means of accelerating its breakdown.

Activated Charcoal

The administration of activated charcoal is rarely initiated by anaesthetists, but as it is routine first-line management following the ingestion of numerous toxins and drugs taken in overdose, the substance may form part of the discussion.

- **Mechanism of action:** activated charcoal adsorbs some, but not all, chemicals and drugs. (Adsorption describes the capacity of solid substances to attract to their surfaces atoms, ions and molecules from a gas, liquid or solution with which they are in contact. Adsorption can be physical, in which the bonding is by relatively weak Van der Waals forces, or chemical. The nature of the chemical bond varies with the adsorbate.) Charcoal is described as 'activated' because the addition of acid and steam to carbonaceous materials results in the formation of ultrafine particles with a large surface area (around 50–70,000 m^2 per 50 g dose).
- **Efficacy:** it may reduce the absorption of some substances by up to 60% and continues to be effective throughout its transit through the bowel. This can be accelerated by the addition of sorbitol, which acts as a hyperosmotic laxative. There are, however, some potential toxins and drugs which are not adsorbed by activated

Pharmacology

4

charcoal. These include alcohols such as ethyl alcohol (alcohol), methyl alcohol (as used in antifreeze) and isopropyl alcohol (as used in hand gels); lithium; heavy metals such as lead and iron and the metalloid arsenic; strongly acidic and basic compounds; and many petroleum- and plant-derived hydrocarbons.

Recreational Drugs and Drugs of Abuse

Commentary

The abuse of recreational drugs is common, and patients may present either because of an adverse reaction, or because, often unwittingly, they have taken or been given an overdose. It can be difficult to identify exactly what substances are involved because street drugs have no quality control, and because these adulterated compounds are often taken in combination. But, as is the case with prescribed drugs, an understanding of their mechanisms of action helps the rational management of overdose.

Core Information

Common drugs of abuse: There are some niche drugs, such as 'GHB' (gamma-hydroxybutyrate) and 'Special K' (ketamine), but the general pattern of drug abuse relates to methadone and heroin (diamorphine), cocaine, ecstasy (MDMA) and alcohol.

Opioids

Methadone and heroin are the main opioids of abuse.

- **Mechanisms of action:** for details see under 'Opiates/Opioids'.
- **Features of overdose:** the features of opioid overdose are well known. The life-threatening complication of opioid overdose is profound central respiratory depression. Patients may be sedated, comatose and bradypnoeic. Hypotension is common, and this may be associated with both tachycardia and bradycardia. The other numerous effects of opioids are of less relative importance. Methadone has a similar spectrum of action to diamorphine, although it is less euphoriant and less sedative. It has a much longer elimination half-life (>24 hours).
- **Management:** the specific opioid antagonist naloxone is the initial drug of choice. The intravenous dose is higher than is used for typical postoperative respiratory depression, being 0.8–2.0 mg, repeated after 2–3 minutes to a maximum of 10 mg. If there has been no response by this stage, then the diagnosis should be reviewed.

Cocaine

- **Mechanisms:** cocaine is an indirect sympathomimetic which blocks the presynaptic re-uptake of noradrenaline. It also exerts central dopaminergic and serotonergic effects.
- **Features of overdose:** these include agitation and disorientation, together with other features of sympathetic hyperstimulation. Hypertension, hyperpyrexia, convulsions

and coma may all be evident. The drug increases myocardial oxygen demand and causes coronary vasospasm. Ventricular fibrillation may supervene.

- **Management:** it would be logical to treat the sympathetic overactivity with α- and β-adrenoceptor blockers, although some authorities dispute the place of β-blockers because of their unopposed α-effects on the circulation. These can be offset by using, for example, phentolamine (5 mg intravenously, repeated as necessary). Otherwise the management of cocaine poisoning is supportive.

MDMA (Ecstasy)

This is a popular recreational drug, which has caused well-publicized deaths among a small number of young people. These deaths are not necessarily related to overdose, although because the drug is illegal, information about quantity, quality and formulation is almost impossible to obtain. The clinical features may therefore be caused by an idiosyncratic reaction.

- **Mechanisms:** 3,4-methylenedioxy methamphetamine (MDMA) is related structurally both to methamphetamine and to mescaline, which is a potent hallucinogen. Amphetamines are centrally acting sympathomimetics which appear to stimulate central aminergic pathways, particularly those mediated by dopamine and noradrenaline. They inhibit re-uptake of neurotransmitter, stimulate its presynaptic release, and act as direct agonists at postsynaptic receptors. These effects occur peripherally as well as centrally. MDMA also acts as an agonist at 5-HT_2 receptors to produce psychotomimetic effects. This may also be partly responsible for the hyperthermia that may be evident.
- **Features of overdose:** ecstasy use is associated with the club scene, and so patients may present having been dancing violently in a hot environment without taking adequate isotonic fluid. They may be delirious or unconscious, with grand mal convulsions. They are frequently diaphoretic and febrile. This hypermetabolic state is associated with a metabolic acidosis, and also with rhabdomyolysis. Disseminated intravascular coagulation may supervene, followed by multi-organ failure.
- **Management:** patients may require full intensive care management, including renal support if indicated. Dantrolene (1 mg kg^{-1} initially) has been used to control hyperpyrexia, although support for its use is not universal.

Alcohol

This may be taken alone in overdose, or as part of a cocktail of substances, and is described in more detail in the immediately preceding section,

Cannabis

Overdose is not a common problem, given that most users in the UK smoke the drug rather than ingesting it. Nor is acute excess directly life-threatening, although the much stronger street preparations are more dangerous than hitherto.

- **Mechanisms:** central cannabinoid receptors (CB$_1$ subtype) exert an inhibitory effect on nociceptive afferents and on transmission via the dorsal horn. Like opioid receptors they are typical G protein-linked receptors, which inhibit adenyl cyclase, hyperpolarize cell membranes by facilitating the opening of potassium channels and decrease neurotransmitter release via calcium channel inhibition. Tetrahydrocannabinol (THC) is analgesic, sedating, anti-emetic, antispasmodic, euphoriant, anxiolytic and bronchodilatory. (These features would actually make the drug ideal pre-operative medication.)

- **Features of acute excess:** the main features are sedation and confusion, although the drug can also cause vasodilatation and tachycardia. Paranoid delusions of the kind that may be seen with hallucinogenic drugs can occur with stronger preparations.
- **Management:** unless patients have complicated cannabis use by concurrent ingestion of other substances, they will usually require only modest supportive therapy.

Supplementary Information

The Anaesthetic Implications of Drug Abuse

There are three main considerations: patients may be under the residual influence of the drug, they may suffer an acute withdrawal syndrome and they may have continued physiological dependence. (Drug-associated co-morbidity such as infection with HIV and hepatitis B and C should also be considered.) It may be very difficult to obtain an accurate history.

- **Opioids:** recent ingestion in a habituated patient will do little more than act as opioid premedication. Withdrawal is characterized by autonomic hyperactivity with clinical features of both sympathetic and parasympathetic stimulation. These include agitation, tachycardia, diaphoresis, vomiting and abdominal cramps. It is important not to precipitate a withdrawal syndrome in the perioperative period by giving inadequate doses of opioid. Postoperative pain requirements should be added to their estimated daily 'maintenance' requirement. PCA doses may need to be increased significantly and must be given via a device that is secure and tamper-proof.
- **Cocaine and amphetamines:** residual sympathetic stimulation will complicate anaesthesia, but its manifestations are easily treated. Cocaine withdrawal is characterized mainly by psychological craving for the drug. This may be mediated by dopamine and/or serotonin, but the use of antagonists is not widespread.
- **Cannabis:** this has many of the properties of a useful drug for premedication, and residual effects may even confer some benefit, as long as these are recognized and the sedation is not compounded by excessive anaesthetic and analgesic doses. A withdrawal syndrome has been described that manifests mainly as restlessness, irritability, insomnia and anorexia.
- **Lysergic acid diethylamide (LSD):** this is a synthetic hallucinogen (natural hallucinogens include mescaline and psilocybin) which is taken orally and which causes visual, auditory and tactile distortions of perception. In some cases the drug can induce transient psychosis, with paranoia and abnormal ideation. The drug is sympathomimetic and also has some analgesic α_2-agonism. Management is generic and supportive.

Drugs Affecting Mood

Commentary

These commonly prescribed drugs are of interest because some have specific implications for anaesthesia. The oral is unlikely to cover all the classes of drugs and may concentrate on one group with only supplementary reference to the others.

Core Information

Anaesthetic implications for one or more of the groups of drugs that are used to treat affective disorders.

Lithium

Lithium (Li^+) is an inorganic ion, which is used prophylactically to control the mood swings of bipolar manic depression. In the acute situation it may help to control mania, but not depression. The drug has a very narrow therapeutic index; it is effective at plasma levels of 0.5–1.0 mmol l^{-1}, produces side effects at >1.5 mmol l^{-1} and may be fatal at a plasma concentration of 3.0–5.0 mmol l^{-1}.

- **Mechanisms:** as an inorganic ion it can mimic the role of sodium in excitable tissue by entering cells via fast voltage-gated channels that generate action potentials. Unlike sodium, however, it is not pumped out of the excitable cell by Na^+/K^+-ATPase and so accumulates within the cytoplasm, partially replacing intracellular potassium. Its therapeutic effect is thought to be mediated by its interference with two of the second messenger systems: cAMP and inositol triphosphate. It may increase 5-HT synthesis in the CNS. Its actions are enhanced by diuretics, which reduce clearance, and by dehydration.
- **Adverse effects and implications for anaesthesia:** side effects include polydipsia and polyuria secondary to ADH inhibition, diarrhoea and vomiting, hypothyroidism, lassitude and renal impairment. Acute toxicity causes cardiac arrhythmias, ataxia, confusion, convulsions and, in extreme cases, coma and death. Plasma levels must be measured before anaesthesia. The drug enhances the effects of all muscle relaxants (both depolarizing and non-depolarizing) and potentiates anaesthetic agents. It has a long plasma half-life and so can be withheld for 2 days preceding surgery. Good hydration is important, as is sodium balance. Low serum sodium increases lithium toxicity, and electrolytes should be restored to normal levels before surgery. NSAIDs may reduce Li^+ clearance and increase plasma levels.

Monoamine Oxidase Inhibitors (MAOIs)

Potentially dangerous interactions led to a fall in the number of patients receiving MAOIs for refractory depressive illness. Recently, however, newer agents have been synthesized, and this class of drugs has enjoyed resurgence. Monoamine oxidase (MAO) describes a non-specific group of enzymes, which is subdivided into two main classes.

- **MAO-A:** this is mainly intraneuronal and degrades dopamine, noradrenaline and 5-HT (serotonin). Inhibition of the enzyme increases levels of amine neurotransmitters, some of which are associated with mood and affect.
- **MAO-B:** this is predominantly extracellular and degrades other amines such as tyramine and dopamine. MAOs have only a minor role in terminating the actions either of noradrenaline at sympathetic nerve terminals (re-uptake is the more important mechanism) or of exogenous direct-acting sympathomimetics.
- **Drugs:** these fall into one of three groups – non-selective and irreversible MAOIs, selective and reversible MAO-A inhibitors, and selective MAO-B inhibitors.
  - **Non-selective and irreversible MAOIs:** drugs such as **phenelzine, tranylcypromine,** and **isocarboxazid** potentiate effects of amines (especially tyramine) in foods. Patients are given strict dietary restrictions because the hazard of hypertensive crisis is real. Such drugs will potentiate the action of any indirectly acting sympathomimetics, although the use of directly acting sympathomimetics is less dangerous. The drugs may also interact with opioids, particularly with piperazine derivatives such as pethidine and fentanyl. Co-administration may result in hyperpyrexia, excitation, muscle rigidity and coma. The mechanism for this reaction is unclear.
  - **Selective and reversible MAO-A inhibitors:** drugs such as **moclobemide** cause less potentiation of amines, and so fewer dietary restrictions are necessary. Vasopressors which have an indirect action, such as ephedrine and metaraminol, should nonetheless be avoided.
  - **Selective MAO-B inhibitors:** the main example is **selegiline,** whose primary use is in the treatment of Parkinson's disease. MAO-B predominates in dopamine-rich areas of the CNS.
- **Implications for anaesthesia:** patients ideally should discontinue these drugs (apart from selegiline, whose sudden withdrawal may exacerbate symptoms) at least 2 weeks before anaesthesia, because the range of interactions is wide and the response is unpredictable. There is an obvious danger in discontinuing treatment in severely depressed patients, and so expert psychiatric opinion should be sought. If emergency surgery cannot be deferred, the anaesthetic management must take into account any likely interactions. This mandates caution with use of extradural or subarachnoid anaesthesia because of the possible need for vasopressors, and caution with the use of opioids. Pethidine should not be used, but morphine is considered to be safe.

Other Antidepressants

The main groups are tricyclic antidepressants (TCAs) such as **amitriptyline, imipramine** and **lofepramine** (which is the safest of the TCAs in overdose); tetracyclic compounds of which the only example in the UK is **mianserin;** and selective serotonin re-uptake inhibitors (SSRIs) such as **fluoxetine** (Prozac), **paroxetine** (Seroxat) and **citalopram.**

- **Mechanisms:** TCAs block the re-uptake of amines, primarily noradrenaline and 5-HT.
- **Implications for anaesthesia:** the effects of sympathomimetic drugs may be exaggerated, and anticholinergic drugs may precipitate confusion by causing the central

anticholinergic syndrome. This is characterized by predictable effects of cholinergic transmission at muscarinic receptors: flushing, pyrexia, mydriasis, drying of mucous membranes, tachycardia, decreased gastrointestinal motility and urinary retention. The central effects are accompanied by alterations in mental state and confusion. Specific treatment is with an anticholinesterase, but this is usually reserved for severe cases of psychosis and/or tachyarrhythmias with haemodynamic instability.

Benzodiazepines
These are anxiolytic and hypnotic.

- **Implications for anaesthesia:** benzodiazepines cause sedation and, when given in combination with other CNS depressants, may be associated with profound respiratory depression.

Drugs Affecting Coagulation

Commentary
Patients presenting for surgery or neuraxial anaesthesia who are receiving anticoagulants and antiplatelet drugs are of obvious interest to anaesthetists. You should be able to formulate a coherent management plan for patients who are receiving these agents. These drugs may limit the options for neuraxial techniques, and so you may also be asked to outline what are considered to be safe intervals between the last dose of a particular agent and the performance of a spinal or epidural block. There are newer models of coagulation, but the traditional model is still ubiquitous, is conceptually somewhat more straightforward and is still likely to predominate in the oral.

Core Information
- **Haemostatic mechanisms:** understanding the actions of anticoagulant drugs requires an appreciation of normal haemostasis. The process of coagulation ends with a haemostatic plug that forms following platelet activation, and which is subsequently reinforced by fibrin. This final step involves the conversion of soluble fibrinogen to insoluble strands of fibrin, in a reaction catalysed by thrombin. Thrombin (factor IIa) is one of several important serine proteases that are present in the coagulation cascade, and is formed from prothrombin (factor II) in the presence of activated factor X. Both coagulation pathways activate factor X, which, as Xa (the suffix 'a' denotes 'active'), converts prothrombin to thrombin.
- **Coagulation pathways and the coagulation cycle:** the traditional 'intrinsic and 'extrinsic' two pathway model of haemostasis has been superseded by an intracellular-based model of coagulation, more akin to a 'coagulation cycle' than a 'coagulation cascade'. If, for example, the intrinsic and extrinsic pathways are genuinely parallel, this does not explain why patients with factor VIII (haemophilia A) or factor IX deficiency (haemophilia B) do not initiate clotting via the alternate

unaffected pathway. The newer model of coagulation suggests that thrombin is generated initially by the extrinsic pathway in a process that involves the activation of factors IX and X by a tissue factor-factor VIIa (TF-VIIa) complex that forms in response to damaged vascular endothelium. Factor Xa binds with prothrombin (factor II) to form thrombin (factor IIa). The amount of thrombin that initially is generated is small, and so this process requires amplification by a number of positive feedback systems in which thrombin activates factors V and VIII. These in turn activate factor IX (to IXa) and X (to Xa) with the generation of more thrombin (IIa). Enzyme complexes, such as prothrombinase, which mediate some of these reactions, further activate platelets and accelerate continued thrombin formation. In the stabilization phase, factor XIII (fibrin stabilizing factor) links fibrin polymers via covalent bonds, while thrombin itself activates an inhibitor of fibrinolysis. (This account is a simplification but should provide sufficient information for the oral.)

- **Coagulation pathways, the traditional 'cascade' model:** the two classically described pathways are the 'intrinsic', or contact, pathway, all of whose components are present within blood, and the 'extrinsic' pathway, in which some components are found outside blood. The intrinsic system is triggered by contact with exposed collagen in endothelium, and the extrinsic system is activated by the release of tissue thromboplastin. The pathways converge on the activation of factor X. The protein coagulation factors are present in blood as inactive precursors, which are then activated by proteolysis, particularly of serine moieties. The cascade is amplified, with each step producing greater quantities of activated clotting factors than the one preceding it. The process in health is held in check by antithrombin III, which neutralizes all the serine proteases involved in the cascade.

Drugs Affecting Coagulation

- **Warfarin:** warfarin is a competitive inhibitor of vitamin K reductase, and so prevents the regeneration of the reduced active form and the addition of the essential carboxyl moiety to the four coagulation factors. It was first isolated from natural coumarins by American researchers after whom the compound was named (Wisconsin Alumni Research Foundation). Its effect takes some days to develop because of the different rates at which the carboxylated coagulation factors degrade. The elimination half-life of factor VII is only 6 hours, whereas that of factor II is 60 hours (the $t_{1/2}$ of factors IX and X are 24 and 40 hours, respectively). The effect of warfarin on the prothrombin time (or international normalized ratio, [INR]) starts at 12–16 hours and lasts for 4–5 days. It is metabolized by the hepatic mixed function oxidase P450 system, and there are a number of drugs which can interfere with its metabolism. Its effects are potentiated by agents that inhibit hepatic drug metabolism. Examples of these are cimetidine, metronidazole and amiodarone. Its effects are attenuated by dietary vitamin K and by drugs such as barbiturates and carbamazepine which induce hepatic cytochrome P450. Some drugs, such as NSAIDs, displace warfarin from binding sites and increase plasma concentrations, but this is of only modest clinical significance.

- **Heparins:** heparin is not a single homogenous substance. Heparins are a family of sulphated glycosaminoglycans (extracted first from liver, hence the name) whose actions are assayed biologically against an agreed international standard. They are therefore usually prescribed in units of activity and not of mass. (One exception is the low-molecular-weight heparin, enoxaparin). Heparin fragments, low-molecular-weight heparins (LMWHs), are much more commonly used than unfractionated preparations. Heparins inhibit coagulation by potentiating the action of antithrombin III (ATIII). ATIII inactivates thrombin and other serine proteases by binding to the active serine site and so inhibits factors II, IX, X, XI and XII. Heparins bind specifically to ATIII. To inhibit thrombin, they need to bind both to the protease enzyme as well as to ATIII, whereas inhibition of factor Xa binding is necessary only to ATIII. The larger molecules of unfractionated heparin bind both to the enzyme and to the inhibitor, but the smaller LMWHs such as tinzaparin, dalteparin and enoxaparin increase the action of ATIII only on factor Xa. (The in vitro effect of unfractionated heparin is measured by the APTT, which is not prolonged by LMWHs.)

Antiplatelet Drugs

- **Non-steroidal anti-inflammatory drugs (NSAIDs).** Aspirin (acetyl salicylic acid) is the original example of this class of drug. Aspirin and the non-selective COX inhibitors such as diclofenac and ibuprofen inactivate the enzyme cyclo-oxygenase (COX) by binding to COX-1 via acetylation of a serine residue on the active site. Aspirin binds irreversibly; the others exhibit competitive antagonism which is reversible. Platelet synthesis of thromboxane (TXA_2), which promotes platelet aggregation, then falls. TXA_2 also reduces the synthesis of prostaglandin PGI_2 (also known as epoprostenol or prostacyclin) in vascular endothelium. This substance inhibits platelet aggregation. The persistent inhibition of platelet aggregation results from the fact that vascular endothelium is able to synthesize new PGI_2, whereas platelets are unable to produce new TXA_2.
- **Clopidogrel.** This is a thienopyridine which binds covalently to the $P2Y_{12}$ ADP receptor on platelet cell membranes, induces a conformational change which renders it inactive and thereby prevents receptor-mediated platelet aggregation. It is a pro-drug which requires hepatic conversion to an active metabolite. Receptor blockade inhibits fibrin cross-linking by preventing activation of the glycoprotein IIb/IIIa pathway. This is a calcium-dependent process that is required for normal platelet aggregation and endothelial adherence. Clopidogrel acts within 2 hours of oral administration, and its irreversible effects last for the lifetime of the platelet (usually 7–10 days).
- **Ticagrelor.** This is a nucleoside analogue which also blocks the $P2Y_{12}$ ADP receptor but at a site separate from that of ADP agonism. Unlike clopidogrel therefore it is a reversible allosteric antagonist.
- **Aspirin (acetyl salicylic acid).** The effect of aspirin is dose-dependent. At the commonly prescribed low dose of 75 mg daily, the drug acetylates serine residues on COX-1 in a reaction that is irreversible. This inhibition blocks the generation by platelets of thromboxane A_2 with a consequent reduction in thrombocyte aggregation and a prolongation of bleeding time. At higher doses, greater than 650 mg daily, aspirin also blocks COX-2, which thereby mediates its anti-inflammatory, antipyretic and analgesic effects.

- **Abciximab.** This is a monoclonal antibody and specific GPIIb/IIa receptor antagonist which inhibits all pathways of platelet activation. It is given by infusion and has a long duration of action, which means that platelet function will not be restored until at least 12 hours after discontinuing the infusion. It provokes an antibody response so repeated administration is not possible. **Eptifibatide** is a shorter-acting non-peptide GP IIb/IIIa antagonist.
- **Direct oral anticoagulants (DOACs):** these drugs which formerly were known as NOACs (novel oral anticoagulants) are now described as 'direct oral anticoagulants' because their action does not depend on other proteins but rather target a specific molecule. (This is in contrast to heparins, for example, which inhibit the action of factors II, IX, X, XI and XII, as described earlier, but do so indirectly via activation of antithrombin III). Compared with warfarin, the DOACs have a more rapid onset and offset of action with more predictable anticoagulation profiles. There are two main classes of DOAC: activated thrombin inhibitors and activated factor X inhibitors.

Direct Thrombin Inhibitors: (Anti-Activated Factor II Inhibitors, Anti-FIIa)

- **Dabigatran.** This a direct thrombin inhibitor whose effects peaks at 2–3 hours with an elimination half-life of 12–14 hours. It is unusual in that it has a specific reversal agent in the form of idarucizimab, which is a monoclonal antibody that restores coagulation to normal within minutes.
- **Bivalirudin.** This is an analogue of hirudin (a natural anticoagulant peptide found in the salivary glands of leeches). Bivalirudin is a synthetic 20 residue peptide which is an irreversible thrombin inhibitor. It is an intravenous preparation.

Activated Factor X Inhibitors (Anti-FXa)

- **Rivaroxaban, apixaban.** These are examples of orally active direct factor Xa inhibitors. The peak effect of rivaroxaban is at 4 hours, and as factor Xa activity takes 24 hours to normalize, the drug can be given once daily. Apixaban has a similarly selective, reversible direct action on factor Xa but needs twice daily dosing.
- **Fondaparinux.** This is a synthetic pentasaccharide that is chemically similar to heparins and which binds to the same high-affinity binding sites on antithrombin III (ATIII) to potentiate its effect on activated factor X. The drug is given subcutaneously.

Supplementary Information and Clinical Considerations

Approach to a Surgical Patient Who Is Receiving Anticoagulants

- **General management:** this will need to be adapted according to the specific clinical situation, but before elective surgery warfarin is usually stopped 4–5 days preoperatively. If the INR remains unacceptably high, then the patient should be given vitamin K (1.0 mg intravenously) and fresh frozen plasma (FFP; 15 ml kg^{-1}). After minor surgery, the warfarin can be resumed on the first postoperative day. After major surgery, anticoagulation should be maintained by heparin infusion (typically at a rate of 1,000–2,000 units h^{-1}) or by subcutaneous low-molecular-weight heparin (LMWH). If necessary, the actions of heparin can be reversed by protamine (1 mg for every 100 units of heparin), whose positive charge neutralizes the negatively charged heparin.

- **Vitamin K:** clotting factors II, VII, IX and X are glycoproteins which contain glutamic acid. The interaction of these factors with calcium, and with negatively charged phospholipid, requires the presence of a carboxyl moiety on their glutamate residues. Reduced vitamin K (named from the German word 'Koagulation') acts as an essential co-factor in this hepatic γ-carboxylation reaction, during which vitamin K is oxidized from the reduced active hydroquinone form to the inactive 2,3-epoxide. In the presence of vitamin K reductase, this process is then reversed.

- **Sample scenario (1):** a 70-year-old man requires inguinal hernia repair. He is on long-term warfarin for atrial fibrillation with an INR of 2.8. Plan: aim for an INR <2.0. Stop warfarin without substituting another anticoagulant and restart normal dose after surgery. There is no need for bridging anti-coagulation in these patients.

- **Sample scenario (2):** a 65-year-old man requires colonic resection. After mechanical mitral valve replacement, his INR has been kept between 3.0 and 4.0. Plan: stop warfarin early enough to allow the INR to fall below 2.0, and follow one of two main options. (1) Heparin: infuse intravenous heparin to maintain activated partial thromboplastin time (APTT) at 1.5–2.5, stop 2 hours prior to surgery and then restart 6 hours postoperatively. Restart warfarin as soon as oral intake is restored. (2) LMWH: for example, tinzaparin 100 units kg^{-1} daily, increasing to 175 units kg^{-1} postoperatively. If surgery is urgent, then a high INR should be reduced by FFP and vitamin K and possibly by prothrombin complex concentrate (PCC). Restart warfarin as soon as oral intake is restored.

- **FFP and PCC.** FFP does not contain sufficient quantities of the vitamin K–dependent clotting factors for complete reversal of warfarin-induced bleeding, although it does reduce the INR. Prothrombin complex concentrate (PCC, Beriplex) contains factors II, VII, IX and X and in a dose of 25–50 units kg^{-1} will correct such acquired coagulation factor deficiencies within 1 hour. A single treatment for a 70 kg patient costs around £550.

- **Surgery:** neurosurgery requires normal coagulation; cataract surgery may be performed safely with an INR of up to 2.5. Some surgeons will sometimes undertake emergency procedures such as hemiarthroplasty in patients whose INR is similarly high. They do so because clinical experience suggests that, contrary to expectation, blood loss under these circumstances is not excessive. Many surgeons would be prepared to perform routine surgery such as day-case arthroscopy on a patient with an INR of 2.0.

Spinals, Epidurals and Antithrombotic Drug Treatment

The number of patients who are receiving antithrombotic treatments is increasing, and with it the number of management dilemmas. When is it and when is it not safe to perform a spinal or epidural block? The incidence of compressive spinal haematoma is extremely low, and so there is unlikely ever to be robust trial data. Hence the information quoted in the following is drawn largely from the recommendations of expert committees such as the Association of Anaesthetists of Great Britain and Ireland (AAGBI) and the European Society of Anaesthesiology (ESA). Nonetheless, evidence or not it does represent a consensus from which few would wish to deviate, unless the risk/benefit analysis in a particular instance makes a compelling case for doing so. There are two intervals to consider, the first being that between the last dose given and the neuraxial block. The second is the interval between the performance of the spinal or epidural, or the removal of the epidural catheter, and the next or first dose of antithrombotic drug. The decision is made more complicated if more than one agent is prescribed.

- **Incidence.** The third National Audit Project (NAP) of the Royal College of Anaesthetists (*Br J Anaesth* 2009, 102: 179–90), which examined major complications of neuraxial blockade, identified eight cases of vertebral canal haematoma, all of which were associated with epidural analgesia. Seven out of those eight had received antithrombotic drugs. NAP 3 estimated an incidence of permanent harm of 1 in 20,000 epidurals and 1 in 140,000 subarachnoid (spinal) blocks.
- **'Safe' intervals.** The following list includes the recommended intervals between the last dose of antithrombotic drug and the performance of a neuraxial block, together with the interval that should elapse before the drugs are restarted, or given *de novo* as the case may be. (If in doubt then commit to the longer, and so theoretically safer, intervals).

LMWHs (prophylactic)	12 hr	2–4 hr
LMWHs (treatment)	24 hr	2–4 hr
Clopidogrel	7 days	No delay needed
Aspirin	None	No delay needed
Coumarins (e.g. warfarin)	INR <1.4	No delay needed
Rivaroxaban	24 hr	2–4 hr
Apixaban	14 hr	2–4 hr
Dabigatran	This is specifically contraindicated by the manufacturer.	
Fondaparinux	36 hr	6–12 hr
Ticagrelor	72 hr	No delay needed
Bivalirudin	10 hr	2–4 hr

- **Vascular surgery.** One special circumstance is in vascular surgery during which some anaesthetists are nervous about siting an epidural catheter in patients who may receive large doses of intravenous unfractionated heparin intraoperatively. There is no prospective evidence which attests to the safety of this practice, but observational studies in large numbers of patients (3,000) have found no increased incidence of epidural haematoma formation.
- **Aspirin and clopidogrel.** Both drugs have an irreversible action of platelet function so it seems curious that a 7-day interval is recommended between the administration of clopidogrel and neuraxial block, whereas no interval at all is mandated for aspirin. The reasons are unclear but are likely to be the result of several large studies, such as the CLASP study which suggests that aspirin is safe in this regard (Collaborative low-dose aspirin study in pregnancy. *Lancet* 1994, 343: 619–29. A total of 1,422 obstetric patients on low-dose aspirin received epidurals without any haemostatic sequelae). Clopidogrel in a dose of 75 mg daily shows between 40% and 60% inhibition at steady state, but the data sheet makes no mention of contraindications to neuraxial

blockade. It is, however, a more potent inhibitor of platelet function than aspirin, and the prohibition seems to be based on the pharmacokinetics of the drug together with the fact that there are no studies as yet which support its safety in the context of neuraxial anaesthesia.

- **Regional anaesthesia.** There are no firm recommendations published in respect of regional blockade and concurrent antithrombotic treatment, mainly because of the heterogeneity of blocks that are performed. Each must be considered on an individual risk/benefit basis. Most major nerve plexuses are in relatively close association with major vessels such as the femoral, popliteal, subclavian or axillary arteries. The routine use of ultrasound however, makes inadvertent vascular puncture a rare event, and the consequences are likely to be much less severe than haemorrhage into the vertebral canal.

Venous Thromboembolism (VTE) Prophylaxis

- **Risk factors for VTE:** the long list includes age (exponential increase); pregnancy (which as a hypercoagulable state increases risk 5×); obesity (3 × increase in risk if BMI exceeds 30); previous positive history; congenital thrombophilic states such as protein C deficiency, or factor V Leiden; thrombotic states such as malignancy (7 × increase) and heart failure; immobility (hence the importance of thromboprophylaxis in critical care); and hormone therapy, including HRT, the oral contraceptive and oestrogen-receptor antagonists such as tamoxifen. Trauma surgery, and lower limb and pelvic surgery also increase risk.
- **Prevention:** these conditions should be tailored to likely risk to include early mobilization, hydration (to minimize haemoconcentration and improve blood rheology), graduated elastic compression stockings, intermittent pneumatic compression devices and pharmacological intervention, usually in the form of low-molecular-weight or unfractionated heparins.

Tranexamic Acid

Commentary

This may not constitute a topic on its own, although interest in, and use of, the drug has increased greatly since the publication of the CRASH-2 trial in 2010, but it may well be included as part of another topic. Tranexamic acid was also the subject of the World Maternal Antifibrinolytic Trial (WOMAN Trial). This large international study was centred on the developing world and examined the impact of the drug when used in women with postpartum haemorrhage.

Core Information

- **Chemistry:** tranexamic acid is a synthetic derivative of the amino acid lysine (chemically it is a stereoisomer, trans 4-[aminomethyl] cyclohexane-carboxylic acid, which explains its UK trade name, Cyclokapron; hexanoic acid also being known as caproic acid).

- **Haemostatic homeostasis.** The balance between coagulation and vascular patency is maintained by fibrinolysis, which is the process by which fibrin clots are degraded. Plasminogen circulates in what is described as a closed conformation, but when binding to clots or to cell surfaces it changes to an open form which makes it susceptible to activation. This occurs under the influence of a number of different enzymes, particularly tissue plasminogen activator (tPA), which cleaves a simple peptide bond in plasminogen to form the serine protease enzyme plasmin. This catalyzes fibrinolysis (with the formation of fibrin degradation products, FDPs).

- **Fibrinolyis.** Under normal circumstances fibrinolysis is a benign process that keeps the circulation patent. In the context of major trauma, however, with hypoperfusion, hypoxia and the up-regulation of tPA, the balance between coagulation and fibrinolysis can be lost such that accelerated fibrinolysis is initiated with the subsequent development of a coagulopathy. Almost 25% of major trauma patients in the UK are coagulopathic on arrival in the emergency department.

- **Actions.** Tranexamic acid has a strong affinity for the five separate lysine binding sites on the plasminogen molecule. This binding both displaces plasminogen from the cell surface and fibrin clot and inhibits its conversion to plasmin. As plasmin is also thought to be a mediator of the inflammatory response via complement and neutrophil activation, its inhibition means that in addition to stabilizing the fibrin clot, tranexamic acid also has an anti-inflammatory action.

- **Dosing regimens.** These vary greatly, but as the drug has a ceiling effect, an initial intravenous dose need not exceed 1,000–2,000 mg. Thereafter and if continued bleeding is a concern, then an infusion of 25–50 mg kg^{-1} 24^{-1} can be started. The drug is available in an oral formulation and given typically in a dose of 1,000 mg 8-hourly.

Supplementary and Clinical information

- **CRASH-2.** The CRASH-2 study, which was published in 2010, randomized more than 20,000 trauma patients to receive either tranexamic acid (1,000 mg stat and a further 1,000 mg over 8 hours) or placebo. (CRASH-1 was a randomized controlled clinical trial of corticosteroids in severe head injury; CRASH-3 is a trial of tranexamic acid for the treatment of significant traumatic brain injury.) The risk of death was significantly reduced in the tranexamic group (mortality was 1.5% lower). It is not clear if the results of CRASH-2 can legitimately be extrapolated to non-trauma surgery, as these are very different populations. Nonetheless a subsequent meta-analysis assessing the effect of tranexamic acid in surgical patients (129 trials involving 10,488 patients) also reported a 37% reduction in blood transfusion (*Br Med J* 2012, 344: e3054) There are also numerous individual studies from sub-specialty surgical areas, in particular major orthopaedic surgery, which have demonstrated its potential benefit in reducing perioperative bleeding.

- **Postpartum haemorrhage.** A Cochrane review published in 2015 assessed 12 trials involving 3,285 patients and concluded that tranexamic acid reduced postpartum blood loss following both vaginal birth and caesarean section (Novikova *et al.*

Tranexamic acid for preventing postpartum haemorrhage. Cochrane Database of Systematic Reviews. 16 June 2015).

- **The WOMAN trial.** The World Maternal Antifibrinolytic Trial was an international randomized double-blind placebo-controlled study of tranexamic acid in the management of postpartum haemorrhage. It recruited more than 20,000 women in 21 countries in the developing world and concluded that tranexamic acid reduces death in women with post-partum haemorrhage with no adverse effects. (WOMAN trial collaborators, Lancet 2017 Open access. April 26th http://dx.doi.org/10.1016/S0140-6736(17)30638-4).
- **Military trauma.** The MATTERs study (Military application of tranexamic acid in trauma emergency resuscitation, *Arch Surg* 2012, 147: 113–19) reported significantly lower mortality rates in casualties given tranexamic acid (6.5% overall and 13.7% in those receiving massive blood transfusion; total number of patients was 896).
- **Thromboembolic complications.** An increase in thrombotic events has remained a theoretical concern, although the evidence is not robust. It seems likely that in the general population there is no increased risk, although more caution may be needed in patients with pre-existing risk factors for venous thromboembolism.
- **In summary.** Tranexamic acid is cheap, safe and reliable. It reduces bleeding in both minor and major injury and surgical trauma, and it has been estimated that were it to be given within an hour of injury, some 128,000 lives might be saved annually, worldwide. If in addition it does reduce deaths from postpartum haemorrhage, currently around 280,000 a year, then its survival benefit will be even more impressive.

Cyclo-Oxygenase (COX) Enzyme Inhibitors

Commentary
The use of non-steroidal anti-inflammatory drugs (NSAIDs) in anaesthetic practice is widespread, but side effects are common and there is continued interest in selective COX-2 inhibitors. The oral is likely to include a discussion of the cyclo-oxygenase enzyme system.

Core Information
- **COX enzymes:** it is now recognized that these exist in at least two isoforms: a 'constitutive' COX-1 enzyme that is present in all tissues and produces prostaglandins, and an 'inducible' COX-2 enzyme which is produced in high concentrations within cells at inflammatory sites. It is present in the brain, uterus, kidney and prostate, but is more or less undetectable elsewhere until induced by tissue damage. (A COX-3 isoform has also been identified, which is thought to mediate pyrexia, but fuller details have not yet been elucidated.)
- **Mechanisms:** COX enzymes catalyze the production of prostanoids, which comprise a family of lipid mediators with numerous diverse biological roles. The preferential substrate for COX enzymes is arachidonic acid. This is a 20-carbon unsaturated

chain which is cleaved from the phospholipid of membranes by phospholipase A_2 (PLA_2). (This exists in at least 10 isoforms. Glucocorticoids inhibit PLA_2 and decrease the induction of COX.) The initial step in prostanoid biosynthesis is the conversion of arachidonic acid to prostaglandin PGG_2 and thence to PGH_2, which is the precursor to all the compounds in the series, including PGE_2, PGD_2, PGF_{2a}, PGI_2 (prostacyclin) and thromboxane (TXA_2). COX enzymes are involved in two different biosynthetic reactions; in addition to catalyzing the production of prostaglandin PGG_2, a secondary peroxidase reaction then converts PGG_2 to PGH_2.

- **Pain pathways:** tissue trauma or inflammation stimulate the release of inflammatory mediators and the enhanced production of prostaglandin PGE_2. (There are four identified PGE_2 receptors: EP_1–EP_4). PGE_2 binds to end-plate receptors and decreases the threshold for neuronal depolarization. This in turn amplifies the afferent input from peripheral nociceptors to the dorsal horn of the spinal cord.

Drugs Which Affect COX Enzymes

- **Indications:** these include acute surgical pain (but note the withdrawal of piroxicam for this indication), treatment of chronic inflammatory conditions, acute gout, dysmenorrhoea and pyrexia.
- **Non-steroidal anti-inflammatory drugs (NSAIDs):** these include non-selective drugs in common use, such as **diclofenac**, **ketoprofen**, **ibuprofen**, **aspirin** and **paracetamol**, as well as the newer selective COX-2 inhibitors (the '-coxib' class), for example, **parecoxib** and **celecoxib**. The beneficial effects of NSAIDs are mediated largely through COX-2 inhibition, whereas adverse effects are related to COX-1 inhibition.
- **Analgesia:** NSAIDs decrease production of the prostaglandins PGE_2 and PGI_2 that sensitize nociceptors to inflammatory mediators such as serotonin and bradykinin. They also exert central effects at spinal cord level, with COX-2 mediating hyperalgesia secondary to increased neuronal excitability. COX-2 inhibition reduces the induction/up-regulation of the enzyme and has been described as 'anti-hyperalgesic' rather than 'analgesic', but the distinction is essentially academic.
- **Antipyretic action:** NSAIDs inhibit prostaglandin production in the hypothalamus. IL-1 release during an inflammatory response stimulates the hypothalamic production of prostaglandin PGEs, which effectively 'reset' the hypothalamic thermostat upwards. PGD_2 in the brain is also involved in temperature homeostasis. COX-2 is induced centrally by pyrogens, with an increase in PGE_2 production.
- **Anti-inflammatory effects:** the inflammatory response is complex, involving a large number of mediators (see under 'Sepsis' in Chapter 3). NSAIDs influence mainly those components in which the products of COX-2 reactions are important. These include vasodilatation, oedema formation and pain. Some NSAIDs (such as sulindac) also act as oxygen free radical scavengers which may reduce tissue damage and inflammation.
- **Antithrombotic effects:** NSAIDs reduce platelet aggregation by inhibiting thromboxane TXA_2 synthesis. This is unaffected by COX-2 inhibitors, which have no antithrombotic effect.
- **Antineoplastic effects:** the regular use of aspirin (and, by extension, any of the NSAIDs) almost halves the risk of colonic cancer. Their potentially protective role

relates to the suppression of COX-2, whose expression is markedly increased in adenocarcinomas as well as in other tumours of the oesophagus and pancreas.

- **Mechanisms of NSAID action:** the drugs affect only the main cyclo-oxygenation step and do not influence the peroxidase conversion stage of prostanoid synthesis. Non-selective drugs act mainly by competitive inhibition of the arachidonic acid binding site. This is reversible, except in the case of aspirin, which irreversibly acetylates hydroxyl groups on serine residues. The -coxib class are non-competitive, time-dependent COX-2 inhibitors, whereas the -oxicam class (meloxicam, tenoxicam) are competitive.

Adverse Effects

These relate mainly, but not exclusively, to the inhibition of the COX-1 'housekeeping' enzyme.

- **Gastrointestinal tract effects:** gastrointestinal complications are common, with gastric damage present in around 20% of chronic users. Prostaglandins decrease gastric acid secretion, increase mucus production and improve the microcirculatory blood flow.
- **Renal effects:** two prostaglandins are important in renal function. PGE_2 has a role in water reabsorption and also mediates compensatory vasodilatation to offset the action of noradrenaline or angiotensin II. PGI_2 also maintains renal dilatation and blood flow, but does so only under circumstances of physiological stress such as hypovolaemia. Concurrent administration of NSAIDs, therefore, can cause acute renal impairment. The situation is made more complex by the fact that COX-2 is constitutively expressed in the kidney. This explains why trials of high-dose COX-2 selective inhibitors have shown an association with hypertension and fluid retention. (The chronic use of NSAIDs may also lead to irreversible analgesic nephropathy.)
- **Respiratory effects:** bronchoconstriction can be triggered in about 10% of asthmatic subjects. This may be due partly to the inhibition of PGE_2-mediated bronchodilatation.
- **Cardiovascular effects:** endothelial COX-1 releases PGI_2 to mediate vasodilatation and inhibition of platelet aggregation. COX-2 can also be expressed in vascular smooth muscle with the release of PGI_2 and PGE_2. COX enzymes may therefore have a cardioprotective function. This may explain the findings of the large VIGOR trial (VIOXX Gastrointestinal Outcomes Research Study), which showed an unexplained increase in the incidence of myocardial infarction in the COX-2 (rofecoxib) group in comparison with the non-selective (naproxen) group. Rofecoxib was withdrawn in 2004, and some years later, in 2010, the Medicines and Healthcare Products Regulatory Agency (MHRA) in the UK concluded that the use of this class of drug increases the thrombotic risk from 8 to 11 events per 1,000 patient years. A similarly small increased risk of arterial thrombosis has also since been identified with diclofenac (following a review in 2013 by the European Medicines Agency's Pharmacovigilance Risk Assessment Committee), with the recommendation that diclofenac, like the COX-2 inhibitors, should be used in the lowest doses for the shortest time possible, and should be avoided in those patients who have pre-existing risk factors for cardiac and thromboembolic events. (Some risk-averse organizations

have responded by banning the use of oral diclofenac completely and have deprived thereby some patients of a useful analgesic.)

- **Effects on haemostasis:** the inhibition of endothelial COX-1 blocks the production of thromboxane A_2, thereby reducing platelet aggregation and prolonging bleeding time. COX-2 inhibitors have no such effect.
- **Effects on bone healing:** the acute inflammatory response to trauma induces COX-2 in osteoblasts, and there is some suggestion that prostaglandin inhibition by NSAIDs compromises bone healing following fracture. The studies, however, are not robust enough to preclude their use, although many orthopaedic surgeons do prefer to avoid them.
- **COX-2 inhibitors:** these drugs have a safer side effect profile in respect of the gastrointestinal system, which is the commonest site of adverse effects, but they are not entirely hazard free in this regard. They should also be used with caution in patients with renal impairment, and there remains concern about cardiovascular effects. As a class of drug the COX-2 inhibitors are associated with an increased risk of thrombotic effects which is dose-dependent.

Magnesium Sulphate

Commentary

When this topic was first asked in the Final FRCA it caused some consternation because most candidates were unaware of its physiological importance and wide range of clinical applications. These are now much better recognized to the point at which the relevance of this subject is unquestioned.

Core Information

Basic Pharmacology and Physiology

- **Mode of action:** many processes are dependent on magnesium (Mg^{2+}), including the production and functioning of ATP (to which it is chelated) and the biosynthesis of DNA and RNA. It has an essential role in the regulation of most cellular functions.
  - It acts as a natural calcium (Ca^{2+}) antagonist. High extracellular Mg^{2+} leads to an increase in intracellular Mg^{2+}, which in turn inhibits Ca^{2+} influx through voltage-dependent Ca^{2+} channels. It is this non-competitive inhibition that appears to mediate many of its effects. It also competes with calcium for binding sites on sarcoplasmic reticulum, thereby inhibiting its release. It acts as a physiological NMDA receptor antagonist.
  - High concentrations inhibit both the presynaptic release of acetylcholine (Ach) as well as post-junctional potentials.
  - Mg^{2+} has an antiadrenergic action; release at all synaptic junctions is decreased and it inhibits catecholamine release.
- **Physiology:** magnesium is the fourth most abundant cation in the body, as well as being the second most important intracellular cation (after potassium). It activates at

least 300 enzyme systems. It affects the activity of neurons, of myocardial and skeletal muscle fibres, and of the myocardial conduction system. It also influences vasomotor tone and hormone receptor binding.

Effects on Systems

- **Central and peripheral nervous systems:** magnesium penetrates the blood–brain barrier poorly, but it nevertheless depresses the CNS and is sedating. It acts as a cerebral vasodilator, and it interferes with the release of neurotransmitters at all synaptic junctions. Deep tendon reflexes are lost at a blood concentration of around 8–10 mmol l^{-1}. High Mg^{2+} levels do not, as once was thought, potentiate the action of depolarizing muscle relaxants. Predictably, however, they do decrease the onset time and reduce the dose requirements of non-depolarizing relaxants.
- **Cardiovascular:** magnesium reduces vascular tone via peripheral vasodilatation thought to be mediated at least partly by the endothelial nitric oxide pathway. It also causes sympathetic block and the inhibition of catecholamine release. It decreases cardiac conduction and diminishes myocardial contractile force. This intrinsic slowing is opposed partly by vagolytic action.
- **Respiratory:** magnesium has no effect on respiratory drive, but it may weaken respiratory muscles. It reduces bronchomotor tone.
- **Uterus:** it is a powerful tocolytic, which has implications for mothers who are being treated with the drug to control hypertensive disease of pregnancy prior to delivery.
- **Renal:** magnesium acts as a vasodilator and diuretic.

Magnesium Toxicity

- **Toxicity**: many of its toxic effects are predictable from its known actions.
  - 0.7–1.0 mmol l^{-1} – normal blood level.
  - 4.0–8.0 mmol l^{-1} – therapeutic level.
  - 15.0 mmol l^{-1} – respiratory paralysis.
  - 15.0 mmol l^{-1} – at these levels SAN and AV block is complete.
  - 25.0 mmol l^{-1} – cardiac arrest.
  - Magnesium crosses the placenta rapidly and so may exert similar effects in the neonate, which may be hypotonic and apnoeic.

Supplementary and Clinical Information

Clinical Uses of Magnesium Sulphate

- **Pre-eclampsia and eclampsia:** magnesium sulphate decreases systemic vascular resistance and reduces CNS excitability. Following the Magpie Trial, its use in the UK to pre-empt eclamptic convulsions is now well established (*Lancet* 2002, 359: 1877–90). A loading dose of 4 g over 5–15 minutes is followed by an infusion at a rate of 1 g hr^{-1} for 24 hours.
- **Tocolysis:** it causes uterine relaxation.
- **Acute arrhythmias:** it is effective at abolishing tachyarrhythmias (particularly ventricular), those induced by adrenaline, digitalis and bupivacaine, and torsade de pointes associated with a long QT interval. A prolonged QTc is itself associated with

hypomagnesaemia. The ECG of hypermagnesaemia shows widening QRS with a prolonged P–Q interval. A typical dose regimen for the emergency treatment of arrhythmias is 2.0 g (8 mmol) infused over 10–15 minutes.

- **Hypomagnesaemia:** this may have endocrine and nutritional causes (normal intake is 0.4 mmol kg^{-1} daily). It may be caused by malabsorption and is also associated with critical illness. Acute decreases may follow subarachnoid haemorrhage.
- **Tetanus:** this is rare in the UK, but magnesium sulphate by infusion is the primary treatment for the muscle spasm and autonomic instability caused by this condition.
- **Epilepsy:** it can be used to control status epilepticus.
- **Subarachnoid haemorrhage:** it has been used to prevent cerebral vasospasm following aneurysmal subarachnoid haemorrhage.
- **Asthma:** magnesium sulphate is a bronchodilator that can be effective in severe refractory asthma. (Initial dose is 25 mg kg^{-1} by infusion, or up to 2 g intravenously over 20 minutes).
- **Analgesia:** as a physiological NMDA receptor antagonist, it has been used as both an epidural and a subarachnoid adjunct to local anaesthetics for postoperative analgesia.
- **Constipation and dyspepsia:** magnesium is a laxative and an antacid.

Tocolytics (Drugs That Relax the Uterus)

Commentary
Tocolysis is indicated either to inhibit premature labour in an attempt to save a threatened fetus, or to attenuate uterine contractions which are compromising fetal oxygenation. Anaesthetists are involved frequently with mothers in these situations, and so you should know about the principles of management. There are a number of drugs which exert a tocolytic effect.

Core Information
There follows the classes of drugs which relax the uterus.

β_2-Adrenoceptor Agonists
- **Drugs:** these include salbutamol and terbutaline. (Ritodrine is no longer available in the UK.)
- **Mechanisms:** the smooth muscle of the myometrium contains numerous β_2-receptors on the outer membrane of myometrial cells. β_2-agonists bind to these specific adrenergic receptors. This stimulation activates adenyl cyclase with the formation of cAMP, the second messenger which in smooth muscle mediates relaxation. (The process is complex, but there is always the risk that more detail may be expected. Smooth muscle contraction depends on the interaction of actin and myosin, an energy-dependent process that is reliant on the hydrolysis of ATP. The interaction of the myofilaments is dependent also on the phosphorylation of myosin by myosin light-chain kinase. This enzyme is activated by calmodulin, which requires

intracellular calcium ions for its activation. Increased cAMP decreases intracellular calcium and thereby inhibits myosin light-chain kinase.)

- **Effects:** the selectivity of β-agonists is limited, and all these drugs have some β_1- as well as β_2-activity. Hypotension, tachycardia and chest pain can complicate their use, as can tachyarrhythmias. Pulmonary oedema has been reported, to which associated high infusion rates may contribute. Patients may become agitated and tremulous. β_2-agonism stimulates glucagon release and hepatic glycogenolysis, which lead to hyperglycaemia. Increased insulin secretion occurs both in response to this rise in blood glucose and to direct β_2-stimulation. Although this maintains glucose homeostasis, the net effect is to lower serum potassium, which moves into cells. β_2-agonists cross the placenta, increase fetal heart rate and can also cause hyperglycaemia and hyperinsulinaemia followed by hypoglycaemia.

Magnesium Sulphate

- $MgSO_4$ is an effective tocolytic.

Calcium Channel Blockers

- **Drugs:** the only drug that is used as a tocolytic is nifedipine.
- **Mechanism:** nifedipine blocks voltage-dependent calcium channels and also antagonizes the release of calcium from sarcoplasmic reticulum.

Oxytocin Antagonists

- **Drugs:** atosiban (Tractocile) is the only available drug of this type.
- **Mechanism:** it is a specific oxytocin antagonist, which has an effect on the pregnant uterus that is similar to ritodrine (now discontinued) but with a better side effect profile. Atosiban inhibits the second messenger release of free intracellular calcium which mediates uterine contraction. It can be used in conjunction with other tocolytics.

Nitrates

- **Drugs:** glyceryl trinitrate (GTN) is the only nitrate used for tocolysis.
- **Mechanism:** effects are mediated via nitric oxide, which relaxes smooth muscle. It is synthesized in the uterus and helps to maintain uteroplacental blood flow. Exogenous GTN is effective transdermally, sublingually or by intravenous infusion. The drug may cause hypotension as well as pulmonary oedema owing to an increase in vascular permeability. It may be less effective after 34 weeks' gestation.

Supplementary Information

Clinical situations in which an anaesthetist rather than an obstetrician might use tocolysis:

- There is no placental blood flow during a contraction, and in a case of fetal distress in which the decision has been made to proceed to operative delivery it is logical to try to relax the uterus. In effect this is intrauterine resuscitation. Inhibiting uterine contractions is also important in situations in which urgent caesarean section is indicated. An example of this is cord prolapse, in which although there may not necessarily be fetal distress, the pressure of the presenting part on the umbilical cord can cut off the fetal blood supply. The disadvantage of using tocolytics for this purpose is the consequent reduction in uterine tone with the potential for postpartum haemorrhage. A rare but serious complication is acute uterine inversion, in which tocolysis is usually necessary before the uterus can be replaced back through the cervix.

Miscellaneous

- Other tocolytics include **ethanol** (ethyl alcohol), which is effective but which may cause maternal intoxication, hypotension and hyperglycaemia. Significant side effects also limit the use of **diazoxide**, which otherwise is another effective agent. Volatile anaesthetic agents cause a dose-dependent relaxation of uterine smooth muscle.

Uterotonics (Drugs That Stimulate the Uterus)

Commentary

Successive reports of the Confidential Enquiry into Maternal Mortality have confirmed that uterine atony is the most important cause of fatal postpartum haemorrhage. A knowledge of the range of drugs that is available is therefore of obvious importance. The list is not very long, and so the oral may also include consideration of postpartum haemorrhage.

Core Information

Normal contractile mechanism of the gravid uterus.

- **Uterine activity:** uterine smooth muscle demonstrates considerable spontaneous electrical and contractile activity. Gap junctions between myometrial cells enhance the spread of electrical activity, and these junctions increase during pregnancy to provide a low resistance pathway. Depolarization takes place in response to the influx of sodium ions, while the availability of calcium ions enhances the response of uterine smooth muscle. These cross the cell membrane to stimulate further release of calcium from the sarcoplasmic reticulum. The uterus contains α_1-adrenergic (excitatory), β_2-adrenergic (inhibitory) and serotoninergic receptors, as well as specific excitatory receptors for oxytocin. These increase in number in late pregnancy (after 37 weeks' gestation).

Uterotonic Drugs
Oxytocins

- **Syntocinon:** this is an oxytocin analogue which is largely free from the arginine vasopressin effects of the endogenous compound.
- **Mechanism of action and effects:** oxytocin acts via specific excitatory receptors, as described previously. In the presence of oestrogen, it stimulates both the force and

frequency of uterine contraction. It also has vasodilator properties which decrease systolic and diastolic pressures, and which provoke a reflex tachycardia. It also appears to have amnesic properties. Its elimination $t_{1/2}$ is between 5 and 12 minutes. Problems associated with oxytocin include hypotension and pulmonary oedema. Retrosternal pain following delivery at caesarean section has been attributed to transient cardiac ischaemia, so the drug is not innocuous. The conventional dose of oxytocin is 5 I.U. given by slow intravenous injection, although in some patients this is supramaximal. In an oxytocin-naïve mother, such as one presenting for elective caesarean section, the ED_{50} for effective uterine contraction has been shown in some studies to be as low as 0.35 I.U. (although in most of these the small bolus dose was followed by an infusion at a rate of 10 I.U. hr^{-1}). The dose is much greater in a mother in whom there has been oxytocin receptor down-regulation as occurs after a long or augmented labour. Higher doses are also required in mothers at less than 37 weeks' gestation, before which time oxytocin receptor expression is minimal.

Ergot Alkaloids

- **Ergometrine:** This is one of the powerful ergot alkaloids derived from the fungus *Claviceps purpurea.*
- **Mechanism of action and effects:** it acts via α_1-adrenergic and also serotoninergic myometrial receptors, but the precise mechanism whereby it mediates its oxytocic effect is not fully understood. It causes uterine contraction. On the already contracted uterus it has little effect, but it is a potent oxytocic if the postpartum uterus is relaxed. Ergometrine also increases blood pressure via arterial and venous constriction. It can cause coronary vasospasm and may even precipitate angina pectoris. It is powerfully emetic, probably through a direct dopaminergic effect on the chemoreceptor trigger zone.

Compound Preparations

- **Drugs:** the main compound preparation is syntometrine, which is a mixture of syntocinon (5 units) and ergometrine (500 μg).
- **Mechanism of action and effects:** the drugs act in combination as already described to cause uterine contraction. The opposing cardiovascular effects of the two drugs in combination minimize the separate cardiovascular effects of each. The preparation is less emetic than ergometrine alone.

Prostaglandins

- **Carboprost:** the main prostaglandin used to counteract uterine atony is 15-methyl $PGF_{2\alpha}$ (carboprost, Hemabate). PGE_2 (dinoprostone, Prostin) is used for induction and augmentation of labour.
- **Mechanism of action and effects:** endogenous prostaglandins are usually synthe-sized and inactivated locally in the tissue in which they are active. PGE_2 and $PGF_{2\alpha}$ mediate strong uterine contractions. The uterus becomes more sensitive to their effects as pregnancy progresses. Exogenous prostaglandins stimulate smooth muscle and can cause diarrhoea and vomiting. $PGF_{2\alpha}$ is also a potent constrictor of bron-chiolar smooth muscle. In addition, this synthetic preparation has hypothalamic

effects which may lead to pyrexia. Flushing and hypotension are common. (It is no longer recommended that carboprost be injected myometrially because of the risk of inadvertent intravenous injection into venous sinuses.)

- **Misoprostol:** this is a synthetic prostaglandin E_1 analogue which is a second-line drug used in postpartum haemorrhage (it is also an abortefacient whose other uses include medical management of miscarriage and induction of labour). It binds directly to myometrial cells to stimulate contraction. It can be given by various routes, including oral, buccal, vaginal and rectal (there is no intravenous preparation). Although randomized controlled trials have not shown it be more effective than oxytocin or ergometrine, 1,000 µg of rectal misoprostol may control postpartum haemorrhage due to uterine atony in situations where those two agents have been ineffective.

Supplementary Information

Causes of postpartum haemorrhage and its predisposing factors.

- **Uterine causes:** atony is the most important cause, and in the UK accounts for one-third of all deaths associated with maternal haemorrhage. The quoted incidence is 0.4 deaths per 100,000 deliveries. Other causes include uterine disruption or inversion, complications of operative or instrumental delivery and retained products of conception. Abnormal placentation (placenta accreta, increta and percreta) occurs in 1 in 3,000 deliveries.
- **Non-uterine causes:** the main causes are genital tract trauma and coagulopathies.
- **Risk factors:** uterine atony is associated with augmentation of labour, with multiple births, with polyhydramnios and with large infants (>4 kg). It is also associated with prolonged labour, with tocolytics and with maternal hypotension. (Ischaemia due to hypoperfusion impairs effective uterine contraction.) Uterine contraction may also be impaired in the morbidly obese.

Drugs Used in Parkinson's Disease

Commentary

The term 'Parkinsonism' or the adjective 'Parkinsonian' refers to the classic triad of rigidity, 'pill-rolling' tremor and bradykinesia. Akinesia is another cardinal feature (difficulty in initiating movement). There are a number of causes, including Parkinson's disease, which refers specifically to the idiopathic disease that particularly affects the extrapyramidal system and which account for around 85% of all cases. As it is a degenerative neurological disease which afflicts primarily the elderly, it is certain that in an ageing population the prevalence will rise from the current estimate of 1% in those greater than 60 years of age. The oral is likely to include the basic pathophysiology of the condition and its pharmacological management. It may also touch on non-pharmacological treatments and implications for anaesthesia and perioperative care.

Core Information

- Parkinson's disease. The underlying disorder in Parkinson's disease is the progressive loss and degeneration of pigmented dopaminergic neurons in the substantia nigra, together with the accumulation of Lewy bodies. (These are abnormal protein aggregates that form within nerve cells and are associated with a number of other neurological conditions, including Lewy body dementia.) Parkinson's disease is a functional disorder of the basal ganglia. These ganglia are found at the base of the forebrain and consist of the striatum (putamen and caudate nucleus), the pallidum, the substantia nigra and the subthalamic nucleus. The functions mediated by the basal ganglia include cognitive and emotional behaviours as well as motor activity. Ganglia connectivity is highly complex, and there is no succinct way of summarizing the diverse inhibitory and excitatory dopaminergic pathways (of which there are five in total and which are incompletely understood), so this is unlikely to be explored any further in a pharmacology oral.

Pharmacological Management
A number of different classes of drugs are available to treat Parkinson's disease.

Dopamine Precursors

- Dopamine precursors provide the greatest symptomatic relief of motor disability. **Levodopa** is the drug of choice, being the amino acid precursor of dopamine. Levodopa crosses the blood–brain barrier, but it is rapidly decarboxylated in the circulation to form dopamine, which does not. Levodopa is therefore coupled with a peripheral decarboxylase inhibitor such as carbidopa (co-careldopa) or benserazide (co-beneldopa). Decreasing the decarboxylation of levodopa to dopamine increases intracerebral concentrations, while the inhibitors themselves do not cross into the brain. Adverse effects are few, but the effectiveness of this treatment wanes with time. When a treated patient is symptom-free, this is known as the 'on' effect; the return of hypokinesia is the 'off' effect. On-off fluctuations may become more marked with time as long-term l-dopa treatment continues. Another treatment option is to deliver the co-careldopa as an intestinal gel preparation and given by infusion down a jejunal tube. By extending the absorption phase in this way the effective concentration of the drug is increased.

Dopamine Receptor Agonists

- These directly activate post-synaptic dopamine receptors and are first-line drugs, particularly in younger patients. They can provide good symptom control either as monotherapy or in conjunction with a monoamine oxidase-B inhibitor. Examples of this class of drug are **ropinirole** and **pramipexole**, which are non-ergot derived dopamine agonists. They have more adverse effects than levodopa, and are more likely to cause psychiatric disorders such as hallucinations and problems with impulse control (which may manifest in behaviours such as hoarding, binge eating, hypersexuality and gambling). Nausea and orthostatic hypotension are more orthodox side effects. **Domperidone** is a peripherally acting dopamine antagonist which is an effective treatment for refractory nausea. Ergot-derived dopamine agonists include **bromocriptine**, **cabergoline** and **pergolide**. These drugs are associated with serious pericardial, retroperitoneal and pulmonary fibrotic reactions and so are now less commonly prescribed. **Apomorphine** is another potent dopamine receptor agonist that is used mainly in advanced disease when the frequency of 'off' periods is increasing. There is no oral formulation, and the drug is usually given by subcutaneous injection. Dopamine agonists may have a neuroprotective action in that they may delay neuronal degeneration, but the data are not conclusive.

Antiviral Drugs

- **Amantadine** is an antiviral agent which in effect acts as a dopamine agonist by potentiating central nervous system dopaminergic responses. It may act to facilitate dopamine (and noradrenaline) release from storage vesicles while also acting as a re-uptake inhibitor, although these mechanisms are more speculative than confirmed. Adverse effects include hallucinations, headache, dizziness and insomnia. It is also associated with disorders of impulse control.

Monoamine Oxidase Inhibitors

- In the human brain dopamine is metabolized by monoamine oxidase-B (MAO-B), and block of this enzymatic reaction increases dopamine concentrations. The drugs are used in the treatment of early disease and offer moderate symptomatic relief with minimal adverse effects. They are also used as adjuvant therapy with levodopa. Examples of these irreversible MAO-B inhibitors are **selegiline** and **rasagiline**. (Unlike selegiline, rasagiline is not metabolized to potentially toxic amines.) Side effects are relatively mild and are mainly limited to headache, nausea and dizziness.

Catechol-O-Methyltransferase (COMT) Inhibitors

- COMT inhibitors block the peripheral metabolism of levodopa and so increase intracerebral concentrations. Examples include **entacapone** and **tolcapone**. They are usually prescribed as adjuvant therapy.

Antimuscarinic Drugs

- Anticholinergic agents are used primarily as second-line drugs to treat tremor that is refractory to dopaminergic medication. They counter the relative central cholinergic excess that occurs as dopamine is depleted. They have little effect on rigidity and bradykinesia. About 50% of patients with tremor who are treated with anticholinergics will benefit, although adverse effects on cognition are relatively common in the typically elderly age group. Examples of this class of drug are **orphenadrine**, **trihexyphenidyl (benzhexol)** and **procyclidine**. Intravenous procyclidine in a dose of 5–10 mg is a very effective treatment for acute dystonic reactions which some patients experience when given antidopaminergic drugs, such as metoclopramide, phenothiazines (e.g. perphenazine, promazine, prochlorperazine) and butyrophenones (e.g. haloperidol, droperidol).

Non-Motor Symptoms

- Parkinson's disease is associated with a number of non-motor symptoms, the most notable of which is depression. Others include daytime somnolence, erectile dysfunction, constipation, excessive fatigue and insomnia. These are mentioned only for completeness, and the range of drugs available to treat these various symptoms are very unlikely to be included in this oral.

Non-Pharmacological Management

- **Deep brain stimulation.** There are non-pharmacological treatments for refractory dyskinaesia which may or may not involve anaesthetists. Historically some patients underwent neuroablative procedures such as thalamotomy, but these have been superseded principally by deep brain stimulation. Under stereotactic control, a small lead is implanted into the targeted area, which can be the thalamus, the globus pallidus or the subthalamic nucleus. Subthalamic stimulation appears to be the most effective. Deep brain stimulation is a neurosurgical procedure and is subject to the same range and incidence of complications (haemorrhage 3–4%, infection 3–5%, serious neurological sequelae 1–2%). The power source for the system is an implantable high-frequency pulse generator which is inserted into a subpectoral pocket similar to that formed for a pacemaker. The procedure is reversible and non-destructive, and pulse generation can be adjusted according to response. There is no single clear explanation as to its precise mechanism of action, and the hypotheses are (or should be) beyond the range of this oral.

Supplementary Information and Clinical Considerations

Anaesthesia and Perioperative Care

- **Medication:** all anti-Parkinson's Disease medication should be continued as long as possible and restarted immediately after surgery where possible. The intestinal gel preparation of co-careldopa may be useful in patients after major surgery. Abrupt discontinuation of therapy may precipitate the very rapid return of symptoms, which may worsen, and there are rare reports of drug withdrawal provoking the neuroleptic malignant syndrome. (This is characterized by pyrexia, excessive muscle rigidity, delirium and autonomic dysfunction.)
- **Associated medical problems:** there are predictable problems associated with the multisystem nature of the disease, which include orthostatic hypotension secondary to autonomic dysfunction, sleep apnoea and ventilatory dyskinesia, excess salivation (sialorrhoea) and dysphagia due to pharyngeal muscle weakness, and the risk of gastro-oesophageal reflux disease leading to the pulmonary aspiration of gastric contents. Depending on the severity of the symptoms and the complexity of surgery, patients may require high dependency level-two postoperative care.
- **Anaesthetic drugs:** Thiopental depletes striatal dopamine, whereas propofol appears to exert an anti-parkinsonian effect. Inhalational agents should be used with caution as they both decrease dopaminergic transmission while inhibiting neuronal release and re-uptake. Neuromuscular blocking drugs are safe but should be used judiciously to ensure that there is no residual effect. Morphine in low doses decreases dyskinaesia but in high doses will worsen it. In addition, the anaesthetist has to be alert to the interactions of some perioperative drugs with those given to treat the disease, and with the effects of some drugs on the central dopaminergic–cholinergic equilibrium. Pethidine should be avoided in patients taking MAO inhibitors; centrally acting

antimuscarinics such as atropine can cause the central anticholinergic syndrome; anti-emetics with an antidopaminergic action may worsen extrapyramidal effects. In view of these various complexities, regional and neuraxial techniques where appropriate may be a better option than general anaesthesia.

Target-Controlled Infusion (TCI)

Commentary

Target-controlled infusion (TCI) for sedation or for total intravenous anaesthesia (TIVA) is now a common technique, but only a small proportion of this oral will be spent on the reasons for its clinical popularity. The remainder of the questioning will relate to the pharmacokinetics of these systems. These can be confusing because of the dissimilar models that are available and the different pump systems that employ them. Experts disagree about some of the fine detail, and so a broad understanding of the differences between the models and the overall concepts should suffice. You are likely to be asked about the differences between the Marsh and Schnider models. Modifications to both means that detailed discussion of each of them would be too lengthy and complex in the context of this oral, hence the following account is necessarily simplified.

Core Information

Pharmacokinetic Principles Relevant to Target-Controlled Infusion (TCI) Systems

- **The TCI systems:** these incorporate a computer-controlled infusion pump (with safety features to prevent the risk of overdose), which is programmed with a pharmacokinetic model specific to the drug that is being infused. A microprocessor computes the infusion rate that is required to maintain a predicted blood concentration and an adequate concentration of drug at the effector site throughout the duration of the procedure. Examples of such drugs include propofol and remifentanil. The uptake kinetics of intravenous agents mean that the infusion rate needs to be changed exponentially to maintain a steady plasma concentration as peripheral compartments fill up and metabolism and elimination begin. When a lower blood concentration is selected, the pump stops infusing and then resumes at a slower rate.
- **Infusion systems:** these include the original Diprifusor in units where it is still available, the Alaris Asena PK system and the Base Primea (Fresenius) system. The pump types are not interchangeable because they use differently modified versions of the pharmacokinetic models. The Alaris offers the original Marsh or the Schnider models, whereas the Base Primea offers a different version of the Schnider and a modified Marsh model. These differences are not academic.
- **Pharmacokinetic modelling:** (Figure 4.5) The decay in blood concentrations following a bolus dose or a continuous infusion of a drug is typically identified by

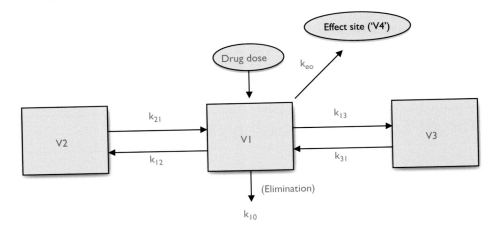

Fig. 4.5 3-compartment pharmacokinetic model.

a three-compartment model, which describes its distribution, redistribution and clearance. At the starting target concentration, a bolus dose fills the central intravascular compartment V1. This is then followed by an initial high-infusion rate which compensates for rapid distribution into the 'vessel rich' compartment V2. Redistribution into the 'vessel-poor' compartment V3 is much slower. Thereafter, the rate decreases to maintain the steady state. The microprocessor employs continuous calculations of the concentrations in the different compartments by employing pharmacokinetic information about the elimination and distribution of the drug. There is of course a fourth additional compartment, V4, which is the effector site – the brain – with a rate constant K_{eo}. The maintenance infusion rate has to compensate for clearance and for redistribution to the peripheral compartments which is governed by different rate constants: K_{10}, which is the elimination rate constant from the central compartment; and K_{12}, K_{21}, K_{13} and K_{31}, which are the rate constants governing movement of drug between the peripheral compartments (V1, 2 and 3). These rate constants are programmed into the infusion device and are either fixed or variable depending on the pharmacokinetic model that is used. In the early phase of drug administration, distribution to other compartments is the most important of the factors which decrease drug effects. With the highly lipophilic propofol, for example, the initial distribution half-life, α, is short (2–3 minutes), whereas intermediate distribution, β_1, takes 30–60 minutes. The terminal phase decline, β_2, is less steep, and takes 3–8 hours. The immediate volume of distribution is 228 ml kg^{-1}, but the steady state volume of distribution in healthy young adults is around 800 litres (up to 10 l kg^{-1}). Propofol is metabolized mainly in the liver, undergoing conjugation to glucuronide and sulphate prior to renal excretion.

- **Plasma and effect-site targeting:** If the plasma concentration is targeted as in the Marsh model there will be an inevitable delay in attaining the effect-site (brain) concentration. Achieving equilibrium with this fourth compartment depends on the pharmacokinetic properties of the drug, the rate constant K_{eo} (from plasma to brain) and the concentration gradient. With effect-site targeting, as in the Schnider model,

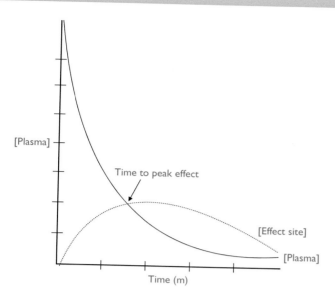

Fig. 4.6 Bioavailability.

the programme increases the blood concentration rapidly and with it the effective concentration gradient, this being the only extrinsic factor over which the anaesthetist has any control. This obviously involves an overshoot in the plasma concentration, and its degree will depend on the size of k_{12} (decline in concentration in the central compartment) and k_{eo}. The latest modification to the Marsh model incorporates a faster k_{eo} so there is a smaller overshoot. If a smaller k_{eo} is determined by the programme (as in Schnider), then there will be a larger plasma overshoot in order to generate the necessary concentration gradient between plasma and brain.

- **Time to peak effect (TTPE):** this is defined by the point at which the decaying plasma concentration curve crosses the rising effect-site concentration curve (Figure 4.6). It is independent of the bolus size.
- **Marsh model:** This made a minor adaptation to a previous pharmacokinetic model by simply changing a factor that increased the volume of the central compartment. (The original Gepts model was derived from the study of only three groups of six patients.) In the Marsh model, the rate constants as described earlier are fixed, but the entered weight alters the size of the three compartments V1, V2 and V3, and the clearances. The estimated plasma concentrations in V1 vary with the patient's weight, whereas the fixed rate constants mean that the estimated rate of decline is the same in all patients. This original Marsh model targets only plasma concentrations.
- **Modified Marsh (1):** This incorporated a rate constant k_{eo} (plasma/effect site) of 0.26 min^{-1} to allow effect-site targeting, and is used in the Alaris pumps.
- **Modified Marsh (2):** This changed the rate constant k_{eo} to 1.2 min^{-1} and is used in the Base Primea pumps.
- **The 'Diprifusor' and 'Open' systems:** The original Diprifusor used the Marsh model for the infusion of propofol and had two main disadvantages. The fixed pharmacokinetic model targeted only plasma concentration, and the pumps could only use

proprietary (and therefore more costly) radio-labeled syringes containing propofol 1% or 2%. In later iterations, the processors incorporated a value for k_{eo} which allowed an estimation of effect-site concentration. Thereafter much more flexible open-target-controlled systems were introduced which could be programmed with different pharmacokinetic models, could use generic drugs and which could target either plasma or the effect site. (The exception is the Alaris pump whose Marsh model allows only plasma site targeting).

- **Schnider model:** This was also based on a small number of patients (24 in total), and incorporates age, gender, weight and height. The size of the compartments V1 and V3 are fixed (4.27 and 238 litres, respectively), as are the rate constants k_{13} and k_{31}. V2 is adjusted according to age along with k_{12} and k_{21}. K_{10} is adjusted according to calculated lean body mass, total body weight and height. The fixed V1 compartment size means that the model assumes the same peak plasma concentration for all patients, regardless of body habitus or age. However, the rate of decrease in plasma concentration as the drugs redistributes into V2 is dependent on age (in contrast to the Marsh model discussed earlier). Weight, height and lean body mass are used to determine the rate of elimination by metabolism (k_{10}) and thereby the rate of propofol infusion to replace that loss. The Schnider model uses a k_{eo} of 0.456 min^{-1} which predicts a TTPE of 1.6 minutes.

- **Infusion pump systems:** here too there are differences which can create confusion. When using the Schnider model, the Base Primea pump incorporates a fixed k_{eo} of 0.456 min^{-1} which results in a TTPE that varies between patients. The Alaris system in contrast incorporates a fixed TTPE that results in a k_{eo} that is individual to each patient.

- **Minto model for remifentanil:** This is a three-compartment model and also uses age, gender, weight and height. K_{eo} is age adjusted, but the very rapid plasma–brain equilibration which is achieved within 5 minutes means that the issue of plasma or effect-site targeting is not important. Its rapid metabolism by non-specific esterases means that its pharmacokinetics are consistent with a duration of action of 5–10 minutes, a very short context-sensitive half-life, and minimal accumulation even after prolonged infusion.

- **TCI in children, Kataria and Paedfusor:** Studies of TCI in children using adult pharmacokinetic modelling showed plasma propofol concentrations that were much lower than predicted by the models. The Kataria model was among those that have been developed to address this problem and has been validated in children from the ages of 3 to 16 years with a minimum weight of 15kg. The Paedfusor model is an adaptation of the Diprifusor Marsh model. (The oral is likely to mention these variants only in passing, as TCI in children is not currently a mainstream technique.)

- **Marsh and Schnider, practical differences:** If a standard 70 kg patient is taken as an example, the Marsh models determine a variable volume for V1, in this example of 15.9 litres, whereas in Schnider V1 this is fixed at 4.27 litres. In practice this means that if the original Marsh plasma target is used the pump will deliver larger volumes of propofol, and in subjects of approximately normal weight this difference in infusion rates will persist until the calculated curves approach each other at around 10 minutes. By 30 minutes after the start of the infusion the models predict the same plasma and effect-site concentrations (assuming that a modified Marsh model is being used). This increase in the mass of propofol delivered in the early stages is more likely to cause hypotension, and because the Marsh models do not incorporate age this may be significant in the elderly. To give an indication of this difference, if the target concentration is set at 4 μg ml^{-1} for a patient weighing 70 kg, Marsh will deliver a bolus of 172 mg, whereas Schnider which will give only 77 mg. Obesity represents a problem for both models. If the Marsh model programmes in the total body weight, then the initial or induction dose will be excessive. Lean body weight can be used (as a guide this only rarely exceeds 70 kg in females and 90 kg in males), but this will then lead to under-dosing during continuous infusion, because the requirement for propofol in the obese during maintenance shows a proportionate increase. Problems with the Schnider model relate primarily to the calculation of lean body mass (LBM). The formula that is used means that LBM increases proportionately with total body weight (TBW) up to a body mass index of 37 kg m^{-2} in females and 42 kg m^{-2} in males. Thereafter it decreases with the result that the calculated k_{10} (the elimination rate constant from the central compartment) increases and with it the infusion rate to match the estimated drug metabolism.

Supplementary Information

- **Context-sensitive half-time (CSHT):** this is the time taken for the plasma concentration to halve after an infusion designed to maintain constant blood levels is stopped. This is different not only for dissimilar drugs but also for the same drug depending on the duration of infusion. The CSHT for remifentanil is about 4.5 minutes after 2 hours of infusion, and 9.0 minutes after 8 hours. Fentanyl in contrast has a CSHT after 2 hours of infusion of 48 minutes, which extends after 8 hours to 282 minutes. The figures for alfentanil are 50 and 64 minutes, and for propofol 16 and 41 minutes. This makes it clear why remifentanil is such a suitable drug for administration in this way (Figure 4.7).
- **Volume of distribution (V$_d$):** the concept of the apparent V$_d$ assumes that a drug is distributed evenly throughout a single compartment. (If, for example, 100 mg of a

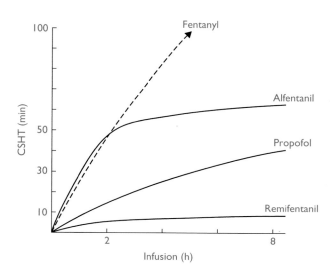

Fig. 4.7 Context-sensitive half-time (CSHT).

drug given intravenously yields a plasma concentration of 1 mg l^{-1}, then the V_d is 100/1 = 100 litres. V_d equals the dose/initial concentration.) Were a drug to remain entirely within the circulation, its V_d would approximate the plasma volume (0.05 l kg^{-1}). Were it to distribute through the extracellular compartment, its V_d would be about 14 litres (0.2 l kg^{-1}). Were it to distribute throughout all fluid compartments, its V_d would approximate to total body water (0.6 l kg^{-1}). If, however, it is sequestrated by ion-trapping, cellular uptake or specific tissue binding, then its V_d will be much larger. The volumes of distribution of drugs used in TCI are useful in explaining their clinical behaviour, being 800 litres for propofol and 30 litres for both alfentanil and remifentanil. V_d is, however, affected by such factors as pregnancy, age and volaemic status.

- **Clearance:** one of several definitions of clearance is the rate of drug elimination per unit time per unit concentration. An alternative (and neat) model-independent method of determining clearance is to divide the dose of drug by the area under its concentration–time curve. The whole body clearance of propofol is 2,500 ml min^{-1}.
- **Target concentration:** this clearly will vary according to the procedure. For 'conscious sedation' a target plasma concentration below 1.0 μg ml^{-1} might prove sufficient, whereas surgical anaesthesia might require upwards of 8.0 or 10.0 μg ml^{-1}. In practice, the range is from around 2.0–8.0 μg ml^{-1}. It is much lower if propofol is used in conjunction with remifentanil. This reflects the considerable pharmacokinetic and pharmacodynamic inter-patient variability. Influences include age, body weight, genetic factors, concurrent disease and administration of other drugs. Alfentanil, for example, reduces the distribution and clearance of propofol.
- **Repeated infusion:** if a patient has to return to theatre soon after TCI has been discontinued, the microprocessor will no longer be storing the pharmacokinetic information. When the TCI is restarted, therefore, the system will deliver another bolus and rapid initial infusion as if there were no residual propofol in the body. The shorter the interval between cessation and resumption, the greater the risk of overdose.

Conscious Sedation

Commentary

Sedation techniques have usually been an afterthought in anaesthetic practice, but reports from various central bodies have brought them into more recent focus. One such was a review of general anaesthesia and sedation in non-hospital dental care that was produced by the chief medical and dental officers in 2000. Entitled 'A Conscious Decision', it ensured that the concept of conscious sedation became more familiar to anaesthetists. It remains of less immediate interest to most, however, because, as we have the experience and skills to manage the situation safely, we tend to be unconcerned should sedation in our hands deepen. There is a continuum from consciousness to anaesthesia along which there is increasing depression of the cardiorespiratory systems which anaesthetists, but not always others, are able to manage. In any discussion therefore there may be a need to repeat the mantra that the same standards of pre-procedural assessment and perioperative monitoring should apply for conscious sedation as for general anaesthesia.

Core Information

- **Conscious sedation:** this is a level of sedation in which the patient remains conscious, although with some likely diminution of cognitive function; retains protective reflexes; and can still respond to commands. It is the particular preserve of dentists, although it is also a skill appropriate for anaesthetists. (The full definition, as accepted by a range of regulatory bodies, including the General Dental Council, is more cumbersome: 'it is a technique in which the use of a drug or drugs produces a state of depression of the central nervous system, which enables treatment to be carried out, but during which verbal contact with the patient can be maintained throughout. The drugs used should have a margin of safety wide enough to render loss of consciousness unlikely. The level of sedation must be such that the patient remains conscious, retains protective reflexes, and is able to respond to verbal commands.') Note that polypharmacy is not proscribed.

- **Indications:** the technique provides anxiolysis and relaxation in patients unable otherwise to tolerate a surgical or medical procedure. It is used commonly for dental treatment, and for surgery performed under local, regional or neuraxial anaesthesia, interventional radiology and endoscopy.

- **Local anaesthesia:** satisfactory conscious sedation for patients is crucially dependent on effective local anaesthesia. The only way that an inadequate block can be overcome is by edging towards deeper sedation and general anaesthesia.

- **Intravenous sedation**
  - **Propofol:** this is usually delivered by TCI although it is possible for patients to administer their own sedation using a system analogous to PCA. Propofol is particularly suitable for TCI because of its short onset of effect, its rapid redistribution and a short CSHT (16 minutes after 2 hours of infusion), which means that accumulation is modest. For conscious sedation, a target plasma concentration below $1.0\ \mu g\ ml^{-1}$ can prove sufficient, but there is considerable inter-individual variability in response.
  - **Midazolam:** this is the commonest used benzodiazepine. It is anxiolytic and hypnotic and potentiates the inhibitory effects of GABA on $GABA_A$ receptors throughout the CNS. It is water-soluble at pH levels below 4, but at body pH the imidazole ring closes and the molecule becomes highly lipophilic. The doses required to achieve conscious sedation are usually small (0.5–1.0 mg increments to a total of about 5 mg). In most patients, higher doses are associated either with sedation that is not 'conscious' or, less commonly, with paradoxical disinhibition. (This is particularly true of benzodiazepine use in children.) Midazolam can also be given orally, nasally and bucally. Bolus dosing by the oral route is unpredictable, but the high bioavailability of intranasal and buccal midazolam (both ~75%) makes it more feasible to use these routes. Overdose is readily treated with flumazenil (Anexate), the specific antagonist which displaces the drug from its binding sites. The normal dose is up to 500 μg titrated against response. Its effective duration of action is 1–2 hours.

- **Inhalation sedation:** also known as 'relative analgesia', this is a technique that produces a maintained level of conscious sedation by the administration of a varying concentration of nitrous oxide in oxygen up to a maximum of 50%. It is used primarily in dental practice. There are some sceptics, but proponents for its use claim that uniquely among single agents it provides analgesia, anxiolysis and mild amnesia while preserving laryngeal reflexes and the maintenance of verbal contact. The sceptics might be wrong. It is possible that at low concentrations of nitrous oxide patients are in Guedel's first stage of anaesthesia – analgesia - and there is some historical evidence to suggest that within a very narrow (but unpredictable) range of concentrations this analgesia can be profound.
- **Ketamine:** some anaesthetists use sub-hypnotic doses of ketamine (<0.5 mg kg^{-1}) as part of a conscious sedation technique (usually in combination with another drug). Ketamine has complex neuropharmacology and there are enough anecdotal reports to suggest that in some hands this technique is ill advised.
- **Complications:** if the sedation remains 'conscious' as defined, then problems such as respiratory depression with hypoxia or hypotension should not occur. Complications usually arise when increased levels of sedation risk the loss of protective reflexes with an unsecured airway. This is more likely to happen when combinations of drugs are used. (In addition, there are the generic complications such as allergic reactions.)

Drugs Used to Treat Diabetes Mellitus

Commentary
Diabetes is a multisystem disorder that gives the anaesthetist the challenge of managing potential co-morbidity while maintaining effective perioperative glucose homeostasis. This question will also focus on an understanding of intermediary metabolism. The incidence of diabetes, particularly of type 2 diabetes, is increasing, as is the range of drugs available to treat it. It is a common and important clinical problem.

Core Information
- Type 1, or insulin-dependent diabetes mellitus, is caused by an absolute deficiency of insulin (10% of patients). Type 2, or non-insulin-dependent diabetes, is caused by a relative deficiency (90% of patients). This comprises either insulin resistance (as in obesity), reduced insulin secretion from the β-cells in the pancreatic islets of Langerhans, or both.

Drugs Used to Treat Type 1 and Type 2 Diabetes Mellitus
Insulin
- This is a major anabolic hormone, which controls not solely carbohydrate metabolism but also intermediary metabolism.
  - **Carbohydrate**: it stimulates glycogen synthesis and inhibits glycogenolysis in the liver while also increasing glucose uptake and utilization in muscle.

— **Fat**: it increases lipid synthesis (fatty acids and triglycerides) and inhibits lipolysis.
— **Protein**: it enhances protein synthesis (hence its abuse amongst bodybuilders) by enhancing amino acid uptake by muscle. It decreases protein catabolism.

- **Mechanisms:** the hormone binds to a specific insulin receptor on the cell membrane. This is a large transmembrane glycoprotein complex, comprising two α-extracellular-binding sites and two β-intracellular and transmembrane proteins.

- **Insulin preparations:** there are numerous formulations whose purpose is to help diabetics stabilize blood glucose levels. **Soluble insulin** (such as human Actrapid) works rapidly, but its action is evanescent. Newer rapidly acting insulin analogues such as **insulin glusiline**, **insulin lispro** and **insulin aspart** work even quicker than soluble insulin and have a shorter duration of action. This allows insulin-dependent diabetics considerable flexibility with regard to their oral intake. These insulins are also used in continuous subcutaneous pump systems. Otherwise bolus injections will control post-prandial blood glucose concentrations and a longer-acting agent will provide continuous background release. Longer-acting preparations are made by precipitating insulin with substances such as zinc and protamine to form an insoluble depot compound from which insulin is more slowly absorbed. **Insulin glargine** is a modified insulin analogue which, because of slow absorption, provides a basal insulin supply to mirror the normal physiological state. **Insulin detemir** and **insulin deglu-dec** are other long-acting recombinant human insulin analogues.

Oral Hypoglycaemic Agents
Biguanides
The only biguanide in routine clinical use is **metformin**.

- **Mechanisms:** biguanides increase glucose uptake and utilization in skeletal muscle while decreasing hepatic gluconeogenesis. They also reduce the plasma concentrations of low-density and very-low-density lipoproteins (LDL and VLDL). Rarely, they may cause a severe lactic acidosis, particularly in patients with impaired renal function. Their precise mode of action is not fully known, but they act only in the presence of residual endogenous insulin.
- **Pharmacokinetics:** metformin has an elimination $t_{1/2}$ of 3 hours. It is excreted renally and will accumulate if renal function is compromised (common in diabetics).

Sulphonylureas
These include tolbutamide (now largely obsolete) and the second-generation sulphonylureas, **glibenclamide** and **glipazide**.

- **Mechanisms:** sulphonylureas promote insulin secretion from β-cells after binding to high-affinity receptors on the cell membrane. They block an ATP-sensitive potassium channel, thereby allowing membrane depolarization, calcium influx and insulin release. They can cause prolonged and severe hypoglycaemia, particularly in the presence of other drugs such as NSAIDs. These can compete for metabolizing enzymes and alter plasma protein binding. These drugs also require residual pancreatic beta-cell activity.

- **Pharmacokinetics:** tolbutamide has a shorter $t_{1/2}$ (6–12 hours) and duration of action (4 hours) than glibenclamide ($t_{1/2}$ 18–24 hours and duration 10 hours) or glipazide ($t_{1/2}$ 16–24 h and duration 7 hours). Some (e.g. glibenclamide) have active metabolites, and these, like the parent compound, are excreted by the kidney. Renal impairment mandates caution with their use.

α-Glucosidase Inhibitors
The only drug of this class that is available is **acarbose**.

- **Mechanisms:** acarbose inhibits intestinal α-glucosidase, which delays the breakdown and absorption of carbohydrates (sugars and starch). Its inhibitory action is maximal against sucrase.
- **Pharmacokinetics:** most of the drug remains within the gut, with only about 1–2% being absorbed systemically. Duration of action varies greatly according to intestinal transit times.

Thiazolidinediones
The primary agent that is available is **pioglitazone** (rosiglitazone was associated with increased cardiovascular mortality).

- **Mechanisms:** the drugs reduce peripheral insulin resistance, enhance glucose uptake by muscle and decrease hepatic gluconeogenesis. Their mechanism of action is complex, but they are agonists at the nuclear PPAR γ-receptor which mediates lipogenesis and uptake both of glucose and of free fatty acids. They also lower LDL concentrations. The thiazolidinediones increase plasma volume and some weight gain is common. Their onset of action develops over weeks, and they should not be used as single-component therapy.
- **Oncogenesis:** pioglitazone has been associated with an increased risk of bladder cancer, particularly with advancing age. The effect is considered to be small and does not outweigh the benefits of treatment, but administration of the drug should be reviewed in any patients with pre-existing risk factors for carcinoma of the bladder.
- **Pharmacokinetics:** time to peak action is 2 hours, and the $t_{1/2}$ for pioglitazone is around 7 hours. It does have a number of active metabolites, with a relatively long $t_{1/2}$ of 24 hours.

Meglitinides
These are analogous in action to the sulphonylureas. The two that have been developed are **nateglinide** (licensed only for use in combination with metformin) and **repaglinide**, which can be prescribed as monotherapy.

- **Mechanisms:** these also promote insulin secretion from β-cells by blocking the ATP-sensitive potassium channel in the cell membrane. The drugs are less potent than the sulphonylureas.
- **Pharmacokinetics:** the time to peak effect is short, at about 55 minutes, and they also have a rapid $t_{1/2}$ of around 3 hours. Inadvertent hypoglycaemia is therefore less likely with their use.

GLP-1 Agonists and DPP-4 Inhibitors

GLP-1 (glucagon-like peptide) is a gut-derived peptide, an incretin, which promotes pancreatic insulin secretion and suppresses the release of glucagon. The compound is metabolized rapidly by the enzyme DPP-4 (dipeptidyl peptidase 4).

- **GLP-1 analogues:** these are synthetic analogues which are resistant to degradation by DPP-4 and include **exenatide**, **liraglutide** and **lixisenatide**. These agents are available in different formulations (exenatide, for example, is available as an ultra-long-acting preparation that is given weekly) but otherwise are given in combination with other hypoglycaemic agents.
- **DPP-4 inhibitors:** these inhibit the breakdown of endogenous GLP-1. Drugs of this class that are available include **saxagliptin**, **sitagliptin**, **linagliptin**, **alogliptin** and **vildagliptin.**

SGLT2 Inhibitors

- **Mechanisms:** these drugs inhibit the Na^+/Glucose co-transporter 2 in the proximal convoluted tubule in the kidney. This has the effect of reducing glucose reabsorption and increasing urinary glucose excretion. Drugs of this class include **canagliflozin** and **dapagliflozin** and can be used either as monotherapy or as part of a combination regimen.

Clinical Considerations

Problems associated with anaesthetizing patients with diabetes mellitus (some 50% of whom will present for surgery) will not be the focus of the oral, and so this account is necessarily cursory. The pre-operative evaluation and perioperative management of patients with diabetes is considerably more complex than this brief summary would suggest.

- **Diabetic morbidity:** as a generalization, type 1 diabetes is characterized by micro-vascular complications, whereas in type 2 it is macrovascular complications that predominate. Type 1 complications therefore include retinopathy, diabetic nephropathy, microangiopathy and peripheral and autonomic neuropathy (with an incidence of 50% in type 1 diabetics as opposed to an incidence of 20% in patients with type 2 disease), with attendant problems such as diabetic gastroparesis and postural hypotension. Morbidity associated with type 2 diabetes include ischaemic heart disease, hypertension, peripheral vascular disease and cerebrovascular disease. Clearly there is much overlap between the conditions. Affected patients may also lose the normal sympathetic response to hypoglycaemia, of which they may remain unaware. Stiff joint syndrome may impair the mobility of the cervical spine and can make tracheal intubation more difficult. Some 20% of diabetics harbour occult infection which may evolve into overt sepsis under the stress of surgery.
- **Perioperative glucose control:** there are numerous different protocols. The main principle of management should be to restore the patient's normal regimen as soon as possible while maintaining adequate glycaemic control in the meantime (blood glucose 6–10 mmol l^{-1}). Tighter control is associated with a greater danger of hypoglycaemic episodes. Major surgery will require postoperative insulin infusion,

either in the form of a GKI regimen (glucose 10% × 500 ml + KCl 10 mmol + Actrapid insulin 15 units) infused at 100 ml h^{-1}, or as a separate infusion (typically using the patient's total daily insulin dose/24 as the starting rate). Variable rate infusions allow much better control and are associated neither with the potential fluid overload or the hyponatraemia that can follow the use of GKI infusions. Giving insulin separately, however, means that there is a greater potential danger of hypoglycaemia. It is important to remember that insulin should always continue to be given no matter how low the measured blood sugar, because without some available insulin then intracellular glucose metabolism will cease.

Chemotherapeutic (Cytotoxic) Drugs

Commentary
Malignancy is common, and patients who are receiving or who have received chemotherapy may present both for cancer-related and non-cancer-related surgery. Most of the implications for anaesthesia are related to the generic consequences of treatment with cytotoxic agents with the only specific concern being the potential toxicity of oxygen in patients who have received bleomycin.

Core Information
The end target of most cytotoxic drugs is DNA and the inhibition of the proliferation of tumour cells. They do this by different mechanisms.

- **Antimetabolites.** These interfere with DNA synthesis, often by acting as false substrates and as competitive inhibitors. Common examples are **methotrexate**, which is a direct folate antagonist; **fluoruracil**, which is a pyridimine antagonist; **mercaptopurine**, which as its name suggests is a purine analogue; and **cytosine arabinose**, which is a competitive inhibitor of DNA polymerase.
- **Alkylating agents.** This is a diverse group of drugs which bind to DNA and suppress its normal function. They include **cisplatin, busulphan, chlorambucil** and the phosphamides (**cyclophosphamide** and **ifosphamide**).
- **Antibiotics.** These are antibacterial agents which have been found to be more toxic to mammalian than to bacterial cells. They work via different mechanisms. Some act primarily by inhibiting topoisomerase enzymes. The complex topography of helical DNA means that it needs to be 'unwound' during the processes of transcription and replication. Topoisomerase I inhibitors (**camptothecins, topotecan**) induce single-strand breaks, and topoisomerase II inhibitors such as the anthracyclines (**daunorubicin, doxorubicin**) are powerful inducers of double-strand breaks. Others such as **bleomycin** exert their effects by generating cytotoxic reactive oxygen species which cause single- and double-stranded breaks in the DNA molecule.
- **Mitotic inhibitors.** These are essentially spindle poisons of which the main examples are the vinca alkaloids, **vincristine** and **vinblastine**.

Supplementary Information and Clinical Considerations

Anaesthetists are not oncologists, and you will not be expected to know the detailed pharmacology of these agents. As a generalization, pre-operative assessment focuses usually on the immediate acute-on-chronic clinical findings and their differential diagnosis. This is with the view firstly of determining if the patient's condition can be improved, and secondly if there are exacerbating perioperative actions that therefore should be avoided. Conditions that are secondary to the effects of chemotherapy are likely to be irreversible, and the management is similar to that of any other chronic systemic pathology. By their very nature the drugs used in the treatment of malignancy are toxic, and so it is no surprise that their adverse systemic effects can be widespread. The more common problems are outlined here.

- **Cardiovascular.** Irreversible cardiomyopathy is associated particularly with anthra-cyclines such as **doxorubicin** (Adriamycin) and **daunorubicin**, but other agents such as the **phosphamides** and **busulphan** can impair myocardial contractility and cause endocardial fibrosis. The final common mechanism appears to be the creation of superoxide anion radicals. The drugs may also cause a range of cardiac arrhythmias, including ventricular tachycardia, prolonged QT interval and torsade de pointes.
- **Renal**. Nephrotoxicity is common with **cisplatin**, occurring in up to 30% of patients, but is also associated with the administration of **methotrexate** and the **phosphamides**. **Carboplatin** is less dangerous. The problem may be exacerbated by under-hydration and the concomitant administration of potentially nephrotoxic drugs such as amino-glycoside antibiotics and non-steroidal anti-inflammatory drugs.
- **Haematological.** Myelosuppression may either be the primary consequence of the disease process or secondary to treatment. Of concern to the anaesthetist is the patient who is anaemic, neutropaenic or thrombocytopaenic. Myelosuppression is a common, but usually reversible side effect of numerous cytotoxic drugs.
- **Hepatic.** Abnormal liver function may result from direct toxicity of the drug or its metabolites. Most have the capacity to impair hepatic function and these include cisplatin, methotrexate and the cytotoxic antibiotics.
- **Neurological.** The vinca alkaloids **vincristine** and **vinblastine** are the most potently neurotoxic agents with central, peripheral and autonomic neuropathic effects. Cisplatin also causes symptoms such as paraesthesia and paresis which are apparent in up to 50% of patients. This potential for neurotoxicity has obvious implications for neuraxial, plexus and peripheral nerve blockade, particularly as in the early stages any neuropathy may be subclinical. The **vinca alkaloids** and **cyclophospha-mide** can in rare cases cause a syndrome of inappropriate anti-diuretic hormone secretion (SIADH).
- **Pulmonary.** In the context of respiratory pathophysiology, it is **bleomycin** that has given rise to the greatest concern, with interstitial pneumonitis and pulmon-ary fibrosis occurring in up to 30% of patients. The specific anaesthetic concern relates to the potential toxicity of higher concentrations of inspired oxygen. The original paper that identified the problem reported a series of only five patients who had been treated with bleomycin and who, having been exposed to an FIO_2 greater than 0.4 during surgery, developed fatal adult respiratory distress syn-drome (ARDS). Thirteen other patients in whom the FIO_2 was restricted to less

than 0.25 survived without any such sequelae. A later study which included a larger number of patients (77) who were given oxygen >40% reported no fatalities and an incidence of minor pulmonary complications in around 25%. Scrupulous fluid balance was thought by the authors to be a more important consideration than the FIO_2. Nonetheless it remains accepted teaching that the inspired oxygen concentration in patients who have been given bleomycin should be restricted to keep the SpO_2 in the region of 92%. Many of the other agents are also toxic to the lung and these include the **vinca alkaloids, cisplatin, busulphan** and **methotrexate**.

- **Tumour lysis syndrome.** This is a potentially fatal complication which occurs when substantial numbers of tumour cells are destroyed rapidly, with the release of toxic metabolites and intracellular ions into the systemic circulation and the development of acute renal failure. It happens usually, but not exclusively, within 48–72 hours of the treatment of non-solid malignancies such as acute leukaemias and non-Hodgkin lymphomas. The metabolic abnormalities include hyperkalaemia, hyperphosphatae-mia from cell lysis, hypocalcaemia secondary to the rise in phosphate concentrations, and hyperuricaemia. Uric acid is the catabolic end product of purine degradation. Critical care with renal, and possibly circulatory and respiratory support is frequently required.

Anaesthetic Implications
Specific anaesthetic considerations are relatively modest, but there are some factors and interactions of which the anaesthetist should be aware.

- **Immunosuppression.** This is a feature both of drugs such as the alkylating agents, and also of the glucocorticoids that may form part of the overall treatment regimen. Scrupulous asepsis is essential.
- **Pseudocholinesterase inhibition. Cyclophosphamide** and some of the other alkylating agents are inhibitors of plasma cholinesterase. This effect can persist for up to 4 weeks, which has implications for the use of drugs such as suxamethonium and mivacurium whose duration of action may therefore be prolonged.
- **Oxygen toxicity.** This is a concern specific to current or past treatment with bleomycin as described previously.
- **NSAIDs.** These drugs are potentially nephrotoxic because they inhibit the prostaglandin-mediated vasodilation of afferent glomerular arterioles and reduce renal blood flow. In addition they reduce the excretion of methotrexate, thereby increasing the risk both of its renal and systemic toxicity.

Bioavailability

Commentary
Bioavailability is a straightforward concept whose value is disputed by some authorities. It is a subject, however, that can fit readily into the time frame of the oral. Ensure that

you can define it and are able to draw simple curves of concentration plotted against time of a drug that is given intravenously and one that is given by some other route. The questioning is likely to revert thereafter to a general discussion of the factors that may affect drug absorption.

Core Information

Definition of the term 'bioavailability' and its measurement.

- Bioavailability is that fraction of the dose of an administered drug that gains access to the systemic circulation, and is therefore available to act at its receptor sites. It is assumed that the bioavailability of an intravenous dose is 100% (or 1.0). Alternatively, bioavailability can be defined simply as the ratio of the effective dose to the administered dose. It has been used most commonly as a measure following oral administration, but it applies equally to drugs given by other routes, of which there are many. These include rectal, vaginal, nasal, ocular, pulmonary, sublingual, extradural, intrathecal and transdermal routes.

- Critics who doubt the usefulness of the term cite the cumbersome American Food and Drug Administration (FDA) definition of bioavailability as 'The rate and extent to which the therapeutic moiety is absorbed and becomes available to the site of drug action.' 'Rate' and 'extent' are separate entities and the expression being 'available to the site of action' is imprecise. Most such definitions are of limited use because they relate bioavailability only to the total proportion of drug that reaches the systemic circulation while ignoring the rate. Clearly, if absorption is complete by 30 minutes, then the clinical effect is likely to be more marked than if that process takes 6 hours. The bioavailability of a particular oral drug is affected both by its formulation and by the physiology of its recipient and so, strictly speaking, it cannot accurately be quantified, except in a particular individual on a given occasion.

- It is nonetheless important to be aware of the concept, particularly in relation to drugs such as digoxin, which have a narrow therapeutic index. Different formulations of digoxin, which contain the same mass of drug, can give rise to plasma levels that vary more than sevenfold. It is also useful to be aware of the bioavailability of drugs that can be given by multiple different routes. That of ketamine, for example, is 20% (orally), 25% (rectally), 50% (nasally), 77% (epidurally) and 90% (intramuscularly).

- **Measurement:** bioavailability is measured by first giving a drug intravenously and then plotting the plasma concentration against time. When the drug has been completely removed from the system, the same agent is administered by a different route and a second elimination curve is plotted. Both curves are continued until they reach the x-axis and the plasma concentration is zero. Bioavailability is given by the ratio of the areas under the curves, $AUC_{non-iv}:AUC_{iv}$ (Figure 4.6).

- **Analysis of low bioavailability:** if bioavailability is low, then urinary or plasma metabolites may indicate broadly the reasons why. High concentrations of metabolites suggest that a drug has undergone extensive first pass metabolism in the liver. Low concentrations suggest either that there is poor gastrointestinal absorption or that significant biotransformation has taken place in the gut.

Supplementary Information

You may be asked about the factors that can influence bioavailability.

- **Physicochemical characteristics:** bioavailability is affected by the physicochemical characteristics of a drug and its formulation. Salts which are highly soluble have a much greater dissolution rate than drugs that are presented as strong acids or bases. Drugs of low lipid solubility, of which acidic and basic salts are an example, are in general absorbed poorly from the gut. Acidic drugs are absorbed better from the stomach, however, because low gastric pH reduces the proportion of drug that is ionized. In the more alkaline environment of the small gut, it is basic drugs whose ionization is reduced and which are therefore absorbed more effectively. There may also be significant interactions within the gut; the absorption of tetracyclines, for example, is prevented if they bind to dietary calcium. Particle size is important, in that smaller particles have a greater surface area:mass ratio and therefore dissolve more rapidly. Formulation in a crystalline form also aids dissolution, as does crystal hydration, anhydrous salts of drugs being more water-soluble. Excipients also affect the rate of absorption, with water repellents such as magnesium stearate decreasing the rate of dissolution. These properties are utilized in slow release and enteric-coated drugs.
- **Physiological factors:** orally and rectally administered drugs are absorbed into the portal circulation where they undergo first pass metabolism by hepatic enzymes. Extensive first pass metabolism clearly reduces bioavailability. Absorption of oral drugs is related to intestinal motility and integrity, as well as the extent to which they are subject to the action of enzymes in the gut wall. Glyceryl trinitrate is an example of a drug that undergoes hydrolysis by enzymes residing in the intestinal epithelium.
- Most of this discussion is relevant for drugs that are given orally. There is probably less extra chemistry and science to discuss in respect of other routes of administration, and there is unlikely to be sufficient time to deal with them in any detail. A logical approach using first principles should be sufficient. Skin, for example, is an effective physical barrier, but lipid-soluble drugs in adequate concentration can be delivered via patches. (Fentanyl, hyoscine, nicotine and sex hormones are examples of drugs that can be given in this way.) Mucous membranes in contrast offer less of an impediment to absorption, because the physical barrier is thinner.

Pharmacogenomics

Commentary

This will not occupy a full question, although the subject is of increasing interest because it has substantial, if expensive, potential benefits. It is discussed briefly here because the vision of matching drugs to the genetic profile of a patient remains largely theoretical despite the numerous genetic polymorphisms that have so far been identified. Much of the research evidence is complex and highly detailed. There are, however, simple examples of known genetic variations in responses to drugs of which it will be useful to be aware. (Pharmacogenomics is effectively the same as pharmacogenetics, but the term emphasizes that the investigation for genetic factors that influence the response to drugs is genome-wide.)

Core Information

- **Definition:** pharmacogenomics is defined simply as the study of the genetic variations which influence an individual's response to drugs. If such variations can be characterized it raises the possibility of tailoring drug therapy for patients across a wide range of conditions, from malignancy to depression.
- **Genetic variance:** pharmacogenomics combines pharmacology with investigation of DNA variations in the human genome. The most common such variations are single nucleotide polymorphisms (SNPs) which are estimated to occur in 1 in around 1,300 base pairs and which may be responsible for the way that an individual responds to drugs, both in terms of efficacy and adverse reactions. There are thought to be at least 11 million such polymorphisms in the human population, and so this is a field of research that will never be exhausted. In respect of therapeutics, the current focus of interest is on the genes that encode the metabolic enzymes that influence the activity of a particular agent. It is also likely that polygenic determinants of drug effects are important, involving both metabolic enzymes and receptors.
- **From complex …** there are more than 30 families of drug-metabolizing enzymes in humans, and it is probable that almost every pathway of metabolism has a genetic variation. Many will be polygenic, such as that affecting the cytochrome P450 CYP3A family. (For details of the cytochrome family nomenclature see under 'Cytochrome(s) P450' in Chapter 3). Almost 75% of Caucasian subjects and 50% of Afro-Caribbean subjects in the United States are unable to express CYP3A5, but this effect is masked by the fact that many of the drugs metabolized by that system are also metabolized by CYP3A4, which is an enzyme that is universally expressed. These pathways of drug metabolism are also complicated by the discovery of single nucleotide polymorphisms in the CYP3A4 gene which mean that its activity varies according to the particular substrate. There is also genetic polymorphism of receptors and of membrane transporters, such as the ATP-binding cassette transporters. Genetic sequence variants affect, for instance, the response to β2-agonists and ACE inhibitors. It is to be hoped that examples like the foregoing are not something that you are likely to be discussing in detail, if at all, but they are included to indicate the range and complexity of the subject.
- **… To simple.** It is more than possible that it was actually anaesthesia that provided the initial stimulus to the developing science of pharmacogenetics some decades ago, following the realization that the inability of atypical cholinesterases to hydrolyze suxamethonium was inherited, with around 1 in 3,500 Caucasian subjects being homozygous for the encoding gene. Also well known to anaesthetists are the variations that patients demonstrate when given codeine. Codeine is effectively a pro-drug whose active metabolite is morphine, formed in a reaction catalyzed by CYP2D6. Some individuals are deficient in this enzyme and will obtain minimal pain relief, in contrast to the ultra-fast metabolizers who have CYP2D6 gene duplication and in whom there may be exaggerated opioid effects. CYP2D6 is responsible for metabolizing – it is said – around a quarter of all the drugs in the British National

Formulary. Some 5–10% of the Caucasian population has CYP2D6 deficiency, and there are numerous mutations in the CYP2D6 gene. The therapeutic implications therefore are clearly very significant.

- **Other examples.** Also identified early was the genetic polymorphism of N-acetyl-transferase, which is a phase II conjugating liver enzyme, and which led to the characterization of 'slow' and 'fast' acetylators. This affects the metabolism of drugs such as the anti-hypertensive agent hydralazine, the anti-tubercular drug isoniazid and sulfonamide antibiotics. Slow acetylators risk toxicity from these agents, and in fast acetylators they may have a suboptimal effect. At least 50% of the UK population lack hepatic N-acetyltransferase and are slow acetylators. The phenotype is an autosomal recessive trait. Genetic profiles are important in oncology; for example, the drug trastuzumab (Herceptin) is effective only in tumours that produce the protein HER2. A gene variant that affects a much greater number of individuals is seen in almost 40% of Chinese, Japanese and Koreans who have an alcohol dehydrogenase enzyme system that is up to 50–100 times more effective in metabolizing ethanol to acetaldehyde. This is then compounded by a relative deficiency in acetaldehyde dehydrogenase which is found in around 50% in the same ethnic groups. These subjects may then exhibit the facial flushing and nausea that is characteristic of acetaldehyde toxicity.

Physics, Clinical Measurement, Equipment and Statistics

Depth of Anaesthesia Monitoring

Commentary

The discovery of anaesthesia transformed the human condition, and unplanned awareness returns a patient to the nightmare that was surgery before anaesthesia and analgesia. Significant advances in the pharmacology and technology of anaesthesia have still not brought reliable means of monitoring its depth much closer, although because awareness is such a serious complication considerable research effort has been dedicated to the search for methods of detection. Some remain research tools or are not yet in widespread use, but you should have some idea about which may in due course find their way into clinical practice. Most current interest centres around bispectral index (BIS) monitoring, with recommendations both from the Association of Anaesthetists and from NICE, which are summarized in the following, and it is likely that the oral will focus more on BIS than on the other technologies.

Core Information

Methods of Determining Depth of Anaesthesia

The list of techniques that has been described is a long one, so in the following description the methods are ranked broadly according to their practicality and utility. Clinical signs are therefore discussed first, not because they are the most reliable, but because every anaesthetist will use them. Some of these sections contain more detail than you reasonably could be expected to have mastered, but they are nonetheless considerable oversimplifications of a scientifically complex subject. (You will, however, need to deliver some of this detail because it will look otherwise as though you are simply reciting a list.)

- **Clinical signs:** in the spontaneously breathing patient who is not paralyzed, awareness may be manifest by purposeful movement. Movement is a reliable indicator of light anaesthesia, although a patient may have no recall.

- **Sympathetic stimulation:** the main clinical signs are tachycardia, hypertension, diaphoresis and lachrymation. Attempts have been made to quantify these objectively by using the PRST scoring system (blood **P**ressure, heart **R**ate, **S**weating, **T**ear formation), but without any real evidence of its benefit. In the absence of other causes, sympathetic signs may be reliable if present, but the main difficulty is that their absence does not exclude awareness.

- **Evoked potentials (EPs):** visual, somatosensory and auditory EPs have been investigated as indicators of the depth of anaesthesia. The few microvolts that are generated by each potential have to be separated from the overall electrical noise that is produced by the brain as a whole. Auditory EPs appear to be the most effective because they are the last to disappear and are the best indicators of anaesthetic depth. The patient's auditory system is stimulated by repetitive clicks at around 6–10 Hz. The electroencephalogram (EEG) is recorded immediately after each stimulus and is amplified, before the auditory EPs are extracted by taking the average of a large number of responses. This is covered in greater detail in 'Evoked Potentials' in the next section.

- **Compressed spectral array:** this is a method of simplifying the EEG in which the signals are subjected to Fourier analysis. Fourier transformation is the mathematical technique whereby complex waveforms are analyzed into their simpler sine wave components. Spectral analysis calculates the total power contained within the different frequencies of cerebral activity over a period of time (known as an epoch). The graph of power against frequency forms a spectral array. As an anaesthetic continues or deepens, each linear plot obtained during successive epochs can be superimposed to give the typical peak and trough, or 'hill and valley', display. This compressed display is what constitutes compressed spectral array. In an anaesthetized patient, power shifts to the lower frequencies.

- **Spectral edge:** this is the frequency above which there is only 5% of the total EEG power. A decrease in the spectral edge frequency accompanies increasing concentrations of anaesthetic agents. The relationship between the two does not appear to be linear, and in the transition between light and deeper anaesthesia there is a poor correlation between spectral edge frequency and drug concentration.

- **Median frequency:** this is another number determined from compressed spectral array, and is the frequency above and below which lies 50% of the total power of the EEG. It may correlate better with drug concentrations, but the spectral array shows a pattern that is not consistent between different anaesthetic agents.

- **Respiratory sinus arrhythmia and R–R interval variation:** this method does have promise, although it is only useful in the presence of an intact autonomic nervous system and healthy myocardial conducting system. Its value is greatly restricted in patients, for example, who are being treated with β-adrenoceptor blockers, who have autonomic neuropathy or dysfunction (common in the elderly), sepsis or who have cardiac conduction abnormalities. It provides a measure of brain stem function, which decreases with increasing depth of anaesthesia.

- **Isolated forearm technique:** this is not strictly a monitor of the depth of anaesthesia, but it is included as a method of detecting awareness that is simple, ingenious and arguably the most effective. It was described originally by Tunstall, who was interested in preventing awareness during obstetric general anaesthesia. An arterial tourniquet isolates the arm from drugs which enter the systemic circulation, and, prior to the procedure, the anaesthetist agrees with the patient the hand signals that they will use to convey awareness. Its practical use is limited both by the considerable degree of cooperation that is necessary and by the fact that after about 20 minutes of tourniquet inflation, ischaemic paralysis supervenes and prevents any further arm movement. Interestingly, only around half of those patients who respond appropriately to the agreed commands have any later recall of having done so, which reflects the complex effects of anaesthesia on memory processing.

- **EEG:** the formal EEG is a highly complex monitor, usually with multiple channels, which is generally regarded as producing too much data to be of any practical use in theatre. The raw EEG demonstrates differing patterns in response to different anaesthetic agents and changes in response to events such as hypoxia and hypercarbia. It also processes a lot of information from the cerebral cortex, which may not in fact be the area most appropriate for examining depth of anaesthesia.

- **Cerebral function monitor (CFM):** this is a processed and simplified EEG which displays only part of the frequency range. It has been used in neurointensive care units as an indirect monitor of cerebral oxygenation. It is of limited value in measuring depth of anaesthesia.

- **Cerebral function analyzing monitor (CFAM):** this is a refinement of the CFM, which separates out the main frequencies of cerebral activity. It is technically easier to use but has a slow response time and may also obtain a disproportionate amount of information from the temporal lobe.

- **Oesophageal contractility:** the amplitude and frequency of contractions of lower oesophageal smooth muscle reduce with increasing depth of anaesthesia. The technique is of limited value because of the high rate of false positive and false negative results.

- **Frontalis (scalp) electromyogram (EMG):** this technique measures the amplitude of the EMG, which decreases with increasing depth of anaesthesia. It is of very restricted benefit if for no other reason than it cannot be used in paralyzed patients.

NICE Recommendations

In 2012, the National Institute for Health and Care Excellence (NICE) published recommendations about depth of anaesthesia monitoring and cited three devices which are described in the following (NICE Diagnostics Guidance [DG6]. Depth of anaesthesia monitors. 2012).

In summary, the committee stated that 'the use of EEG-based depth of anaesthesia monitors is recommended as an option during any type of general anaesthesia in patients considered at higher risk of adverse outcomes. This includes patients at higher risk of unintended awareness and patients at higher risk of excessively deep anaesthesia. The Bispectral Index (BIS) depth of anaesthesia monitor is therefore recommended as an option in these patients.' They went on to comment that 'although there is greater uncertainty of clinical benefit for the E-Entropy and Narcotrend-Compact M monitors than for the BIS monitor . . . they are broadly equivalent.' The report also recommended depth of anaesthesia monitoring in all patients receiving total intravenous anaesthesia (TIVA).

- **Bispectral analysis and bispectral index (BIS):** this is another modification of the EEG, in which there is analysis of the phase and power relationships between the numerous frequencies. The term 'bispectral' describes the phase and power relationships between any two frequencies in the EEG. The bispectral index is a number generated from these phased and power frequencies that are the components of the EEG, and in essence compares frequency harmonics in the frontal EEG. The dimensionless scale of 0 (cortical electrical silence) to 100 (normal cortical electrical activity) has been derived from EEG recordings in volunteers and patients undergoing transitions between consciousness and unconsciousness. A bispectral index score of between 40 and 60 suggests surgical anaesthesia. The details of the calculation algorithm remain a commercial secret. The device has a variable response time, with a lag that is usually around 25 seconds, but which can extend for as long as 4 minutes. It appears to be accurate in respect of hypnotic drugs, both inhalational and intravenous, but reflects less well the synergistic sedative effects of opioids when used as part of 'balanced anaesthesia'. Nitrous oxide and ketamine produce different EEG changes and so also limit the usefulness of BIS. The BIS number will reduce if a patient is given muscle relaxants. This is usually attributed to their effect on the EMG, but it is possible that deafferentation may also contribute, with some loss of proprioceptive and muscle input through the reticular activating system. BIS has no predictive value for any particular individual's threshold for loss of consciousness.

  No authoritative body has yet endorsed the routine use of the processed EEG (pEEG), probably because the evidence base is not sufficiently robust. The B-Aware randomized controlled trial in 2,463 patients reported an 82% reduced risk of awareness in a population identified as being at high risk (Myles *et al. Lancet* 2004, 363: 1757–63), but the subsequent B-unaware study of 2,000 patients showed no difference between subjects monitored with BIS and with those managed according to a MAC-based protocol. The authors' conclusion was unequivocal: 'Our findings do not support routine BIS monitoring as part of standard practice' (Avidan *et al. NEJM* 2008, 358: 1097–1108). The same primary investigator headed up the BAG-RECALL trial which compared BIS of 40–60 to age-adjusted MAC values of 0.7–1.3 and in the 6,041 patients found no difference (Avidan *et al. NEJM* 2011, 365: 591–600).

- **E-entropy.** In the context of depth of anaesthesia monitoring, entropy is defined as a measure of irregularity in a signal. In the awake subject the EEG shows very irregular patterns which become more ordered as anaesthesia deepens. The E-entropy device is another form of processed EEG, but it also incorporates signals from the frontalis muscle EMG (fast frontalis EMG: FEMG), which gives a more rapid response (<2 s). The monitor uses a proprietary algorithm to process the EEG and EMG signals to produce two separate values to indicate the depth of anaesthesia. One is a rapid reaction to facial muscle activation which may occur in response to external stimuli and lightening of anaesthesia (response entropy, RE); the second is a slower response based on the processed EEG and which purports to assess the cerebral effect of anaesthetic agents (state entropy, SE). The scales are similar to those of the BIS monitor; RE ranges from 0 (cortical silence) to 100 (full wakefulness) and SE from 0 to 91. The target value similarly is 40–60.

- **Narcotrend.** This is another device that processes the raw EEG using spectral analysis, and via the application of complex proprietary algorithms derives a visual classification which ranges from A (full wakefulness) through E (appropriate anaesthetic depth) to F (deep hypnosis).

Supplementary and Clinical Information

Awareness, or accidental awareness during general anaesthesia (AAGA) to give it its full title, is an enduring concern both of anaesthetists and patients. The fifth National Audit project of the Royal College of Anaesthetists and Association of Anaesthetists of Great Britain and Ireland (NAP 5) reported an overall incidence of awareness of 1 in 19,000 but a much higher incidence in selected groups; 1 in 8,000 patients given neuromuscular blockers and a disconcertingly high 1 in 670 patients undergoing caesarean section. It therefore remains a problem.

- **Definitions:** awareness can be 'explicit' or 'implicit'. Explicit awareness is defined by spontaneous or prompted recall of intraoperative events, which may or may not include pain. Implicit awareness is a less specific concept and is defined by some degree of cortical perception but without conscious recall.
- **Causes:** its causes lie in equipment and its (mis)use, in pharmacology and its application and, very rarely, in the physiology of patients.
- **Equipment and apparatus:** awareness may result from a failure of the apparatus to deliver adequate concentrations of anaesthetic agent. The anaesthetic machine must deliver an accurate fresh gas flow via an appropriate breathing system using a vaporizer. For patients receiving TIVA, an accurate syringe driver is required, together with a reliable system of infusion tubing. Awareness may result if there are failures in any part of these systems. Such failures include leaks, faulty or empty vaporizers, a misconnected or disconnected breathing system, inaccurate pumps, misplaced venous cannulae and occluded infusion tubing.
- **Use of equipment and apparatus:** awareness may result from a failure of the anaesthetist to use the equipment properly. Circle systems can present a particular difficulty.
- **Monitoring:** failure to monitor the concentrations of inspired and expired volatile agents may result in inadequate anaesthetic agent being delivered. TIVA is more difficult to monitor in this respect because the effect site concentrations are calculated rather than measured directly.
- **Pharmacology:** awareness, by definition, results from inadequate anaesthesia. The dose of induction agent may have been inadequate, as may be the alveolar concentration (it is important to remember that the MAC value that is quoted is only the MAC_{50}) or the computed blood concentration in target-controlled infusion (TCI). Awareness is not prevented by hyperventilation, by the use of nitrous oxide and oxygen alone, nor by the use of opioids. Muscle relaxant drugs are not anaesthetics, and anaesthesia should not be discontinued until their effects have been reversed fully.
- **Physiology:** very rarely, a patient may be 'resistant' to anaesthetic agents. Alcohol and other drugs of abuse are convenient scapegoats, but the evidence is unconvincing. Similarly, high anxiety is frequently cited as the reason that some patients may need larger than normal induction doses. In any of these situations the anaesthetist

should be alert to the clinical signs indicative of inadequate anaesthesia. On occasion, a patient may be so moribund (or so inadequately resuscitated) that adequate anaesthesia may be incompatible with maintaining cardiac function.

- **Airway problems and bronchoscopy:** during a difficult intubation, the effects of the induction agent may wear off before those of the muscle relaxant. Awareness is also a potential problem during some anaesthetic techniques for rigid bronchoscopy (such as those using insufflation or injectors). Cardiac bypass is another technique in which the likely incidence of awareness is higher.
- **Sequelae:** it is very unusual to cause physical morbidity as a result of cardiovascular stresses provoked by being aware, although it is a theoretical possibility. Much more common are manifestations of a post-traumatic stress disorder (PTSD), whose typical features may include nightmares, insomnia, panic attacks and agoraphobia. Patients with PTSD will need considerable support, explanation and counselling.

Evoked Potentials

Commentary

Evoked potentials (EPs) are one means of monitoring the depth of anaesthesia, and they are also used to assess spinal cord function during surgery. The first usage remains confined mainly to research centres and the second to specialist centres, yet the topic is of some general anaesthetic interest. The underlying neurophysiology and the signal processing are too complex to explore in a short oral examination, and a broad knowledge of the principles should suffice.

Core Information

- An evoked potential (EP), also known as an evoked response (ER) or event-related potential (ERP), is an aspect of EEG monitoring. The signal in the EEG is produced when an individual receives a visual, auditory or somatosensory stimulus, and the EPs are detected by an electrode which is positioned over the primary receiving area for that sensory modality. Somatosensory evoked potentials (SSEPs), for example, are recorded from electrodes positioned over the sensory cortex.
- The potentials are only a few microvolts in amplitude and so are swamped by the noise of the global EEG. Each can measure from as low as 0.1 μV up to around 2 μV, compared with the EEG background amplitude of 10–300 μV. These low potentials are extracted from the EEG by a process of computer averaging. The patient is subjected to a large number of repeated stimuli, and the EEG is recorded during a fixed period after each one. It is then amplified before the EPs are extracted by taking the average of this large number of responses.
- **Auditory evoked responses (AERs):** the processed signals comprise a series of peaks and troughs, which represent the response time or 'latency'. This has been mapped most thoroughly in respect of auditory ERs, which produce a series of waves as the repetitive 6–10 Hz stimulus activates pathways from the cochlea to the cortex.

(The separate waves relate to their anatomical origin.) Neither the brain stem response (0–10 ms latency) nor the late cortical response (50–500 ms latency) correlates with depth of anaesthesia. It is examination of the waveform of the middle latency section (10–50 ms latency) which provides this information. (It originates in the auditory cortex.) This mid-latency region contains two troughs separated by a peak. The amplitude and latency of the peak (Pa) and second trough, or nadir (Nb), are analyzed. Signals beyond around 100–1,000 ms represent the late cortical response which arises from the frontal cortex and association areas.

- **Visual evoked potentials (VEPs):** these are produced in response to a pulsed flash of light and elicit mainly a cortical response. They are more variable than auditory EPs and so give more qualitative than quantitative information.
- **Somatosensory evoked potentials (SSEPs):** as described, these are potentials of very small amplitude which are measured by electrodes over the sensory cortex. Traditionally it was assumed that if sensory pathways were intact, as in spinal surgery for example, then motor pathways will not have been damaged. This does not always hold true.
- **Motor evoked potentials (MEPs):** these are large amplitude potentials which are generated by stimulation of the motor cortex and measured by needle electrodes placed in selected muscles. Their absence suggests damage to the corticospinal tract whose integrity is essential for the motor response. In contrast to SSEPs, motor evoked responses are suppressed by volatile anaesthetic agents at MAC values greater than 0.5, and so total intravenous anaesthesia may be indicated for spinal surgery. An alternative is to test cord function by means of epidural motor EPs, which are relatively unaffected by anaesthetic agents.

Supplementary and Clinical Information

- **Anaesthetic depth:** EPs have been investigated as indicators of the depth of anaesthesia. Visual and somatosensory EPs show less promise than auditory evoked responses.
- **Spinal surgery:** EPs are used to monitor spinal cord function, which can be compromised by distraction during scoliosis surgery. Historically, patients were subjected to the intraoperative wake-up test, during which anaesthesia was lightened (with appropriate analgesia) to the point at which the subject could respond to a request to move both arms and legs. (Arm movement excludes the possibility of neuromuscular blockade.) This technique actually worked better than it may sound to those who have never seen it done, but it is nonetheless crude in comparison to somatosensory and motor EPs. As described earlier, the potentials are of very low amplitude, and the signal is averaged. The latency and amplitude are measured, usually by electrodes which monitor the cerebral cortex. Somatosensory potentials are also depressed by high-concentration volatile agents, although not at normal concentrations, and by high-dose opioids (such as fentanyl in doses greater than 50 $\mu g \ kg^{-1}$), but the normal clinical use of these drugs does not compromise the technique. Hypoxaemia and hypoperfusion of the cord are confounding factors which may influence the response. They decrease its amplitude but do not have any effect on its waveform.
- **Neurology:** EPs are used to aid the diagnosis of a number of neurological conditions. These include multiple sclerosis and other demyelinating diseases, tumours in the posterior fossa, in which auditory EPs are useful, and global head injury.

Pulse Oximetry

Commentary

Pulse oximetry has been widely available in the UK since the late 1980s, and rapidly became established as probably the single most important form of monitoring in anaesthetic practice. Accordingly, a broad understanding of how the technique works will be expected, with particular reference to its limitations and potential sources of error.

Core Information

The Rationale for the Use of Pulse Oximetry

- The clinical recognition of cyanosis is very variable between observers. Experimental studies in volunteers breathing various hypoxic mixtures have suggested that up to 25% of observers will be unable to detect cyanosis even at oxygen saturations as low as 75%, and that conversely some 10–15% will claim that cyanosis is present at saturations of greater than 91% (and in some cases as high as 100%). This variability is compounded by factors such as the type and intensity of ambient light and the patient's skin pigmentation. In addition, the generation of cyanosis is said to require around 50 g l^{-1} of deoxygenated haemoglobin in the capillary bed (this figure was derived originally from calculations by Lundsgaard and Van Slyke which are almost a century old, but subsequent investigations confirmed a figure of between 40 and 50 g l^{-1}), and so the clinical detection of oxygen desaturation will vary according to the patient's haemoglobin concentration. If the haemoglobin is 150 g l^{-1}, cyanosis will be discernible at an oxygen saturation of around 80%. If, however, the patient is anaemic, with a haemoglobin of around 90–100 g l^{-1} then they will not become cyanosed until their saturation falls to around 65%. A very anaemic patient may not demonstrate cyanosis at all.

Principles of the Pulse Oximeter

- Oxygenated haemoglobin (HbO_2) and deoxygenated haemoglobin (Hb) have differential absorption spectra.
- At a wavelength of 660 nm (red light), HbO_2 absorbs less than Hb, hence its red colour.
- At a wavelength of 940 nm (infrared light), this is reversed and Hb absorbs more than HbO_2. At 800 nm – the isobestic point – the absorption coefficients are identical.
- The pulse oximeter uses two light-emitting diodes which emit pulses of red (660nm) and infrared (980nm) light every 5–10 μs from one side of the probe. The light is transmitted through the tissue to be sensed by a photocell on the other side.
- The output is submitted to electronic processing, during which the absorption of the blood at the two different wavelengths is converted to a ratio, which is compared to an algorithm produced from experimental data.

- Oximetry aims to measure the saturation in arterial blood, and so the instrument detects the points of maximum and minimum absorption (during cardiac systole and diastole). It measures the pulsatile component and subtracts the non-arterial constant component before displaying a pulse waveform and the percentage oxygen saturation. Hence, strictly defined, it is measuring the Sp (plethysmographic) O_2 rather than the Sa (arterial) O_2.

Potential Sources of Error and Limitations of the Technique

- Pulse oximetry is calibrated against healthy volunteers, which means that calibration against dangerously hypoxic values has not been possible. The instruments are less accurate at SpO_2 values below 70%. (You can use this fact to reassure colleagues who are less composed than you in the face of a patient's saturation that otherwise seems alarmingly low.)
- Interference by ambient light. This can occur if light is bright and direct, but the pulsed nature of the emissions is intended to allow detection of, and compensation for, any ambient light.
- Loss of the pulsatile component. This occurs in conditions of hypoperfusion, hypothermia and peripheral vasoconstriction, when there is a narrow pulse pressure, arrhythmias which distort the points of maximum and minimum absorption, or venous congestion. These are all common reasons for a poor signal.
- Movement artefact or electrical interference (neither are major problems).
- Infrared absorption by other substances, such as nail varnish or nicotine staining.
- More significant errors are associated with absorption by abnormal haemoglobins and other compounds:
  - **Carboxyhaemoglobinaemia:** this is seen in heavy smokers or in CO poisoning. COHb has a similar absorption coefficient to HbO_2 and will give an abnormally high SpO_2 reading of about 96%.
  - **Jaundice:** bilirubin has a similar absorption coefficient to deoxygenated Hb and will give abnormally low saturation readings.
  - **Methaemoglobinaemia:** metHb has absorption similar at both wavelengths and gives a saturation reading of around 84%.
  - **Dyes.** Various dyes in the circulation such as methylene blue or disulphine blue give falsely low readings.

Problems in Interpretation

- Pulse oximetry does not detect respiratory failure. A high FiO_2 may mask ventilatory failure by ensuring high SpO_2% readings despite a rising CO_2.
- The slope of the oxygen–haemoglobin dissociation curve means that there is a lag of 20 seconds or more between any drop in arterial oxygen tension and the resultant fall in oxygen saturation.
- In very anaemic patients SpO_2% readings may show high saturations, although oxygen delivery to the tissues may be impaired.
- The amplitude of the pulse waveform is not a reliable indicator of the pulse volume. Many instruments automatically augment the trace to fill the display.

- As a general point of discussion (should there be time to spare), it can be argued that pulse oximetry may not actually be the most useful single monitor, were anaesthetists to be restricted to one. The amplitude of the pulse waveform is not a reliable indicator of the pulse volume. In contrast to end-tidal CO_2 measurement, pulse oximetry gives information some of which can be obtained by clinical observation, although clinical recognition of cyanosis is unreliable. The examiner might ask what single, theoretical monitoring device you would use, were you to be allowed only one. An answer might be a device that reliably measured the state of cerebral oxygenation. (If cerebral oxygenation is maintained, then none of the other monitored indices really matter.) One such is the use of near infrared spectroscopy.

Measurement of CO_2

Commentary

The capnograph is an essential monitor which is used in all but the briefest of anaesthetics. Capnography is also now viewed as an essential standard in every area where there are intubated patients or patients with laryngeal mask airways in place. There is not a vast amount to ask about the principles of the commonest method of CO_2 measurement (infrared absorption), and unless you are unfortunate enough to encounter an examiner who has a passion for Raman scattering, the oral is likely to concentrate equally on clinical uses. Make sure that you are able to interpret the range of capnograph traces that you may commonly encounter. It will help if you can draw them.

Core Information

Methods of Measuring End-Tidal CO_2

- **Infrared absorption:** this is the main method of measuring CO_2 in the operating theatre.
- Its principle is that a molecule will absorb infrared radiation (wavelength 1–40 μm) as long as it contains at least two different atoms. This applies to CO_2, as well as to N_2O and to all other inhalational agents.
- The system comprises an infrared source, a filter to ensure that only radiation of the desired wavelength is transmitted, a crystal window (glass absorbs infrared), a sample chamber and a photodetector.
- The fraction of radiation absorbed is compared with a reference gas (so regular calibration against zero and known CO_2 concentrations is essential) before the value is displayed.
- The infrared wavelength absorbed varies with the gas, thereby allowing its identification. For CO_2, this absorption is maximal at 4.28 μm. There is some overlap between CO_2 and N_2O for which modern instruments can compensate; collision broadening would otherwise falsely elevate the CO_2 readings.

- **Colorimetric:** carbonic acid forms from CO_2 and water and will change a pH-sensitive colour indicator. This principle is used in portable devices intended to confirm correct tracheal tube placement in emergency situations in which formal capnography is not available.
- **Mass spectrometry:** this technique is extremely accurate, has a very rapid response time and allows the simultaneous measurement of different compounds. The instruments, however, are very large and expensive and are not used for routine gas monitoring in the UK. The gas sample is introduced into an ionization chamber in which some of its component molecules pass through an electron beam and become charged. The ionized particles are then accelerated out of the chamber into a strong magnetic field, which deflects the particles according to their mass.
- **Raman effect:** the interaction of electromagnetic radiation with a molecule may result in a partial, as opposed to a complete, transfer of energy. Intermolecular bonds absorb the energy, and some is then re-emitted at different wavelengths. There is usually a decrease in wavelength which is characteristic of the individual molecule.

Supplementary and Clinical Information

Information that can be obtained from a capnograph trace (Figure 5.1).
- **Cardiovascular information:** CO_2 production can occur only if the patient has a cardiac output. A falling CO_2 may indicate a decreasing cardiac output, a sudden fall may be a sign of pulmonary embolus and a flat trace will be seen if there is complete

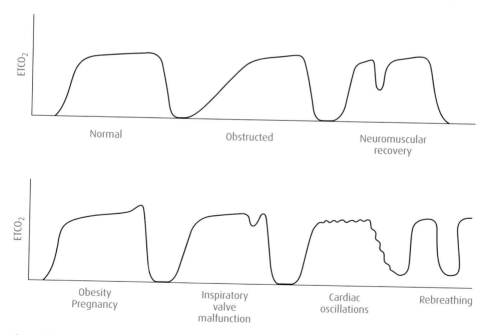

Fig. 5.1 Capnography waveforms (capnograms). $ETCO_2$, End-tidal CO_2.

circulatory arrest. Normal end-tidal CO_2 usually reassures the anaesthetist that ventilation is adequate.

- **Respiratory information:** there are many possible variations of a capnograph trace, some of which may be quite subtle, such as the waveform you may see with intermittent malfunction of an inspiratory valve, or the small rise at the end of the rising plateau phase that may be seen in obese and pregnant patients. (This is attributed to fast- and slow-emptying alveoli with different time constants.) You are more likely to be asked about the traces which convey more commonly important information.
  - **No CO_2 trace:** this may indicate oesophageal intubation, tracheal tube displacement or disconnection of the breathing system.
  - **Low or falling end-tidal CO_2:** this may be due to overventilation if IPPV is being used, or to hyperventilation in a patient breathing spontaneously.
  - **High or rising end-tidal CO_2:** this may be caused by inadequate ventilation, respiratory depression, rebreathing or exhaustion of the soda lime. It may rarely be a sign of a hypermetabolic state, of which the most extreme example is malignant hyperpyrexia, in which there is a massive increase in CO_2 production.
  - **Abnormal capnography waveforms:** a slow upstroke and slowly rising plateau indicates chronic or acute airway obstruction. The obstruction can be anywhere in the system – either in the upper or lower airway or in the breathing circuit. A trace that shows inspiratory dips in the waveform may be indicating partial recovery from neuromuscular blockade. A raised baseline indicates rebreathing.

The Fuel Cell (Oxygen Measurement)

Commentary

It is a little difficult to know why this question continues to appear, given that fuel cell oxygen analyzers are no longer widely in use. The subject may broaden to include other methods of measuring oxygen concentrations, although there is no obvious clinical angle to leaven the science. A few examiners may be excited by the topic; most will be rather less enthusiastic and so do not worry if the oral seems a bit flat at this stage. It will probably be because the examiners will be depressed more by the line of questioning they are constrained to follow than by your answers.

Core Information

Methods of Measuring Oxygen
The Galvanic Fuel Cell

- A reliable method of analyzing oxygen in the common gas outlet of the anaesthetic machine is fundamental to patient safety.
- The fuel cell is similar in principle to a polarographic (Clark) oxygen electrode. It comprises a lead anode and a gold mesh cathode bathed in an electrolyte solution.

At the anode, lead reacts with hydroxyl ions to produce electrons. At the cathode, oxygen reacts with the electrons and water, and generates hydroxyl ions.

- The current flow is proportional to the partial pressure of oxygen. The response time is around 30 seconds.
- The fuel cell produces its own voltage and needs no other electrical source. Protecting it from oxygen (air) during the periods when it is not in use will prolong its life. Its function is not affected by water vapour.
- Fuel cells are bulky, heavy and are not robust. They may also be affected by the accumulation of nitrogen that occurs if nitrous oxide is passed though the cell.

The Clark Electrode

- The Clark electrode consists of a silver/silver chloride anode and platinum cathode bathed in an electrolyte solution. A small potential is applied across the electrodes and the current measured. The electrode works in an analogous way to the fuel cell, in that current flow is proportional to the oxygen tension at the cathode. The Clark electrode measures oxygen in a blood sample from which it is separated by a plastic membrane.

Paramagnetic Oxygen Analyzer

- Oxygen is paramagnetic, with unpaired electrons in the outer shell, which means that it is drawn into a magnetic field. (Most other gases are diamagnetic.) The traditional paramagnetic analyzer comprises a chamber containing a nitrogen-filled glass dumb-bell, which is suspended on a wire and allowed to rotate within a non-uniform magnetic field. When oxygen enters the chamber, it is attracted by the magnetic field and displaces the dumbbell. The degree of rotation is proportional to the amount of oxygen present. Modern analyzers comprise two chambers separated by a pressure transducer. One is a reference chamber containing 20.93% oxygen (air); the other contains the sample to be measured. Both chambers are then subjected to a changing magnetic field, which increases the activity of the oxygen molecules. This agitation changes the pressure in each chamber; the oxygen partial pressure difference is proportional to the pressure difference across the transducer. These analyzers are very accurate and have a rapid response time which allows breath-by-breath measurement.

Mass Spectrometry

- This technique is accurate, has a very rapid response time and allows the simultaneous measurement of different compounds, including oxygen.

Supply of Medical Gases

Commentary

Conceptually this is not a difficult question, and it requires of you no judgement and little science. It requires simply facts, and facts which are mostly of modest clinical relevance, albeit of some general interest. (The question is not a very good discriminator, so you might as well learn the basic information, repeat it gratefully to the examiner and hope that the next subject about which you are asked is rather more enticing.)

Core Information

The supply of medical gases (oxygen, nitrous oxide, Entonox and medical air) to a typical hospital.

- **Central gas supply**
  - Piped gas (oxygen, nitrous oxide, Entonox and medical air) is supplied through high-quality copper pipelines. The outlets have a non-interchangeable coupling in the form of a Schrader-type valve. The hoses from the gas outlet to the anaesthetic machine are colour-coded. Gas is supplied at a pressure of 4 bar, apart from the medical gas that is used to drive surgical instruments which is supplied at 7 bar.
  - The gases may come from a manifold of large cylinders. They may be arranged in banks of cylinders, each of which should contain enough gas to supply a hospital for at least 2 days.
  - Oxygen is usually supplied from a liquid oxygen source. Liquid oxygen is stored below its critical temperature ($-118\ °C$) at around $-160\ °C$ and at a pressure of 7 bar, which is the vapour pressure of oxygen at that temperature. The low temperature is maintained both by a vacuum insulated shell and by the fact that as the oxygen evaporates, its temperature will fall. The contents of the storage device can be determined either by weight or by pressure gauges, which measure the pressure difference between the top and bottom of the liquid oxygen.

- **Gas cylinders**
  - The cylinders on an anaesthetic machine are usually size 'E', which contain 680 litres of oxygen, 1,800 litres of nitrous oxide and 680 litres of medical air. Designed to withstand very high pressures (they are tested to 250 bar), they are made of molybdenum, chromium steel, manganese and high-carbon manganese steel. (Cylinders for domiciliary oxygen can be made of lightweight aluminium alloy.)
  - Their features include colour coding (which is not international; oxygen cylinders in the UK are black with white shoulders, whereas in the USA they are green), a pin index system to ensure attachment only to the correct yoke and information about the contents of the cylinder. The coloured plastic collar indicates the date of the last cylinder test (the interval is between 5 and 10 years). The bodok seal is a neoprene washer enclosed within an aluminium surround which provides a gas-tight seal between the cylinder head and the yoke.

- **Cylinder contents**
  - Oxygen is stored as a gas at a pressure of 13,700 kPa (137 bar).
  - Nitrous oxide is in a mixed liquid and vapour phase whose pressure is 4,400 kPa.
  - Entonox is a 50:50 gas mixture of oxygen and nitrous oxide at a pressure of 13,700 kPa.
  - Medical air is stored in cylinders of high tensile steel at a pressure of 13,700 kPa. Larger cylinders (which contain 4,600 litres) are designed for a higher maximum working pressure of 23,000 kPa.

- **Oxygen concentrators**
  - These provide an alternative method of providing oxygen, although their low flow rates ($4\,l\,min^{-1}$) and pressures (70 kPa) mean that they are more commonly used to provide domiciliary supplies for individual patients.
  - They comprise zeolite-containing columns. Zeolites are hydrated aluminium silicates which are ion-exchangers and molecular sieves. The flow of air into the cylinders is directed so that nitrogen and water vapour are absorbed from one cylinder, and absorbed gas from the other is extracted by a vacuum pump. Every 30 seconds a solenoid valve switches the flow to ensure a constant flow of 95% oxygen to the reservoir. The remaining 5% is argon, which appears to have no adverse effects. (Although in higher concentrations it has the same effect as xenon in stimulating erythropoietin release.)
- **Medical air:** this can be supplied from a central compressor or from cylinders. It must be dry, free from particulate matter, including the mineral oils used to lubricate the compressor, and free from bacteria. The air is, therefore, desiccated and filtered.

Supplementary Information

Miscellaneous Definitions; Safety; Safe storage; Supply Failure

- **Critical temperature and pressure:** the critical temperature of a gas is the temperature at which it cannot be liquefied no matter how great the pressure that is applied (oxygen: $-118.6\,°C$, nitrous oxide: $36.4\,°C$, xenon: $16.6\,°C$). The critical pressure of a substance is the pressure required to liquefy a gas at its critical temperature.
- **Filling ratio:** this is the mass of gas used to fill a cylinder divided by the mass of water needed to fill the cylinder completely. It applies to gases that are stored in the liquid phase, and for nitrous oxide, it is 0.75. If the cylinder is to be used in hotter climates, this is reduced to 0.67. An overfilled cylinder that is exposed to high ambient temperatures will generate dangerously high pressures.
- **Safe storage:** this is largely common sense. Cylinders should be kept in a secure and dry environment, free from extremes of temperature. Full and empty cylinders should ideally be kept in separate areas to avoid the risk of substitution. Large cylinders are usually stored upright; smaller ones may be laid horizontally.
- **Entonox:** this is a 50:50 N_2O/O_2 mixture. Cylinders should be stored flat to prevent the risk of delivering 100% nitrous oxide when the cylinder is first used.
- **Nitrous oxide:** you may be asked what happens when a nitrous oxide cylinder empties. In theory, the pressure, which is the vapour pressure, should remain constant until the liquid phase is exhausted, after which the pressure would fall to zero as the cylinder emptied. In practice, because the temperature of the liquid nitrous oxide falls as it vaporizes, the cylinder pressure also drops. The pressure returns to 4,400 kPa only if the gas flow ceases and the cylinder is allowed to return to room temperature.
- **Gas supply or oxygen failure:** failure of the liquid oxygen source triggers supply from a reserve manifold of large oxygen cylinders, which are also remote from the site of delivery to the patient. There should also be reserve cylinders available in theatre. Should there be a complete failure of oxygen delivery, the anaesthetic machine should discontinue the flow of nitrous oxide and entrain air.

The Anaesthetic Machine

Commentary
This topic may be asked in various ways. The oral may deal with overall safety features, or it may concentrate on prevention of barotrauma or hypoxia. A structured approach should allow you to answer the question adequately, from whichever direction it is approached. It is a core subject, but not one which is difficult. The safety features of the anaesthetic machine are numerous, and you will have little time to do more than list them.

Core Information
- The modern anaesthetic machine delivers accurate mixtures of anaesthetic gases and inhalational agents at variable, controlled flow rates and at low pressure. It accomplishes this via a number of features that are best described by tracing the gas flow through the system from the cylinder or pipeline to the fresh gas outlet.
- **Gas pipelines:** these are colour-coded for the UK, but there is no international consistency. A Schrader coupling system ensures that the pipeline connections are non-interchangeable. Reducing valves reduce the pressures to 400 kPa (4 bar). The pipeline hose connection to the rear of the anaesthetic machine is permanent. The threads are gas-specific (NIST – non-interchangeable screw thread), and a one-way valve ensures unidirectional flow.
- **Gas cylinders:** these are also colour-coded for the UK, but here too there is no international standard. They are made from molybdenum steel alloy. They are robust and undergo rigorous regular hydraulic testing (as does the cylinder outlet valve). A pin-index system, which is unique to each gas, prevents connection to the wrong yoke, and side guards on each yoke ensure that the cylinders are vertical. Bodok (**bo**nded **d**isk) seals ensure a gas-tight fit. A Bourdon pressure gauge indicates cylinder pressure.
- **Pressure regulators:** primary pressure regulators/reducing valves decrease the high cylinder pressures to 4 bar, and a relief valve is located downstream in case of regulator failure. Adjustable pressure-limiting (APL) valves are part of the breathing system rather than the anaesthetic machine itself, but are designed to minimize the risk of barotrauma by venting gas when a pre-set pressure is exceeded. When fully closed, the APL will open at a pressure of 60 cmH$_2$O.
- **Flow restrictors:** these are placed upstream of the flowmeter block and protect the low-pressure part of the system from damaging surges in gas pressure from the piped supply. They may sometimes be used downstream of the vaporizer back bar to minimize backpressure associated with IPPV.
- **Flow control valves:** these govern the transition from the high-pressure to the low-pressure system, and reduce the pressure from 4 bar to just above atmospheric as gas enters the flowmeter block.
- **Oxygen failure and interlock devices:** systems vary, but a British Standard specifies that the failure alarm should be powered by the O$_2$ supply pressure in the machine

pipeline and activated by a pressure reduction to below 2 bar. In most systems the gas mixture is then vented, and an audible warning tone is activated. The same valve opens an air-entrainment valve so that the patient cannot be exposed to a hypoxic mixture resulting from failure of O_2 delivery. An interlock system between the O_2 and N_2O control valves prevents the administration of a hypoxic mixture. The machine cannot deliver a nitrous oxide concentration greater than 75%.

- **Emergency oxygen flush:** O_2 is supplied direct from the high-pressure circuit upstream of the vaporizer block and provides 35–75 l min^{-1} (if the O_2 flowmeter needle valve is opened fully, it delivers about 40 l min^{-1}). Both methods may cause barotrauma in vulnerable patients.
- **Flowmeters:** these are constant pressure variable orifice flowmeters (Rotameter is a trade name) which are calibrated for a specific gas. Accuracy is to within 2.5%. The tubes have an antistatic coating to prevent sticking, and there are vanes etched into the bobbin to ensure rotation. In the UK the oxygen knob is always on the left, is larger, is hexagonal in profile and is more prominent than the others. (This is said to be because Boyle, who designed one of the original anaesthetic machines, was left-handed). This position does, however, put the patient at risk of breathing a hypoxic mixture if there is damage to a downstream flowmeter tube. Thus, modern O_2 flowmeters feed distal to other gases should there be a proximal leak. CO_2 has disappeared from most machines; where it is still delivered, it is usually governed to prevent a flow of greater than 500 ml min^{-1}. Not all modern machines use flowmeters; some control gas flow by microprocessors and produce an electronic display.
- **Vaporizers and back bar:** the most common vaporizers are temperature-compensated variable bypass devices which allow accurate and safe delivery of the dialled concentrations. A locking mechanism on the back bar prevents more than one vaporizer being used at the same time. A spring-loaded non-return valve on the back bar prevents retrograde flow caused by the pumping effect of IPPV. A pressure relief valve on the downstream end of the back bar protects against increases in the pressure within the circuit.
- **Common gas outlet:** this receives gases from the back bar and from the emergency O_2 flush. It has a swivel outlet with a standard 15-mm female connection.

Clinical Applications
Protection from barotrauma: the key features from the preceding list include

- Pressure-reducing valves, both pipeline and cylinders.
- Flow restrictors.
- Flow control valves.
- Pressure relief valves downstream of the vaporizer back bar.

Protection from hypoxia: the key features from the preceding list include

- Gas pipelines, colour coding and NIST connections.
- Gas cylinders, colour coding and pin indexing.
- Oxygen failure devices.
- Interlock system.
- Emergency oxygen flush.

Flowmeters

Commentary
There are few anaesthetics given which do not involve the use of at least one flowmeter, although microprocessor-controlled gas flow is becoming more widespread as older anaesthetic machines are replaced. It is important, nonetheless, to be aware of how traditional flowmeters function as well as of the potential sources of inaccuracy. This is a predictable and straightforward question, but it is fairly thin, and so you will be expected to know the basic physics.

Core Information
The physical principles which underlie the function of flowmeters.

- A flowmeter is a variable orifice, fixed pressure difference device, which gives a continuous indication of the rate of gas flow. ('Rotameter' is actually a trade name which continual use has given generic status.)
- A bobbin floats within a vertical conical glass tube, supported by the gas flow which is controlled by a needle valve.
- At low flows the orifice around the bobbin is an annular tube, and the gas flow is laminar. Flow rate through a tube is related to the viscosity of the gas and the fourth power of the radius.
- At higher flows and further up the tube, the area of the annular orifice is larger in relation to the bobbin and the flow is turbulent. Flow rate through an orifice is related to the density of the gas and the square of the radius.
- These factors mean therefore that flowmeters have to be calibrated for the specific gases that they are measuring. They are not interchangeable for different gases. They are accurate to $\pm 2.5\%$.
- The pressure across the bobbin at any flow rate remains constant, because the force to which it gives rise is balanced exactly by the force of gravity acting on the bobbin.

Further Features
- The bobbin is designed with small slots or fins in its upper part so that it will rotate centrally within the gas stream without touching the flowmeter tube. This is to prevent its sticking to the sides because of dirt or static electricity.
- To prevent the accumulation of static charge, tubes have either a conductive coating or a conductive strip at the back.
- The flowmeter blocks are designed to ensure that the bobbin remains visible at the top of the tubes, even when the gas flow is at its maximum.

Supplementary Information
Potential sources of inaccuracy.

- Accumulation of dirt or static electricity (despite the design features mentioned).
- A flowmeter block may not be vertical; the bobbin must not impinge on the sides of the tube.

- Back pressure on the gas flow may still be a problem on some anaesthetic machines, although this is normally prevented by a spring-loaded non-return valve.
- Cracked seals or tubes may provide a source of error. Oxygen is often the last gas to be added to the mixture that is delivered to the back bar, although some modern flowmeter blocks are designed to deliver oxygen downstream of the other gases should there be a proximal leak.

Laminar and Turbulent Flow

Commentary

Precise physical principles underlie the concepts of laminar and turbulent flow, and the oral is likely to concentrate more on these than on their practical implications. Factors which influence flow are important in relation to intravenous fluid therapy and to the administration of inhaled gases, but their relevance is obvious, and the potential for discussion is relatively limited. Examiners tend to view this as a straightforward and predictable question. They do not expect candidates to have much difficulty with it, and so you should know the topic well.

Core Information

- **Flow:** flow is the amount of a fluid (gas or liquid) passing a point in unit time.
- **Laminar flow**
  - This describes the situation in which a molecule of the given substance maintains a constant spatial relationship to all the others that are flowing in the same layer, or lamina, down the tube. The flow is greatest in the centre of the tube, being approximately twice the mean flow, whereas at the walls of the tube the flow reduces almost to zero.
  - A number of factors influence flow; these include the pressure differential between the ends of the tube ($P_1 - P_2$), the radius of the tube (r), the length of the tube (l) and the viscosity of the fluid (η).
  - These factors have been combined (together with a proportionality constant $\pi/128$) to derive the Poiseuille–Hagen equation:

$$\text{Flow rate} = (P_1 - P_2) \times r^4 \times \pi/128 \times l \times \eta.$$

  - This applies only to an ideal or Newtonian fluid, which is defined as any fluid that demonstrates a linear relation between the applied shear stress and the rate of deformation. A flowing liquid can be visualized as a series of parallel laminae. If the flow is to double, therefore, it must overcome a resistive force that is twice as great. Water is a Newtonian fluid, but blood is not.
  - Fluids resist flow because of the phenomenon of viscosity. Viscosity describes the frictional forces which act between the layers of the fluid as it moves down the tube. (Its units are Pascal seconds.)

- **Turbulent flow:** this describes fluid flow in which the orderly arrangement of the molecules is lost and the fluid swirls and eddies, thereby increasing the resistance. In contrast to laminar flow, in which flow is directly proportional to the pressure differential (ΔP), when the flow is turbulent, then fluid flow is proportional to the square root of the differential ($\sqrt{\Delta P}$).
- **The transition from laminar to turbulent flow**
  - This is given by the Reynolds number, which is an index derived from a combination of linear velocity (v), the density of the fluid (ρ), the diameter of the tube (d) and the viscosity of the fluid (η). Reynolds number = $v\rho d/\eta$.
  - When the Reynolds number exceeds 2,000, turbulent flow supervenes. (This information has been obtained empirically from in vitro experiments.)
  - Critical flow and critical velocity refer to the situation in which the Reynolds number is 2,000, and the flow is liable to become turbulent.
  - Any local increase in velocity, such as occurs in the angles or constrictions of a breathing system, is likely to change gas flow from laminar to turbulent, with a resultant increase in resistance and the work of breathing.

Supplementary Information and Clinical Considerations

The practical relevance of laminar and turbulent flow.

- **Gas flow:** turbulent flow increases resistance, and so it is important to minimize angles and constrictions in breathing systems. Increased velocity may increase turbulence, which can be of significance, for example, in a hyperventilating asthmatic patient. In an infant with bronchiolitis, a small decrease in the calibre of the airways due to inflammation and oedema may critically impair the capacity of the exhausted baby to maintain effective ventilation. (These are some of several possible examples.)
- **Fluid flow:** the Poiseuille–Hagen equation is well known to anaesthetists because of its clinical relevance. The flow of fluid via an intravenous infusion will double if the driving pressure is doubled or if the length of the cannula is halved. Fluid resuscitation through long central venous catheters therefore may not be effective. Flow, however, in theory will increase by 16 times if the internal diameter of the cannula is doubled. (In practice, the increase may not be quite as impressive; a typical 14G cannula of 2.20 mm [external] diameter has a flow rate of 315 ml min^{-1}, in contrast to an 18G cannula with a diameter of 1.30 mm through which distilled water flows at 100 ml min^{-1}.) The difference remains significant enough, however, to mandate the use of short, wide-bore cannulae for rapid restoration of circulating volume.
- **Laminar flow operating theatres:** the typical orthopaedic operating theatre in the UK will have a (costly) laminar flow system, which describes a body of air within the demarcated area which moves with uniform velocity along parallel flow lines and in a single direction. These systems can generate 300 air changes an hour compared with up to 25 an hour in conventionally ventilated turbulent air theatres. Accepted wisdom has it that laminar flow reduces surgical site infection, particularly when prostheses are inserted, as in hip and knee arthroplasty. This confidence may be misplaced. While there are some small single-centre studies which do demonstrate reduction in infection rates, there equally are some very large surveys (80–100,000 patients) which have

demonstrated the opposite. Data from national joint registry and hospital infection surveillance systems have revealed statistically significantly greater deep infection rates in laminar flow theatres. (Isolation surgical suits also make no difference.) The reasons are unclear, but it is speculated that one factor is the greater use of forced air warming blankets. What are of proven benefit are the administration of appropriate antibiotic prophylaxis and maintaining patient normothermia.

Vaporizers

Commentary

Vaporizers, volatile agents and circle systems are of obvious clinical relevance, but this being the science section of the exam it is the basic principles which will dominate the questions. The oral should follow a relatively predictable course, including the 'trick' question about the use of vaporizers at altitude.

Core Information

Classification of Vaporizers

- There are three main types of vaporizer. The variable bypass plenum vaporizer is the commonest in routine use. These have a high internal resistance which requires the delivery of fresh gas flow at above atmospheric pressure. They are calibrated specifically to a single agent and are one-directional. The measured gas flow plenum vaporizers have the same basic characteristics but deliver vapour directly to the fresh gas flow (see the following). Draw-over vaporizers are simple low-resistance devices in which the fresh gas flow is at atmospheric pressure. These portable devices are used in field anaesthesia and rarely if ever in the modern hospital setting.

Physical Principles of Vaporization and the Problems for Vaporizer Design

- **Saturated vapour pressure (SVP):** standard vaporizers have to overcome the fact that the SVP of volatile agents at 20 °C is many times greater than that required to produce anaesthesia. (The SVP of sevoflurane is 22.7 kPa, and so its maximum achievable concentration is 22.4% [22.7/101.325]. For desflurane, with an SVP of 89.2, the figure is 88%). Vaporizers have to be designed to allow the addition of a controlled amount of volatile anaesthetic agent to the fresh gas flow, having changed the liquid to a vapour. This is done by streaming the fresh gas flow (FGF).
- **Splitting ratio:** as the FGF enters the vaporizer it is split into two streams; approximately 20% passes into the vaporization chamber while the rest enters a bypass chamber. The gas leaving the vaporizing chamber should be fully saturated with vapour. This is achieved by increasing the available surface area by the use of wicks or a series of baffles. These are variable bypass vaporizers.

- **Desflurane:** the physical properties of desflurane require a more complex vaporizer, one that is designed like no other in current use. At 23.5 °C, the boiling point of desflurane is close to room temperature. Small changes in operating theatre temperature could therefore cause large changes in the SVP of desflurane, with an increase in vapour output. To control this accurately, the vaporizer is heated to 39 °C. This produces a gas under pressure (200 kPa) which is then injected into the FGF. This design obviates the need for any temperature compensation devices. (It is technically easier to heat a vaporizer than to cool it, which would be the alternative technique.) This is an example of a measured flow vaporizer.
- **Latent heat of vaporization:** as a liquid vaporizes so its temperature falls, and compensation for this change is essential. If there is no such compensation, then the SVP of the agent and its delivered concentration will also fall. Vaporizers are made of material with high thermal conductivity, which supplies energy for the heat of vaporization by allowing heat to flow from the vaporizer into the anaesthetic in its liquid phase. The splitting ratio must also be altered as the temperature changes, hence the design of the bimetallic strip (which contains two metals with different coefficients of thermal expansion), which allows more gas into the vaporizing chamber as the temperature drops.
- **Calibration:** vaporizers are calibrated for individual agents, and should one inadvertently be filled with a different volatile anaesthetic then it will deliver either excessive or inadequate vapour concentrations depending on the respective vapour pressures. If a volatile with a high SVP (such as desflurane, 89.2 kPa) is used in a sevoflurane vaporizer (SVP 22.7 kPa), then vapour output will be high. If the situation is reversed, then vapour output will be low. Even if the SVP differences are small, the effect is still significant; isoflurane (SVP 32.5 kPa) in a halothane vaporizer (SVP 32.1 kPa) will deliver a concentration that is 25–50% higher than is dialled up.

Supplementary Information

Potential Problems

- **Flow rate dependence:** modern vaporizers function independently of flow rates between 0.5 and 15 l min^{-1}. Outside these limits they will deliver less than the dialled concentration.
- **Overfilling:** volatile agent may get directly into the bypass chamber if the vaporizer is overfilled, leading to the delivery of dangerously high concentrations.
- **'Pumping' effect:** if a ventilator produces cyclical changes in the pressure in the back bar, this may force gas back into the vaporizing chamber and saturated gas in the vaporizing chamber back into the bypass channel. The forward flow as the ventilator cycles then increases the concentration of delivered vapour. This occurred with minute volume divider ventilators, which are now used much less commonly.
- **'Pressurizing' effect:** this occurs if the overall pressure in the vaporizer is raised (as happens in large vaporizer chambers at high flows). When the gas reaches the common outlet it expands to atmospheric pressure, with a lowering of the effective concentration.
- **Monitoring:** it is obvious that accurate analysis of inspired and end-tidal anaesthetic agents will minimize these theoretical risks.

Effects of Changes in Barometric Pressure

You may be asked a number of miscellaneous questions which may include the use of vaporizers at altitude or under hyperbaric conditions, the characteristics of the desflurane vaporizer and the use of vaporizers inside and outside circle systems.

- **Effects of altitude on variable bypass vaporizers.** At altitude the atmospheric pressure is reduced, but the SVP of the volatile agent remains unchanged. The actual output of vapour in volumes percent increases, but the partial pressure remains the same. For example, if the vaporizer is being used at an altitude where the barometric pressure is half that at sea level (380 mm Hg), then the vapour output will double, and 3.0% sevoflurane as dialled up will deliver 6.0%. (This would be at the improbable height of 6,000 metres). Sevoflurane 3.0% at sea level delivers a partial pressure of 22.8 mm Hg (0.03×760), which is the same as at 6,000 metres (0.06×380). As it is the partial pressure of the agent and not the concentration that is responsible for anaesthesia, the vaporizer can be used in the same way at altitude as at sea level. The same applies to vaporizers used under hyperbaric conditions.

- **Effects of altitude on measured flow vaporizers.** The heated desflurane vaporizer generates a vapour pressure of 200 kPa inside the chamber whatever the ambient atmospheric pressure. Hence 10% desflurane as dialled up will deliver 10% at any altitude. Thus an alveolar partial pressure at sea level of 76 mm Hg (0.1×760) will be halved to 38 mm Hg at 6,000 metres (0.1×380), and so the concentration would have to be increased accordingly.

- **Effects of altitude on Bourdon pressure gauges:** these are calibrated at atmospheric pressure at sea level, and so at increasing altitude the gauges will over-read. The very high pressures in gas cylinders relative to atmosphere, however, means that this potential error is of little clinical consequence.

- **Effects of altitude on flowmeters:** at altitude, the lower density of atmospheric gases means that standard variable orifice constant differential flowmeters will under-read (by around 20% at an altitude of 3,000 metres).

- **Position of vaporizers in the circuit**
  - **VOC (vaporizer outside circle):** plenum vaporizers (in which positive upstream pressure drives the gas) have high internal resistance, are unsuitable for use within circle breathing systems and deliver volatile agent from the back bar of the anaesthetic machine. At low flows, large changes in the dialled concentration are reflected only very slowly within the circle system. A change in FGF rather than vapour concentration may be necessary to effect a more rapid change in the depth of anaesthesia.
  - **VIC (vaporizer inside circle):** drawover vaporizers (in which a subatmospheric pressure generated distal to the vaporizer either mechanically or by the patient's spontaneous respiration, draws the gas through the system) have minimal resistance to flow and can be used within a circle. At low flows the vapour concentration rises, because rather than being diluted it is being added to each inspiration. If the minute volume is large, then the risk of delivering very high concentrations of volatile agent is increased.

Anaesthetic Breathing Systems

Commentary

This is a standard topic, which will inevitably involve a discussion either of the circle system or of the Mapleson classification. Alternatively, you might be asked to talk about both, which means that you will not have to go into the subject in any depth. You may be asked to draw some of the different arrangements, and a useful way of dealing with this request is to give a commentary as you draw the components. If you do this, you will not find yourself sitting at the table drawing in silence while the examiners watch, and it will allow you to demonstrate that you understand how these breathing systems behave. Analysis of the behaviour of the systems can be complex, and so you are more likely to be asked about those (such as the Magill attachment and the circle system) that can be explained within the time available.

Core Information

- **Principles of use of a circle system**
  - **Closed:** the circle system can be used as a genuine closed circuit in which expired gases and volatile agents recirculate. No more oxygen is added than is required for the patient's metabolic demand, and CO_2 is removed by passage of the gases through soda lime. Volatile anaesthetic agents enter the system via vaporizers that can be sited either outside (VOC) the circuit or, much less commonly, within the circuit (VIC) as a drawover vaporizer. In a truly closed system delivering only basal flows, it is important to realize that prolonged anaesthesia with nitrous oxide can cause hypoxia. Consider a situation in which 1.0 l min^{-1} is being delivered, 0.25 l of which is oxygen. At the end of one tidal volume breath this basal oxygen will be absorbed, leaving the alveoli filled with 100% N_2O which will dilute the next breath. Equilibrium takes a long time to achieve, however, and N_2O uptake is still 100 ml h^{-1} after 2 hours. It is prudent, nevertheless, to flush out the system periodically. (At the beginning of anaesthesia there is the opposite problem. The rapid N_2O uptake of 450 ml min^{-1} reduces the partial pressure in the system with the risk of inadequate anaesthesia.)
  - **Semi-open (also referred to as semi-closed):** in this arrangement, the circle is used with a higher than basal FGF with the excess gas being vented through the pressure relief spill valve. Under these circumstances the concentrations of gases and volatile agent in the fresh gas supply are closer to those in the circle and can be changed more quickly. This represents a compromise between economy and ease of use.
- **Practical considerations:** the total volume of the system, including the breathing hoses, the air in the absorber, reservoir bag and the patient's FRC, is around 5 litres. Immediate delivery of low flows at 1.0 l min^{-1} would clearly result in inadequate anaesthesia. An additional factor which reduces anaesthetic partial pressures in the breathing system is the very rapid uptake of N_2O (if used) and volatile agent during the early part of the anaesthetic. This means that high flows must be used for the first 5–10 minutes. A VOC will always show a higher concentration than is being inspired (unless equilibrium has been reached), and rapid changes can only be initiated by a

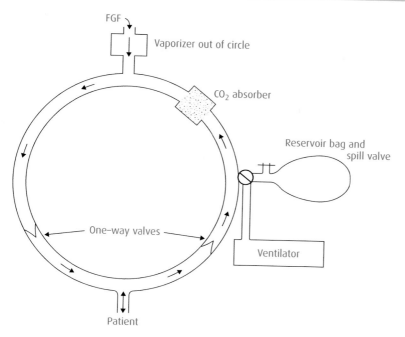

FGF

Vaporizer out of circle

CO_2 absorber

Reservoir bag and
spill valve

One-way valves

Ventilator

Patient

Fig. 5.2 Schematic arrangement of a circle system.

reversion to high flow. If a fully closed system is used, then monitors which measure inspiratory gas and volatile concentrations as close to the patient as possible must be used, and the system should be flushed at regular intervals to minimize the risk of dilutional hypoxia.

Typical components of a circle system.

- **Circle system:** the fresh gas flow, together with volatile anaesthetic (if used), enters the inspiratory limb and travels through a one-way non-return valve to the patient. Expired air enters the expiratory limb and passes through a second non-return valve. Excess gas (mixed expired air) is vented through the pressure relief valve on the reservoir bag, with the remainder passing through the CO_2^- absorbing soda lime and back into the inspiratory limb (Figure 5.2).

You may be asked in more detail why the components are arranged in this way, and what would be the effects of altering their positions in the system. There are numerous potential combinations, but you should be able to answer most variations of this question if you have understood the basic principles of the circuit. (For example, were the pressure relief valve and reservoir bag to be sited between the patient and the inspiratory one-way valve, then rebreathing would occur.)

Advantages and disadvantages of the circle system

- **Advantages:** the circle is very efficient in terms of conservation of gases, heat and moisture. It is therefore more economical and less polluting than semi-closed systems.

- **Disadvantages:** the circle is simple in outline theory but much more complex in detailed execution. The uptake and excretion of the different components within the system can vary greatly, and it is essential to monitor the FiO_2, CO_2 and agent concentration within the circle. The system is slow to react to changes in the inspired volatile concentration. If nitrous oxide is used in a closed system, then hypoxia is a potential risk as described earlier. Should soda lime be allowed to dry it may react with the CHF_2 group of desflurane, isoflurane and enflurane to produce carbon monoxide.

You may be asked to compare the behaviour of the circle breathing systems with those systems categorized by Mapleson.

The Mapleson Classification

There are apparently more logical ways of analyzing breathing systems, but this classification has become hallowed by tradition and familiarity, and shows little sign of being superseded. (Mapleson was Professor of Medical Physics in Cardiff who, in 1953, published his analysis of the behaviour of the various combinations of the valve, tubing, reservoir bag and FGF that were used in breathing systems.) Strictly speaking, these should always be described as breathing *systems* rather than *circuits*, but common usage makes the term permissible, although technically incorrect.

- **Classification:** the systems were classified as A to F, and they all potentially allow rebreathing. They are 'semi-closed' ('semi-open' in the USA) and supply more gas than the patient needs, with the excess being vented to the atmosphere. If rebreathing of CO_2 does occur, a healthy patient who is breathing spontaneously will respond by increasing alveolar ventilation which will rise, by up to 20 times if necessary, to keep the $PaCO_2$ normal. These systems are defined therefore in terms of the FGF that is needed to maintain an unchanged $PaCO_2$ in the face of unchanged ventilation.
- **Mapleson A:** this is most commonly used in the form of the Magill attachment and comprises a reservoir bag into which the FGF is directed, a length of corrugated tubing (which is resistant to kinking) and, at the patient end, an adjustable pressure-limiting (APL) valve (Figure 5.3).
  - **Spontaneous respiration:** the system is very efficient. At the end of inspiration the valve is closed and the reservoir bag is emptying. During expiration, the FGF is filling the reservoir bag, while expired air (dead space gas and then alveolar gas) is passing into the tube. Hence the pressure in both the reservoir bag and the breathing system increase to the point at which the valve opens and vents expired air. The FGF continues to flow down the tube. At an FGF equal to the alveolar

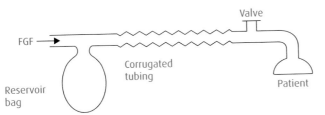

Fig. 5.3 Mapleson A breathing system. FGF, Fresh gas flow.

ventilation, it is alveolar gas and not dead space gas that is expelled preferentially. This analysis is based on the assumption that there is no longitudinal mixing of dead space and alveolar gases, and Mapleson recommended that the FGF should equal the minute ventilation. (Subsequent investigation suggested that 70% of minute ventilation, i.e. the alveolar ventilation, would be adequate.)

— **Controlled ventilation**: if controlled ventilation is used, the circuit loses all its economy. Fresh gas is vented during inspiration, while during expiration the valve tends to close, and all expired air passes back into the system which selectively retains expired air. To prevent rebreathing the FGF should be at least twice the minute ventilation.

— **Co-axial versions**: co-axial versions, of which the commonest is the Lack system, function in the same way. Early narrow co-axial systems effectively reduced the capacity of the outer expiratory limb to store gas, and hence expired gas could reach the reservoir bag. Increasing the dimensions solved this problem, but at the cost of increasing the bulk of the system.

- **Mapleson B and C:** the Mapleson C comprises an APL at the patient end with the FGF entering just proximally. A short length of tubing connects this to the reservoir bag which, in the classic 'Waters' circuit, includes a CO_2-absorbing canister. The Mapleson B includes a length of corrugated tubing between the FGF and the reservoir bag. The Mapleson C circuit is used in resuscitation and in areas such as theatre recovery. Both systems allow mixing of expired air with the FGF, which must approximate three times minute ventilation to flush the system and prevent rebreathing. A Mapleson B circuit nevertheless is still more efficient than the Mapleson A during controlled ventilation (Figure 5.4).

- **Mapleson D, E and F:** these systems all function as T-pieces, being inefficient for spontaneous respiration but efficient for controlled ventilation. Analysis of their behaviour is much more complex than that of the Mapleson A system, although, as a simplification, they require up to three times the minute ventilation to prevent rebreathing during spontaneous respiration (150–200 ml kg^{-1}) but only 70 ml kg^{-1} to achieve normocapnia during IPPV. Analysis is complicated by, amongst other factors, the influence of the respiratory pattern. The respiratory cycle is a sinusoidal waveform, and, in order to prevent rebreathing, the FGF must equal or exceed the

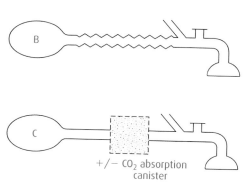

Fig. 5.4 Mapleson B and C breathing systems.

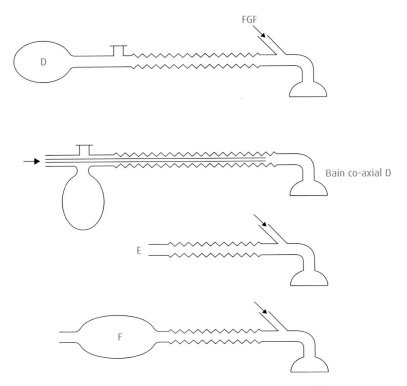

FGF

D

Bain co-axial D

E

F

Fig. 5.5 Mapleson D, E and F breathing systems. FGF, Fresh gas flow.

peak inspiratory flow rate (PIFR). At end-expiration, alveolar gas has moved into the expiratory limb where it mixes with the FGF, and, to prevent rebreathing, the FGF should approach three times the minute ventilation. If, however, there is an expiratory pause, some alveolar gas will be expelled by the FGF and theoretically the flow rate can be decreased (Figure 5.5).

— **Mapleson D:** the Bain circuit is the co-axial version of the Mapleson D circuit.
— **Mapleson E:** this is the original Ayre's T-piece. It can allow both rebreathing of CO_2-containing gas as well as entrainment of ambient air. There is no reservoir bag and expiratory resistance is negligible.
— **Mapleson F:** this differs from the E only in that it has a reservoir bag, added by Jackson-Rees (who was a paediatric anaesthetist in Liverpool) to allow controlled ventilation. The system has no valves and so there is minimal expiratory resistance, hence its traditional use in paediatric anaesthesia. Effective scavenging is difficult from both the E and F systems.
• **Humphrey ADE system:** the Humphrey block is located at the common gas outlet and exists in both parallel and co-axial versions (of equal efficiency). It comprises an APL valve, a pressure relief valve, a reservoir bag, a ventilator port and a lever for selection of spontaneous ventilation (in the A mode) or controlled ventilation (in D/E mode).

- **Monitoring:** it is worth commenting that, although it is important to understand the functional behaviour of these breathing systems, the modern ability to measure the concentrations of gases and volatile agents has removed many of the potential hazards posed by imprecision of the analyses and by inter-patient variability.

Soda Lime

Commentary

This question appears in the Final FRCA, although it is a topic that you may already have encountered in the Primary. The potential clinical problems with the use of soda lime are almost entirely theoretical, but there will be insufficient time for a discussion of low-flow anaesthesia, which, logically, is where the oral should lead. The subject is conceptually not difficult, and so this is another one of those questions about which you will just have to know some of the facts. It is worth remembering the formula for the chemical reaction, not for its intrinsic utility, but because if you are struggling with a particular topic examiners will often ask a straightforward factual question as a way of trying to restore your confidence and get you back on track.

Core Information

The composition of soda lime and its mode of action.

- Soda lime is used to absorb CO_2. The discovery is not recent; it has been known for more than two centuries that CO_2 is absorbed by strong alkali (caustic soda).
- Its main use is to allow the rebreathing of exhaled gases within breathing systems. This is most commonly the circle system, although it was also used in the original Waters circuit. To-and-fro breathing was allowed by the insertion into the system of a small soda lime canister.
- Its chemical constituents are calcium hydroxide ($Ca[OH]_2$) 80%, sodium hydroxide (NaOH) 2% and water (H_2O). (Potassium hydroxide [KOH] was previously added as an accelerator, but this is one of the strong alkalis which are implicated in the formation of carbon monoxide and Compound A and so was removed by the manufacturers, who also reduced the level of NaOH from around 4% down to 2%).
- Also added are silicates in trace amounts which harden the granules which otherwise would disintegrate into powder. An indicator dye is present which changes the colour of the soda lime as it is progressively exhausted. This is either phenolphthalein (the colour changes from red to white) or, less commonly, ethyl violet (the colour changes from white to purple). As these colour changes are in opposite directions, it is clearly important to know which dye is being used.
- Soda lime is formed either into granules whose size is 4–8 mesh (mesh describes the number of openings per inch in a uniform metal strainer) or into spheres. The more uniform the shape, the greater the likelihood of uniform flow through the canister.

The size of the granules or spheres is a compromise between providing the largest surface area for absorption without providing excessive resistance to flow.
- Under ideal conditions, 1 kg can absorb up to 250 litres of CO_2.
- In the presence of water and with NaOH as an activator, the chemical reaction can be summarized as follows:

$$\text{Full equation}: CO_2 + H_2O \rightarrow H_2CO_3$$

$$2H_2CO_3 + 2NaOH + Ca(OH)_2 \rightarrow Na_2CO_3 + CaCO_3 + 4H_2O + \text{Heat}$$

$$\text{Simple equation}: CO_2 + Ca(OH)_2 \rightarrow CaCO_3 + H_2O$$

- Partially exhausted soda lime may regenerate on standing, with the migration of unused hydroxide ions from the core to outer areas. The colour may also revert; however, its absorptive capacity in this state is minimal.

Other Compounds That Can Be Used to Absorb CO_2
- **Barium lime (Baralyme):** this consists of calcium hydroxide $(Ca[OH]_2)$ 80% and barium hydroxide $(Ba[OH]_2)$ 20%. Water is incorporated into the structure of Ba $(OH)_2$. The chemical reaction is similar to that of soda lime, although it is less efficient.
- **Amsorb:** this compound (developed in Belfast) contains $Ca(OH)_2$, calcium chloride and two setting agents. Its absorption capacity is comparable to other agents, but its use is associated neither with carbon monoxide (CO) nor compound A formation.

Reactions between CO_2 Absorbents and Anaesthetic Agents
- **Carbon monoxide (CO):** modern anaesthetic machines continue to deliver a fresh gas flow of 200 ml min^{-1} of oxygen even when the flowmeters are turned off. If the machine goes unused for some time, then this constant flow may dry out a canister of soda or barium lime. Under these circumstances, the reaction of the desiccated absorbent with the CHF_2 group of isoflurane, enflurane or desflurane can produce high levels of CO.
- **Compound A:** sevoflurane reacts with strong monovalent hydroxide bases, such as those which are used in soda lime and barium lime CO_2-absorbers, to produce a number of substances, including compound A. (The reaction with barium lime is about five times more rapid than with soda lime.) Of the degradation products (compounds A, B, D, E and G), only compound A, a vinyl halide, has been shown to have any toxicity. However, the dose-dependent renal damage noted in rats has never been seen in humans. Amsorb appears to be safer in this respect. Compound A production is substantially reduced if the absorbent is cooled.
- **Trilene (trichloroethylene):** of historical interest, and included just in case the topic should arise, is the reaction between the volatile agent trilene and soda lime. This produced dichloroacetylene, which is a potent neurotoxin that affected particularly the trigeminal and facial nerves.

Scavenging

Commentary

This topic is dull, but it is hard to argue with the importance of minimizing pollution within the theatre environment, and so scavenging is something that you will have to know about, even though the direct clinical implications are only modest.

Core Information

- **Scavenging system:** the basic arrangement comprises collection, transfer, receiving and disposal systems.
  - **Collection system:** this is usually a shroud that is connected to the APL or expiratory valves of the ventilator via a 30-mm connector (which prevents confusion with components of the breathing system).
  - **Transfer system:** this comprises wide-bore tubing to remove the gases.
  - **Receiving system:** this is a reservoir system, which is protected against excessive pressures by valves. The positive pressure relief valve is set at 1,000 Pa (1 kPa); the negative pressure relief valve is set at −50 Pa (0.05 kPa).
  - **Disposal system:** subatmospheric pressure to eject the gases is generated by a fan which develops a low-pressure high-volume system which can vent 75 l min^{-1}. Other ejector systems include vacuums and venturi devices. Passive extraction is used only in areas where this level of sophistication is unaffordable, but whatever the system, the exhaust is simply vented to atmosphere where the pollution becomes someone else's problem.
- There are two main types of system: **passive** and **active**.
  - **Passive systems:** the components of the system are as described earlier, and the gases are vented to atmosphere either by the patient's spontaneous respiratory efforts or by the mechanical ventilator.

    The 'Cardiff Aldasorber' is another passive device which comprises a canister containing charcoal particles that absorb halogenated volatile anaesthetic agents. Absorption does not render the agents inert; if the canister is disposed of by incineration, the inhalational agents are released to atmosphere. This device does not absorb nitrous oxide.
  - **Active systems:** the basic components of the system are again as described , but the vacuum created by a fan or a pump in the disposal system draws the anaesthetic gases through the system. It is important that the negative pressures so generated cannot be transmitted to the patient.

Supplementary Information

- **Purpose of scavenging:** the safe removal of waste theatre gases is a health and safety issue and, since 1989, with the government introduction of Control of Substances Hazardous to Health (COSHH), has been a legal requirement. It is only the local environment that is protected, because the gases are pollutants that are vented unchanged to atmosphere. Most are potent greenhouse gases.

- **Staff health issues:** some studies have identified increased risks of spontaneous abortion in women exposed to trace concentrations of anaesthetic gases, and also that male anaesthetists were more likely to father daughters than sons. There was, in addition, the suggestion of an increase in haematological malignancies. The association is not strong, because other studies have not replicated these data. Moreover, many millions of general anaesthetics are given annually in the developed world and were this to be a real problem, then its provenance would be a lot more obvious.

Other Means of Minimizing Operating Theatre Pollution
- Theatre air changes (at least 15 times per hour).
- Substitution of total intravenous anaesthesia (TIVA) and regional anaesthesia for inhalational anaesthesia.
- Use of low- and ultra-low-flow breathing systems.

Maximum Permitted Exposure Levels
These maxima are expressed as an 8-hour time-weighted average. The practical relevance of knowing these numbers is elusive, and it also seems suspicious both that there is such a big variation in levels between the UK and the USA, and that in the UK the permitted maxima are all multiples of 10. This looks more like number preference than science, and so the evidence underlying these permitted levels may not therefore be robust.

- Permitted maxima
    - **Nitrous oxide:** 100 parts per million (ppm) (25 ppm in the USA).
    - **Isoflurane and enflurane**: 50 ppm.
    - **Sevoflurane and desflurane:** 50 ppm. As yet there are no maximum limits; COSHH states that their similarity to enflurane means that 50 ppm would be appropriate.
    - **Halothane:** 10 ppm.
    - **USA:** in America, the permitted maximum for all halogenated volatiles is 2 ppm.

The Gas Laws

Commentary
This is the kind of question that you thought you had left behind when you passed the Primary FRCA exam, but it does reappear in the Final. It will not be asked of you in any greater detail, and the examiners are expecting you to list each gas law and indicate their relevance to anaesthetic practice.

Core Information

The Gas Laws

- **Boyle's law**
  - This is the first perfect gas law. It states that at a constant temperature, the volume of a given (fixed) mass of gas varies inversely with the absolute pressure. It can be expressed the other way round, namely that at a constant temperature, the pressure of a given mass of gas is inversely proportional to the volume. Pressure (P) × volume (V), therefore, is a constant.
  - (This law was described in 1662 by Robert Boyle [1627–1691], born in Ireland as the youngest of 14 children, but who lived and studied in England and who was one of the founders of the scientific method.)
- **Charles's law**
  - This is the second perfect gas law. It states that at a constant pressure, the volume of a given mass of gas varies directly with the absolute temperature (T). The relationship is linear, which means that at absolute zero that fixed mass of gas would have no volume.
  - (This law was described in 1787 by Jacques Charles [1746–1823], a French physicist who constructed the first gas balloon and who later made an ascent to an altitude of greater than 10,000 feet.)
- **Universal gas law**
  - Boyle's Law and Charles's Law can be combined to give the universal gas law, in which $P \times V = T \times n$R, where R is the universal gas constant (8.1 J K^{-1} mol^{-1}) and n is the number of moles of a gas.
- **Gay-Lussac's law**
  - From the equation $PV = nRT$ it is evident that, for a fixed mass of gas at constant volume, the pressure varies directly with temperature.
  - (The enunciation of this relationship is attributed to another physicist [and balloonist], Joseph Gay-Lussac [1778–1850]. In some texts this is described as the 'third perfect gas law'.)
- **Dalton's law of partial pressures**
  - This states that the pressure that is exerted by each gas in a mixture of gases is the same as it would exert if it alone occupied the container.
  - (This law was described in 1801 by John Dalton [1766–1844], an English chemist from Manchester. He also did early work on colour blindness, which for a while became known as Daltonism.)
- **Henry's law**
  - This states that the amount of gas that is dissolved in a liquid at a given temperature is proportional to the partial pressure in the gas in equilibrium with the solution.
  - (This law was described in 1801 by William Henry [1774–1836], an English chemist and physician. He also identified as methane the gas known as 'firedamp' that was responsible for the death of miners.)
- **Avogadro's law**
  - This states that equal volumes of gases at the same temperature and pressure contain the same number of molecules. This also means that 1 g molecular weight

of any gas occupies the same volume (22.4 litres at standard temperature and pressure, STP, which is 273.15 K (0° C) and 101.325 kPa).
— (The law was described in 1811 by Amadeus Avogadro [1776–1856], an Italian professor of mathematical physics who lived and worked in Turin. This theory went unremarked for more than 50 years, partly due to the scepticism and opposition of scientists such as Dalton.)
- **Combined gas laws:** the gas laws can be combined so that

$$P_1 \times V_1/T_1 = P_2 \times V_2/T_2.$$

Supplementary Information and Clinical Applications

It would be more logical were you to be asked to give examples of the anaesthetic relevance of the gas laws as you describe them. In practice, however, this discussion tends to be deferred until the second part of the oral. The reason for this is probably that if a candidate spends a lot of time struggling to identify the clinical application of the first one or two gas laws, then they may not have a chance to give the examiner the rest of the list that is expected.

Some practical applications include the following.

- **Boyle's law:** (At constant T, PV is a constant; so $P_1 \times V_1 = P_2 \times V_2$.)
  — This can be used to calculate the volume of gas remaining in a cylinder. A size E oxygen cylinder has an internal volume of 10 litres, and so contains 10 litres (V_1) at 13,800 kPa (P_1). (Remember that this is absolute pressure, so 100 kPa of atmospheric pressure must be included.) At atmospheric pressure (P_2) there will therefore be 1,380 litres of oxygen (V_2) available from the cylinder.
- **Dalton's law of partial pressures:** (The pressure exerted by each gas in a mixture is the same as if it were alone.)
  — This is relevant for the partial pressure of gases in any mixture, whether it be in a cylinder or within the alveoli.
  — Dalton's law explains why the settings on variable bypass vaporizers do not have to be altered when used at altitude.
- **Henry's law:** (The amount of gas that is dissolved in a liquid at a given temperature is proportional to the partial pressure in the gas in equilibrium with the solution.)
  — This has relevance for hyperbaric therapy. At atmospheric pressure and breathing air, the O_2 solubility coefficient (0.003 ml dl^{-1} $mmHg^{-1}$) means that the dissolved oxygen content is about 0.26 ml dl^{-1}. In a patient breathing 100% oxygen, this increases to 1.7 ml dl^{-1}, and at three atmospheres in a hyperbaric chamber it reaches 5.6 ml dl^{-1}. At this level of pressure, therefore, dissolved oxygen can make a significant contribution to delivery. If nitrogen is present in the gas mixture then it will pass into the tissues, only to come out of solution in the form of bubbles if the pressure decreases too abruptly. This is the cause of decompression sickness.
- **Avogadro's law:** (Equal volumes of gases at the same temperature and pressure contain the same number of molecules.)
  — This can be used, for example, to calibrate a vaporizer. The molecular weight of sevoflurane is 200, 1 mole is 200 g and will occupy 22.4 litres at STP. Imagine,

therefore, a vaporizer containing 40 ml of sevoflurane, which is 0.2 mol occupying 4.48 litres at STP. If this is vaporized fully into oxygen of volume 224 litres, then the resulting concentration will be 4.48/224 or 2%.

Gases and Vapours

Commentary

This is another area that could be seen more properly as being the province of the Primary exam, but subjects related to gases, vapours and pressures will be viewed inevitably as appropriate for discussion. Oral questioning on these subjects can be haphazard, and you may be asked for a number of definitions before moving on to one or more disparate topics, amongst which may be partial pressure, saturated vapour pressure (SVP), vaporizers, water vapour and humidification.

Core Information

There is no obvious clinical entry point for this topic and so you may be asked first for some definitions.

- **Gas:** a gas is a substance above its critical temperature.
- **Vapour:** a vapour is a substance below its critical temperature.
- **Critical temperature:** this is defined as the temperature above which a gas cannot be liquefied, no matter how great is the pressure that is applied.
- **Critical pressure:** this is defined as the vapour pressure of the substance at its critical temperature. It is the pressure needed to liquefy the gas at its critical temperature.
- **SVP:** a saturated vapour is one that is in equilibrium with its own liquid, so the number of molecules entering the liquid phase equals those entering the vapour phase. If the temperature rises, more molecules enter the vapour phase and the vapour pressure rises. The SVP is the maximum partial pressure that can be achieved at a given temperature. The relationship of SVP and temperature is nonlinear. You could be asked the maximum concentration of one or other of the volatile agents that can be obtained at 20 °C. The SVP of sevoflurane at this temperature is 22.7 kPa; its maximum concentration is therefore 22.7/101 or approximately 22.5%.
- **Boiling point:** when the SVP is the same as the ambient pressure, the liquid boils and the vapour concentration at the surface of the liquid is 100%. Hence the boiling point is the temperature at which the vapour pressure of a liquid equals the ambient temperature above it. The boiling point will therefore decrease as the ambient pressure falls, for example, during ascent to altitude.
- **Latent heat:** when any substance changes from a liquid to a vapour or from a solid to a liquid, heat must be supplied despite the fact that this change of state takes place at a constant temperature. This is the latent heat of vaporization (if the change is from a liquid to a vapour) or the latent heat of fusion (if the change is from a solid to a

liquid). In any particular homogenous fluid the molecules do not possess identical kinetic energy. Those with a higher velocity escape the surface of the liquid and are vaporized, thus the mean kinetic energy of the remainder diminishes and the liquid cools. The latent heat of vaporization is defined as the additional heat that is required to convert a given mass of liquid into vapour at the same temperature. Conversely, heat is generated as vapour condenses back to a liquid.

- **Pseudocritical temperature:** in a mixture of gases there is a specific critical temperature, the pseudocritical temperature, at which the gas mixture may separate into its different constituents. The only stored gas mixture in common use in anaesthesia is Entonox (50% O_2: 50% N_2O). The critical temperature of N_2O is 36.5 °C, but the interaction with oxygen lowers this to −5.5 °C (its pseudocritical temperature). Thus, below −6 °C, liquefaction of nitrous oxide takes place. This is potentially dangerous because, although at this point the N_2O has about 20% oxygen dissolved in it, as the oxygen-rich supernatant is drawn off, the oxygen in the liquid comes out of solution, leading eventually to the delivery of a hypoxic mixture.

Clinical Applications

- **N_2O cylinders:** the critical temperature of N_2O is 36.5 °C, and so under normal circumstances in temperate climates it is stored in a liquid phase with its vapour above it. In the UK the filling ratio (the mass of gas in the cylinder divided by the mass of water that would completely fill the cylinder) is 0.75, to allow for expansion and to limit increases in pressure. As the liquid expands it compresses its vapour, some of which then condenses back to a liquid and restricts the pressure rise. In hotter climates the filling ratio is 0.67. If an N_2O cylinder is used continuously, it will cool as it vaporizes and the saturated vapour and gauge pressures will drop. If the gas is turned off, then both will be restored to normal as the cylinder rewarms. The belief that the gauge pressure will remain unchanged until the moment just before the cylinder empties is therefore a misconception.
- **Oxygen supplies:** liquid oxygen must be kept at a temperature lower than its critical temperature of 118 °C (see under 'Supply of Medical Gases'.)
- **Vaporization of volatile anaesthetic agents:** see under 'Vaporizers'.
- **Water vapour and humidification:** see under 'Humidification (of Inspired Gases)'.

Pressure

Commentary

Pressures and their measurement are so much part of anaesthesia that it is not surprising to find them appearing as examination topics. The oral may start with any one of the disparate clinical implications before moving on to the underlying principles of definition and measurement. Alternatively, some of the basic science outlined in the following may form part of questioning on one of many potential subjects.

Core Information
Definitions and methods of measurement.

- **Definitions:** pressure is defined as force per unit area, force being that which changes or tends to change the state of rest or motion of an object. The unit of force is the newton (N), 1 N being that force which will accelerate a (frictionless) mass of 1 kg at 1 m s^{-2} (in a vacuum). The SI unit of pressure is the pascal (Pa), 1 pascal being a force of 1 N acting over an area of 1 m^2. Gravity gives any mass an acceleration of 9.81 m s^{-2}, so the force acting on 1 kg is 9.81 N. 1 N is therefore equivalent to 102 g. This is a small pressure, hence the use of the kilopascal (kPa) as the main unit of physiological pressure. Higher pressures are still quoted in bar (1 bar = 100 kPa = 1 atmosphere).
- (The relationship between force and pressure explains why a small syringe can generate far higher pressures than a larger one. The pressure developed is force divided by area. The smaller the area represented by the plunger in the syringe, then the greater is the pressure generated for a given applied force; hence a 2 ml syringe is much more effective than a 10 ml syringe in flushing a blocked intravenous catheter.)
- **Absolute pressure and gauge pressure:** an empty gas cylinder has a gauge pressure of zero, but the ambient pressure inside the cylinder is 1 atmosphere. Absolute pressure, therefore, is given by the gauge pressure plus atmospheric pressure.
- **Measurement**
  - **Liquid manometry:** the pressure in the column is equal to the product of the height of the column, the density of the liquid and the force of gravity. The width and shape of the column have no effect on the pressure reading. Surface tension provides a potential source of error in columns less than 10 mm in diameter, but in the clinical context of central venous pressure measurement, in which trends are commonly more important than absolute numbers, this is not significant.
  - **Aneroid gauges:** examples include the Bourdon gauge for high pressures, which comprises a flattened coiled tube which unwinds as pressures increase.
  - **Diaphragm gauges:** these are used for many physiological pressures. Pressure changes cause movement in a flexible diaphragm, and these are either read directly or transduced. Electromechanical devices are probably the commonest, employing wire strain gauges whose resistance changes in response to pressure. The sensing diaphragm can also be incorporated as one plate of a capacitor, the other being fixed. The charge that is carried varies with the separation of the plates.

Clinical Applications
- **Non-invasive blood pressure:** automatic machines utilize the oscillometric principle. The movement of the arterial wall is transmitted to the cuff, and the pressure changes are sensed by a transducer. Above systolic pressure and below diastolic pressure, the oscillations are minimal. As the cuff deflates automatically to systolic pressure, oscillations begin and increase in amplitude until mean blood pressure is reached, after which the amplitude decreases until the diastolic pressure point is reached. The fluctuations are analyzed by a microprocessor prior to being displayed digitally.
- **Invasive blood pressure:** see under 'Intra-arterial Blood Pressure Measurement' in the next section.

- **Central venous pressure:** see under 'Central Venous Pressure and Cannulation' in Chapter 3.
- **Intravascular pressures – Laplace's law:** in a tube, such as the aorta, the transmural pressure gradient is given by the wall tension divided by the radius ($P = T/r$). For a sphere the relationship is $P = 2T/r$. This pressure relationship explains why an expanding aortic aneurysm is increasingly likely to rupture as the aorta dilates, and why a reservoir bag on a breathing circuit does not cause barotrauma to normal lungs if it is allowed to distend by tightening the valve.
- **The Venturi principle:** flowing gas contains potential energy (from its pressure) and kinetic energy (associated with its flow). At a constriction, the flow, and hence the kinetic energy of the gas, increases. The total amount of energy must remain constant, and so the potential energy, and hence the pressure, decreases, allowing the entrainment of gas or fluid.
- **Intracranial pressure:** see under 'Intracranial Pressure' in Chapter 3.
- **Intrapleural pressures:** see under 'Pneumothorax' in Chapter 3. **Intraocular pressure:** see under 'Intraocular Pressure' in Chapter 3. The normal value is 10–22 mmHg, and its prime determinants are choroidal blood flow and volume (influenced by $PaCO_2$, venous drainage, hypoxia), the formation and drainage of aqueous humour, and external pressure on the globe by contraction of extraocular muscles and of the orbicularis oculi muscle (or by orbital local anaesthetic or retrobulbar haemorrhage). Coughing, straining or vomiting will transiently increase the pressure by 40 mmHg or more.

Intra-Arterial Blood Pressure Measurement

Commentary

Invasive arterial blood pressure monitoring is a routine part of modern anaesthetic and intensive care practice, and so the questioning is likely to include clinical aspects such as indications and complications. The rest of the oral will concentrate on the physics that underlies the behaviour of a measurement system. You will not, however, be asked to discuss Fourier analysis of complex waveforms; time constraints will not allow it, and it would take the questioning too far away from applied clinical science. Make sure, however, that you can draw the main arterial waveforms, because these are relevant to clinical practice.

Core Information

The components of a system for direct blood pressure measurement and the generation of the arterial waveform.

- The basic system for invasive blood pressure measurement consists of a parallel-walled intra-arterial cannula, a column of saline which is in continuity with blood, and a transducer (a device that converts the mechanical energy into an electrical signal that is processed and displayed on a monitor). The column of saline is pressurized to 300 mmHg and incorporates a manual flushing device.

- The fluid-filled catheter is in direct contact with the diaphragm of the transducer. Movement of this diaphragm is associated with alteration in the length of a strain gauge, which in some transducers is in the form of a wire resistor in a Wheatstone bridge circuit. (This contains four resistances, one of which is a strain gauge, another of which is variable. The variable resistance can be altered so that when $R_1/R_2 = R_3/R_4$ there is no current flow.) Most transducers include four strain gauges, comprising the four resistances of the bridge. The resistances of two gauges at opposite sides of the bridge are designed to increase as the pressure increases, whereas the resistances of the other two decrease. This gives rise to a larger potential change, with a deflection in the galvanometer that is amplified and displayed as a pressure.

- This whole system oscillates at the frequency of the arterial pulse, which is the fundamental frequency (the first harmonic). The arterial pressure waveform, however, comprises a series of sine waves of different frequencies and amplitude. For the system to reproduce the amplitude and phase difference of each harmonic to produce an accurate waveform, it requires a frequency response that is around 10 times the fundamental frequency (the heart rate). If the heart rate is 150 beats per minute, the frequency response would need to be $(150 \times 10)/60 = 25$ Hz. The more rapid the rate of pressure change, the greater the number of harmonics. In practice, this means that the system requires a flat frequency response between 0.5 and 30 Hz.

- To reproduce the arterial waveform accurately, any recording system must also reproduce the amplitude and phase difference of each harmonic in the waveform. The system, therefore, needs a high resonant (or natural) frequency, which can then be optimally damped.

- This natural frequency is the frequency at which any system will resonate, and at which amplification of the signal will occur. If this frequency lies within the range of frequencies that comprise the pressure waveform, then that signal may be distorted by the superimposed sine wave that will be generated.

- The resonant frequency of the pressure-measuring system can be manipulated by altering the characteristics of its components. It is directly proportional to the diameter of the catheter, and is inversely proportional to the square root of the compliance or elasticity of the system, to the square root of the length of tubing and to the square root of the density of the fluid within the system. This has clinical relevance, because stiffening the diaphragm of the transducer, shortening the length of the intra-arterial cannula or increasing its diameter, will lift the resonant frequency out of the frequency response range.

- **Damping.** If there is no damping, the system oscillates at its natural frequency. If the system is overdamped, the recorded signal falls slowly to the baseline. This can occur when there ceases to be free communication between the column of blood and the diaphragm of the transducer. A large air bubble, for example, will absorb pressure due to its compressibility, while clot or debris will restrict the pressure transmission even more effectively. The whole waveform trace is flattened as a result. If the damping is adjusted so that the output signal falls more rapidly to the baseline, but without any overshoot, then the system is described as being critically damped. (The 'damping factor' gives a quantitative assessment of the degree of damping. A critically damped system is said to have a damping factor of 1.0.) With critical damping, the amplitude is registered accurately but the speed of response is too slow.

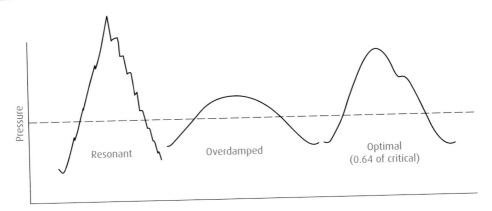

Fig. 5.6 Arterial waveforms.

The best compromise between speed and accuracy is when the system is optimally damped, which is at 0.64 of critical. An underdamped waveform will increase systolic and decrease diastolic pressures (damping factor of <0.64), whereas an overdamped signal (damping factor >1.0) will decrease both (Figure 5.6). The mean arterial pressure in both instances will (largely) be unchanged.

Supplementary Information and Clinical Considerations

- **Indications:** these are not difficult to define. Direct intra-arterial blood pressure monitoring (IABP) gives beat-to-beat information which is particularly useful in patients with actual or potential cardiovascular instability. It is used routinely in the critically ill, both to measure pressures and to allow arterial blood gas analysis. It is helpful in high-risk patients undergoing surgery, and in patients facing high-risk surgery. Many anaesthetists would also regard its use as mandatory whenever intravenous vasoactive drugs are used to manipulate the blood pressure, particularly in hypotensive anaesthesia. It may also be indicated in very obese patients whose size makes other methods of blood pressure monitoring inaccurate.

- **Information provided by direct IABP monitoring:** this is not confined purely to numbers (Figure 5.7). The slope of the systolic upstroke gives some indication of the contractile state of the myocardium, and the maximum rate of rise of left ventricular pressure (dP/dt max) can be calculated. The area under the curve up to the position of the dicrotic notch gives an indication of stroke volume, and the position of the dicrotic notch on the downstroke of the waveform reflects systemic vascular resistance. In the presence of peripheral vasoconstriction, the dicrotic notch is high; if there is vasodilatation, then it moves lower down the curve. Pressure changes during IPPV can also be significant; a systolic pressure variation between the maximum and minimum recorded during the respiratory cycle of more than 10 mmHg suggests at least a 10% reduction in circulating volume.

- **Complications:** vascular damage distal to the cannula may follow because of direct occlusion, of later occlusion due to thrombosis or as a result of inadvertent intra-arterial injection. Disconnection is a potential hazard; fatal exsanguination could occur should it go unrecognized. Long-term cannulation, as is common in intensive care patients, may also be complicated by infection.

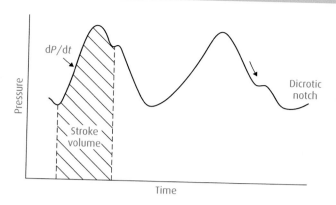

Fig. 5.7 The arterial pressure waveform.

Measurement of Organ Blood Flow

Commentary

This question may no longer stand alone, but details of these methods of determining flow may form part of questions on other topics. Examiners are likely to concentrate more on those methods that are useful clinically, such as Doppler ultrasonography and techniques based on the Fick principle.

Core Information

Determination of organ blood flow.

- **Direct cannulation and measurement:** this is possible, but impractical in any clinical context.
- **Doppler ultrasonography:** the Doppler effect describes the change in the frequency of sound (including ultrasound) if either the emitter or the receiver is moving. If a noise source, for example a siren, moves towards a listener, the wavelength of the sound decreases, its frequency increases, and so its pitch rises. This principle is utilized in Doppler ultrasonography, in which ultrasound is directed at a diagonal from one crystal and is sensed by a second crystal as it reflects off red blood cells. The frequency of these reflected waves increases by an amount that is proportional to the velocity of flow towards the receiving crystal. It is difficult to calibrate a Doppler ultrasound probe to provide accurate quantitative measurements because determinations of vessel calibre may be inaccurate, and the shape of the flow profile may not be uniform. Nonetheless, the technique can provide some assessment of the adequacy of flow, particularly after vascular surgery to the carotid arteries or to vessels of the lower limb. It can also be used to give a non-invasive determination of cardiac output by measuring velocity in the arch of the aorta and relating it to aortic diameter. Transcranial Doppler ultrasonography can be used to give a measure of flow through large cerebral arteries.

- **Doppler equation:** (if you are asked this it may not be as malevolent as it sounds. The examiner may be assuming that a straightforward factual question will either give you some confidence or restore it after a shaky start.)

$$Fd = 2FtVCos\theta/C$$

Fd is flow; Ft is transmitted Doppler frequency; V is the speed of blood flow; $Cos\theta$ is the cosine of the blood flow to beam angle; C is the speed of sound in tissue.

- **The Fick principle:** this is the basis of several methods which are used to measure both cardiac output and regional blood flow. It underlies thermal and chemical indicator dilution tests, renal clearance estimations and measurement of cerebral blood flow. It has been described as an application of the law of conservation of matter, in that the uptake or excretion of a substance by an organ or tissue must be equal to the difference between the amount entering the organ (arterial flow $\times$ concentration) and the amount leaving the organ (venous flow $\times$ venous concentration). Rearrangement of this relationship gives the familiar formula, namely that blood flow to an organ = rate of uptake or rate of excretion of a substance/ arteriovenous concentration. If oxygen is used as the substance, for example, then cardiac output is given by:

$$CO = VO_2 (ml\ min^{-1}) / Arterial\ O_2 content\ (CaO_2 - Venous\ O_2 content\ (CvO_2)$$

The Fick principle applies only to situations in which the arterial supply presents the only source of the substance that is taken up.

- **Indicator dilution methods:** this was the commonest method in clinical use during the era in which pulmonary artery catheters were popular. The thermodilution technique for measuring cardiac output involves both injection and sampling carried out via a catheter in the right side of the heart. Cold fluid (such as glucose 5% at 0 °C) is injected into the right atrium, and the temperature change is detected by a thermistor at the distal end of the flotation catheter in the pulmonary artery. The recorded temperatures generate a concentration against time dilution curve analogous to that which would be seen had a chemical indicator been used. The equation that is used is as follows: Flow (cardiac output) = 'heat dose' $\times$ 60/average concentration (AUC) $\times$ time (s). The injectate–blood temperature difference multiplied by the density, specific heat and volume of the injectate gives the numerator (the heat dose). The area under the curve (AUC) multiplied by the density and specific heat of blood gives the denominator. The potential complexity of these calculations means that the cardiac output determinations are computer generated.

- **Electromagnetic flowmeters:** if a conductor (such as blood) flows at right angles to a magnetic field, then an electromotive force is induced which is perpendicular to the magnetic field and to the direction of fluid flow. The induced voltage is proportional to the strength of the field and to the velocity of blood flow. A determination of the diameter of the vessel allows calculation of flow.

- **Para-amino hippuric acid (PAH) clearance:** the clearance of PAH is used to determine renal blood flow, also using the Fick principle. PAH is not utilized or excreted by any other organ apart from the kidney, and so the peripheral venous PAH concentration will equal the arterial. Renal PAH uptake is given by the product of the urinary PAH concentration [U] and urinary volume (V). The final simplified equation is the same as that for PAH clearance: Renal blood flow = $[U] \times V/[P]$ Where $[P]$ is plasma PAH concentration. This actually measures plasma flow, because blood is not filtered at the glomerulus and the volume from which PAH is removed is plasma. Blood flow can thereafter be calculated if the haematocrit is known.

- **The Kety–Schmidt method:** this is an adaptation of the Fick principle which is used to make a global determination of cerebral blood flow (see under 'Cerebral Blood Flow' in Chapter 3).
- **PET and SPECT scanning:** positron emission tomography (PET) is a technique which monitors the uptake by different areas of the brain of 2-deoxyglucose labelled with a positron emitter. Scintillography and SPECT scanning use radioactive xenon to trace regional blood flow, with or without enhancement by CT or MR imaging.

Measurement of Cardiac Output

Commentary

Devices that determine cardiac output (CO) are popular; whether this popularity is deserved remains contentious. Certainly there are experienced anaesthetists and intensivists who believe that the ability to measure CO neither improves nor affects outcome. This debate is unlikely to occupy much of the oral, although the PACMAN study may warrant brief discussion. As there are now several different methods available, you are more likely to be asked to give a brief description rather than a detailed analysis. Moreover, many of the equations that are applied are quite complex; for example, determination of blood flow velocity using Doppler ultrasound is given by (v) velocity = Doppler shift (Fd) x speed of ultrasound in tissue (c) (1,540 m s^{-1}) / 2 $\times$ ultrasound frequency (Fo) $\times$ the angle of the ultrasound beam in relation to the blood flow (Cosθ), yet this is only part of the calculation. There is unlikely to be the time to explore this science in any detail.

Core Information

- **Cardiac output (CO):** delivers oxygen to tissues. Its prime determinants are heart rate (HR) and stroke volume (SV), in turn influenced by venous filling (preload), systemic vascular resistance (afterload) and myocardial contractility. Low CO states predict adverse outcomes both in the critically ill and in patients undergoing major surgery.
- **Pulmonary artery flotation catheter (PAC):** although the use of the PAC has all but disappeared from most critical care units, it is still regarded as the most accurate method of determining CO and is the one against which other techniques are judged. The principles of measurement are described under 'Measurement of Organ Blood Flow' in the immediately previous section.
- **Oesophageal Doppler monitor (ODM):** this non-invasive ultrasonic device measures the velocity of blood flow in the descending thoracic aorta. The shift in

frequency is proportional to the velocity of ejected blood. The device generates a velocity/time waveform to which is applied a calibration factor derived from the patient's height, weight and age. The SV is then derived from the flow velocity, ejection time and aortic area. (A second transducer measures the cross-sectional area of the aorta.) The useful indices that the ODM produces are the CO, the SV and the corrected systolic flow time (FT_c). The FT_c is normally between 330 and 360 ms and is an indicator of volaemic status; a low (short) FT_c is associated with inadequate filling. Softer and smaller probes introduced nasally allow this technique to be used in the awake patient. Flow through the descending aorta is only around 70% of the total CO (the remainder is distributed through the subclavian arteries to the head, neck and upper limbs), but the device corrects for this proportion.

- **ODM and NICE:** in 2011, NICE published guidance for oesophageal Doppler monitoring during surgery and explicitly named the Deltex Medical CardioQ-ODM as the recommended device. NICE cited reductions in postoperative complications, reduced length of stay and a saving of around £1,100 per patient. The recommendation has been roundly criticized, and not without reason, as they were based on relatively few (eight) small trials, not all of which reported length of stay. One astringent commentator also noted that the main differentiation between controls and the study group was the intraoperative infusion of around 500 ml of colloid and queried whether such a modest intervention could really save more than a thousand pounds per patient. The point is well made.
- **Transoesophageal echocardiography (TOE):** (see under 'Ultrasound'. This technique also uses Doppler ultrasound. The TOE probe allows 180° views of the heart, and not only measures CO but also gives a range of information about ventricular function, wall motion abnormalities and valvular anatomy. It is however very operator-dependent.
- **Pulse contour analysis:** it has long been recognized that arterial pressure changes during respiration may be an indicator of volaemic status, and that a systolic pressure variation between the maximum and minimum recorded during one cycle of IPPV of more than 10 mmHg suggests at least a 10% reduction in circulating volume. Pulse contour analysis examines the arterial waveform, quantifies the SV and calculates the stroke volume variation (SVV). It is used both in LiDCO and PiCCO. As the devices are utilizing the arterial waveform, an optimal trace is essential for accurate determination.
- **Lithium dilution (LiDCO):** this is a bolus indicator dilution method of measuring CO. After intravenous injection of a small dose of lithium (0.15 mmol), the plasma concentration is measured by an ion-selective electrode attached to the arterial line. The resulting concentration/time curve allows the calculation of CO (given by dose × 60/mean concentration [AUC] × time [s]). LiDCO can be used in combination with pulse contour analysis to provide continuous readings of CO, SV and SVV. (The technique cannot be used in patients who are receiving therapeutic lithium, nor in the first trimester of pregnancy.) LiDCO correlates well with invasive thermodilution catheter derived measurements.
- **Pulse contour CO (PiCCO):** this technique uses a thermodilution technique in conjunction with pulse contour waveform analysis. Cold saline is injected through into a central vein, and temperature is measured by a thermistor in an arterial

cannula sited in a large artery (such as the brachial or femoral). This thermodilution CO measurement calibrates the system, after which the arterial waveform is analyzed to produce beat-to-beat determinations of SV, SVV and a continuous measure of CO. (It is also claimed that PiCCO can provide information about other volumetric parameters: global end-diastolic volume [GEDV], intrathoracic blood volume [ITBV] and extravascular lung water [EVLW]. You will not be asked how it does so.) PiCCO also correlates well with PA catheter–derived measurements.

- **Thoracic electrical bioimpedance:** as the name suggests, this technique involves measuring the resistance to current flow through the thorax. This resistance changes both with the respiratory cycle and with pulsatile blood flow. High-frequency low-amplitude alternating current is emitted and sensed via electrodes on the neck and lower chest wall. Changes in impedance are detected as blood distends and then leaves the aorta. These changes allow continuous determinations of CO, SV, contractile state and SVR. The technique tends to overestimate CO.

Supplementary Information

Evidence to Support the Use of These Devices

- The short answer is that there is none. The closest attempt to provide some evidence came in the form of the multicentre Pulmonary Artery Catheters in Patient Management (PACMAN) study which investigated whether the use of PA catheters reduced hospital mortality in the critically ill (it was published in 2005). More than 1,000 critically ill patients were randomized either to receive a PAC or to a control group in which management did not involve a PAC but could include the use of other devices to measure CO. There was no overall evidence of benefit or harm. (The 10% complication rate related largely to central venous access rather than the PAC itself.) The study was not flawless; there were, for example, no objective inclusion criteria, only the opinion of a clinician that a PAC was indicated. The fact that 80% of the patients in the no-PAC group had CO measured by a different means was potentially confounding, and sceptics were quick to point out that the outcomes in the other 20% of patients who had no CO measurement at all were very similar to those in patients who had PACs. Definitive evidence, therefore, will come only from one or more randomized controlled trials which compare CO measurement against none.

Jugular Venous Bulb Oxygen Saturation (SjVO$_2$)

Commentary

Jugular venous bulb oxygen saturation (SjVO$_2$) provides a measure of global cerebral oxygenation and finds uses in neurosurgery, in neurotrauma and in cerebral monitoring during cardiac surgery. This is an area of specialist practice which you may well not have encountered. An answer based on first principles will compensate for any lack of direct experience.

Core Information

- **SjVO$_2$** is an indirect indicator of cerebral oxygen utilization: when O$_2$ demand exceeds supply, then O$_2$ extraction increases and SjVO$_2$ falls (desaturated at <50%). Conversely, when supply exceeds demand the SjVO$_2$ rises (luxuriant at >75%). Bulb O$_2$ saturation can be used as a specific measure of global cerebral oxygenation, but it cannot provide information about smaller focal areas of ischaemia.
- **AjvDO$_2$**. The difference in oxygen content between arterial and jugular venous blood (AjvDO$_2$) is given by CMRO$_2$/CBF (cerebral metabolic rate for O$_2$/cerebral blood flow). The normal value is 4–8 ml O$_2$/100 ml of blood.
- If AjvDO$_2$ is <4, supply is luxuriant; if >8 it suggests ischaemia.
- **Factors decreasing SjVO$_2$:** an increased oxygen demand (as in seizure activity or pyrexia) or a decrease in supply (leading to a fall in SjVO$_2$ and rise in AjvDO$_2$) results from raised intracranial pressure (ICP), severe systemic hypotension, hypocapnia (<3.75 kPa), arterial hypoxia, seizure activity and cerebral vasospasm. During rewarming after profound hypothermia, the SjVO$_2$ may be below 40%, reflecting maximal O$_2$ extraction. It will also fall in response to any increase in metabolic demand. A decrease in SjVO$_2$ always indicates potential cerebral dysfunction.
- **Factors increasing SjVO$_2$:** a decreased O$_2$ demand or increase in supply (leading to a rise in SjVO$_2$ and fall in AjvDO$_2$) results from decreased metabolic demand (such as occurs with hypothermia or sedation), brain death (in which there is minimal demand), an increased blood supply, hypercapnia and arterial hyperoxia. Loss of cerebral autoregulation will increase blood flow and SjVO$_2$ will rise, as it will if blood has been shunted past capillary beds by high intracranial pressure. Thus an increase in SjVO$_2$ may also herald cerebral damage.
- SjVO$_2$ can be used to guide therapeutic interventions in the brain-injured patient, such as the use of moderate hyperventilation, osmotic diuretics and cerebrospinal fluid drainage.

Measurement of SjVO$_2$

- SjVO$_2$ is usually measured via an intravascular catheter which is threaded retrogradely up the internal jugular vein as far as the superior jugular bulb. (The jugular bulb is a dilatation at the origin of the vein, and lies just below the posterior part of the floor of the tympanic cavity.) The normal value is 55–75%.
- A fibreoptic catheter uses reflectance oximetry (as in pulmonary arterial catheter monitoring of mixed venous saturation) to provide continuous SjVO$_2$ monitoring. As with pulse oximetry, the apparatus uses the light absorption spectra of haemoglobin and deoxyhaemoglobin.
- Catheter placement can be facilitated by locating the vessel using ultrasound, and is verified by lateral skull X-ray, which should confirm the tip lying at the level of, and medial to, the mastoid process.
- Alternatively, a sample may be taken directly from the jugular bulb and the oxygen saturation measured by co-oximetry.

SjVO$_2$ Measurement: Problems

- It is an invasive technique which carries all the generic complications of a catheter that is inserted into a complex circulation (the tip lies just below the base of skull).

- As with all such devices, there can be rapid protein deposition at the tip which may interfere with sampling.
- If the catheter is not precisely positioned in the jugular bulb but lies too low it may also sample venous blood draining from face or the scalp.
- As described earlier, SjVO2 provides a measure of global cerebral oxygenation but gives no information about focal areas of ischaemia or damage.

Measurement of Cerebral Oxygenation (Near Infrared Spectroscopy)

Commentary

If there is one physiological variable that should be maintained during anaesthesia it must be cerebral oxygenation. It is also the variable that is measured directly least often but instead is inferred from other forms of indirect monitoring such as pulse oximetry, arterial blood pressure and capnography. A reliable non-invasive monitor of cerebral oxygenation would render these less important, on the general assumption that if the brain is being perfused with oxygenated blood then other systems will also function. There are such non-invasive devices available, and it remains somewhat surprising that they have not found their way into mainstream anaesthetic practice. The physics of optical spectrophotometry are too detailed to be encompassed within the time frame of the oral, but the following simplified account should provide the necessary information.

Core Information

Near infrared spectroscopy (NIRS) is based on physical principles similar to those which underlie pulse oximetry, and it can be used in the same way to measure the oxygen saturation of peripheral tissues. However, its particular value lies in its ability to provide a non-invasive measure not only of cerebral oxygenation but also of other deeper structures that are usually inaccessible, such as the spinal cord and the splanchnic circulation.

- A 'niroscope' is essentially an optical spectrophotometer that uses wavelengths in the near infrared range, from 700 to 1,100 nanometres (nm). This utilizes the fact that tissues, including those of the bony cranium, allow penetration of light at these wavelengths to depths as great as 8 centimetres. Visible light, in contrast, with wavelengths that range from 450 to 700 nm, is able to penetrate little more than 1 cm of tissue due to much greater attenuation by absorption, reflectance and scattering.
- Absorption is a function of the nature of the molecules in the pathway of the emitted light. At wavelengths greater than 1,300 nm, water absorbs all photons within a few millimetres, whereas at the shorter wavelengths of visible light, the absorption bands of haemoglobin and increased scattering prevent onward transmission. Reflectance is variable, depending mainly on the angle at which the light beam strikes the surface.

- Scattering of light occurs when the beam is deviated by the material that it encounters, and will depend on the wavelength and the refractive indices of the particles. This scattering of photons will increase the distance they travel, known as their pathlength, and thereby their absorption by tissue. Up to 80% of light in the near infrared spectrum is scattered in this way, which makes the provision of quantitative information more difficult.

- The instruments use laser diodes to generate infrared (IR) light and employ reflectance-mode spectroscopy. The light is emitted and received by optodes (the term used in this context for optical sensors). The transmitter and receiver are on the same side but are separated by around 5 cm. This is because the pathway of IR light from the emitter, through the tissue, and back to the detector is elliptical; and its maximal penetration is proportional to the separation between the two. This is variously quoted as being one-third to one-half of that distance.

- The emitted IR light is absorbed by chromophores, of which oxygenated haemoglobin (HbO_2) and deoxygenated haemoglobin (Hb) are two such species with absorption spectra of 800–850 nm and 650–800 nm, respectively. Others include cytochrome P450 enzymes, myoglobin (mainly in the frontalis muscle) and bilirubin (of significance only in jaundiced patients). Each different chromophore has a specific absorption, or extinction, coefficient which is expressed as a function of wavelength. The selected wavelengths generally are between 700 and 850 nm, which is the range within which the absorption spectra of HbO_2 and Hb show maximal separation.

- Cerebral oxygen saturation is determined by application of the Beer-Lambert law, which put at its simplest states that the concentration of a substance can be measured by the amount of light that it absorbs. Expressed more formally it means that attenuation or absorbance, 'A', is equal to the product of the absorption or extinction coefficient 'ε' of the substance (which varies with its nature and the wavelength of the incident light); 'L', which is the photon pathlength; and 'c', which is the concentration of the absorbent substance. Thus $A = \varepsilon \times [c] \times L$ which after rearrangement gives: [**concentration**] $= A / \varepsilon \times L$ which thereby allows determination of oxygen saturation.

- The available devices can determine changes in oxygenated and deoxygenated haemoglobin but are unable to distinguish between arterial and venous concentrations. The distribution of haemoglobin in cortical tissue is approximately 70% in the venous system and 30% in arterial blood. Hence a 'normal' rSO_2 is not 96% or greater as would be expected from a peripheral oximeter probe, but is between 55% and 80%, and so trend monitoring is of more value than absolute values. A value below 50%, or a fall of 20% from baseline suggests cortical hypoxaemia. One potential difficulty is that in non-metabolizing or dead brain, HbO_2 may be sequestered in veins and capillaries which will lead to misleadingly normal rSO_2 values. This is more likely to be a problem when cortical oxygenation is being assessed after brain injury than during surgery when a falling rSO_2 will indicate hypoperfusion or hypoxia before cell death has occurred.

Supplementary Information and Clinical Considerations

- Much of the work on cerebral oxygenation has related to cardiac surgery, but a systematic review that was published in 2014 looked at changes in regional (cerebral) oxygen saturation (rSO_2) in non-cardiac surgery and found significant falls in one-lung ventilation during thoracic surgery, in major abdominal surgery, in carotid end-arterectomy with arterial cross-clamping, in hip surgery and in laparoscopic surgery performed in the reverse Trendelenberg (head-up) position. The review also noted 'pronounced cerebral desaturation during shoulder arthroscopy in the beach chair position' (H.B. Nielsen. Systematic review of near infrared determined cerebral oxygenation during non-cardiac surgery. March 2014, http://dx.doi.org/10.3389/fphys.2014.00093).

- The clinical importance of maintaining cerebral oxygenation is self-evident, and the studies so far done would seem to illustrate two important realities. The first is that silent cerebral cortical desaturation can occur without any obvious perturbations of routine systemic vital signs such as heart rate, arterial blood pressure and peripheral oxygen saturation. The second is that such episodes of desaturation do appear to correlate with the development of postoperative cognitive dysfunction.

- Given that routine monitoring may be falsely reassuring, it is difficult to know exactly how specifically to manage anaesthesia during those higher-risk procedures. But if the beach chair position for shoulder surgery is taken as an example, there should be a high index of suspicion for any factors that might potentially lead to cerebral hypoperfusion. Hence, in addition to maintaining cardiac output, volaemic status, normocapnia and an adequate haemoglobin concentration to ensure oxygen delivery, the anaesthetist should perhaps tolerate only minimal divergence from the patient's baseline levels. (These can readily be determined in the anaesthetic room in the sitting position prior to the induction of anaesthesia.)

Renal Replacement Therapy (RRT)

Commentary

Renal support with haemofiltration or haemodiafiltration is a common intensive therapy intervention. Many critically ill patients develop acute kidney injury, and so you will be expected to have some familiarity with the principles of management. Remember again that if your examiners do not work in intensive care units, then your experience and knowledge may be more recent than theirs.

Core Information

Indications for Renal Replacement Therapy (RRT)

- **Indications:** these have widened from the original primary indication, which was for acute kidney injury accompanied by a metabolic acidosis, hyperkalaemia or uraemia. Isolated uraemia is a problem usually only when the urea concentration is high enough to cause clinical symptoms such as vomiting, diarrhoea, pruritus or mental disturbance. Renal replacement therapy can also be used to manage volume overload and to clear some drugs and poisons from the circulation. It can have a role in the acute management of severe hypothermia; veno–venous systems using counter-current blood warmers can raise core temperatures by up to 2 °C per hour.

Principles of Haemofiltration (HF)

- The filters used in HF are in effect literal renal substitutes.
- In the normal kidney the glomerulus filters water, ions, negatively charged particles of molecular weight of less than 15,000 and neutral substances of molecular weight up to about 40,000. Renal corpuscular channels have negatively charged pores, which oppose the passage of negatively charged plasma proteins such as albumin.
- The normal glomerular filtration rate (GFR) is 125 ml min^{-1} (7.5 l h^{-1}).
- Tubular reabsorption reduces the filtrate of 180 l day^{-1} to about 1.0 l day^{-1}, and the process salvages many of the filtered ions and other particles (by diffusion and mediated transport). Tubular secretion is the means whereby larger molecules and protein-bound substances (such as drugs and toxins) are eliminated.
- In the HF system, arterial pressure (usually assisted by a peristaltic roller pump) delivers a flow, if necessary, of more than 200 ml min^{-1} to the semi-permeable membrane in the filter. Water and low-molecular-weight substances (up to 20,000) cross the membrane (which is acting as the 'glomerulus'). This process creates a pressure gradient rather than a concentration gradient, with the bulk flow of water taking solute with it (by convective mass transfer).
- Urea and creatinine will be removed, as will electrolytes and some drugs and toxins. Plasma proteins and all formed blood components remain within the circulation.
- Tubular reabsorption is mimicked by the direct infusion of balanced electrolyte solution, with concentrations adjusted as necessary. The volume infused will depend on the clinical situation. If the patient is not volume-overloaded, then infusion will be at the same rate as the filtration rate, plus a component for maintenance fluid. If fluid removal is indicated, then negative balance is easily achieved by decreasing the infusion rate.
- HF is an efficient means of treating fluid overload, but in comparison with the kidney is very inefficient at removing solute. Very high volumes of ultrafiltrate (upwards of 15 l day^{-1}) are required to remove urea, creatinine and other products of metabolism.
- The '**dose**' of renal replacement therapy. This can be specifically defined as the rate of clearance of a marker solute, indexed to body weight, but in clinical practice the 'dose' of continuous RRT (CRRT) is essentially the flow rate of the effluent (which consists of the ultrafiltrate and the dialysate). A number of studies have investigated the effect of dose on mortality without showing any consistent benefit of higher-intensity regimens. In practice the standard dose rate is around 20–30 ml kg^{-1} h^{-1}, although there is local variation between units. Some, for example, may initiate higher doses in patients with sepsis.
- Pre- or post-dilution. The fluid reinfusion to restore volaemic status can be instituted before or after the filter. If before (pre-dilution), the dilution decreases the concentration of solutes to be filtered and so it is less efficient, but the risk of filter failure is lowered. During HF, protein particles accumulate on the inner surface of the hollow fibre filtration tubes leading to impairment of function within 24 hours. A more dilute solute slows this process. Post-dilution clears solute more efficiently and a

smaller volume of replacement fluid is required (whose only advantage is perhaps the marginal cost benefit). The limiting factor in the rate of post-dilution ultrafiltration is blood flow; if the rate is too great, then end-filtrate haematocrit will also be too high. This means in practice that the typical standard dose rate of ~25 ml kg^{-1} h^{-1} may be impossible to achieve.

- Haemodiafiltration is much more efficient at removing solute. A dialysis solution is passed across the filter in a counter-current fashion so that solute can be removed both by convection (as in HF alone) and by diffusion down the concentration gradient.

Supplementary and Clinical Information

- **CRRT in sepsis:** the inflammatory mediators and cytokines that are produced in sepsis have a range of molecular weights from around 5,000 to 50,000, and so their effective removal is limited by the standard size of filtration membranes which allow the passage of compounds of molecular weight up to 20,000. Experimental high cut-off membranes have shown promise in animal models and may in due course be available for clinical use.
- **Complications of RRT**
  - **Fluid mismanagement:** very large volumes are both filtered and infused, and the potential scope for error is high. Fluid overload is possible, but more common is hypotension secondary to the transient hypovolaemia that may occur with ultrafiltration. This may be compounded by any impairment in myocardial reserve.
  - **Metabolic derangement:** high-intensity CRRT can contribute to hypophosphataemia and hypomagnesaemia, together with loss of some vitamins and amino acids.
  - **Coagulation problems:** blood clots in extracorporeal circulations and produces diffuse thrombi on the artificial surfaces unless the system is anticoagulated, usually with heparins or prostacyclin. Inadequate coagulation leads to problems with the circuit as the filter clots, but this is not immediately dangerous to the patient. An iatrogenic coagulopathy may be much more hazardous.
- **Other Complications**
  - **Cannulation complications:** these are generic, but apply to the insertion of any wide-bore line into a central vein. Renal replacement therapy requires a large bore double lumen catheter inserted into the jugular of femoral veins. The subclavian vein is usually avoided because of the risk of thrombosis, which would compromise arteriovenous fistula formation should acute kidney injury progress to chronic renal failure.
  - **Air embolus:** this is always a potential danger with the use of relatively complex extracorporeal circuits.
  - **Antibiotic concentrations:** CRRT has varying effects on the excretion and concentration of antibiotics depending on the treatment in use. Ideally blood levels should be measured so as to ensure appropriate dosing.
  - **Heat loss:** this is a potential problem associated with the large fluid shifts.
  - **Disconnection:** HF requires wide-bore dedicated arterial and venous lines.
  - **Filter failure.** Filters may clot unless the system is adequately anticoagulated.

Temperature and Its Measurement

Commentary

The maintenance and control of body temperature are of evident importance in clinical anaesthetic practice. (It is a little more difficult to see how an intimate knowledge of thermistors and thermocouples is especially helpful, but this will form the bulk of the science component of the question.)

Core Information

Methods of measuring temperature.

- Heat is an energy form related to the activity, or kinetic energy, in the molecules of the particular substance. Temperature is a way of quantifying the thermal state of a substance.
- **Units of measurement:** the SI unit is the Kelvin (K), which equals Celsius (°C) plus 273.15. As 1° C is the same as 1 K, the unit is used universally in medicine.
- Most of the body heat content (66%) lies within the central core compartment comprising the brain and the organs of the trunk, whose temperature is maintained between 36.5 and 37.5 °C. The remaining 33% is accounted for by the periphery, the temperature of which can undergo much wider fluctuation. It is essential, therefore, to measure core temperature.
- There are three main types of device for measuring temperature: electrical, non-electrical and infrared.
- **Electrical**
  - **Thermistor**: a small bead of a semiconductor material, usually a metal oxide, is incorporated into a Wheatstone bridge circuit. The resistance of the bead decreases exponentially as the temperature rises. These beads are both robust and very small, and are used in the tips of pulmonary artery flotation catheters and in arterial lines for thermodilution measurements. They are very accurate (±0.1 °C).
  - **Thermocouple**: if two dissimilar metals are joined, a small potential difference develops which is proportional to the temperature of the junction. (This is known as the Seebeck effect.) Another junction between the metals is necessary to complete an electrical circuit, although another temperature-dependent voltage will develop at this junction. The metals that are used commonly are copper and a copper/nickel alloy. When the thermocouple is used as a thermometer, one of the junctions forms the temperature probe, while the other is kept at a constant temperature and acts as a reference. Thermocouples are stable and also accurate to ±0.1 °C.
  - **Resistance thermometer**: these are based on the principle that electrical resistance in metals (usually platinum) shows a linear increase with temperature. These systems are not used clinically.
- **Non-electrical**
  - **Mercury and alcohol thermometers**: volume increases with temperature. Like all thermometers, these are calibrated against fixed points, such as the triple point (at which water, water vapour and ice are in equilibrium) and boiling point of water.

— **Dial thermometers**: these may use a coil comprising two metals with differential coefficients of expansion. As the temperature changes, the coil tightens and relaxes, and an attached lever moves across a calibrated dial.

- **Infrared**
  — **Tympanic membrane and non-contact (forehead) thermometers**: the living body emits infrared radiation, whose intensity and wavelength vary with temperature. This property is utilized in tympanic membrane and non-contact thermometers. These use pyroelectric sensors, which comprise an electrically polarized substance whose polarization alters with temperature. This change can be used to generate an electrical output, which is proportional to the temperature. Their response time is very rapid compared with other types of clinical thermometer. The tympanic membrane is the favoured site in anaesthesia because it offers the most accurate indication of cerebral temperature.

Supplementary Information and Clinical Considerations

The clinical consequences of hypothermia are covered in more detail under 'Heat Loss' in the next section, and so the following is an outline summary.

- **Cardiorespiratory effects:** oxygen consumption increases and cardiac output decreases. Arrhythmias and myocardial ischaemia are more likely. The oxygen–haemoglobin dissociation curve shifts to the left and reduces oxygen delivery. Blood viscosity increases.
- **Coagulation:** platelet function is impaired, intraoperative blood loss increases and transfusion requirements rise.
- **Metabolic effects and effects on drugs:** within a few degrees of normal core temperature, metabolic rate decreases by 6–7% for each 1 °C fall (this is a generalization which applies to the initial drops in temperature, because the relationship is not linear). Enzymatic reactions and intermediary metabolism are slower at core temperatures below 34 °C. Drug actions are prolonged, especially those of muscle relaxants. Glucose utilization decreases and hyperglycaemia can result. Metabolic acidosis may supervene.
- **Surgical outcome:** hypothermia compromises immune function and increases postoperative infection rates. Wound healing is adversely affected and hospital stay may be extended.

Heat Loss During Anaesthesia

This is covered in more detail in the immediate next section

- **Radiation (50%):** the body is an efficient radiator, transferring heat from a hot to cooler objects.
- **Convection (30%):** air in the layer close to the body is warmed by conduction, rises as its temperature increases and is carried away by convection currents.
- **Evaporation (20–25%):** moisture on the body's surface evaporates, loses latent heat of vaporization and the body cools.
- **Conduction (3–5%):** this occurs only if the patient is lying unprotected on an efficient heat conductor.

- **Respiration (10%):** heat loss is via evaporation and the need to heat inspired air.
- **Anaesthesia:** this causes vasodilatation and also affects central thermoregulation.

Heat Loss

Commentary
This topic incorporates some basic science and is also of clinical importance, given evidence of the morbidity that is associated with perioperative heat loss.

Core Information

Mechanisms by Which Patients Lose Heat during Anaesthesia
- **Radiation:** this is the most important mechanism and may account for at least 50% of heat loss. The body is a highly efficient radiator, transferring heat from hot to cooler objects. The process is accelerated during anaesthesia if the patient is surrounded by cool objects and prevented from receiving radiant heat from the environment. Further heat loss will also occur if the body is forced to heat cold infused fluids up to 37 °C. (Infusion of crystalloid 30 ml kg^{-1} at room temperature will decrease core temperature by around 0.5 °C.)
- **Convection:** this accounts for up to 30% of heat loss. Air in the layer close to the body is warmed by conduction, rises as its temperature increases and is carried away by convection currents. The process is accelerated during anaesthesia if a large surface area is exposed to convection currents (particularly in laminar flow theatres).
- **Evaporation:** this accounts for some 20–25% of heat loss. As moisture on the body's surface evaporates, it loses latent heat of vaporization and the body cools. This is a highly developed mechanism for heat loss in health, but undesirable during surgery. It is accelerated during anaesthesia if there is a large moist surface area open to atmosphere (especially in major intra-abdominal surgery, intrathoracic surgery, reconstructive plastic surgery and major orthopaedic surgery).
- **Conduction:** this is not a significant cause of heat loss during normal circumstances, accounting for only 3–5% of the total. Heat loss by this mechanism increases during anaesthesia only if the patient is lying unprotected on an efficient heat conductor such as metal table.
- **Respiration:** heat loss occurs due to evaporation and the heating of inspired air. This amounts to around 10% of the total, but it can be minimized during anaesthesia by the use of heat and moisture exchangers.

Supplementary Information and Clinical Considerations
The clinical consequences of hypothermia. (This question is directed at mild falls in perioperative temperature rather than profound hypothermia, although if you have covered the basic ground then the questioning may extend to the latter.)

- **Mild perioperative hypothermia**: This is defined by a fall in core temperature of 1–3 °C, and is common during anaesthesia. General anaesthesia not only causes vasodilatation and a diversion of core blood to the periphery, but it also decreases the threshold at which thermoregulatory vasoconstriction is activated. This leads to the rapid fall in temperature of 1–1.5 °C that is seen in many patients undergoing even short procedures. The development of hypothermia is triphasic; after the initial drop the second phase begins at around an hour during which, as surgery continues, patients lose heat more slowly via the mechanisms described in the following. Typically, this is of the order of 1 °C over 2–3 hours. Usually the temperature reaches a plateau at this point which is where the lowered vasoconstriction threshold is activated, and where heat loss is compensated by metabolic heat production.

- **Severe hypothermia**: This occurs either as a result of environmental exposure or when a patient's body temperature is deliberately lowered to allow specialized forms of surgery. In deep hypothermic circulatory arrest, the core temperature may be reduced as low as 15 °C for aortic arch replacement or cerebral aneurysm repair.

- **Cardiorespiratory effects:** oxygen consumption increases during mild hypothermia, although it may increase by 500% during shivering as a patient rewarms. Cardiac output is decreased and hypothermia increases the incidence of arrhythmias. The oxygen–haemoglobin dissociation curve shifts to the left, increasing oxygen affinity and reducing oxygen delivery. Blood viscosity increases and, with it, the risk of intravascular sludging. Studies have suggested that a drop in core temperature to around 35 °C is associated with a 6% incidence of myocardial ischaemia or arrhythmia (1% in control groups).

- **Coagulation:** the most significant effect of hypothermia is the impairment of platelet function such that intraoperative blood loss increases and with it the need for blood transfusion (demonstrated, for example, in patients undergoing total hip replacement).

- **Metabolic effects and effects on drugs:** metabolic rate decreases initially by around 6–7% for each 1 °C drop in core temperature from normal. (This fall is not linear but exponential. At 15 °C, for example, a further 1 °C drop results in a decrease in $CMRO_2$ of only 1%.) Enzymatic reactions are slowed, and all the reactions of intermediate metabolism are affected at core temperatures lower than 34 °C. The effects of most drugs therefore are prolonged, particularly neuromuscular blocking agents whose duration of action at 35 °C is extended by around 50%. MAC of inhaled anaesthetics decreases by 5% for each 1 °C drop in core temperature below normal. Hypothermia leads to a progressive acidosis. Renal and hepatic function is depressed, but diuresis can result from the failure of active reabsorption of sodium and water. Hyperglycaemia may occur as glucose utilization falls.

- **CNS effects:** there is a progressive deterioration in mental function to the point at which the EEG will record no cerebral activity. This occurs at a core temperature of around 18 °C. (The brain is still metabolically active and will exhaust energy substrate after around 25 minutes.)

- **Surgical outcome:** wound healing is adversely affected both because of the reduction in subcutaneous wound tissue oxygenation and because of direct impairment of neutrophil function. Thus, hypothermia compromises immune function and leads to a threefold increase in the risk of postoperative infection and prolonged hospital stay.
- **Prevention:** patients can be prewarmed with forced air warming if necessary, and during surgery heat losses owing to the mechanisms described earlier can be minimized by the use, for example, of insulated operating table warmers, heat and moisture exchangers in the breathing system, warm air blankets, warmed infused fluids and protection of the head. (A litre of crystalloid infused at room temperature lowers core temperature by 0.25 °C, which was the figure arrived at following the original study. Elsewhere a slightly unrealistic figure of 0.5° C is commonly quoted.)
- **Beneficial effects of hypothermia:** any decrease in metabolic rate is accompanied by a drop in oxygen demand which may benefit particularly those organs with high consumption such as the brain and myocardium. Aerobic metabolism may therefore continue longer in the face of compromised oxygen supply. Enzyme activity is reduced with a consequent fall in synthetic activity, but this also applies to the formation of inflammatory mediators.

Severe Hypothermia

- The examiners are much less interested in the generic approach (investigation of any underlying cause after attention to Airway, Breathing and Circulation) than in specific details of rewarming.
- Passive warming is effective only when the patient's own heat-generating mechanisms are intact. Moderate and severe hypothermia require active warming. Techniques include the use of external heat sources (forced warm air blankets, radiant heaters) and internal warming. This can be via the use of warm intravenous, intragastric and intraperitoneal fluids, as well as by bladder irrigation via a urinary catheter. The most efficient, but most invasive method, of rewarming is cardiopulmonary bypass. This can raise the core temperature by around 1 °C every 5 minutes. Although other extracorporeal systems such as haemofiltration units lack rapid flow rates, veno–venous systems using counter-current blood warmers can raise core temperatures by 2 °C an hour. The rate of rewarming is important. While there is some evidence to support rapid rewarming, particularly after rapid onset hypothermia (such as sudden immersion), it is more usual to raise the core temperature gradually, by 1 °C an hour. Rapid rewarming in brain-injured patients is associated with worse outcomes and recommended rates as low as 0.25 °C an hour have been recommended. Even slow rewarming is associated with significant problems, including persistent temperature variation between organs, reperfusion injury and 'rewarming shock', which is characterized by acute metabolic acidosis as the patient vasodilates too rapidly for the rate of fluid replacement. It would appear therefore that it is not possible to generalize about optimal warming rates as there are substantial differences according to the clinical context.

Scoring Systems

Commentary

This question nominally appears under the guise of a clinical measurement topic and has understandably disappointed some candidates of whom it has been asked, who have felt that it amounts to reciting little more than a list. The oral can even start with a discussion of MEWS, which as a simple ward-based assessment tool may seem a topic somewhat distant from rigorous basic science. There are now numerous scoring systems that have been developed, particularly in critical care, but also for general assessment and for specific medical conditions. More than 50 systems have been described in the context of critical care, trauma and the emergency department. What follows is a selection of the many which are now available. After you have given one or more of these a mention, the oral is likely to focus on those of more mainstream importance such as POSSUM and APACHE.

Core Information

- **Modified Early Warning System (MEWS).** As the name suggests, MEWS scoring aims to allow early identification of clinical deterioration and to prevent delayed intervention. (It is so named because it is a modification of a previous system originally described by Morgan and colleagues in 1997.) It is a simple ward-based scoring system that is determined from the standard observation chart. A score of 0, 1, 2 or 3 is assigned to the six routine physiological variables of respiratory rate, heart rate, systolic pressure, temperature, urine output and neurological status. The lowest score is therefore 0 and the highest possible is 18. A score of 4 or more usually triggers referral initially to an appropriate medical professional, usually the ward doctor. There are many local variations.

- **PEWS, MEOWS, NEWS.** These are all further variations of MEWS. **PEWS** is the Paediatric Early Warning System used in patients below the age of 16 and in whom the reference ranges are quite different, particularly in much younger children; it is not simply a modification of the adult system. Most PEWS systems have different charts for infants, pre-school (1–4 years), school age (5–12 years) and teenage (12–15 years). Here too there are many local variations in the way that the scores are determined. Typically, PEWS looks at 'Respiratory' (rate, recession, accessory muscles, tracheal tug), 'Cardiovascular' (colour, capillary refill, tachycardia of >30 above normal rate) and 'Behaviour' (alert, sleeping, irritable, lethargic). **MEOWS** is the Modified Early Obstetric Warning Score for use in parturients and which usually uses similar parameters to MEWS. **NEWS** is a National Early Warning Score which is an attempt by the Royal College of Physicians to introduce a standardized set of criteria, so far without universal adoption.

- **Glasgow Coma Score (GCS).** This is almost too familiar to include, but is an assessment of conscious state based on eye opening (1–4), verbal response (1–5) and motor response (1–6), giving a minimum score of 3, which is either deep coma or death, and a maximum of 15, which is full consciousness. It is included as part of several other scoring systems. A simplified version which is also useful in children is the **AVPU** score which determines whether a patient is **A**wake, responding to **V**oice, responding to **P**ain, or **U**nresponsive.

- **Wilson score (prediction of difficult intubation).** This is a simple tool for airway assessment with a point assigned to each of five variables: weight, craniocervical mobility, mouth opening, retrognathia and prominent overbite. It has minimal inter-observer variation and so is more reliable in that respect than the Mallampati test, but although the sensitivity of the Wilson scoring system is high, its specificity is low.

- **Global Registry of Adverse Coronary Events (GRACE).** The registry enrolled more than 100,00 patients between 1999 and 2009 and developed a risk calculator to allow clinicians to assess the future risk of myocardial infarction or death in patients with acute coronary syndrome (ACS) (see under 'Myocardial Blood Supply' in Chapter 2). The scoring system utilizes eight variables: age, heart rate, systolic blood pressure, serum creatinine, cardiac arrest at hospital admission, ST segment deviation, elevated markers of myocardial injury and the Killip class. (This is a classification of heart failure ranging from 'None' to 'Cardiogenic shock'.) It categorizes patients into levels of risk for immediate management and determines the probability of in-hospital death and at 6 months, 12 months and 3 years after admission. GRACE 2.0 also gives the combined risk of death or myocardial infarction at 1 year.

- **Apfel score (risk of postoperative nausea and vomiting).** The Apfel score estimates the likelihood of PONV according to the number of predisposing factors. These are previous history, non-smoking, female gender and administration of opioids. The incidence of PONV in relation to the number of factors is quoted as 0–10%, 1–20%, 2–40%, 3–60% and 4–80%. This suggests that a non-smoking female undergoing, say, routine day-case orthopaedic surgery, would have a 40% likelihood of PONV. Clinical experience suggests that this would seem improbably high, but validations of the various models suggest that they can be useful.

- **Ranson score for predicting outcome of acute pancreatitis.** This scoring system estimates mortality based on laboratory values on admission with some repeated at 48 hours. It gives one point to each of the following 11 values: white blood cell count >16,000; age >55 years; glucose >10 mmol/L on admission; aspartate aminotransferase (AST) >250 i.u. l^{-1}; lactate dehydrogenase (LDH) >350 i.u. l^{-1}; at 48 hours: haematocrit fall of >10%; increase in urea concentration by >1.4 mmol l^{-1}; serum Ca^{2+} <2.0 mmol l^{-1}; base deficit >4; fluid requirements of >6 l within 48 hours; PaO2 <8 kPa. A total of 5–6 points predicts a mortality of 40%; at 7–11 points this rises to 80%. (Ranson scoring has been used for several decades, but the Computed Tomography Severity Index appears to be a better predictor).

- **Model for End-Stage Liver Disease: MELD scoring.** This is another organ-specific scoring system that can be used to assist decision-making around liver transplantation. The formula is complex, although it only uses three indices: bilirubin concentration, prothrombin time and creatinine concentration ($3.78 \times$ [bilirubin] + $11.2 \times$ INR + $9.57 \times$ [creatinine] + 6.43), and it yields a round number which allows a prediction of 3-month mortality in hospitalized patients. If the score is 40 or more, for example, predicted mortality is greater than 70%.

- **POSSUM and P-POSSUM.** This is the **P**hysiological and **O**perative **S**everity **S**core for the en**U**meration of **M**ortality and **M**orbidity. P-POSSUM (Portsmouth-POSSUM) is a modification. The scores are calculated using an equation which combines weighted variables both of physiological and operative data. These are too detailed to be discussed in detail in the oral, but the 12 physiological variables consist of age, cardiac signs, respiratory history, pulse rate and systolic blood pressure, Glasgow Coma Score, haemoglobin concentration, white blood cell count, urea, sodium, potassium and the ECG. The six operative variables are severity, multiple procedures, malignancy, peritoneal soiling, total blood loss and the CEPOD mode of surgery (elective, urgent, emergency). These variables were combined into a formula which subsequently was judged to overestimate the risk of mortality, particularly in lower-risk patients. For completeness and to indicate its complexity, the predicted risk of mortality is given by: $= -7.04 + (0.13 \times$ physiological score) $+ (0.16 \times$ operative severity score). In due course, the equation was modified by a group in Portsmouth using linear analysis but using the same variables, and hence the scoring system became referred to as 'P-POSSUM': mortality $= -9.065 + (0.1692 \times$ physiological score) $+ (0.1550 \times$ operative severity score). This still appears to overestimate mortality, and the two systems are probably broadly comparable. The model has been adapted to sub-specialty areas of surgery such that there are V-POSSUM and CR-POSSUM scores for vascular and colorectal surgery, respectively.

Scoring Systems in the Critically Ill

There are multiple critical care scoring systems of which APACHE is the most widely used. However, their function can be misunderstood. They are not intended to allow a prediction of morbidity and mortality in an individual patient, tempting though it may be to use them in that way. It reflects the paradox of evidence-based medicine in that the likelihood of mortality associated with a specific score relates to an overall population of similarly ill patients and not to the individual. A patient may have an APACHE II score consistent with a predicted mortality of greater than 70% but which may in that particular case be completely unreliable. With that caveat in mind some of the critical care scoring systems are outlined here.

- **APACHE.** This is the **A**cute **P**hysiology **A**nd **C**hronic **H**ealth **E**valuation score which has had further iterations since its introduction in 1981. APACHE II (1985) reduced the number of variables from 34 to 12 and altered some of the weightings, for example, giving higher weightings for acute kidney injury. The score is measured during the first 24 hours of admission to critical care. Each variable is scored between 0 and 4; a total of 25 is predictive of 50% mortality, which rises to 80% with a score of 35 or greater (total range is 0–71). (It is unlikely that the examiners will want specific details about the component variables, but they may ask for a summary of the 12. These are temperature, mean arterial pressure, heart rate, respiratory rate, A-a DO_2 ($FiO_2 > 0.5$) or PaO_2 ($FiO2 < 0.5$), arterial pH, serum Na^+, serum K^+, serum creatinine, haematocrit, white cell count and Glasgow Coma Score. Also incorporated are age and chronic health problems, including hepatic cirrhosis, New York Heart Association class IV, severe chronic obstructive pulmonary disease, on renal dialysis and immunocompromise. APACHE III was a further refinement that was released in 1991 and which both increased the number of physiological variables to 20 and developed substantially more complex weightings. It is said to perform marginally better than APACHE II, but because the programme is proprietary and therefore expensive it has not superseded the previous iteration.

- **SAPS II. Simplified Acute Physiology Score.** This is another point-scoring system which assesses a total of 17 variables during the first 24 hours after admission: 12 physiological; age and type of admission (elective, emergency, medical); and three medical disease variables: AIDS, haematological malignancy and metastatic malignancy. SAPS 3 was developed in 2005 using a totally different model. Variables were identified using a database of almost 17,000 critical care patients from some 35 countries, and predictably complex statistical techniques were used to weight them and provide an estimate of hospital mortality. SAPS 3 also provides equations that are specific to several different geographical regions, but these do not, for example, include the Asian subcontinent, Africa or China. Both SAPS II and SAPS 3 are considered to have an acceptable level of 'discrimination' (i.e. predictive accuracy).

- **MODS. Multiple Organ Dysfunction Score.** This was developed in 1995 to describe organ dysfunction in the context of critical care. A score of 0–4 is allocated to each of six organ systems (Respiratory: PaO_2/FiO_2; Cardiovascular: HR × CVP/MAP; Renal: [creatinine]; Hepatic: [bilirubin]; Haematological: [platelet]; Neurological: Glasgow Coma Score). Scores are repeated daily. It is a relatively reliable predictor of length of stay in critical care and of patient mortality.

- **SOFA. Sequential Organ Failure Assessment.** SOFA takes the same six variables and scores the worst values on each day, usually for 72 hours. The main difference between MODS and SOFA is that the latter includes therapeutic measures, whereas MOD scoring is independent of treatment. The two are similar in respect of reliability.

- **LOD score. Logistic Organ Dysfunction score.** This was described in 1996. It is calculated during the first 24 hours after admission and takes the same six organ systems, assigning one to three levels of dysfunction for each (1, 3 or 5 points). It uses logistic regression techniques to yield a global score that summarizes the combined effects of multiple organ dysfunction, and unlike the other organ dysfunction scoring systems, predicts mortality. Most studies appear to suggest that its accuracy is high.

- **ICNARC.** This is the **I**ntensive **C**are **N**ational **A**udit and **R**esearch **C**entre which in effect was established following a national study of APACHE II scoring in UK critical care units. It describes itself as a national centre for comparative audit and research in intensive care, in the context of which the various scoring systems and their evaluation have obvious relevance. ICNARC also looks at data such as the standardized mortality ratio. This is the ratio of the observed mortality rate to the expected mortality rate and takes into account the severity of illness (using scoring systems as described previously) and the differences in case mix.

Humidification (of Inspired Gases)

Commentary

This is a standard subject. Artificial humidification of dry inspired gases is important in the context both of anaesthesia and intensive care, and so you will be expected to know about the different methods that are commonly used. Although the methods of measurement are of limited clinical relevance, they may still be introduced as a means of bulking out what is not a very complex topic.

Core Information

The physical principles and main methods of humidification.
Humidity is expressed in one of two ways.

- **Absolute humidity:** this is defined by the mass of water vapour that is present in a given volume of air. The SI unit is $g\ m^{-3}$. Absolute humidity is temperature-dependent; at 20 °C it is 17 $g\ m^{-3}$, whereas at 37 °C it is 44 $g\ m^{-3}$ (for example in alveolar gas).
- **Relative humidity:** this is the ratio of the mass of water in a given volume of air to the mass of water in the same volume were it to be fully saturated. It is usually expressed as a percentage.

Methods of Humidification

- **HME (heat and moisture exchange) filter:** This is a widely used method, which is passive, and which cannot therefore attain 100% efficiency, but which may reach 70%. The HME contains a hygroscopic material within a sealed unit. As the warm expired gas cools, so the water vapour condenses on the element, which is warmed both by the specific heat of the exhaled gas and the latent heat of the water. Inhaled, dry and cool gas is thus warmed during inspiration, during which process the element cools down prior to the next exhalation. Problems include moderate inefficiency with prolonged use, increased dead space, increased resistance and infection risk.
- **Circle systems:** the absorption of CO_2 by soda lime generates water and heat (see under 'Soda Lime'), and so within a circle breathing system the humidity will rise, although the process is relatively slow, taking up to an hour.
- **Water bath (cold):** this system is passive, in that dry gases bubble through water at room temperature. It is inefficient (~30%) and becomes even more so as the loss of latent heat of vaporization cools the water further.
- **Water bath (warm):** this system is active, in that dry gases bubble through water which is heated, usually to 60 °C (to inhibit microbial contamination). These can achieve efficiencies of greater than 90%. They are more complex devices, and there is a risk of thermal injury to the patient (which is minimized by thermostats).
- **Cascade humidifier:** this is a variation on the warm water bath. Gas is allowed to bubble through a perforated plate; this process maximizes the surface area which is exposed to water.
- **Nebulizers:** these can also be used as active humidifiers. A high-pressure gas stream is directed onto an anvil and entrains water which then breaks into droplets. There are also ultrasonic devices in which water is nebulized by a plate that vibrates at ultrasonic frequencies. These are not in common use as humidifiers because they can deliver gas with greater than 100% relative humidity and may therefore overload the pulmonary tree with fluid.
- **Droplet size:** droplets of 1 micron (μm) will be deposited in the alveoli. This is optimal. Smaller droplets may simply pass in and out with the respiratory cycle.

Larger droplets (5 μm) risk being deposited in the trachea, which may help loosen secretions, but will not humidify the distal airways (nor deliver a drug dose effectively). Larger droplets still, of 20 μm and above, will not travel further than the upper airway and may condense out in the equipment tubing itself.

Supplementary Information and Clinical Considerations

Methods of measuring humidity. (In common with most you will probably never have done this, and so you should not have to take this part of the subject very far.)

- **Hair hygrometer:** the hair, which is linked to a spring and pointer, elongates as humidity increases. It is accurate between relative humidity measurements of about 30% and 90%.
- **Wet and dry bulb hygrometer:** this is a cumbersome technique. The temperature difference between two thermometers relates to evaporation of water round the wet bulb, which in turn relates to ambient humidity. The figure is calculated from tables.
- **Regnault's hygrometer:** this is a more accurate technique in which air is blown through ether within a silver tube. The temperature at which condensation appears on the outer surface is the dew point, which is the temperature to which air must be cooled, at constant pressure, to become fully saturated. The ratio of the saturated vapour pressure (SVP) at the dew point to the SVP at ambient temperature gives the relative humidity. The result is determined from tables.
- **Transducers:** as a substance absorbs atmospheric water, there is a change either in capacitance or in electrical resistance.
- **Mass spectrometer:** this is very accurate and has a rapid (breath-by-breath) response time. The equipment is expensive.

Clinical Relevance of Humidification

- The normal physiological process in health sees inspired air warmed to 37 °C and fully saturated at the isothermic saturation boundary which is typically about 5 cm below the carina. The upper respiratory mucosa contains pseudostratified columnar ciliated epithelium with goblet cells that maintain the mucus layers. Beyond the terminal bronchioles, the lining contains many fewer goblet cells and has a simple cuboidal epithelium. This structure is less able to sustain the efficient humidification of the upper airway. Tracheal intubation moves the isothermic saturation boundary distally and so delivers gases to parts of the respiratory tract that are less able to humidify them if they are dry.
- The consequences of failure to humidify gases include drying and keratinization of parts of the tracheobronchial tree, reduction of ciliary activity and impairment of the mucociliary escalator. In addition, there may be inflammatory change in the ciliated pulmonary epithelium, drying and crusting of secretions, mucus plugging, atelectasis, superimposed chest infection and impaired gas exchange. If this is prolonged, then respiratory tract changes can include necrosis of the epithelium and squamous cell metaplasia. Finally, heat loss may occur via latent heat of vaporization as dry anaesthetic gas is humidified in the respiratory tract. This can be important in children. After 90 minutes of ventilation with non-humidified gases, the core temperature of anaesthetized children has been shown to drop by 0.75 °C.

- Particular patients at risk include those undergoing prolonged anaesthesia and those with pre-existing respiratory disease in whom the impairment of important pulmonary defence functions will be more significant. Those at the extremes of age are at risk (neonates, infants and the elderly), as are all intensive care patients.
- Over-humidification. This is also deleterious and is associated with a reduction in the viscosity of mucus, surfactant dilution and bronchial infiltration by neutrophils. This leads to effects as adverse as those caused by under-humidification, including retention of secretions, atelectasis, decreasing pulmonary compliance and a widening A-aO$_2$ gradient.
- It is also of some importance to maintain the relative humidity of the operating theatre environment at an appropriate level. High humidity is uncomfortable, and low humidity increases the risk of static sparks.

Filters

Commentary

The topic of filters seems scarcely enough to furnish adequate material for a whole question, but it is part of the syllabus and can be asked as part of another subject such as humidification, epidural analgesia, blood transfusion and cell salvage. Some of the following material does appear elsewhere but is repeated here for convenience.

Core Information

- **HME (heat and moisture exchange) filters:** This is a widely used method, which is passive, and which cannot therefore attain 100% efficiency, but which may reach 70%. The HME contains a hygroscopic material within a sealed unit. They have a pore size of 0.2 μm to filter bacteria, viruses and particles, this function does not depend on two-way gas flow which is essential for their function as humidifiers. As the warm expired gas cools, so the water vapour condenses on the element, which is warmed both by the specific heat of the exhaled gas and the latent heat of the water. Inhaled, dry and cool gas is thus warmed during inspiration, during which process the element cools down prior to the next exhalation. Problems include moderate inefficiency with prolonged use, increased dead space, increased resistance and infection risk.
- **Leucocyte depletion filters (LDFs):** These filters are fibreglass with a 40 μm pore size and are used to remove white blood cells and other particles and aggregates; in obstetric use, they remove particulate components of amniotic fluid, particularly fetal squames and lamellar bodies. The filters work not only by passive sieving of matter and adherence to the material surface but also by the presence of an electric charge. This is usually negative. They do, however, have the propensity to cause profound hypotension, and the Food and Drug Administration (FDA) in the USA has put out an alert to this effect. When platelets or Factor VIII adhere to the surface, their exposure to this negative charge is associated with significant bradykinin production.

(Bradykinin is an inflammatory mediator, a vasoactive nonopeptide which binds rapidly to the vascular endothelium and mediates vasodilatation and hypotension via G protein-coupled receptors. It has a short half-life of around 15 seconds and is metabolized in passage through the lung.) If the LDF is being used for cell-salvaged blood, it is safe to remove the filter and continue reinfusing the cell-salvaged blood. If it is being used to infuse stored blood, then a micro-aggregate filter should be considered instead.

- **Blood transfusion filters:** The standard blood giving set has a filtration pore size of 170 μm. This is too large to filter some of the particles and micro-aggregates that form in stored blood after around 5 days. These aggregates consist of leucocytes, fibrin and platelets and vary in size between 10 and 200 μm. The specific characteristics of a micro-aggregate filters vary with the manufacturer, but typically the pore size ranges between 10 and 400 μm. The screen medium is usually polyester with a large surface area (40–160 cm^2). There is no good evidence to support their routine use.
- **Epidural catheter filters:** These are used to prevent the inadvertent injection of microscopic glass particles and to prevent the access of bacteria or viruses to the epidural space. The precise dimensions vary with the manufacturer, but a typical product is of low volume (0.8 ml), with a hydrophilic membrane to which bacteria adhere and a pore size of 0.2 μm. Luer lock devices are still widely available despite the recommendation by the now-defunct National Patient Safety Agency (NPSA) that they should be replaced on safety grounds by non-Luer connections. Most manufacturers recommend that syringes no smaller than 10 ml should be used for injection in order to prevent the disruptively high pressures that otherwise can be generated during injection.

Lasers

Commentary

The subject of lasers reappears in the exam mainly because of safety issues. In practice, and with one exception, these concerns are modest; clearly staff and patients must be protected from potential harm, but the actual precautions required to achieve that aim are not complex. The exception is in ENT surgery where there is risk of instant conflagration if a laser beam hits an unprotected endotracheal tube. This aspect of the subject will not extend to 8 minutes of questioning, however, hence the need for you to familiarize yourself with aspects of the basic science.

Core Information

- 'LASER' is an acronym: **L**ight **A**mplification by **S**timulated **E**mission of **R**adiation.
- A laser produces an intense beam of light, which is monochromatic (of a single wavelength or colour). The beam is coherent, with photons in phase, and is collimated, with the photons in almost parallel alignment so there is negligible divergence.

- It is produced by directing an energy source such as an intense flash of light or a high-voltage discharge into a lasing medium. Atoms within the medium absorb the photons of absorbed energy, which drive their electrons to a higher energy level. As the excited atom falls back to its stable state, it emits a photon of energy. If this is reflected back to encounter another excited atom, then another photon will be emitted which is parallel to, and in phase with, the first. Multiple reflection by mirrors back into the lasing medium is used to generate a chain reaction which then produces an intense parallel beam of light. The energy of the laser radiation is given by the equation $E = h \times v$, where E is the energy, h is Planck's constant, and v is photon frequency, which therefore is the only determinant of the energy of the beam.
- The wavelength of the light is dependent on the lasing medium that is used. It is the wavelength that determines the depth of tissue penetration. The lasing medium may be a gas, such as carbon dioxide, argon or helium; a solid such as neodymium: yttrium-aluminium garnet (Nd:YAG); or a liquid. There are many varieties of laser; some relevant examples are outlined in the following. The output of continuous wave lasers is measured in watts (power); that of pulsed lasers is measured in joules (energy).
  - **CO_2 lasers**: these produce infrared light (10,600 nm) whose energy is absorbed by water, which is vaporized. These lasers penetrate tissue no further than 200 μm and so are used for cutting superficial tissues. The beam simultaneously coagulates blood vessels.
  - **Argon**: blue–green argon laser light (480 nm) penetrates between 0.5 and 2 mm and is absorbed maximally by red tissues. It is used, for example, to treat diabetic retinopathy and skin lesions such as port wine birthmarks.
  - **Nd:YAG**: these lasers produce energy in the near infrared spectrum (1,064 nm) and penetrate tissues deeply between 2 and 6 mm. The beam is invisible to the human eye and so is guided by a low-power laser light. At lower power it denatures protein molecules; at higher power it vaporizes tissue and can be used for the surgical removal and debulking of large tumours.
  - **Excimer lasers**: these are 'cold' ultraviolet lasers which do not heat tissues but which break chemical bonds in protein molecules. Their main use is in refractive corneal surgery.

Clinical Considerations

Practical safety implications for the use of lasers in theatre.

- The main danger is to the eyesight of theatre personnel. The non-divergent beam of laser light, even when reflected, may be focused by the lens of the eye onto the fovea and cause irreversible blindness. Distance offers no protection. Other parts of the retina may also absorb the energy, as may the lens and the aqueous and vitreous humours. This does not apply to CO_2 lasers, which will not penetrate that far but which may still be responsible for damage to the cornea and lens.
- Staff should be issued with goggles which protect specifically against the wavelength that is being generated, and, ideally, surgical instruments should have a matt finish to minimize the likelihood of reflection.
- There is a specific hazard associated with laser surgery to the upper airway. A normal PVC tracheal tube will ignite within a few seconds should it be exposed directly to a

laser beam. Stainless steel foil has been used to protect tubes, but there are specially designed tracheal tubes available for use with laser surgery on the upper airway. Although these have flexible metal bodies (either stainless steel or aluminium), they still have cuffs and pilot balloons which should be filled with saline as a precaution. Air/oxygen gas mixtures are safer than nitrous oxide/oxygen mixtures, and ideally the FiO_2 should be kept at no greater than 25%. Surgical swabs or packs can also ignite, and so these must be kept moistened with saline.

Magnetic Resonance Imaging

Commentary

Magnetic resonance (MR) scanning has become the prime imaging technique for numerous soft tissue conditions, and for diseases which affect the CNS. But despite this status, few anaesthetists have wide experience of anaesthetizing patients in this environment, although in some specialist centres MR scanning is being incorporated into the neurosurgical operating theatre environment. The physics that underlies MR imaging (MRI) is also formidable. Why then does the topic continue to reappear in this part of the exam? It may be because the underlying science is elegant, and because the consequences of ignorance are potentially so disastrous.

Core Information

- MRI requires the generation of very strong magnetic fields, typically up to 3.0 tesla. The devices use superconducting magnets which are cooled by immersion in liquid helium at a temperature of 4.2 Kelvin. It complements computerized tomography (CT) in providing high-quality images of soft tissue.
- MRI is based on the principle that, when a cell nucleus with an unpaired proton is exposed to an electromagnetic field, it becomes aligned along the axis of that field. A charged and spinning nucleus generates a magnetic field and acts itself like a small magnet. The aligned nuclei can then be displaced by brief exposure to another magnetic field, generated at right angles to the first. This provokes the phenomenon of nuclear precession, in which the nuclei rotate around an axis different from that around which they are spinning. When the electromagnetic field is removed, the nucleus resumes its original position, and as it relaxes to this position it emits low radiofrequency (RF) radiation. This signal, which is very small, is converted by sophisticated computer technology into an image. The rate at which the nucleus relaxes to its original position varies with the nature of the tissue. (This explanation is simplistic, but this is the FRCA, not the FRCR, and it would be hard to explain why any more detailed exposition is necessary for anaesthetic practice.)
- MR reports usually refer to T_1 and T_2 views. 'T' is a relaxation time constant, T_1 being the image generated a few milliseconds after the electromagnetic field is removed, and T_2 is an image generated slightly later. Nuclei in hydrogen take longer to decay to their original position. In practice, this means, for example, that in a T_1

view, fluid will be dark (as minimal signal is generated), whereas in the T_2 view, fluid will be white.

- The tesla is the unit of magnetic flux density. Should you be asked, 1 tesla (T) is equal to 1 weber m^{-2}, a weber being the SI unit of magnetic flux. It is equal to the magnetic flux that in linking a circuit of one turn produces in it an electromotive force of 1 V as it is uniformly reduced to zero within 1 second. The Earth's magnetic field is approximately 1 gauss. 10,000 gauss equal 1 tesla. (It will be a very peculiar examiner who really wants to know the answer to these questions, but you may as well be prepared.)
- Intravenous contrast agents are sometimes used, typically gadolinium chelates, which shorten nuclear relaxation rates, particularly in T_1 imaging. In patients with impaired renal function these chelates (and other exposure to gadolinium) uniquely can cause the rare condition of nephrogenic systemic fibrosis (nephrogenic fibrosing dermopathy), which is characterized by fibrosis of skin and internal organs.

Supplementary Information and Clinical Applications
The implications of delivering anaesthesia or sedation in an MR scanner.

- **Practical problems:** there are practical difficulties in relation to the physical environment. The patient is enclosed within a narrow tube to which access is limited. The scanner is noisy (>85 decibels) and some patients may be very claustrophobic. Scanning may be prolonged, with complex examinations lasting as long as 1–2 hours.
- **Magnetic field:** at a magnetic field strength of approximately 50 gauss (indicated within the scanning room as a contour marked as the '50-gauss' line), all ferromagnetic items will be subject to movement and will also interfere with the generated image. Items typically affected include hypodermic needles, watches, pagers, mobile telephones, stethoscopes, anaesthetic gas cylinders and ECG electrodes. If these items are close to the field they will become projectile objects.
- **Anaesthesia delivery:** anaesthetic machines which contain ferrous metals (there are non-magnetic machines and cylinders available) must remain outside the 50-gauss line. The machine requires very long anaesthetic tubing and long leads.
- **Patient access:** this is very restricted, and in particular the head and airway are completely inaccessible during scanning. All airway devices must be checked for the presence of any ferromagnetic material: the one-way valve on the pilot balloon of some cuffed endotracheal tubes contains a small spring, as do laryngeal mask airways.
- **Anaesthetic monitoring:** the field may induce current within electric cabling. The consequent heating may lead to thermal injury. Long sampling leads for gas analysis extends delay. Standard ECG electrodes cannot be used. An oesophageal stethoscope may be useful. Pulse oximetry probes are non-ferrous, but a distal site should be used and cable should be insulated. (Severe burns due to induction heating have been reported with standard pulse oximeters.) Non-invasive blood pressure cuffs must have plastic connections as well as long leads to the machines, which must be outside the 50-gauss line. Gas analysis, airways pressure and respiratory indices are usually displayed at the anaesthetic machine, and so again the main problem is delayed sampling time (up to 20 seconds) owing to long tubing.

- **Pacemakers:** cardiac pacemakers and implantable defibrillators require special consideration, as they will malfunction in fields greater than 5 gauss.
- **Infusion pumps:** these may fail if the field strength exceeds 30 gauss.
- **Implants and foreign bodies:** most patient implants (such as orthopaedic prostheses) are non-ferrous. Surgical clips and wires may be magnetic, but their presence does not usually contraindicate MR scanning, as they become embedded in fixed fibrous tissue. Exceptions are intracranial vascular clips. Metal foreign bodies are likely to be ferrous. Non-ferrous items may heat.
- **Generic problems:** there are the generic problems of anaesthetizing patients in remote, unfamiliar and isolated areas. Many more children than adults require general anaesthesia for MR scanning.
- Should you have either exhausted the information here or struggled to provide the information, then you may be asked how you might set up an anaesthetic service for MR scanning. You may not have much time on this, and so a few generic platitudes about the undesirability of a remote location, of the need for training, the use of protocols and the importance of safety issues should be enough to see you through.

Ultrasound

Commentary
The use of ultrasound in anaesthesia and critical care is now routine. Intensivists are performing ultrasound scans of the thorax and abdomen and using bedside echocardiography, and general anaesthetists are using ultrasound not only to guide central venous cannulation and peripheral nerve blockade but also to derive perioperative information about cardiac function. As there are so many important clinical applications, you will not become involved in mathematical discussions about the Doppler equation, but, as with all these physics-based questions, you will have to demonstrate that you know enough about the basic principles of ultrasound to inform your use of the devices.

Core Information
- **Principles of ultrasound:** sound waves which exceed the threshold of human hearing (around 20,000 Hz) are described as ultrasonic. Medical ultrasound uses frequencies of 2–15 MHz. These waves are generated by applying a high-frequency alternating voltage to the two sides of a piezo-electric crystal transducer (which deforms when a voltage is applied to it). This changes the thickness of the crystal, which then emits ultrasonic radiation of the same frequency as the applied potential difference. The crystal also transduces the reflected waves back into an electrical signal from which a computer-generated cross-sectional image can be displayed. The signals are unable to penetrate bone or gas-filled structures, including the lung, and so ultrasound studies of these structures are not possible. Reflected signals are strongest from the interface between tissues of different

density, such as air and blood, and when the structure being examined is perpendicular to the angle of the beam.

- **Images of tissues:** tissue that is highly reflective (hyperechoic) appears white. (Examples include bone and fascial planes.) Weakly reflected waves (hypoechoic) are darker. (Examples include muscle and fat.) Nerves can be either hyperechoic or hypoechoic. The cervical nerve roots in the neck, for example, are hypoechoic and appear dark, but by the time they have formed divisions at the lateral border of the first rib are hyperechoic and white. Blood does not reflect (anechoic) and so blood vessels appear black. Air–tissue interfaces reflect strongly.
- **Frequency effects:** the higher the frequency the better the resolution of the image, but this is at the expense of tissue penetration. Lower frequencies will produce images from deeper structures, but their definition is less good.
- **Attenuation of ultrasound:** this can be expressed as the 'half-power distance', which is the depth at which the sound is halved. This depth is 3,800 mm for water and less than 1 mm for air and lung. Sound is attenuated by bone (2–7 mm) and also by muscle (6–10 mm).
- **Velocity:** ultrasound moves through tissue at 1,540 m s^{-1}. This rapid transmission and reception of pulses of sound allows the generation of dynamic images.
- **2-D images:** these are generated by probes which comprise an array of parallel piezo-electric elements that are activated in sequence, rather than simultaneously. This wavefront can, in practice, scan a 90° sector of tissue, with the reflected echoes processed into a two-dimensional picture.
- **Doppler effect and colour Doppler:** the Doppler effect describes the change in the frequency of sound and ultrasound if either the emitter or the receiver is moving. Colour flow Doppler is able to display blood flow in real time, using three basic colours. Blood flow towards the transducer is red, whereas that away from the transducer is blue. It is clearly important not to assume that these colours indicate arterial and venous blood. The colour green can be added when blood flow velocity exceeds a preset limit. In areas of turbulent flow, such as may occur across a diseased cardiac valve, all three colours may be displayed.

Supplementary and Clinical Information

Clinical uses of ultrasound in intensive care and anaesthesia.

- **Critical care:** ultrasound scans of the abdomen and thorax can identify fluid collections, which can then be drained under ultrasound guidance. Cranial scanning is routinely used in neonatal intensive care to detect intraventricular haemorrhage and midline shift.
- **Echocardiography in critical care:** echocardiography is increasingly popular in critical care to assess cardiac function. Imaging can be structural, identifying, for example, pericardial effusion or abnormalities of ventricular wall and cavity size, and it can be haemodynamic, utilizing Doppler techniques to view blood flow through the valves and cardiac chambers.
- **Central venous cannulation:** ultrasonic-guided cannulation is now routine, particularly for the internal jugular route.

- **Air embolism:** the interface between air and blood generates a strong reflected signal, and a Doppler probe over the praecordium is sensitive enough to produce ultrasound images from bubbles as small as 2 mm in diameter.
- **Ultrasonic devices:** the principles of ultrasound can be used in gas flowmeters, in cleaning devices and in humidifiers.
- **TOE:** modern TOE probes allow $180°$ views of the heart, and the absence of large tissue masses between the probe and the myocardium allows for well-defined ultrasound images. It has specialist cardiac uses such as the assessment of valvular heart disease, the diagnosis of bacterial endocarditis, the identification of atrial thrombus and the investigation of congenital heart disease. It can identify aortic atherosclerosis, aortic dissection and disease, and can assess paracardiac masses. For the general anaesthetist, its main value lies in the intra-operative determination of left ventricular preload and function, the diagnosis of acute left ventricular dysfunction and myocardial ischaemia, and the detection of air embolism. (Complications are mainly mechanical, and relate to the passage and presence of a firm probe within the thin-walled oesophagus with the consequent risk of perforation. The reported complication rate is very low; in one [early] series of 10,419 awake patients there were only two cases of bleeding.)
- **Oesophageal Doppler monitoring (ODM):** see under 'Measurement of Cardiac Output'.
- **Regional nerve blockade:** ultrasound-guided regional anaesthesia (UGRA) is now regarded by many as a technique that is faster, safer and more efficacious than either landmark or nerve-stimulator assisted methods. The evidence for these assumptions is absent, and the controlled trials to support this view may be a long time coming. As the complication rate of nerve blocks is already low, the numbers of patients required to demonstrate a difference are impractically large. Few would argue, however, with the intuitive proposition that if the needle tip is visible and if the local anaesthetic is seen spreading circumferentially around the nerve, then more successful and safer blocks seem likely. Nerve fascicles themselves are dark, whereas supporting connective tissue tends to be brighter and more hyperechoic. This is a generalization because the varying structure of the fascia which invests a particular nerve means that the same nerve may have a different ultrasound appearance along its course. Superficial nerves and plexuses are more suitable for UGRA than those sited more deeply. The sciatic nerve in the buttock, for example, is a large structure that is nonetheless difficult to identify because of attenuation of the beam by surrounding gluteal muscles. The advancing needles are best displayed if they are parallel to the probe face; at angles greater than $45°$ they become difficult to see. In central neuraxial techniques, ultrasound-assisted location may help confirm the depth to the epidural space, the midline or the spinal level, but real-time guidance is more difficult given that both spinals and epidurals are two-handed techniques, and so its use is not yet routine.
- **Gastric emptying.** Ultrasound can also be used to assess gastric contents (which is of particular interest in obstetric and emergency anaesthesia) by scanning the gastric antrum. Its value is limited by a high false negative rate of up to 25%, and so it is not currently possible to state unequivocally that the stomach is empty, but the false positive rate is low and so it does allow a broad assessment of risk.

- **The cricothyroid membrane.** The high failure rate of emergency front-of-neck access has been attributed largely to the inability accurately to locate the cricothyroid membrane. Ultrasound of the neck prior to induction of anaesthesia provides the most reliable means of identification.

Videolaryngoscopy

Commentary

This oral may touch on the various guidelines that are produced by the Difficult Airway Society (DAS), although videolaryngoscopy does not figure strongly in these, and it does not feature at all in the 2015 obstetric airway algorithms. Nonetheless, the use of these devices is increasingly common, hence their appearance in the exam. The underlying physical principles are limited, but the laryngoscopes themselves do differ in design, and this has formed the basis of some of the questions around this topic.

Core Information

- **Conventional direct laryngoscopy:** direct laryngoscopy has been a core anaesthetic skill since Janeway devised the precursor of modern laryngoscopes in 1913. It remains the gold standard in as much as it may provide an uninterrupted view of the laryngeal inlet, but it is nonetheless a technique of some complexity. It requires the alignment of the oral, the pharyngeal and the tracheal planes into a single visual axis from the incisors to the glottis; and laryngoscopy and tracheal intubation will be made more difficult by anything which impedes that process. Such factors include limited mouth opening, prominent upper incisors, a pronounced overbite, macroglossia, an arched palate, an infantile epiglottis and a high anterior larynx. But even in a normal airway the attainment of a Cormack and Lehane Grade 1 view (in which the whole glottis is visible) may require considerable physical manipulation, including occipital extension, neck flexion, external laryngeal pressure and substantial lifting forces imposed by the laryngoscope blade in the vallecula.
- **Videolaryngoscopy:** this can mitigate some of these factors. It is not necessary to obtain a direct visual axis, and videolaryngoscopes allow the glottis to be seen indirectly. This can minimize potentially traumatic airway manipulation with less movement of the head and cervical spine, and with much lower lifting forces.
- **Basic design:** the various available devices have different features, but in terms of the physical principles all simply use forms of video camera technology to allow an indirect view of the glottis. High-resolution digital cameras at the tip of the laryngoscope blade can produce high-definition images, either on a small screen attached to the device itself or on a larger monitor. The proximity of the camera to the glottis provides a much wider angle of view than is typical when a $15°$ direct laryngoscope is used.
- **Classification of videolaryngoscopes.** This is evolving as newer models are introduced; however, one accepted classification of these devices is into:

Macintosh-modified, tube/guide channel and angulated blade laryngoscopes. An open access systematic review published in 2012 cited more than 25 different models in their search terms, which suggests that obtaining uniform data for comparison is likely to be very difficult. The devices outlined here are examples of just three of those that are available.

- **Macintosh-modification.** An example of this design is the McGrath Mac, which essentially integrates video technology with a conventional Macintosh laryngoscope. This design means that the device can give an indirect view but can also be used to obtain a direct view of the glottis in the traditional way. (It can also be classified as an angulated blade device.)
- **Tube/guide channel.** An example of this design is the Airtraq. These devices have a guide channel with a preloaded tracheal tube. The Airtraq has a small video screen attached to the handle but the camera can be attached to a monitor as desired.
- **Angulated blade.** An example of this design is the GlideScope. The angulated blade is designed to allow a video view of the glottis with minimal manipulation of the head and neck, although a greater tilt of the handle may be necessary with greater potential risk to the upper incisors. The tracheal tube is preloaded with a curved stylet which takes it round the natural hypopharyngeal curve. Once the tube is at the glottis the stylet is removed, the tube straightens, and as it does so it advances into the trachea automatically without the need for any further downward movement of the tube.

Supplementary and Clinical Information

- **Evidence of benefit:** the currently available videolaryngoscopes are different in design, as are the groups of medical professionals in the studies which have reported their use, so there are as yet no unequivocal data to support their introduction into routine practice. The main outcome measures are successful intubation, first-time intubation and time to tracheal intubation. In a group of unselected patients, intubation using direct laryngoscopy will be straightforward in 95%, so it is no surprise that videolaryngoscopy is no better than direct laryngoscopy. In patients in whom difficult intubation is suspected and in unexpected difficult laryngoscopy, videolaryngoscopes increase the proportion of Cormack and Lehane Grade 1 views. (Not all the devices are the same and so this is a generalization. It would be unreasonable were an examiner to start asking about the specific differences say between the Pentax AWS and the V-MAC models). It is also the case that, although Cormack and Lehane grades correlate well with the ease or otherwise of intubation after direct laryngoscopy, that may not be so with videolaryngoscopy in which a good view of the glottis is not necessarily associated with success. Many of the studies give no accurate assessment of the competence and experience of the operators, and this also limits the conclusions that can be drawn. Hence, these conclusions are limited essentially to the fact that the devices can certainly improve the laryngeal view that is obtained, especially with non-experts, and especially in cases with Cormack and Lehane grades 3 and 4. Whether or not this translates to a higher success rate in tracheal and in difficult tracheal intubation has yet to be established. Despite the lack of uniformity in the studies, however, the overall impression given by the enthusiasts for the technique is that the videolaryngoscope is an easier device to master than the traditional laryngoscope, that it can provide a better view and that in due course it may well become the default means by which the trachea is intubated.

- **Difficult Airway Society (DAS) Guidelines 2015.** Airway guidelines invariably involve quite detailed algorithms which it is not practicable to reproduce during an oral. You might, however, be asked to outline your approach to an unanticipated difficult intubation. The 2015 DAS guidelines are the most recent (at the time of writing), but it is possible that in due course the updates will have more emphasis on newer technologies. Otherwise, in summary, the steps of the basic algorithm can be described as follows. (As always any algorithm should always be considered in context. Unanticipated difficult intubation will require different management if it occurs in a leaking aortic aneurysm or a category one caesarean section rather than an elective laparoscopic cholecystectomy.)
- **1. Attempted laryngoscopy and tracheal intubation.** On the assumption that the patient is in the optimal position for laryngoscopy, that the appropriate blade is being used and that neuromuscular paralysis is adequate, the algorithm suggests manoeuvres such as external laryngeal pressure, the removal of cricoid pressure in cases where it is being employed, the use of a bougie and a maximum of three plus one attempts (the last by a more experienced clinician if available). These attempts can include the use of a videolaryngoscope. Multiple failed attempts risk airway trauma and the development of a 'Can't intubate, can't oxygenate' (CICO) scenario.
- **2. Rescue via second-generation supraglottic airway device (SAD).** Should laryngoscopy fail, the guidelines recommend the use of a second-generation SAD such as a Pro-Seal or LMA Supreme. (These airways include features such as oesophageal drainage tubes, posterior inflatable cuffs and integral bite blocks.) Again, three attempts with or without a change of device are recommended. During these steps oxygenation and anaesthesia must be maintained throughout.
- **3. Actions after successful SAD ventilation.** Should SAD insertion and ventilation be successful, the options thereafter depend on the surgical context and the risk and benefits of proceeding. Alternatives are (i) to proceed without intubation, (ii) attempt to intubate via the SAD, (iii) continue to a surgical airway or (iv) allow the patient to awaken.
- **4. Actions after failed SAD ventilation.** Should SAD ventilation fail, then the anaesthetist should revert to facemask ventilation using a two-handed, two-person technique as necessary. If oxygenation is maintained by this method then the patient should be allowed to awaken.
- **5. Actions after failed facemask ventilation.** This CICO scenario should be managed by emergency front-of-neck access.

Peripheral Nerve Stimulators

Commentary

There are two types of peripheral nerve stimulator: those which assess the degree of neuromuscular blockade and those which are used to aid accurate needle placement in regional analgesia. The discussion will probably centre round one or other of the devices rather than both. Neither is unduly complex electrically, and the oral is likely to focus equally on practical and clinical aspects of their use.

Core Information

Nerve Stimulation for Assessment of Neuromuscular Block

It is now considered mandatory to use a peripheral nerve stimulator to assess the degree of residual muscular blockade after any neuromuscular blocking drugs have been given.

Assessment

- **Clinical signs:** grip strength, the generation of a tidal volume of between 15 and 20 ml kg^{-1}, the ability to keep the head lifted from the pillow for 5 seconds and the capacity to retain a tongue depressor gripped between the teeth are cited as useful, if crude indicators of recovery from neuromuscular block.
- **Nerve stimulators:** the degree of block can be assessed using a battery-operated nerve stimulator that is capable of delivering different patterns of square wave monophasic pulses of uniform amplitude. (A biphasic pulse or one that lasts longer than 0.5 ms may give misleading results either by causing direct muscle stimulation or by eliciting repetitive firing.) The threshold current, which is the current required to elicit a detectable muscle response, is around 15 mA. In order to ensure recruitment of all the muscle fibres, a supramaximal impulse is delivered, typically of around 50–60 mA (if transcutaneous electrodes are being used). From Ohm's law any increase in resistance (secondary to cool or greasy skin, for example) requires an increase in voltage to maintain a constant current. Modern nerve stimulators change the internal voltage to maintain a constant current over a range of different resistances. The different patterns of stimulation include the following.
- **Single twitch:** a single supramaximal stimulus is delivered once every 10 seconds (0.1 Hz). A decrease in twitch height will be apparent only after 75% or more receptors are blocked and will disappear at 90% occupancy, so this is of limited use in monitoring non-depolarizing block. It can be used for assessing block caused by depolarizing relaxants (which do not exhibit fade or post-tetanic facilitation).
- **Train-of-four (TOF):** four identical supramaximal stimuli are delivered at 2 Hz and repeated every 10 seconds. The number of twitches observed corresponds approximately to the percentage receptor blockade (0 twitches = 100% blockade, 1 twitch = 90%, 2 twitches = 80%, 3 twitches = 75%, 4 twitches = <75%). The ratio of twitch heights can be quantified to give an objective measure of block. The $T_4:T_1$ ratio must be 90% before it can be assumed that protective airway reflexes are intact.
- **Double burst stimulation (DBS):** two tetanic bursts at 50 Hz and separated by 750 ms are applied every 20 ms. The muscle response is detectable as two twitches which show a more exaggerated fade than that of the TOF. DBS is more sensitive at detecting residual block, which makes it of particular value at the end of surgery.
- **Tetanic stimulation:** stimuli of 50 or 100 Hz for 5 seconds may produce fade in situations when the twitch response after TOF or DBS has returned to normal. It is therefore a more sensitive means of detecting low levels of receptor blockade. Fade is also seen with phase II block. It is followed by post-tetanic potentiation if single

twitch stimulation is given within 2 minutes. Tetanic stimulation cannot be used in the conscious patient who may be aware of marked residual discomfort even if the stimulus has been applied during anaesthesia.

- **Post-tetanic count (PTC):** a tetanic stimulus as described earlier is followed by single stimuli at 1-second intervals. Tetany triggers supranormal acetylcholine release (post-tetanic facilitation) which transiently overcomes the neuromuscular blockade. The twitches which result comprise the post-tetanic count. The technique is used to monitor significant degrees of block (for example, in neurosurgery during which any patient movement could be disastrous), and a PTC of less than 5 indicates profound block. A PTC of greater than 15 approximates to two twitches following TOF stimulation, at which point pharmacological reversal should be possible.

- **Mechanomyography, electromyography** and **acceleromyography:** these methods allow much more accurate measurement of neuromuscular blockade during onset and offset of effect. **Mechanomyography** measures the isometric contraction force in the adductor pollicis following ulnar nerve stimulation. **Electromyography** records the electrical activity of the stimulated muscle immediately prior to contraction. It determines the amplitude of the signal, usually the sum of the compound muscle action potentials. **Acceleromyography** uses a small piezoelectric transducer to measure the isotonic acceleration of the muscle (isotonic describes a change in muscle length without any change in tension). If mass remains constant, as it clearly does, then from Newton's second law (force = mass × acceleration) the force of contraction can be calculated. Whether or not such (relatively expensive) accuracy is necessary during routine clinical practice remains contentious, and at present these instruments are used mainly in research.

- **Clinical practicalities:** the sensitivity of muscle groups to non-depolarizing muscle-blocking drugs varies considerably (but is similar across mammalian species), and so recovery in one particular set does not necessarily confirm adequate overall reversal. The motor nerves that are usually stimulated are the ulnar nerve at the wrist – evoking a response in the adductor pollicis, and the facial nerve in the region of the temporo-mandibular joint – evoking a response in the orbicularis oculi muscle around the eye. The diaphragm is the most resistant muscle of all and requires up to twice the dose for the same effect as the adductor pollicis. The muscles of facial expression and of the larynx are much less resistant. These sites of stimulation are useful therefore because block of orbicularis oculi is a better indicator of laryngeal muscle block than adductor pollicis, which itself is slow to recover and better reflects the degree of any residual diaphragmatic paralysis.

Nerve Stimulation for Location of Peripheral Nerves

Ultrasound-guided nerve blockade is now commonplace, but the peripheral nerve stimulator is still useful, either for supplementary confirmation of needle placement or as a safety device to minimize the risk of neurapraxia or intraneural injection.

- The device should maintain a constant current despite the changes in resistance that the needle will encounter as it penetrates tissues of different densities. This is perhaps the most important characteristic. These resistances in the external circuit can vary from around 1–20 kΩ (kOhm), so were the device to deliver a constant voltage the current could vary 20-fold.

- It should have a linear output which can easily be varied.
- The output should be monophasic so that the current flows in one direction only. It is usually a rectangular waveform, but there is no evidence that this is better than any other.
- It should have the facility to alter the frequency of the stimulus delivered (usually 1–2 Hz).
- It should have a clear digital display across the current range from 0.1 to 5.0 mA.
- It should have a short pulse width of 50–100 s, which provides better discrimination of the distance between the needle and the nerve. The shorter the pulse width the greater the change in stimulation strength as the needle advances.
- It should incorporate an indicator that shows the integrity of the electrical circuit.
- It should be battery operated (for patient safety), have a battery-level indicator, low resistance clips and be robust.
- **Electrodes:** the negative electrode should be attached to the stimulator needle rather than the positive. In this situation, the current flow towards the needle produces an area of depolarization which readily triggers an action potential. This requires only 25% of the current that is needed if the polarity is reversed. If the anode is used, the current produces a zone of hyperpolarization immediately around the needle tip, with an area of depolarization encircling it.
- **Pulse duration – rheobase and chronaxie:** the rheobase is the minimum current required to stimulate a nerve, while the chronaxie is the duration of current stimulus required to stimulate that nerve at twice the rheobase. This has some clinical relevance because different nerves have different chronaxie, and this is a means of quantifying their excitability. Large A motor fibres have shorter chronaxie (0.05–0.1 ms) than the fibres subserving touch and pain (A and C fibres with chronaxie of 0.15 and 0.4 ms, respectively). This means that, in an awake patient, it is possible to use a short pulse duration to stimulate motor fibres without eliciting pain.
- **Thresholds:** techniques vary; some anaesthetists start with a relatively high current of up to 2.0 mA, whereas others stay below 1.0 mA. As the needle approaches the likely site of injection, the current should be reduced to about 0.5 mA; at this stimulus the needle tip will be 1–2 mm from the nerve. This is a broad consequence of Coulomb's (inverse-square) law in that the minimum current needed to stimulate a nerve is directly proportional to the square of the distance from that nerve. In theory, therefore, if the distance between needle and nerve is halved the stimulatory current will be reduced to an eighth. If you are eliciting a vigorous twitch at a low current, say of around 0.2 mA, then you will be very close to, or even in, the nerve. The use of ultrasound, however, has demonstrated that in practice the relationship may not be so reliable as a needle sometimes may be in close proximity to a nerve but yet a current of more than 1.0 mA will elicit no motor response.
- **Injection:** a small amount of local anaesthetic will abolish the twitch by physical displacement. This has been demonstrated experimentally using saline and air. If the twitch does not disappear on injection, it suggests that the needle may be intraneural and so should be withdrawn slightly.

Characteristics of Stimulator Needles

- **Insulated or non-insulated:** most needles are insulated (with Teflon coating) apart from the uncovered tip through which the current passes. You should be aware that non-insulated needles can also be used effectively because the current density remains greater at the tip of the needle than down the shaft. False positives are more common, however, because there can be some nerve stimulation at the level of the shaft.
- **Long bevel, short bevel or side-ported:** the choice of needle is contentious. A long-bevelled needle is sharp, penetrates tissues readily and so reduces the appreciation of fascial planes. Should it penetrate a nerve, however, the clean cut may actually cause less damage either than a short-bevelled (30°) or pencil-point needle with a proximal side hole. Increasing experience with ultrasound is showing that even when an effective twitch has been elicited these 'atraumatic' needles may deliver the local anaesthetic too far from the nerve. They may also produce a less clear ultrasound image.
- **Sizes:** there are numerous sizes, depending on the manufacturer, but common lengths include 30, 50, 90, 100 and 150 mm. Most are 22G.
- Nerve stimulators complement, but do not obviate, the need for accurate anatomical knowledge. The rationale for their use is twofold.
  - **Efficacy:** their use has been reported to double the success rate of some blocks (pre-ultrasound). Their value may in due course be reduced to that of providing confirmation that an ultrasound-guided needle is correctly placed.
  - **Safety:** their use removes the need to elicit paraesthesia. Paraesthesia occurs only when the advancing needle touches a nerve, and some chronic pain specialists believe that paraesthesia is associated almost invariably with later dysaesthesia. A low current setting of around 0.2–0.3 mA will warn the anaesthetist that the needle is too close to a nerve.

Electrical Safety

Commentary

In general, patients are well protected from electrical danger, and for most anaesthetists this topic will remain only theoretical. Electricity does appear as a subject, but its main application, apart from biological potentials, relates to safety.

Core Information

Basic Definitions

- **Electricity:** this is the flow of electrons, which is driven by potential difference (the voltage) through a conductor past a given point per unit time. This current is measured in amperes.

- **Resistance:** this is the resistance along a conductor to the flow of current. It is not frequency-dependent. Resistance is measured in ohms.
- **Ohm's law:** this states that the electrical potential (V) = current (I) × resistance (R).
- **Impedance:** the impedance is the sum of all the forces impeding electron flow in an AC circuit. Unlike resistance, it is dependent on frequency and includes resistors, capacitors and inductors. (Insulators are high-impedance devices; conductors are low-impedance devices.) Impedance through capacitors and inductors is related to the frequency at which AC reverses direction. Impedance is also measured in ohms (volt/ampere).
- **Lethal current:** the relationships described previously explain how dangerous currents can be generated. Ohm's law determines the magnitude of the current that flows, $I = V/R$. An individual standing on an antistatic floor may have an impedance of 20 kΩ or more, and so, should he or she touch a live enclosure, the current flow will be 240/20,000, or 12 mA. Wet hands or fluid on the floor may reduce the impedance to 2 kΩ, and so the current, 240/2,000, becomes potentially lethal at 120 mA. This is not enough to blow the fuse and the circuit remains live.

Risks to Patients within the Operating Theatre

Patients can become part of an electrical circuit in two ways

- **Direct connection (resistive coupling):** if any part of the body is directly in contact with an electricity source or with an earthed object, then current may pass through the patient to earth. This can be caused either by faulty equipment or by leakage currents. As all electrical equipment is at a higher potential than earth, current seeks to flow to earth through a circuit of which a patient may form part. Medical equipment is well insulated and these leakage currents are usually small, but they do still carry the risk of microshock.
- **Indirect connection (capacitive coupling):** in some circumstances, the body can act as one plate of a capacitor. If DC is applied to a capacitor such as a defibrillator, current continues to flow only until the positive plate reaches the same potential as the electrical source. If, however, AC is applied, then the plates alternate polarity at the same frequency as the current. The repetitive pattern of charge and discharge sets up a current flow across the gap with the effective completion of the circuit. A patient on an operating table can therefore act as one plate of a capacitor while the theatre light with its 50 Hz AC supply forms the other.

Minimizing Risks

Use of appropriate (and well-maintained) equipment.

- **Identification:** equipment designed for medical use is generally of high specification with an identifier to show the grade of protection that it offers.
  - *Class I:* offers basic protection only. Any conducting part that is accessible to the user, such as the casing, must be connected to earth, and must be insulated from the main supply. (Such equipment has fuses on the live and neutral supply in the equipment, as well as on the live wire in the mains plug.)

— *Class II:* this equipment has reinforced, or double, insulation that protects all the parts that are accessible. It does not require an earth.

— *Class III:* this equipment uses safety extra low voltage (SELV) which does not exceed 24 V AC. There is no risk of gross electrocution, but microshock is still possible.

— *Type B:* such equipment has low leakage currents; 0.5 mA for class 1B and 0.1 mA for class IIB.

— *Type BF:* type BF is the same as type B, except that the piece of equipment that is applied to the patient is isolated from all its other parts.

— *Type CF:* this is class I or II equipment which is considered safe for direct connection to the heart. Leakage currents are extremely low, being 0.05 mA per electrode for class ICF equipment and 0.01 mA per electrode for class IICF.

Other Precautions

- **Common earth:** voltage differences between multiple pieces of medical equipment increase the risk of leakage currents which may flow from the higher to the lower potential via the patient. This risk is minimized if the equipment is connected to a common equipotential earth point via a single cable.
- **Isolated (floating) circuits:** in these circuits the equipment that is mains-powered is separated from the patient circuit by an isolating transformer (comprising primary and secondary coils that are insulated from each other). AC from the primary (earthed) mains supply induces current in the secondary coil, which means that although the patient circuit is live, it remains earth-free.
- **Earth leakage circuit breakers (ELCB):** these devices do not protect against short circuits or overloading (appropriate fuses are still required), but they do cut off the electrical supply to faulty equipment in the presence of current leakage. There are different types, but in simplistic terms each consists of a tripping coil which, when activated by excessive current, trips a relay which interrupts the supply.

Clinical Applications

The effects of electric current within the body.

- **Effects of electricity:** at 1 mA a subject will feel tingling and at 5 mA definite pain. At 15 mA there is tonic contraction of muscles, which at 50 mA involves all the muscles of respiration. At 100 mA ventricular fibrillation supervenes.
- **Electrocution:** this can happen should a patient become part of an electrical circuit. The main problem is the fibrillatory potential of the current, which, if applied externally, need reach only 50–100 mA. Such current disrupts the normal function of cells, causing muscle contraction, respiratory paralysis and ventricular fibrillation. The current frequency is also important, with 50 Hz (the frequency of alternating current [AC] in the UK) being optimally lethal. AC at 50 Hz can generate high voltages economically and can readily be transformed, but it will interfere with ion flux across all cell membranes and force ions in both directions. (The ion pump can cope better with direct current [DC] voltages.) Higher frequencies are much less dangerous and above 100 Hz have no fibrillatory potential. In electrocution, there is additional thermal injury, caused as the electrical energy dissipates through tissues.

The severity of the electrical burn is directly proportional to the current density and its duration of application.

- **Microshock:** gross electrocution by externally applied energy requires currents of around 100 mA, but very much lower currents in the region of 50–100 µA can induce ventricular fibrillation if they are applied directly to the ventricle. This rare phenomenon is known as microshock. It can occur only with a combination of factors that arise in specialized situations in which the patient accidentally becomes part of an electrical circuit. Microshock requires an electrical contact applied directly over a small area of the myocardium and which can be earthed through the patient. Faulty equipment, even with very low leakage currents, but which is connected to intracardiac devices such as pacing wires or catheters, is capable of delivering this microcurrent directly to the ventricle and inducing fibrillation. Someone holding a pacing wire in one hand while touching the leakage source with the other may inadvertently complete the circuit and electrocute the patient. The risk is lessened in this instance by wearing gloves, and in general by the use of earth-free mains supply.

Defibrillation

Commentary
This is primarily a question about the physics of electrical defibrillation. There has been recent interest in different waveforms, and this may extend the science questioning, but not so far that you will not be asked about the clinical implications. Resuscitation is a core anaesthetic skill.

Core Information
The electrical principles underlying defibrillation; the basic circuit and its components (Figure 5.8).

- **Capacitance:** a capacitor consists of two plates that are separated by an insulator and which will store electrons after the application of a potential difference. Capacitance is the ability to hold electric charge. Its units are coulombs, C. One coulomb is the amount of electric charge which passes a point when a current of 1 A flows for 1 s.
- **Defibrillator circuit:** a potential of between 4,000 and 6,000 V is applied across the capacitor to produce a store of electrons. (The selected voltage is varied by means of a variable transformer.) When the defibrillator is activated, this stored charge is released as a pulse of current across the patient's heart. This stored energy is by convention expressed in joules rather than volts. (One joule is the work required to move a charge of 1 C through a potential difference of 1 V [$J = V \times C$].) Not all of this energy is delivered; the inductance coil (inductor) in the output circuit decelerates the rapid discharge of the capacitor to give a shock that is slowed to 4–10 ms. This duration gives the optimal chance of synchronous myocardial depolarization. (The displayed energy is that delivered, not that stored.)

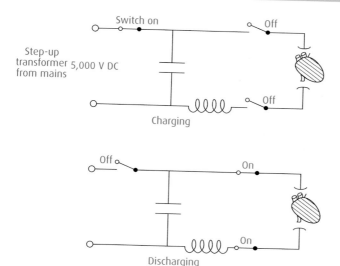

Fig. 5.8 Defibrillator circuit.

- **Impedance:** the efficiency of the applied shock is greater if transthoracic impedance is minimized by the use of conductive gels, firm paddle pressure, and by defibrillation from front-to-back rather than from sternum to apex. (Impedance is the sum of all forces impeding electron flow in an AC circuit.)
- **Waveforms:** the current pulse described previously is monophasic, travelling in the positive direction only. A monophasic pulse can have two waveforms (exponential current decay and a damped sine wave), which are of similar efficacy. In a defibrillator that uses a biphasic waveform, the current is reversed halfway through the discharge to move both in a positive and a negative direction. (There are also two biphasic waveforms: truncated exponential decay and rectilinear.) Biphasic shocks are not only more effective than monophasic, but they also cause less myocardial injury. Their use is now becoming widespread.

Supplementary Information and Clinical Considerations

- **Atrial and ventricular fibrillation:** in health, the sinus impulse is conducted evenly and concentrically to all parts of the atria and thence to the ventricles. When atrial fibrillation (AF) supervenes, the excitation and recovery of different parts of the atria becomes uncoordinated, with various areas at different stages of excitation and recovery. It is similar with ventricular fibrillation (VF). The changing amplitude of the ECG reflects electrical activity, but depolarization is chaotic and unable therefore to generate any cardiac output.
- **Effects:** in AF, there is loss of the atrial contribution to ventricular filling, which is usually around 20%. In addition, the risk of thrombus formation is substantially increased. A fibrillating ventricle produces no cardiac output.
- **Causes:** these are numerous and the examiner will not want you to do more than suggest the most significant. Common causes of AF include ischaemic heart disease and acute critical illness, particularly sepsis. (Other cited causes such as mitral

stenosis and thyrotoxicosis are rare.) VF is caused by myocardial disease, both ischaemic and myopathic, by hypoxia, by profound hypothermia, by electrolyte imbalance, by some drugs and by electrocution.

The Electrical Management of Fibrillation

- **Atrial fibrillation (AF):** refractory AF is treated by the application of a DC shock, which is synchronized to the peak deflection of the 'R' wave of ventricular depolarization on the ECG. The risk of inducing VF is very high during repolarization (as shown by the 'T' wave on the ECG). This is why the 'R-on-T' rhythm is particularly dangerous.
- **Ventricular fibrillation (VF):** this can be treated either by mechanical defibrillation or electrical defibrillation. The application of mechanical energy in the form of a praecordial thump (sometimes known as 'thumpversion') may convert VF to a viable rhythm only if it is applied very early. It normally achieves only around 5–10 joules of mechanical energy. In electrical defibrillation, a defibrillator delivers a charge across the chest which causes simultaneous depolarization of myocardial cells. If the procedure is successful, there is a short refractory period after which there is resumption of normal pacemaker activity with myocardial contraction and a stable rhythm.

Surgical Diathermy

Commentary

Diathermy is used widely and is in essence a surgical instrument. The anaesthetist, unfair though it seems, may in practice be blamed should a patient suffer a burn owing to malpositioning of the plate. Diathermy may also interfere with monitors and can disrupt pacemaker function, and so it is a topic on which some basic knowledge is expected.

Core Information

- Diathermy is used widely in surgical practice, both for coagulation and for cutting, and relies on the heat generated as an electric current passes through a resistance that is concentrated in the probe itself.
- Heat generation is proportional to the power that is developed, typically 50–400 W. Heat is proportional to I^2 (current)/A (area).
- A high-frequency sine waveform is used for cutting, typically 0.5 MHz.
- A damped waveform is used for coagulation, typically 1.0–1.5 MHz.
- High frequency is necessary because muscle is very sensitive to DC and to AC at low frequencies. Mains frequency is low, at 50 Hz, which is a frequency that is particularly efficient at precipitating VF. Very high-frequency current has minimal tissue penetration and passes across the myocardium without ill effect.
- Burning and heating effects can occur at all frequencies.

- There are two types of diathermy:
  - **Unipolar:** there are two connections to the patient; the neutral (or indifferent) patient plate, and the active coagulation or cutting electrode. Current passes through both, but the current density at the active electrode is very high and generates high temperatures. At the patient plate, the current density is dispersed over a wide area and heating does not occur. The patient plate, and hence the patient, is kept at earth potential, which reduces the risks of capacitor linkage (in which diathermy current may flow in the absence of direct contact). Modern diathermy machines incorporate isolating capacitors to minimize the problem. An alternative is to use an earth-free or floating circuit.
  - **Bipolar:** in this instance the current is localized to the instrument; it passes only from one blade of the forceps to the other. Bipolar diathermy uses low power, and this limits its efficacy in the coagulation of all but small vessels. The circuit is not earthed.

Supplementary and Clinical Information

Risks of Diathermy

- There is a risk of thermal injury at the site of the indifferent electrode (the diathermy plate) which must be in close and even contact with a large area of skin, ideally an area that is well perfused and so which will dissipate heat. Adhesive and conductive gels are useful. If the area of contact is small, the current density increases to the point at which a burn is probable.
- Thermal injury at a metal contact site may occur if the plate is detached or malpositioned. The diathermy current may flow to earth through any point at which the patient is touching metal (such as the operating table, lithotomy poles or ECG electrodes) and cause a burn.
- The plate should not be placed over an area where there is a metal prosthesis in place (usually the hip). Metal has a low resistance in comparison with tissue, and so the current will flow preferentially through the prosthesis, generating a potentially dangerous current density.
- The instrument may be activated when it is not in contact with the tissue to be cut or coagulated.
- The circuit may be completed via a route that does not include the indifferent electrode; this may also result in a burn.
- Alcoholic skin preparation solutions have ignited after diathermy activation.
- Diathermy may interfere with cardiac pacemaker function. The indifferent electrode should be sited as far distant as possible from the pacemaker, and bipolar diathermy should be used wherever possible. If the use of unipolar diathermy is unavoidable, it should be deployed in short bursts. Cutting diathermy causes more of a problem than coagulation. Implantable cardiac defibrillators (ICDs) are increasingly common. In emergency surgery these can be protected from the effects of surgical diathermy by the application of a magnet which will deactivate the ICD but not the pacing function.
- Diathermy may interfere with monitoring devices. This problem can be minimized by the use of electrical filters.

Physics, Clinical Measurement, Equipment and Statistics

- Diathermy may lead to ischaemia and infarction of structures supplied by fine end-arteries. Classic examples include the penis (hence unipolar diathermy must be avoided in circumcision) and the testis, which has a vulnerable vascular pedicle.

Point of Care Tests (and ROTEM)

Commentary

This is likely to be an oral which focuses most on thromboelastography, but it may be introduced by a general question about the point of care tests with which you are familiar (and possibly about their broad principles of measurement). Some of these are described in the following outline, but you are likely to move through these and on to ROTEM fairly quickly.

Core Information

Blood Glucose

- There are various devices available for measuring blood glucose which range from colorimetric strips to more sophisticated handheld meters. The simple strips are usually impregnated with glucose oxidase which converts glucose to gluconic acid with the production of hydrogen peroxide. They also contain a chromogen (such as ortho-toluidine, for example) which changes colour when oxidized by the hydrogen peroxide produced in the first reaction. Electronic glucometers use the same initial oxidation reaction, but the strips also contain an electrode together with potassium ferricyanide which is converted to ferrocyanide by combination with gluconic acid. The electrode oxidizes the ferrocyanide and generates a current which is proportional to the blood glucose concentration. (It is common in the UK to refer to a point of care glucose measurement as a 'BM'. This has nothing to do with glucose itself, but stands for 'Boehringer Mannheim', which was the company that first produced the strips.)

Haemoglobin

- The commonest device in use in the UK is probably the Hemocue, for which a drop of blood is collected into a microcuvette. Within the cuvette there takes place a modified azide-methaemoglobin reaction. Erythrocytes are haemolysed by sodium deoxycholate. This releases haemoglobin which is converted by sodium nitrite to methaemoglobin, which then combines with sodium azide to form azidemethaemo-globin. The absorbance of this compound is measured at 570 and 880 nm (which effectively corrects for any turbidity in the sample), and the device converts this to display as a haemoglobin concentration.

Arterial Blood Gases

- Some of the information produced by arterial blood gas analyzers is from direct measurement, but a number of the indices are derived. The details of

CHAP
5

measurement are beyond the scope of the oral, but arterial pH, for example, is measured by a pH electrode which compares the potential developed at the electrode tip with a reference potential, with the voltage being directly proportional to the hydrogen ion (H^+) concentration. The $PaCO_2$ electrode is a pH electrode whose tip is covered by a semi-permeable membrane. CO_2 and H_2O combine in the space between the electrode and the membrane to produce H^+ ions whose concentration is proportional to the partial pressure of CO_2. Oxygen diffuses across a plastic membrane to a gold wire or platinum cathode in a rod which is immersed in a phosphate buffer with KCl. The application of 600–800 mV reduces O_2 to two hydroxyl ions: $O_2 + 2H_2O + 4e \rightarrow 4(OH^-)$, which creates a current flow between the cathode and the silver/silver chloride anode and whose magnitude is proportional to the PaO_2.

Electrolytes and Others

- Devices such as the 'i-Stat' have different diagnostic cartridges which can measure sodium, potassium and calcium; urea and creatinine; and lactate. They can also assess the activated clotting and prothombin times (ACT and PT) and can measure some cardiac markers, including brain natriuretic peptide (BNP). (The measurement methods are too diverse to be discussed in an oral such as this.)
- HIV status. There is a point of care test for HIV, which measures antibodies to HIV-1 and HIV-2, as well as the P24 antigen which is a viral protein that comprises most of the human immunopathic viral core. The test has a sensitivity and specificity greater than 99%.

Coagulation

- **Thromboelastography (TEG).** This is the commonest and most sophisticated technology that is currently used for point of care coagulation testing. Despite many years of prior usage, a company in the USA in the 1990s contrived to make 'TEG' a registered trademark. Undeterred, other manufacturers simply renamed it 'thromboelastometry' (TEM) and developed the ROTEM system, which is probably the one with which most UK anaesthetists will be familiar. (The term 'TEG' will be used in the following in the original sense and is not a reference to the Haemonetics Corporation.)
- **Principle of measurement.** A cylindrical pin is inserted into the cuvette which holds the blood sample, leaving a 1 mm gap between the side wall and the rotating pin, which rotates alternately clockwise and anti-clockwise. As long as the blood does not clot, this movement is unrestricted, but with increasing clot firmness the rotation of the pin begins to reduce. Pin rotation is inversely proportional to the integrity of the clot. It is detected optically and the decelerating rotations are processed by an integrated computer before generating the familiar ROTEM traces.

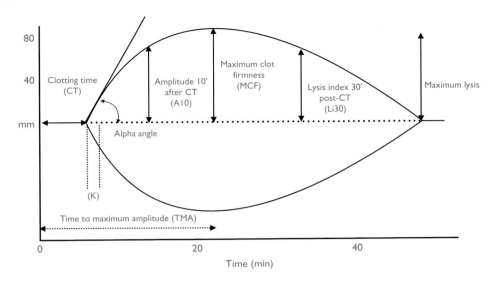

Fig. 5.9 ROTEM: normal coagulation profile.

- **Normal TEG trace.** Figure 5.9 shows a normal coagulation pattern, in which clot amplitude is plotted against time. 'CT' is the clotting time, which is the time from the beginning of the test to the start of fibrin formation. (This interval is also known as 'R' for reaction time.) 'A10' is the amplitude at 10 minutes after CT and is an index of clot strength. 'MA' is maximum amplitude, and 'TMA' is time to maximum amplitude. This is the coagulation phase. The decrease in clot amplitude thereafter is the phase of fibrinolysis, which can be prolonged. 'A30', which gives the percentage decrease in amplitude at 30 minutes after maximum amplitude, can therefore be used to determine the degree of fibrinolysis. 'K' (kinetics) is the amplification phase of the cell-based model of coagulation and is the time taken to reach a specific level of clot strength, which is an amplitude of 20 mm. Alpha, α, is the angle of the slope between 'CT' and 'K' and is used to assess the rate of clot formation. This allows an earlier assessment to be made without waiting for completion of the full process.
- **The ROTEM.** The addition of various activators or inhibitors to the blood sample gives information similar to formal laboratory tests. The INTEM tests the intrinsic pathway and provides similar information to the Activated Partial Thromboplastin Time (APTT). The EXTEM tests the extrinsic pathway and provides information similar to the Prothrombin time (PT). The FIBTEM uses an inhibitor of thrombocyte function and by removing the platelet contribution to coagulation allows an assessment of fibrinogen function.
- **Abnormal patterns.** In general, rather than specialist anaesthetic practice, the clinician will usually be using thromboelastography in the context of acute

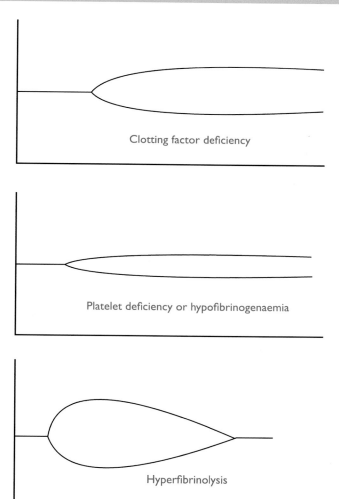

Fig. 5.10 Abnormal ROTEM patterns.

major haemorrhage: surgical, traumatic and obstetric. Put at its simplest, TEG will identify the contribution to a coagulopathy of four main factors, alone or in combination. These are (1) low levels of clotting factors, (2) reduced platelet activity, (3) low concentrations of fibrinogen and (4) accelerated fibrinolysis. The main patterns of ROTEM abnormality are shown in Figure 5.10.

- **Limitations.** The ROTEM is not able to give information about every clotting derangement. It does not detect the effect on coagulation of low-molecular-weight heparins or warfarin, and it is also insensitive to the effect of platelet inhibitors such as clopidogrel and aspirin.

Biological Potentials

Commentary

It is difficult to make the topic of biological potentials overtly clinical, and the questioning is likely to revert quite rapidly to the equipment that is necessary for their capture. It may seem as though the subject has no obvious narrative and the oral may feel unstructured. There should be sufficient information in the simplified details that follow to allow you to discuss it convincingly.

Core Information

- There is a negative resting potential across the membrane of excitable cells of around 90 mV. When the interior depolarizes, an action potential is generated that leads to a wave of depolarization that spreads along a neuron or across a contracting muscle. These electric potentials are transmitted through overlying tissues and can be detected by electrodes on the skin.
- Biological potentials differ both in magnitude and in frequency. The signals are also greatly attenuated as they pass through tissue. The myocardium generates local potentials at the skin of only around 0.5–2.0 mV, with a frequency range of 0.5–100 Hz. The brain produces much smaller potentials of some 50 µV, with a more restricted frequency range of 1–60 Hz. Muscle potentials range from 100 µV up to 30 mV depending on the size of the motor unit and with a wide frequency range of between 1 and >1,000 Hz. (These potentials are detected by the ECG, the EEG and the EMG, respectively.)

Capture, Amplification and Display

- **Detection:** the small electrical potentials are detected by skin electrodes. These are not simply passive devices, and their characteristics are important. When metal contacts an electrolyte solution, it forms an electrochemical half-cell which generates a potential. This potential may not only be detected by the amplifier but can also alter the characteristics of the electrode in a process known as polarization. This distorts any signal being captured. The problem is largely theoretical because modern electrodes whose surfaces use a metal which is in contact with one of its own salts (such as Ag:AgCl) do not cause polarization, and they produce a stable electrode potential that does not distort recordings.
- **Amplification:** these small potentials require amplifiers with a high degree of discrimination, which can minimize distortion by electrical noise emanating either from the patient or from the environment. It is easy to see how the potential differences produced by the heartbeat could interfere with the much smaller differences produced by cerebral neuronal activity, and how both could be swamped by AC mains voltage at 50 Hz. Typically, biological amplifiers are differential; that is, they measure the difference in electrical potential between two sources. Any input that is common to both is eliminated, and the difference in input to both is amplified. This capacity of a differential amplifier to eliminate the signals that are common to

both inputs is known as the common-mode rejection ratio (CMRR). (It is defined as the ratio of the magnitude of the differential gain to the magnitude of the common mode gain. For a biopotential amplifier, the CMRR should be at least 1,000:1.)

The design of amplifiers is such that they can exploit the dissimilarities between biological potentials. The ECG signal is many times larger than that of the EEG, but it is in phase. Highly discriminating instruments are able to attenuate in-phase signals and amplify out-of-phase signals, thereby ensuring that the EEG can be recorded free from interference. Similarly, the generally much higher frequency of muscle potentials can also be eliminated. (Modern instruments offer multiple filters for signal processing.) In addition to a high CMRR, the amplifier should have a high input impedance (>5 ohms). In combination with good electrode contact and minimal attenuation of the input signal, this ensures both truer recording of the potential and protection of the patient from electrocution. (In modern equipment, both the CMRR and input impedance are much higher than the figures quoted.)

Amplifiers must also have the appropriate bandwidth; that is, the ability to amplify the signal constantly across the range of frequencies that are involved. They also require adequate gain so that very small biological potentials can be captured. (Gain is the ratio of the voltage at the amplifier output to the voltage at the signal input.) Some instruments can demonstrate drift; this is a change in amplifier output even while the input potential remains constant. This is a function of the alteration in resistance of semiconductor materials in response to temperature changes. It is less problematic in amplifiers designed for AC potentials.

- **Recording and display:** there are a number of historical and rather cumbersome devices based on galvanometers which the oral should bypass. They are adequate for recording slow analogue signals but not for those of higher frequency. These signals are best displayed by a cathode ray tube (CRT). The cathode produces a stream of electrons which passes between two sets of charged plates before striking a phosphorescent screen. The charged electrons will be repelled from the negative plate and attracted to the positive with the degree of deflection being proportional to the charge. The x axis plates move the electron beam horizontally, whereas the y axis plates move it vertically. As the beam reaches the right-hand side of the screen, the charge reverses and restores it to the left. The beam has negligible inertia, and thus the CRT has a very high frequency response suitable for the display of all biological potentials.

Osmosis

Commentary

This is a fairly circumscribed topic which fits readily into the time frame of this oral. Although its main interest lies in clinical disorders which disrupt plasma osmolality, you may spend more time on the basic definitions and concepts, none of which is that complicated.

Core Information

- **Definition:** osmosis describes the process of the net movement of water molecules due to diffusion between areas of different concentration.
- **Osmolarity and osmolality:** osmolarity is the number of osmoles (or mosmoles) of solute per litre of solution, Osm l^{-1}, and is influenced by temperature. Osmolality is the number of osmoles per kilogram of solution, Osm kg^{-1} and, because it is temperature-independent, removes a source of potential inaccuracy.
- **Estimation of osmolality:** there are a large number of formulae for calculating plasma osmolality, and there is at least one review that has evaluated the 36 that have so far been described. Many are cumbersome:

$$\text{Osmolality} = 1.89 \times [Na^+] + 1.38 \times [K^+] + 1.08 \times [\text{Glucose}] + 1.03 \times [\text{Urea}] + 7.47$$

It is therefore more practical to make a rapid estimation using the widely accepted simple formula which sums the major solutes:

$$\text{Osmolality} = [2 \times Na^+] + [\text{Glucose}] + [\text{Urea}] \left(\text{all in mmol } l^{-1}\right)$$

Some formulae include potassium ions: $[2 \times Na^+] + [2 \times K^+] + [\text{Glucose}] + [\text{Urea}]$
   The plasma osmolality is kept constant in health, at around 290 mosmol kg^{-1} H_2O. More than 99% of the osmolality of plasma is due to electrolytes, with the contribution of plasma proteins (the oncotic pressure) being less than 1% (1 mosmol is equivalent to 17 mmHg or 2.26 kPa).
- **Osmolar gap:** this is the difference between the measured osmolality and the calculated osmolarity of the sample. Its clinical relevance lies in the fact that it may identify an osmotically active substance, such as ethyl alcohol, that is not normally present in plasma, and so can help to differentiate the cause of a metabolic acidosis.
- **Osmotic pressure:** an effective concentration gradient of water can be produced between two compartments separated by a semi-permeable membrane (permeable to water but not to solute). The movement of water into such a compartment will increase the pressure and/or volume of the compartment. This movement can be opposed by increasing the pressure in the compartment, and the pressure needed to prevent osmosis is defined as the osmotic pressure exerted by the solution. (If one compartment contains 22.4 litres and 1 mol of solute at 0 °C, it will exert an osmotic pressure of 1 atmosphere, or 101.325 kPa.)
- **Calculation of osmotic pressure:** the van't Hoff equation is based on the recognition that dilute solutions behave in a similar way to gases, hence: osmotic pressure = n (number of particles) × (concentration/molecular weight) × R (universal gas constant) × T (absolute temperature) (P = n × [–] × R × T).
- **Measurement of osmotic pressure:** this is measured by an osmometer, which utilizes one or more of the colligative properties of a solution. (These depend on the osmolality and are depression of freezing point, elevation of boiling point, reduction in vapour pressure and exertion of osmotic pressure.) Osmometers utilize the fact either that 1 mol of a solute which is added to 1 kg of water will depress the freezing point by 1.86 °C, or that the molar concentration of a solute causes a directly proportional reduction in the vapour pressure of the solvent (Raoult's law). (Such devices have the advantage of requiring smaller samples than the freezing point

osmometer.) The measurement of change of 1 mosmol requires apparatus capable of recording a temperature change of 0.002 °C.

- **Oncotic pressure:** the oncotic pressure is the contribution made to total osmolality by colloids (hence the alternative term 'colloid osmotic pressure', COP). The plasma oncotic pressure, at 25–28 mmHg, is only about 0.5% that of total plasma osmotic pressure, but it is significant because it is the major factor in the retention of fluid within capillaries. Albumin is responsible for about 75% of the total COP.
- **Measurement of oncotic pressure:** the colloid osmotic pressure can be measured by an oncometer, which comprises a semi-permeable membrane which separates the plasma sample from a saline reference solution. The change to the oncotic pressure can readily be transduced and measured.
- **Tonicity:** in contrast to osmolality, which measures all the particles in a solution, tonicity refers only to those particles which exert an osmotic force. Urea and glucose are freely permeable and so are not included. (The exception is in diabetes mellitus when glucose does not pass into cells and so becomes osmotically active. Urea can exert a local osmotic effect because it does not cross the blood–brain barrier, and so a high urea may cause intracranial dehydration and a reduction in ICP.)

Supplementary and Clinical Information

Conditions That Result in Derangements of Osmolality

- **Syndrome of inappropriate antidiuretic hormone (ADH) secretion (SIADH):** this is defined by the non-osmotic release of ADH with consequent water retention and hypotonicity. Its causes are numerous, but include intracranial tumours and pulmonary malignancy and infection. Treatment is via water restriction and, in chronic cases, with the use of demeclocycline (a tetracycline) which blocks ADH action in the kidney.
- **ADH:** this increases conservation of water and sodium in the distal renal tubules via a mechanism mediated by cAMP. Osmoreceptors in the supraoptic nuclei of the hypothalamus have a mean threshold of 289 ± 2.3 mosmol kg^{-1}. Above this plasma level, ADH release is stimulated. (The kidneys should be able to produce a urine osmolality of at least 1,000 mosmol kg^{-1}.)
- **Diabetes insipidus (DI):** this also has many causes and can be neurogenic (with deficiency of ADH synthesis or impaired release) or nephrogenic (with renal resistance to the action of ADH). It is characterized by massive diuresis and hypovolaemia. Neurogenic DI is treated with desmopressin (an ADH analogue) in a dose tailored to allow a mild diuresis to avoid the complication of water intoxication. Chlorpropamide potentiates the effects of endogenous ADH and also sensitizes distal tubules.
- **Glycine intoxication (TUR syndrome) with hyponatraemia:** this may follow excessive absorption of irrigating fluid during transurethral procedures (usually prostatectomy). Treatment is with administration of normal saline and judicious diuretic. Rapid restoration of normal sodium (for example, by the use of hypertonic saline) is associated with central pontine myelinosis.
- **Water intoxication:** this follows excessive intake of water, usually self-inflicted (29% of the finishers in one Hawaiian Ironman Triathlon were hyponatraemic), but is also associated with iatrogenic infusion of large volumes of glucose solution. The decrease

in plasma osmolality inhibits ADH secretion, but it can still cause potentially fatal electrolyte disturbance.

- **Hyperosmolar states:** the commonest hyperosmolar state is that of hyperglycaemic non-ketotic hyperosmolar coma, secondary to type 2 diabetes and precipitated by any dehydrating illness or reduction in insulin activity. (The serum osmolality is typically >320 mOsmol kg^{-1}) (see under 'Diabetic Ketoacidosis (DKA and HONK)' in Chapter 3.) Hyperosmolarity can also be iatrogenic following, for example, the administration of mannitol to neurosurgical patients.

Parametric and Non-Parametric Data

Commentary

Statistics questions usually start quite simply and frequently end up simply, for the reasons outlined in the Introduction. It may feel as though you are just being asked to give a series of definitions, but the examiners will be using your answers to discern whether you do understand the basic differences between types of data. You might at some stage be given a straightforward theoretical trial to discuss, but you will not be expected to perform any statistical calculations. The oral may divert to include systematic reviews, meta-analysis or the design of clinical trials.

Core Information

You will be asked to describe the difference between parametric and non-parametric data, and during the course of that description, to explain the terms that you are using.

- **Parametric data:** these are quantitative data that have a normal (Gaussian) distribution. In such a distribution the mean (average of all the results), the median (the value above and below which contains equal numbers of results) and the mode (the most frequently occurring value) are all the same. The variation around the mean is given by the variance, σ^2, the square root of which is the standard deviation (SD), σ. The Poisson and binomial distributions are parametric but are unlikely to be discussed in any detail in the oral for the reasons outlined previously.
- **Non-parametric data:** these do not have a normal distribution and the typical bell-shaped curve is replaced by one which may, for example, be skewed in either direction or may be bimodal (with two peaks). The data can sometimes be transformed mathematically so that they assume a normal distribution and can be analyzed by parametric tests. This may be desirable because parametric statistical tests are more powerful than non-parametric.
- **SD:** this provides a convenient way of describing the spread around the mean, with 68% of a population falling within ±1 SD, 96% within ±2 SD, and 99% within ±3 SD of the mean. The information can be expressed the other way round, namely that 95% of the values will be included within 1.96 SDs of the mean.
- **Standard error of the mean (SEM):** this is used to determine whether the mean of the sample reflects the mean of the population. It is calculated by dividing the

standard deviation by the square root of the degrees of freedom (SEM = SD/$\sqrt{n}$). It is not normally SD/$\sqrt{n-1}$, because standard deviation is calculated from sample data as the unbiased estimator of the population SD. In effect, SEM is the SD of the mean, thus 68% of sample means lie within ±1 SE of the true population mean, 96% within ±2 SE, and 99.7% within ±3 SEs.

- **Confidence intervals:** this concept is linked to the SEM. A sample mean will lie beyond 1.96 SEs only 5% of the time, and so we can be 95% confident that the sample mean does reflect the population mean. They have the advantage that they are expressed in the same units as the measurements, rather than as a probability value.
- **Parametric tests:** these include Student's t-test and analysis of variance (ANOVA). ANOVA and not the t-test should be used if there are more than two groups. The data are considered paired if they derive from the same patient. For example, blood pressure measurements before and after laryngoscopy would be analyzed using a paired t-test. If different but very well-matched patients are entered into separate limbs of a trial, then paired statistical tests may also be used.
- **Non-parametric tests:** these are applied to quantitative data which do not have a normal distribution. These include the Wilcoxon signed rank test for paired data and the Mann–Whitney U test for unpaired data. If there are more than two groups, then the corresponding tests are the Friedman (paired) and Kruskal–Wallis (unpaired).
- **Qualitative data:** these data (for example, ASA grades, pain scores, operation type) are usually analyzed using the Chi-squared test.

Examples

You may be asked what statistical tests you might use in a particular trial, for example, in a comparison of two anti-hypertensive agents.

- These are quantitative not qualitative data, and are likely to be normally distributed. (There are formal tests for normality, but if the mean and median are the same and the range of measurements spans around 5 SDs, then the data are probably parametric.)
- The data may be unpaired if two groups of patients are being studied, but will be paired if the anti-hypertensive drugs are being given sequentially to the same individuals.
- An appropriate test, therefore, would be Student's t-test (paired or unpaired as discussed), or ANOVA (also paired or unpaired).
- A P value of less than 0.05 may be the level at which the null hypothesis is disproved (i.e. confirming that there is a difference between the treatments), but this means nevertheless that there is up to a 5% probability that this observed difference could have arisen entirely by chance. This is the type I or alpha error (false positive).

The discussion may widen to include the potential errors in data interpretation from clinical trials, meta-analysis and levels of evidence.

- **Levels of evidence:** these have been defined as follows.
  — *I:* evidence from at least one review of multiple randomized controlled trials (RCTs).
  — *II:* evidence from at least one well-designed RCT.

— *III*: evidence from well-designed trials without randomization or matched controls.

— *IV*: evidence from well-designed non-experimental studies from more than one group.

— *V*: opinions based on clinical evidence, on descriptive studies or on the reports of expert committees.

Systematic Review and Meta-Analysis

Commentary

Systematic review is seen as providing the strongest level of evidence in support of, or refuting, a specific proposition, although independent reviews of the reviews suggest that 30–50% of them have significant flaws. They may include meta-analyses. The oral may include interpretation of a typical forest plot.

Core Information

- **Systematic review.** A systematic review aims to identify all relevant studies on a particular subject and to then aggregate and interpret the data. The Cochrane Collaboration gives the following definitions, the first being directed at the lay public: 'A systematic review summarizes the results of carefully designed healthcare studies and provides a high level of evidence on the effectiveness of healthcare intervention'.

    The definition for professionals is more detailed and specific: 'A systematic review is a review of a clearly formulated question that uses systematic and explicit methods to identify, select and critically appraise relevant research, and to collect and analyze data from the studies that are included in the review. Meta-analyses may or may not be used to analyse and summarize the results of the included studies'. (Cochrane 2014)

    The descriptor 'systematic' is justified only by quite stringent criteria. It must address a clearly formulated question; must search extensively to identify relevant studies; must assess the quality of those studies; and must summarize the evidence, using statistical methods including meta-analysis as appropriate, either for the whole review or for sub-groups. Interpretation of the findings should characterize heterogeneity and, if necessary, assign more weight to well-conducted studies, while assessing the risk of any forms of bias. Such reviews typically involve a number of different researchers who assess the data independently of each other. The process sounds as though it should produce robust and sound conclusions, but independent analysis suggests that there can be substantial flaws in more than 50% of reviews. The Cochrane Injuries Group Albumin Reviewers concluded in 1998, for example, that albumin increased mortality in critically ill patients. The patient populations were very disparate and even included neonates, and subsequent subgroup analysis suggested that in some of those groups albumin actually improved survival.

- **Meta-analysis.** This is a technique that aggregates the data from a number of individual RCTs with the aim of confirming or refuting an effect that the smaller studies have been unable to do. In effect, it combines the results of individual studies and applies techniques of statistical analysis to obtain a more accurate judgement of effect. Hence, whereas a systematic review aims to answer a defined question by summarizing the evidence that fits pre-determined eligibility criteria, meta-analysis uses statistical tools to summarize those results.

— *Advantages:* meta-analysis can produce a conclusion (synthesis) from a number of trials which may even have had contradictory findings. The power and significance of the overview can be increased by this synthesis of the individual results, and may allow a definite conclusion to be drawn even when individual studies conflict.

— *Problems:* meta-analyses are the tools of statisticians and epidemiologists and are not without drawbacks. They are subject to 'publication bias', as negative studies are much less likely to be published than positive ones. They may also be affected by double counting, which may occur when the same data are incorporated into more than one trial report. Their credibility is also tested severely if the populations in the RCTs are different. Even if the populations are similar, the trial designs may be very different, with matched subgroups being too small to permit formal meta-analysis.

- **Forest plots:** these are the graphical representation of the effect sizes and confidence intervals from a meta-analysis (Fig. 5.11). Each individual trial (which is usually listed on the left of the plot) is represented as a line, with the centre box representing the mean effect size of the study. The size of this box represents the weight that is given to the study. The ends of each line define the 95% confidence intervals. The wider the confidence intervals, the less reliable are likely to be the results. The centre

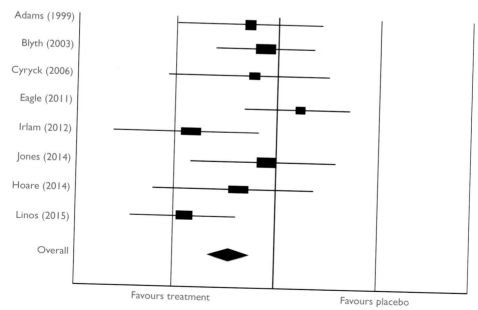

Fig. 5.11 Forest plot.

of the graph is the zero mark, to the left of which is the side favouring treatment, to the right of which favours the control. A summary effect size appears at the base of the plot in the shape of a diamond. If the entire diamond falls to one side or the other, the question is answered unequivocally. If part of the diamond touches the centre line, then the overall combined result is not statistically significant. Forest plots usually also contain other information, including numerical weightings, risk ratios and a score for heterogeneity, but you are unlikely to have to explore these aspects in detail, and so they do not appear the figure.

- **Cochrane Collaboration**. Cochrane, as it is now called, produces systematic reviews of primary research in human health care which are updated in the light of any new research. Independent assessments of Cochrane reviews suggest that although up to 30% may have significant problems, this nonetheless means that they remain the most reliable source of aggregated data that is available.
  - *Recommendations:* these are linked to levels of evidence: **A**, level I studies; **B**, level II or III studies; **C**, level IV studies; and **D**, level V evidence or inconsistent or inconclusive studies of any level.

Design of a Clinical Trial for a New (Analgesic) Drug

Commentary

Drugs are at the core of the specialty of anaesthesia, and so you should not find it unreasonable to be asked about the broad principles that underpin RCTs. The subject is not too difficult, and you should be able to work out the important aspects of this kind of research even if you do not have the information readily to hand. It is inevitable that statistics will form part of the discussion. You will always do well to start simply when the subject of statistics arises, because a demonstration that you understand the basic concepts will usually be sufficient to get you through. This question could be asked in the pharmacology part of the oral, but it is more logically a clinical measurement question.

Core Information

Designs of clinical trials for new drugs (for example an anaesthetic or analgesic agent).

- A clinical trial for a new agent is carried out during phase II or phase III of the drug's development. (Preclinical development involves animal studies into aspects such as safety, efficacy and mutagenicity. Phase I involves small group studies of fewer than 100 healthy volunteers, looking at pharmacokinetics, pharmacodynamics and adverse effects. Phase II recruits larger numbers of patients, typically 200–300, in which the findings of the phase I studies are refined. Phase III involves still larger numbers of patients, usually in the thousands, who are entered into definitive RCTs.

Phase IV occurs after the drug has been licensed for use, and involves post-marketing surveillance of its effects in much greater numbers of individuals.)

- **Ethics committee approval:** no clinical trial can proceed without the approval of an appropriately constituted ethics committee, which will include laypeople amongst its members. The scrutiny of applications by these committees is increasingly rigorous, and in essence each committee seeks to preserve the full protection of the rights of every potential participant. Individuals must receive full information about all aspects of the trial before they consent, and they must be free to withdraw at any stage without compromising their future care. Committees will examine particularly intently any trial in which financial inducements are involved.

- **Trial design:** the best-designed clinical trials seek to answer a single simple question: in the case, for example, of a novel painkiller, whether this new analgesic is superior to established treatments. It is essential to have a control in the study, which in this instance would be an analgesic in clinical use that was of proven benefit. Trial design must therefore involve defining endpoints for efficacy, and must also ensure that data relating to adverse effects are collected. The use of placebos in trials of analgesics is considered to be unethical, and so the drugs in all limbs of the trial will be pharmacologically active.

- **Subject selection:** it is important that the groups are matched as far as possible. Such matching should include age, gender, American Society of Anesthesiologists (ASA) status and racial characteristics. Exclusion criteria must also be established. If the drug is to be used for treatment of chronic pain, then the trial can be a double-blind crossover trial (see the following) in which the patient can act as his or her own control. Sufficient time must elapse between administrations of the two drugs to ensure that the first one the patient has received is no longer exerting any effect.

- **Sample size:** the conclusions of any trial can be erroneous. The study can determine either that there is a difference between treatments when none exists, or it can determine that there is no difference between treatments when a difference does in fact exist. The first (false positive) conclusion is known as a type I error. The second (false negative) conclusion is a type II error. The probability of avoiding a type II error and missing a significant difference between treatments is known as the power of the trial. In other words, the power of a study is its ability to reveal a difference of a particular size. The power calculation allows the investigator to determine the sample size necessary to demonstrate this difference. It is calculated from $1-\beta$, where β is the type II error. Trials are usually designed with a power of 80% ($\beta = 0.2$) or better, 90% ($\beta = 0.1$). The investigators must also decide the magnitude of the difference that is sought.

- **Randomization:** randomization of patients to one or other limbs of the trial is intended to remove bias. The bias may be unconscious or hidden. Patients may not have been allocated randomly to an operating list, for example, and so assigning alternate patients to trial groups might be unreliable. Simple methods such as tossing a coin are valid, although it is more common to use computer-generated randomization.

- **Blinding:** it is ideal for the trial to be double blind, so that neither the patient nor the investigator knows to which group they have been assigned. This is of particular importance when the outcome data are subjective, as in a comparison of analgesic drugs or techniques.

- **Data collection:** obvious considerations apply to the scrupulous collection of data. Inherent variation can be avoided by minimizing the number of investigators involved in the process.

- **Statistical evaluation:** the appropriate statistical tests must be chosen for the question that is being asked. In this case the null hypothesis is that there is no difference between new analgesic A and established analgesic B. The tests of statistical significance aim to define whether the null hypothesis has been disproved; in other words, that there is a difference between drugs A and B, and at what level of probability. The investigators must also decide whether the data are continuous and normally distributed, in which case a parametric test is appropriate. If the data do not follow a normal distribution, then a non-parametric test should be used. The evaluation of an analgesic would almost certainly involve the use of visual analogue scales, about which statisticians may disagree. Some argue that response to pain is a biological variable with a normal distribution; others contend that the data are not normally distributed and that non-parametric tests should be applied.

- **Clinical and statistical significance:** trial data will be cited according to the strength of its statistical significance, although clinical significance is more important. The bigger the sample size, the more likely it is that a small effect will be statistically significant, even though clinically its impact may be negligible.

Clinical Trials: Errors in Interpretation of Data

Commentary

This is not a topic about flaws in the design of clinical trials but rather about potential problems with statistical analysis. It may not be asked as a sole question but may instead form part of a discussion about the design of clinical trials or in the context of a specific study that may be cited. Many of the terms and definitions are similar and do need precise enunciation so as to avoid confusion of both candidate and examiner.

Core Information

The Null Hypothesis and Types of Error

- **Null hypothesis:** this is the assumption made at the start of any investigation that there is no difference between the populations, treatments and samples that are being compared. Tests of statistical significance aim to disprove the null hypothesis at a given level of probability. This is usually 0.05 (which means that there is a 5% likelihood of the difference occurring purely due to chance).

- **Types of error**
  - *Type I or α error*: in this case the null hypothesis is wrongly rejected, and a difference is found when there is none. This is a false positive. The likelihood of a

type I error is reduced by requiring a higher probability value (making P smaller), by increasing the sample size, or both. By convention, a 5% probability of making a type I error is accepted, and the confidence level is given by $(1 - \alpha)$.

— *Type II or β error*: in this instance the null hypothesis is wrongly proved, and so no difference is found when one does in fact exist. This is a false negative. Type II errors are easier to avoid than type I, and their commonest cause is a sample size that is too small. They may also occur if there is a wide variation in the study population or if differences that may be clinically significant are quantitatively quite small. Type II errors are linked with the power of the study. More leniency is allowed in respect of type II errors, such that a 10% or 20% probability of an error is accepted. A study is adequately powered, therefore, if β is equal to or less than 0.2.

- **Power:** the 'power' of a study is the measure of its likelihood of detecting a difference between groups if a difference really does exist. It is also defined by $(1 - \beta)$ where β is the probability of a type II error. The power of a trial is the probability of avoiding a type II error, and so it is clear that underpowered studies may reject treatments that in fact may be effective. The determination of the numbers needed is also a reflection of the minimal clinically important difference, which is set by the investigator. It is probably not important, for example, to detect a 5% reduction in systolic blood pressure, but it may be very important to identify a 5% reduction in mortality. Were a study to miss such a fall in mortality, then it might lead to the abandonment of a therapy that could save 50 lives for every 1,000 patients treated.

Methods of Quantifying the Value of a Clinical Test

- **Sensitivity:** this is a measure of how good is a clinical test at excluding false positives and is defined by the proportion of positives that are correctly identified by the test. It is determined by the proportion of patients who test positive in relation to the numbers who actually are positive.
- **Positive predictive value:** this is an alternative means of determining whether an abnormal result predicts a genuine abnormality. It is defined by the numbers of patients who both test positive and who are genuinely positive as a proportion of the total of correct positive tests.
- **Specificity:** this is a measure of how good is a clinical test at excluding false negatives and is defined by the proportion of negatives that are correctly identified by the test. It is determined by the proportion of patients who test negative in relation to the numbers who actually are negative.
- **Negative predictive value:** this is an alternative means of determining whether a normal result precludes a genuine abnormality. It is defined by the numbers of patients who both test negative and who are genuinely negative, as a proportion of the total of correct negative tests.
- **Statistical and clinical significance:** it is erroneous to equate statistical with clinical significance. Statistics are essentially measures of probability; clinical judgement must thereafter inform their use.

Index

a wave, 179

AAGA. *See* accidental awareness during general anaesthesia

abciximab, 385

abdominal compartment syndrome, 80

abdominal obesity, 238

abdominal wall

anterior, 87–8

blocks, 87–8

nerve supply, 87

abducens nerve, 17

abduction, of laryngeal muscles, 45

abnormal placentation, 198

abnormal pupillary signs, 24–5

abnormal respiratory patterns, 136

absolute humidity, 481

absolute pressure, 457

absorption atelectasis, oxygen toxicity and, 165–6

acarbose, 412

acceleromyography, 495

accidental awareness during general anaesthesia (AAGA), 425

ACE inhibitors. *See* angiotensin-converting enzyme inhibitors

acebutolol, 361–2

acetylcholine, 31, 232

metabolism of, 353

acquired immunity, 277–9

acquired resistance, to local anaesthesia, 107

acromegaly, 28

ACT. *See* acute trauma coagulopathy

ACTH. *See* adrenocorticotrophic hormone

actinomycin D, 350

activated charcoal, 376–7

activated factor X inhibitors, 385

activated protein C (APC), 178

active scavenging systems, 451

acute coronary syndrome (ACS), 65–6

acute myocardial ischemia, 65–6

acute trauma coagulopathy (ACT), 187

adduction, of laryngeal muscles, 45

adductor canal block, 121

adductor longus, 118

adenohypophysis, 27

adenosine, 357

ADH. *See* antidiuretic hormone

adrenaline (epinephrine), 246, 337–8, 367–9

β-adrenoceptor agonists, 395–6

β-adrenoceptor blockers, 346, 359–60, 362

specific uses for, 362

adrenocortical suppression, 301

adrenocorticotrophic hormone (ACTH), 27–8, 110, 242–3

AER. *See* auditory evoked response

AF. *See* atrial fibrillation

ageing

airway and, 240

autonomic nervous system and, 240

cardiovascular system and, 240

CNS and, 240

coexisting disease, 241

gastrointestinal system and, 240–1

physiology of, 240–1

renal system and, 241

respiratory system and, 240

agglutinogens, 189

air embolism, 22, 471, 490

airway, 248

access, prone position and, 216–17

ageing and, 240

supraglottic, device, 493

thyroid disease and, 258

airway pressure release ventilation (APRV), 145

albumin, 255

alcohol, 82, 376

overdose, 376

withdrawal, 348

alfentanil, 324

alkalinization, local anaesthetics, 336

alkylating agents (cytotoxics), 414

allergic reactions, 193

local anaesthesia and, 334

Index

intra-arterial blood pressure (cont.)
  measurement, 458
  monitoring, 460
intra-arterial injection, 102–3
intracranial pressure (ICP), 218–19
  cerebral blood flow and, 225
  clinical features of, 221
  factors influencing, 219–20
  impaired drainage and, 220
  management of, 221–2
  mass lesions and, 219
  measurement of, 220
  pathophysiology, 220
  symptoms and signs, 221
  volume increases and, 219–20
intraocular pressure, 26, 229–31, 458
  definition, 229
  determinants, 229–30
  effects of anaesthesia, 230–1
  lowering, 231
  measurement of, 230
intraoperative atrial fibrillation, 359
intraparenchymal monitors, 220
intrapleural catheters, 60–1
  placement, 22
intrapleural space, 131–2
intrapulmonary alveolar rupture, 132
intrathecal septae, 107
intrathecal spread
  barbotage and, 106
  baricity of drug and, 105–6
  drug dose and, 105
  gender and, 106
  injection level and, 105
  patient age and, 106
  patient height and, 106
  patient position and, 106
  pregnancy and, 106
  vasoconstriction and, 106
intravascular volume, 20–1
  CVP and, 180–1
intravenous immunoglobulin (IVIG), 256, 269
intravenous induction agents, 225
intravenous iron supplementation, 196
intravenous sedation, 409–10
intraventricular catheters, 220
intrinsic sympathomimetic activity (ISA), 361–2
inverse ratio ventilation, 145
iPACK block, 121–2
IPPV. See intermittent positive pressure ventilation

iron
  dose regimens, 196
  intravenous supplementation, 196
  oral supplementation, 196
  side effects of, 196–7
ISA. See intrinsic sympathomimetic activity
ischaemia
  acute lower limb, 116
  conditions, 55
  delayed cerebral, 15
  HBOT for, 163
  perioperative, 360–1
ischaemic preconditioning, 303–4
isocarboxazid, 381
isoflurane, 293, 306, 313–15
  cardiovascular system and, 307
  CNS effects, 306
  exposure levels, 452
  kidneys and, 307
  liver and, 307
  physicochemical characteristics, 306
  respiratory system and, 307
isolated (floating) circuits, 499
isolated forearm technique, 422–3
isomerism, 292–3
isoprenaline, 369
i-Stat, electrolyte measurement, 505
IVIG. See intravenous immunoglobulin

jaundice, 281–2, 429
  causes of, 282
  liver and, 76
  perioperative complications of, 282–3
  postoperative, 283
jugular venous bulb oxygen saturation (SjVO$_2$), 466
  factors decreasing, 466
  factors increasing, 466
  measurement, 466–7

Kataria model, TCI, 406
ketamine, 293, 296–8, 343, 410
  as antidepressant, 299
  bladder, 299
  cardiovascular system and, 298
  chemistry, 297
  clinical uses, 299
  CNS and, 298
  doses, 297
  induction agents, 298–9

liver (cont.)
   in drug biotransformation, 75
   in erythropoiesis, 76
   in immunological functions, 76
   isoflurane and, 307
   jaundice and, 76
   lipid metabolism, 75–6
   metabolism of nitrogenous compounds, 75
   portal area, 74
   portal triads, 74
   protein synthesis, 75
   sevoflurane and, 303
   traditional microscopic architecture, 74
   xenon and, 308
lixisenatide, 413
local anaesthesia
   acquired resistance to, 107
   action, 328
   adjuvants, 337
   alkalinization, 336
   allergic reactions and, 334
   barriers to, 329
   basic structure, 327
   binding, 333
   carbonation, 336–7
   cardiovascular system and, 335
   CEA under, 42–3
   CNS and, 335
   drug action, 336
   drug dosage, 332–3
   duration of, 337–8
   for eye surgery, 25–6
   for foot, 125
   frequency dependence, 341
   impulse propagation, 328
   innate resistance to, 107
   in intercostal nerve blocks, 70
   for nasotracheal intubation, 37
   new formulations, 338
   normal action potential, 327
   onset and duration, 335–6
   pulmonary sequestration, 334, 341
   resistance to, 330–1
   sensory-motor dissociation, 341
   structure-activity relationships of, 329
   toxicity, 332–5
LODS. See Logistic Organ Dysfunction Score
Lofepramine, 381
Logistic Organ Dysfunction Score (LODS), 480
long saphenous vein, 116

lower limb blood supply, 114–15
   arterial, 115
   venous drainage, 115–16
lower limb ischaemia, acute, 116
lower limb revascularization, 117
lower thoracic region, 126–9
LSD. See lysergic acid diethylamide
lumbar csf volume, 107
lumbar lordosis, 105
lumbar paravertebral block, 58
lumbar plexus block, 85–6
   technique, 86
lumbar region, 126–9
   cross-sectional view of, 127–9
lumbar sympathectomy, indications, 85
lumbar sympathetic block
   complications, 85
   technique, 85
lumbar sympathetic chain, 84
   anatomy of, 84–5
lung. See also one-lung anaesthesia
   barrier function, 151
   bronchopulmonary segments of, 49–50
   drug metabolism and, 151
   failing, 142–3
   filtration functions of, 151
   immune function of, 151
   injury, acute, 142
   metabolic functions of, 150
   neuroendocrine functions, 150–1
   non-respiratory functions of, 150
   as vascular reserve, 151–2
   volume, 139
lung-protective ventilation, 143
luteinising hormone, 18–19, 27–8
lymphatic clearance, decreased, 155–6
lymphocytes, 277
lymphopoiesis, 77
lysergic acid diethylamide (LSD), 379

macrolides, 351
macrophages, 277
magnesium, 262, 337
magnesium sulphate, 147, 343, 357, 393
   cardiovascular system and, 394
   clinical uses, 394–5
   CNS and, 394
   pharmacology, 393–4
   respiratory system and, 394
   toxicity, 394

Index

Printed in the United States
by Baker & Taylor Publisher Services